IFMBE Proceedings

Volume 44

Series Editor

Ratko Magjarevic

Deputy Editors

Fatimah Binti Ibrahim
Igor Lacković
Piotr Ładyżyński
Emilio Sacristan Rock

For further volumes:
http://www.springer.com/series/7403

The International Federation for Medical and Biological Engineering, IFMBE, is a federation of national and transnational organizations representing internationally the interests of medical and biological engineering and sciences. The IFMBE is a non-profit organization fostering the creation, dissemination and application of medical and biological engineering knowledge and the management of technology for improved health and quality of life. Its activities include participation in the formulation of public policy and the dissemination of information through publications and forums. Within the field of medical, clinical, and biological engineering, IFMBE's aims are to encourage research and the application of knowledge, and to disseminate information and promote collaboration. The objectives of the IFMBE are scientific, technological, literary, and educational.

The IFMBE is a WHO accredited NGO covering the full range of biomedical and clinical engineering, healthcare, healthcare technology and management. It is representing through its 60 member societies some 120.000 professionals involved in the various issues of improved health and health care delivery.

Simona Vlad · Radu V. Ciupa
Editors

International Conference on Advancements of Medicine and Health Care through Technology; 5th – 7th June 2014, Cluj-Napoca, Romania

MEDITECH 2014

Springer

Editors
Simona Vlad
Faculty of Electrical Engineering
Technical University of Cluj-Napoca
Cluj-Napoca
Romania

Radu V. Ciupa
Faculty of Electrical Engineering
Technical University of Cluj-Napoca
Cluj-Napoca
Romania

ISSN 1680-0737 ISSN 1433-9277 (electronic)
ISBN 978-3-319-07652-2 ISBN 978-3-319-07653-9 (eBook)
DOI 10.1007/978-3-319-07653-9
Springer Cham Heidelberg New York Dordrecht London

Library of Congress Control Number: 2014939994

The IFMBE Proceedings is an Official Publication of the International Federation for Medical and Biological Engineering (IFMBE)

Printed on acid-free paper

Springer is part of Springer Science+Business Media (www.springer.com)

Foreword

The 4th Conference on Advancements of Medicine and Health Care through Technology - MediTech2014 aims to provide opportunities for the Romanian professionals involved in basic research, R&D, industry and medical applications to exchange their know-how and build up collaboration in one of the most human field of science and techniques. The conference is intended to be an international forum for researchers and practitioners interested in the advance in, and applications of biomedical engineering to exchange the latest research results and ideas in the areas covered by the topics (hardware/software technologies, medical devices/instrumentation, biosignal and image processing, biomaterials, biomechanics, biotechnologies, etc.).

Another objective is to improve communication and encourage collaboration among all health care professionals through the presentation and discussion of the new research and current challenges.

Biomedical engineers work at the intersection of engineering, the life sciences and healthcare. These engineers take principles from applied science (including mechanical, electrical, chemical and computer engineering) and physical sciences (including physics, chemistry and mathematics) and apply them to biology and medicine.

It is well known that the improvement of quality of life is possible only through research and innovation. Of course, this can be achieved by an efficient use of information and management systems and biomedical technology.

Frequently however, the implications of technologies in terms of increasing recurrent costs, additional required support services, change in medical practice and training needs are underestimated. As a result, the widespread irrational use of technologies leads to a wastage of scarce resources and weakens health systems performance. To avoid such problems, a systematic and effective Health Technology System must be developed and introduced, requiring the support and commitment of decision makers of all levels of the health system.

All papers submitted for presentation went through a review process and were evaluated by two reviewers (whose effort and hard work reflect their commitment and dedication to the profession). Those individuals whose papers were chosen for presentation at the conference submitted manuscripts to be published in these *Proceedings*.

Sincere appreciation and gratitude are expressed to members of the Scientific Advisory Committee for their diligent efforts in effecting a most timely and provocative conference. To document the current thinking in such a publication is most important and should serve as a useful guide for others working in the field.

Professor Radu V. Ciupa
MediTech2014 Conference Chair

Organization

Organizers

Romanian National Society for Medical Engineering and Biological Technology

Partners

Technical University of Cluj-Napoca
Iuliu Hatieganu University of Medicine and Pharmacy Cluj-Napoca
Medical University of Vienna
The University of Sheffield

Conference Chair

Radu V. Ciupa	Technical University of Cluj-Napoca, Romania

Honorary Committee

Aurel Vlaicu	Technical University of Cluj-Napoca, Romania, Rector
Alexandru Irimie	Iuliu Hatieganu University of Medicine and Pharmacy Cluj-Napoca, Romania, Rector; Corresponding Member of the Romanian Academy of Medical Sciences
Radu Munteanu	President of the Romanian Academy of Technical Sciences, Cluj-Napoca subsidiary, Romania

Scientific Advisory Committee

Marcela Achim (Romania)
Radu Badea (Romania)
Corina Botoca (Romania)
Remus Brad (Romania)
Simion Bran (Romania)
Macarie Breazu (Romania)
Mariana Brumaru (Romania)
Alexandru Gh. Catana (Romania)
Lelia Ciontea (Romania)
Radu Ciorap (Romania)
Radu V. Ciupa (Romania)
Hariton Costin (Romania)
Cecilia Cristea (Romania)
Vanessa Diaz-Zuccarini (UK)
Gabriele Dubini (Italy)
Winfried Mayr (Austria)
Dan D. Micu (Romania)
Ioan Mihu (Romania)
Petru Mircea (Romania)
Alexandru Morega (Romania)
Mihaela Morega (Romania)
Marius Muji (Romania)
Calin Munteanu (Romania)
Mihai S. Munteanu (Romania)
Andrew Narracott (UK)
Sever Pasca (Romania)
Traian Petrisor (Romania)
Dan Pitica (Romania)
Petre G. Pop (Romania)
Catalin Popa (Romania)

Sorin Dudea (Romania)
John Fenner (UK)
Mircea Giurgiu (Romania)
Horia Hedesiu (Romania)
Mihaela Hedesiu (Romania)
Sorin Hintea (Romania)
Rodica Holonec (Romania)
Rod Hose (UK) (Romania)
Cornel Iancu (Romania)
Beriliu Ilie (Romania)
Ioan Jivet (Romania)
Matthias Krenn (Austria)
Mircea Leabu (Romania)
Patricia Lawford (UK)
Eugen Lupu (Romania)
Dan Mandru (Romania)
Dan V. Rafiroiu (Romania)
Marius N. Roman (Romania)
Horatiu Rotar (Romania)
Janez Rozman (Slovenia)
Corneliu Rusu (Romania)
Robert Sandulescu (Romania)
Dan I. Stoia (Romania)
Mihai Tarata (Romania)
Vasile Topa (Romania)
Mirela Toth-Tascau (Romania)
Mircea Vaida (Romania)
Kari Vehmaskoski (Finland)
Simona Vlad (Romania)
Laurian Vlase (Romania)
Daniel Volovici (Romania)

Local Organizing Committee

Radu Badea
Mihaela Cretu
Felicia Loghin
Victoria Man
Petru Mircea
Marius Muji
Mihai S. Munteanu
Anca I. Nicu
Dan V. Rafiroiu
Marius N. Roman
Simona Vlad

Table of Contents

Health Care Technology

Medical Devices, Measurement and Instrumentation

Medical Imaging, Image and Signal Processing

Modelling and Simulation

Molecular Bioengineering, Biomechanics

Making Existing Buildings Accessible

N. Cobîrzan and S. Pălăcean

Technical University of Cluj-Napoca, Faculty of Civil Engineering, Cluj-Napoca, Romania

Abstract– **Depending on their functionality, buildings are designed to be durable, constantly influencing the inhabitants' quality of life. Therefore the great majority of older or disabled people who are owning their dwellings, find themselves in the position to sell them and buy new ones, adapted to the own needs. These persons also face serious difficulties in using public places and buildings that are not made accessible – a situation currently encountered in Romania.**

The paper presents the main aspects concerning the retrofitting of a worship building in Cluj-Napoca in order to ensure the unrestricted access to all category of people.

Keywords— **accessibility, structural rehabilitation, elevator, universal design, disability**

I. Introduction

The idea of making the built environment accessible emerged in the mid 60ies as a consequence of the demands formulated by disabled people [1].

In Romania there are 700,736 persons with disabilities out of which only 16,815 are institutionalized, the rest of 683,921 living in the own dwellings [2]. 20.26% of the latter [2] are people with physical disabilities who need assistance to be able to use the own dwellings and/or to move inside public spaces and respectively inside the public buildings (education institutions, churches, theatres, office buildings) [3], [4].

The lack of elevators, access ramps, tactile markings for warning at stairs/ramps end or the missing handrails on both sides of stairs, as well as the high steps or the narrow doors are current problems encountered in most of the public buildings in Romania.

According to the government Emergency Order 102/1999 regarding the special protection and integration in labour of disabled people [5], or Law no. 448/2006 regarding the protection and the promotion of disabled people's rights [6], all the buildings belonging to public institutions, culture, sports or leisure should have been adapted to the needs of disabled people, thus becoming accessible for all.

In spite of the legislation in force at that time, only few public buildings have been made accessible: some of the banks, city halls, museums.

Even at the present, the most important cathedrals and many churches in Cluj-Napoca do not have access ramps at the entrances (Fig. 1).

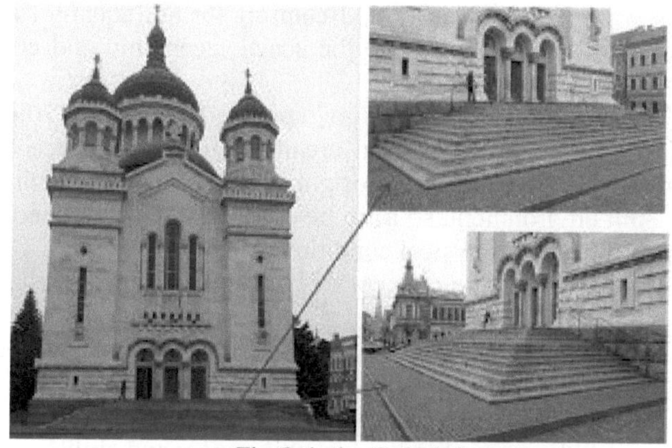

a. The Orthodox Cathedral

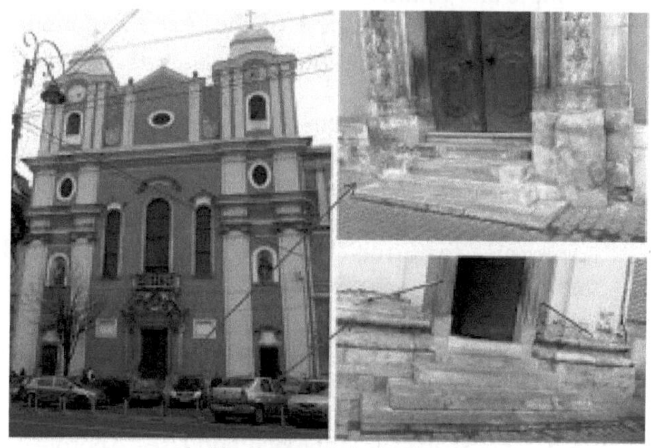

b. The Roman-Catholic Church

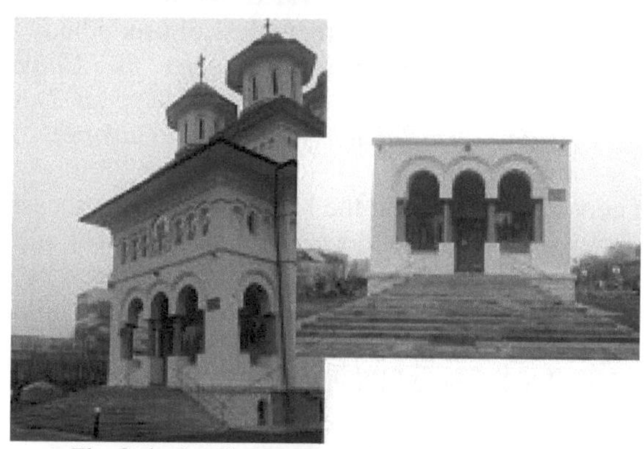

c. The Orthodox Church "The Saint Archangel Michael"

Fig. 1 Some important worship buildings in Cluj-Napoca

S. Vlad and R.V. Ciupa (eds.), *International Conference on Advancements of Medicine and Health Care through Technology*, IFMBE Proceedings 44,
DOI: 10.1007/978-3-319-07653-9_1, © Springer International Publishing Switzerland 2014

An accessible environment is not only favourable for disabled, but also for many other users (pregnant women, elderly people and families with small children or diseased persons) and may prevent the isolation, facilitating their social integration.

In order to eliminate discrimination, it is necessary to enforce and expand the application of the law regarding accessibility to any kind of building, regardless its destination. This will provide security and comfort for all, equally[1], as well as the chance to enjoy the social, economic and cultural benefits of the society.

The term "Universal Design" appeared in the mid 70ies being used by the American architect Ronald L. Mace to describe a new concept in designing products and planning the built environment, so as to be used by all easily, regardless of the age or physical condition.

The principles the concept of Universal Design is relied on are the following:

- „Equitable Use - The design is useful and marketable to people with diverse abilities;
- Flexibility in Use -The design accommodates a wide range of individual preferences and abilities.
- Simple and Intuitive Use - Use of the design is easy to understand, regardless of the user's experience, knowledge, language skills, or current concentration level.
- Perceptible Information- The design communicates necessary information effectively to the user, regardless of ambient conditions or the user's sensory abilities.
- Tolerance for Error- The design minimizes hazards and the adverse consequences of accidental or unintended actions.
- Low Physical Effort-The design can be used efficiently and comfortably and with a minimum of fatigue.
- Size and Space for Approach and Use- Appropriate size and space is provided for approach, reach, manipulation and use regardless of user's body size, posture, or mobility."(*The Center for Universal Design (1997). The Principles of Universal Design, Version 2.0. Raleigh,NC: North Carolina State University*)[7]

The concerns for making the built environment accessible were intensified in the last decades at both, global and national level, this resulting from numerous researches performed by professionals in multidisciplinary domains (architects, engineers etc.) in cooperation with representatives of disabled people [4,8,9,10,11,12].

[1] Resolution 2001/1 of the Commission of Ministers in the Council of Europe regarding "Universal Design" or "Design for All".

II. CASE STUDY

The building making the subject of the present study (Fig. 2) is a Pentecostal church located in the Eastern part of the City of Cluj-Napoca and was designed in 1996.

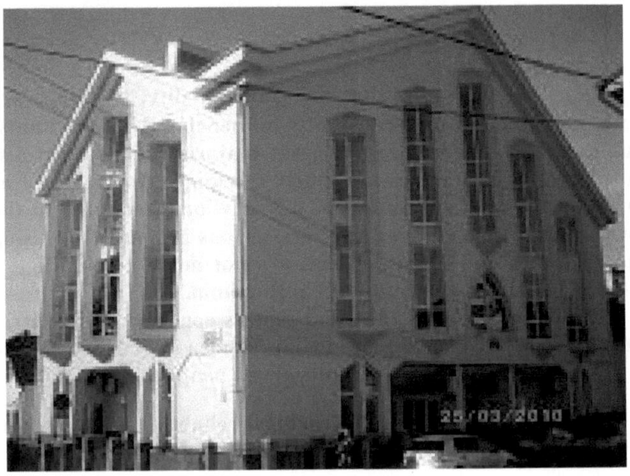

Fig. 2 "Hope" Pentecostal Church

The resistance structure (hall type) consists of masonry loadbearing walls strengthened with reinforced concrete columns and tie-beams (Fig. 3).

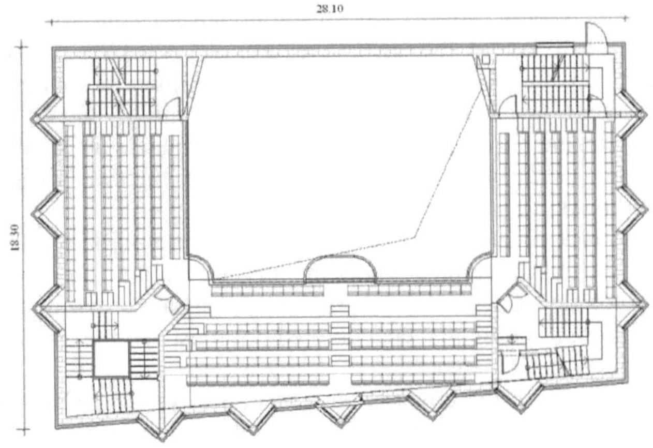

Fig. 3 First floor – the original plan

The horizontal loadbearing elements – encased floors and balconies supported by crossed beams are made of reinforced concrete cast in situ.

The building has a high semi-basement (the meeting hall, auxiliary spaces, toilets), ground floor (the big hall with 1,000 places) and two more partial floors developed as balconies following three of the building sides (Fig. 3 and 4).

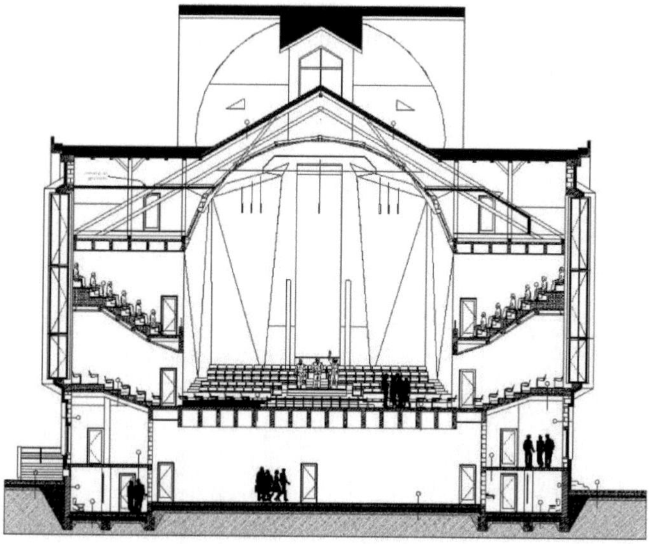

Fig. 4 Cross section

The attic floor is shared in spaces with adequate functionality for a worship place. The roof framing is made of timber bars joint with metallic bolts.

The vertical circulation is performed through four staircases designed such a way as to ensure the proper and secure access and evacuation of all the people from inside the building.

Taking into consideration that the building was designed when the elaboration and application of the regulation concerning accessibility of disabled people was at the very beginning, this aspect has not been considered in the design phase.

The problem of accessibility in public spaces started to be brought under regulation beginning with 2001, together with the elaboration of the norm NP 051/2001 [10] that provided a series of solutions close to the exigencies of the European standards in the field.

In the present case study, with the occasion of some changes necessary to be made inside the building in 2012, it has been also decided to perform the appropriate adjustments for making the building accessible. In this respect, the following solutions were considered:

- building an exterior ramp, starting from the sidewalk level, for ensuring the access of disabled people in wheelchairs inside the building;
- installation of an elevator within the space limited by the stairs, ensuring the vertical circulation among the different building floors;
- installation of a stair elevator;
- design and execution of an accessible toilet according to the rules established by the regulations in force.

The proposed solution of installing a stair elevator was not viable because the necessary space for the transfer from and to the wheelchair was not adequate. Also, in case of fire the stair elevator could compromise the effectiveness of evacuation for the rest of the persons.

By analyzing the feasible technical-economic solutions in this case, it appeared that the optimal decision would be to install an elevator within the space limited by ramps, in one of the 4 staircases of the building (Fig. 5).

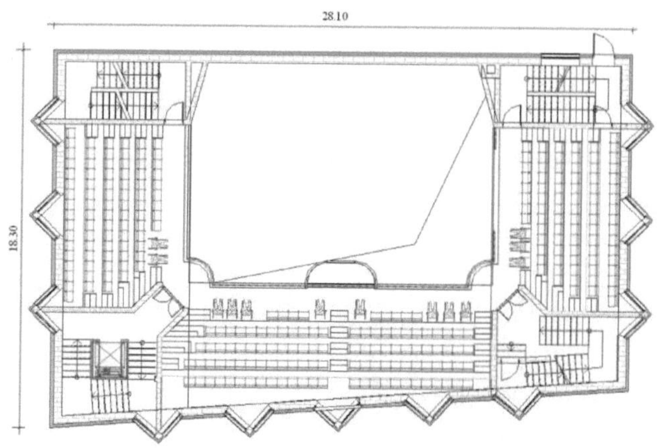

Fig. 5 First floor plan – proposed solution

In order to build the supporting elements of the elevator a spatial structure made of metallic bars, connected to the stair ramps and landings with anchors has been designed (Fig. 6).

The foundation of this structure was built of reinforced concrete tank having the slab of 1.0 m high and 30 cm thick.

The dimension in plan of the elevator's cage is 1,700 x 1,700 mm and the cabin is 1,000 x 1,250 x 2,100 mm.

The enclosure of this cage was made with plasterboards, complying with the details provided by the producer for fire protection. The electric elevator has a capacity of 450 kg (6 persons) and the control panel is also provided with vocal commands facilities and Braille inscriptions.

The investment amounted at 29,000 Euro, of which 7,000 Euro for the metallic structure and 22,000 Euro for the elevator.

Besides motoric disabled people, the elevator is also useful for other categories of users like pregnant women, aged and visually impaired persons [9].

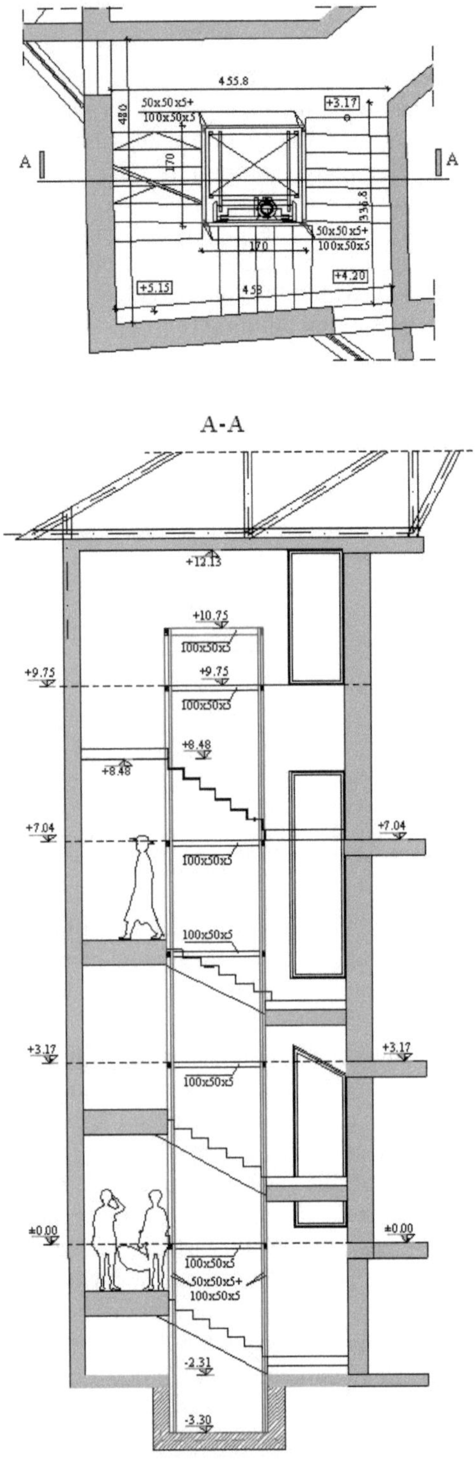

Fig. 6 Section through the elevator cage

The elevator cage ready, connected horizontally with the stairs loadbearing elements as previously mentioned, is shown in Fig. 7.

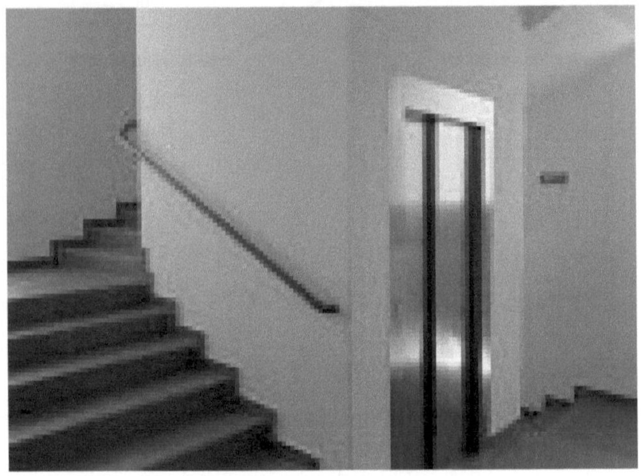

Fig. 7 The finished elevator cage

In order to ensure the necessary space for wheelchair users, the first two rows of chairs have been removed (Fig.8).

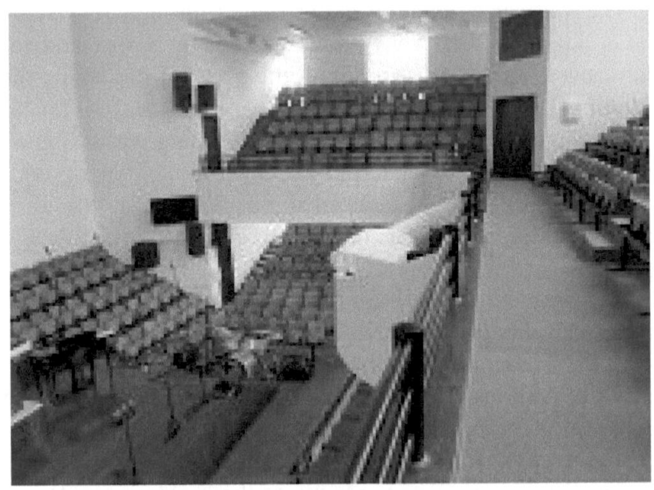

Fig. 8 Floor plan after the removal of two rows of chairs

The design of the accessible toilet (Fig. 9) was made in compliance with the requirements imposed by the Romanian regulation NP 051-2001 [10] referring to the minimal dimensions in plan.

The distance between the back wall and the WC was chosen such a way to facilitate the slipping through from the wheelchair, standing at the side of the WC. The location of the accessible toilet is shown in Fig.9 (next to the elevator) and some details in Fig. 10.

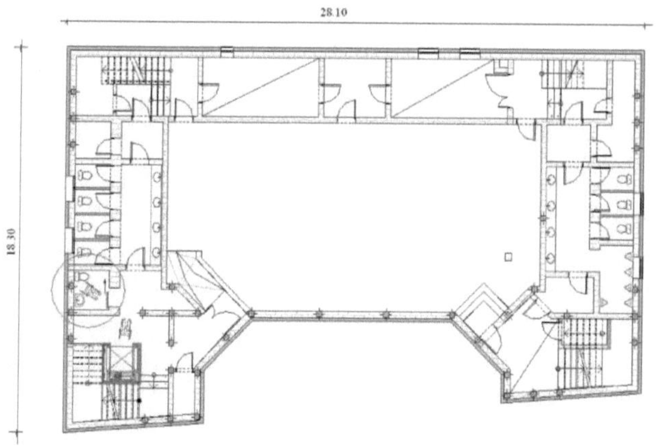

Fig. 9 Semi-basement plan with elevator and accessible toilet

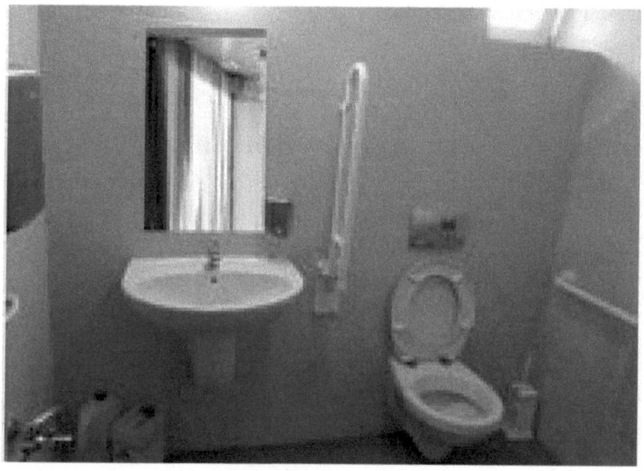

Fig. 10 The accessible toilet finished

In order to provide comfortable access within the building, the existing fence (Fig.11) has been removed and an exterior access ramp was built (Fig. 12).

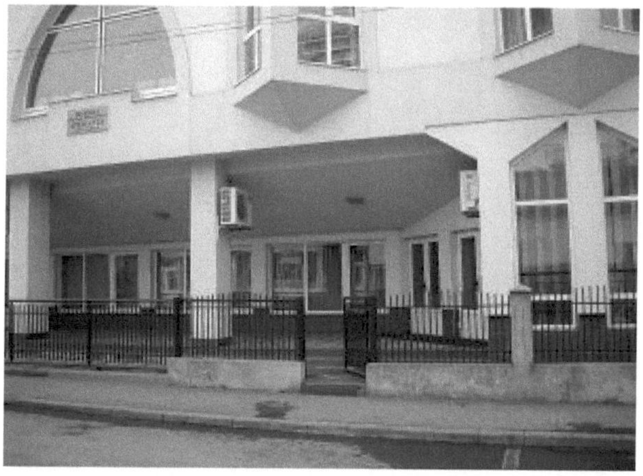

Fig. 11 Front view: the former entrance

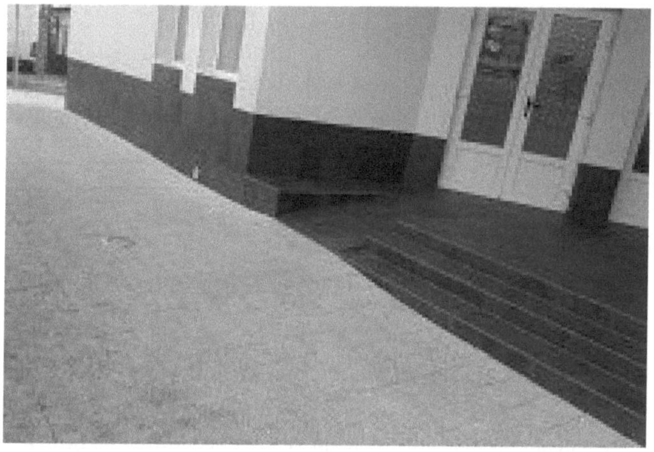

Fig. 12 New entrance with access ramp and the fence removed

III. Conclusions

A building that may not be used by all, is not fulfilling the purpose for which it was built.

The responsibility for taking into consideration the entire human life cycle and to consider the fact that disability is a normal state of life that may occur at any time, goes to the designer.

The number of new constructions is relatively small compared to that of the existing buildings, therefore making these buildings accessible is of major importance and should be stimulated [13].

In most of cases there are no serious barriers in making existing buildings accessible and even if there are, such problems may be successfully solved by good professionals.

Besides the advantages for disabled, making the built environment accessible undeniably creates advantages for a larger category of users (e.g. aged persons) by increasing the comfort in service.

The universal, adaptable elements generally are not more expensive than the traditional ones, if incorporated by the designers in the initial conceptual phase. The designer should raise the clients' awareness not only on the costs of the accessible building but also on the costs implied by ignoring in the long term an important segment of the population.

In the extent in which the construction industry and manufacturing sectors will answer the needs of ageing population and the requirements of attached regulations, the collocation of "beneficial for disabled and elderly persons" will be replaced by "beneficial for all", as a marketing strategy for planning.

Acknowledgment

The study and the research were carried out in the "Hope" Pentecostal Church from Cluj-Napoca, for which the authors are grateful to all the authorities.

Conflict of Interest

The authors declare that they have no conflict of interest.

References

1. Barnes C., (2013) Understanding disability and the importance of design for all, Journal of Accessibility and Design for All, CC) JACCES, 2011 – 1(1): 55-80. ISSN: 2013-7087
2. Autoritatea Naţională pentru Persoanele cu Handicap (National Autority for disable people) at http://www.anph.ro
3. Access improving the accessibility of historic buildings and places, National disability authority (NDA), Published by the stationary office, Dublin 2011, ISBN 978-1-4064-2319-8.
4. Hamzat T.K., Dada O.O. (2005), Wheelchair accessibility of public buildings in Ibadan, Nigeria, Asia Pacific Disability Rehabilitation Journal, Vol. 16 No. 2
5. Ordonanta de Urgenta 102/1999 privind protecţia specială şi încadrarea în muncă a persoanelor cu handicap (Emergency Order 102/1999 regarding the special protection and integration in labour of disabled people)
6. Legea nr. 448/2006 privind protectia si promovarea drepturilor persoanelor cu handicap (Law no. 448/2006 regarding the protection and the promotion of the rights of peoples with dissability).
7. The Center for Universal Design (1997). The Principles of Universal Design, Version 2.0. Raleigh,NC: North Carolina State University, at http://www.ncsu.edu/ncsu/design/cud/about_ud/udprinciplestext.htm
8. Abdul Kadir S.Jamaludin M., (2012) Applicability of Malaysian Standards and Universal Design in Public Buildings in Putrajaya, ASIAN Journal of Environment-Behaviour Studies, volume 3, Number 9
9. AWARD - Accessible World for All, Respecting Differences, Leonardo da Vinci Programme, Project nr.07/0227-L/LLP-LdV-TOI-200–HU_001 at http://constructii.utcluj.ro/award/
10. Indicativ: NP 051/2001 Normativ pentru adaptarea cladirilor civile si spatiului urban afferent la exigentele persoanelor cu handicap (Code for adaptive of buildings and urband space to disable peoples requirements), Institutul de Proiectare, Cercetare si Tehnica de Calcul in Constructii, IPCT-SA (Institute for Design, Research and Computation Techniques in Constructions).
11. Practice Guidebook for Adaptive Re-use of and Alteration and Addition Works to Heritage Buildings, 2012, Buildings Department Hong Kong (available online: Practice Guidebook for Adaptive Re-use of and Alteration and Addition).
12. Rimmer J.H. (2011), Building a future in disability and public health, Disability and Health Journal 4 (2011) 6e11.
13. Konkolla M., Koivu H. (2003), Accessible Homes, Finnish Association of People with Mobility Dissabilities/ Disable Persons Planning Service, Helsinki.

Author: Nicoleta Cobîrzan
Institute: Technical University of Cluj-Napoca, Faculty of Civil Engineering
Street: 15 Daicoviciu Street
City: Cluj-Napoca
Country: Romania
Email: Nicoleta.Cobarzan@cif.utcluj.ro

A Proposal for a Driving System of a Four DOF Rehabilitation Exoskeleton

B. Chetran, O. Tătar, S. Noveanu, and D. Mândru

Technical University of Cluj-Napoca, Department of Mechatronics and Machine Dynamics, Cluj-Napoca, Romania

Abstract— **The paper presents a proposal of a four degrees of freedom (DOF) upper limb rehabilitation exoskeleton and its control system which is designed for the control of the serial mechanisms angular position. It contains as an extension, a module for driving of a braking system with smart fluids. The proposed control system is suitable for active and passive exercises. The rehabilitation system is developed for rehabilitation training at home, without a supervision of a qualified person during exercises.**

Keywords— **upper limb, rehabilitation, exoskeleton, driver, electrorheologic fluid**

I. INTRODUCTION

As a result of the increasing number of peoples with physical disabilities, the robot-assisted therapy systems are being used in more effective rehabilitation processes. The rehabilitation robotic systems are coming with great advantages regarding the repeated movements during goal-directed tasks, the evaluation of different physiological and functional parameters during rehabilitation exercises, wide range and variety of exercises, improving motivation and promoting home exercises and training, [1], [2]. The exoskeleton systems are smart, wearable robotic exercisers which provide physical support for limbs segments and allow exercises with active and passive movements.

Presently, different exoskeletons for upper limb are developed. These are designed as assistive devices in performing physical tasks or as rehabilitation trainers. The assistive exoskeletons are portable, able to retrieve a part of total force exhibited on the human body segments. The rehabilitation exercises for the entire upper limb are in most cases developed as stationary equipment. Those developed to be portable are in most cases designed as devices for some specific upper limb movements, [2].

II. THE DEVELOPED EXOSKELETON AND THE IMPOSED CONSTRAINTS

In our previous work, based on anatomical and biomechanical considerations, the structural synthesis of the mechanisms for upper limb wearable exercisers was given, initial design of a family of such exercisers was emphasized and an original Matlab model of upper limb – wearable exerciser ensemble was described, [3].

Our efforts were focused on the development of the mechanical structure of an upper limb rehabilitation exoskeleton (Fig.1). The following constrains are considered: the linkage adapts to the anthropometric dimensions, the mechanical structure sustains the upper limb segments during passive exercises but can be also used for active movements; the angles and torque should be adjusted during or before exercises; the chosen actuators are 12 V DC motors with gear boxes and the braking modules for active exercises are clutches with smart fluids (electro / magneto-rheological fluids ERF/MRF), [4].

The simulations concerning the torque during passive exercises reveal the average value of around 24 Nm exerted in the humeral joint. The chosen DC motor can develop this torque at 12V with consumption current of 25A.

For the assessment of the rehabilitation process, the control system of the exoskeleton must be able to quantify the movement angles, speed, acceleration and torque on each joint.

III. THE COMAND AND CONTROL SYSTEM

The quadrature encoder for angle measurement is easy to implement on the mechanical structure. Signals received are digital and are not influenced by external parasite frequencies. The disadvantage is given by the complexity of electronic diagram and the software that should be able to read all the time the encoder. For that it must be allocated a controller for each encoder that should communicate with the master controller.

The quadrature encoder consists from a Q9864 optical switch with two channels (a LED light source and two phototransistors) and a slot disk mounted on the joint shaft.

This construction was adopted in order to be capable to read the movement during both passive and active exercises. The sensitivity is set by the slots number and for the final prototype will be less the one degree.

Another method to read the angles is to use on each joint, variable resistors. In comparison with the encoders the variable resistor are cost effective, are simpler are available in a variation of forms and sizes. As disadvantages can be mentioned that the output signals are analogic and are distorted by the digital signals on the PCB (printed circuit board). The electronics should contain low pass filters and the PCB should be developed with a good ground plane design.

S. Vlad and R.V. Ciupa (eds.), *International Conference on Advancements of Medicine and Health Care through Technology*, IFMBE Proceedings 44,
DOI: 10.1007/978-3-319-07653-9_2, © Springer International Publishing Switzerland 2014

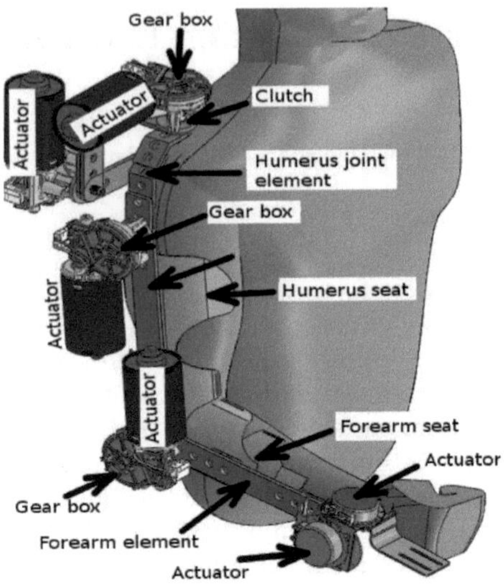

a.

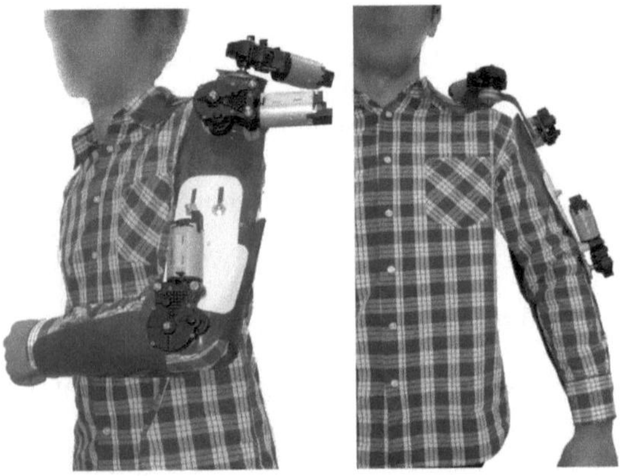

b.

Fig. 1 a The 3D CAD model of the exoskeleton, b. - The developed exoskeleton

Electronic gyroscopes can also be used as angle measurement systems. These components come with an integrated controller that has the capacity to communicate via I2C. The disadvantages are represented by their price.

The force sensors are required in order to measure the amount of force developed over the upper limb during exercises. Also, force sensors act as a safety measurement to protect both the upper limb and mechanical structure to overload. The force sensors come in different sizes and forms and with different active elements. The ones choose to measure the forces during exercises are square shape resistive sensors. The total surface area is 4.47 cm^2 and it will be mounted in specific areas between the upper limb segments and the exoskeleton links. The values read from these sensors can be used also for torque computation.

A. Sensors and Controllers

The control system (Fig. 5) must be able to perform different parallel tasks like: reading four position sensors and controlling the motors speed at a time. The controller can perform such tasks only in serial mode. A serial control system can cause delays in controlling the actuator position or speed, situation unaccepted for rehabilitation robotic systems. By adopting a master – slave structure the control system can provide parallel control of sensors and actuators.

An Atmel AVR microcontroller system was chosen to control the exoskeleton structure. The master controller is ATMega 328 which communicates on I2C interface with all other controllers. A serial communication with an external PC is required on the same controller. All sensors must be read by their specific programmed controller as follow:

- Quadrature encoders read by ATTiny 2313; one controller for each encoder, (Fig. 2);
- Gyroscope sensors communicate directly with the master controller via I2C, (Fig. 3).
- Resistive force sensors read by ATMega32 controller via ADC Port. In order to extend the number of force sensors a multiplexer will be used, if necessary, (Fig. 4).

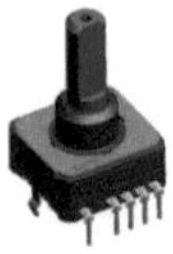

Fig. 2 Quadrature encoder

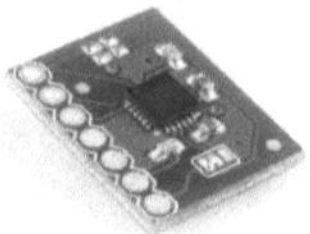

Fig. 3 Gyroscope ITG 3200

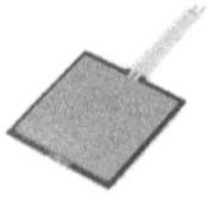

Fig. 4 Force sensor

The quadrature encoders have to be independently read by one controller in order to generate a stop signal precisely when the required position was achieved. The read program should be as short as possible otherwise steps are misread. If encoder sequence is included into the master controller program creates disadvantages like: when one encoder is read, the program is looped only in this sequence and the controller is disabled by the other tasks.

The signal *A* of each quadrature encoder is connected on pin PD2 and the signal *B* to the PD3 pin of one ATTiny2313 controller. The PD2 and PD3 pins are the external interrupts pins. The controller is programmed with the external interrupts are enabled and read on rising edge. When the signal *A* rises from 0 to logical 1 (+5V) then the pin PD3(encoder signal *B*) is state checked; if the value of the pin is 0 then the rotation direction is clockwise and if the value of the pin is logical 1 then the rotation is counterclockwise. Each time when the *A* signal rises an variable is incremented or decremented according with the direction.

Reading angles by aid of variable resistors are also a good alternative. Here the potentiometers are read by an

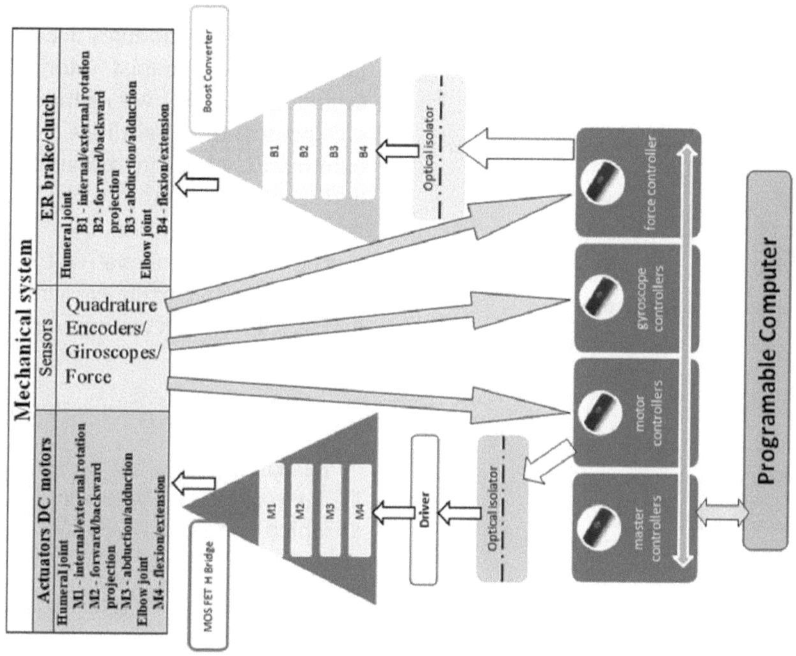

Fig. 5 The control block diagram of the exoskeleton

ATMega 32 microcontroller on analog port. The potentiometer wiper has to be connected on the joint shaft. The voltage drop on the variable resistor is read by the analog comparator port PA0 to PA3 one pin for each potentiometer. In this case is not required to have different controllers for each sensor. The values are read independently of each port and the value is compared with the zero set value or start position.

Force sensors are read in the same manner as the variable resistors for angles measurement. The controller used is another ATMega 32. The scope of using another controller is to have the possibility to control the ERF or MRF brake.

The ERF brakes are driven by boost converters, one for each brake. When the force rises to a desired value, the ERF force controller must maintain the force value by controlling the voltage on the ERF brake. Another case is to use MRF brakes. In this case the brakes are controlled by a magnetic field generated by a coil, [6]. The coil is drove by a BD239 transistor controlled in pulse width modulation (PWM) by the force controller, (Fig. 5).

B. Motors and Brakes Drivers

The DC Motors are drove by the controller ATTINY2313 that read the encoder, (Fig.6). The according PWM signals are software set with the desired values received from PC. Pins PB7 and PB6 are set high according with the desired direction. The direction signals are feeding the inputs of L293 motor driver. The L293 motor driver, receive the PWM signals and generate outputs according with the direction and the PWM signals, (Fig.7). These signals are controlling the H bridge transistors in order to amplify the current up to 25 A required by the DC motors, (Fig. 8), [6]. Fig. 9 shows the force controller and the electrical diagram of the ERF brake amplifier circuit. The ERF brake is varies the output torque in respect with the intensity of the electric field applied on the ERF. The field intensity is given by the boost converter output. The output is adjusted in respect with a desired value by the PWM signal that triggers the Q1 switch, [7]. Because of the high voltage obtained an optocoupler is used to separate the control board by the high voltage board. The Boost converter PWM signal is generated by the same controller used for reading the force sensors.

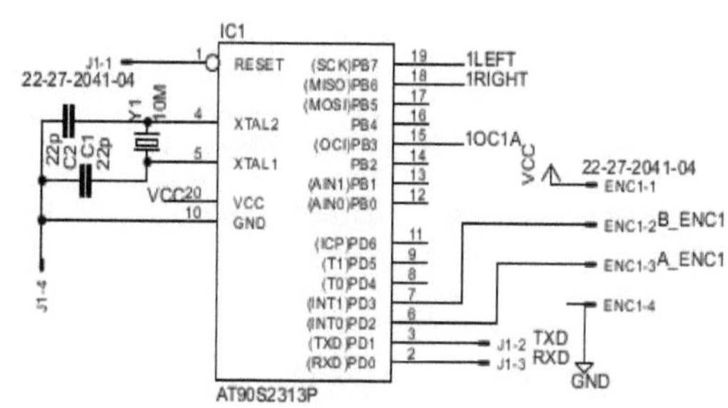

Fig. 6 The motor and quadrature encoder controller

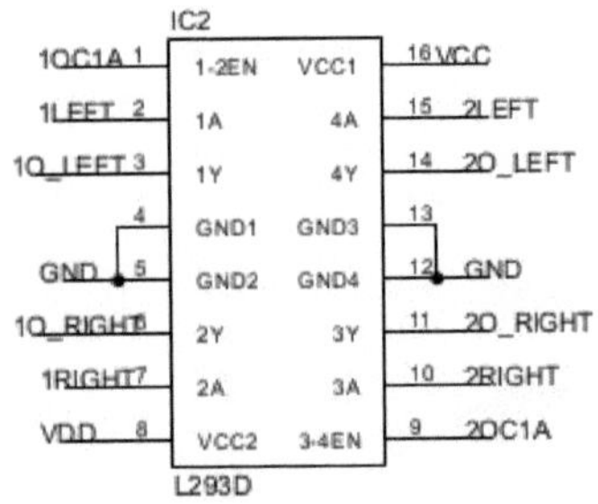

Fig. 7 L293 motor driver connections

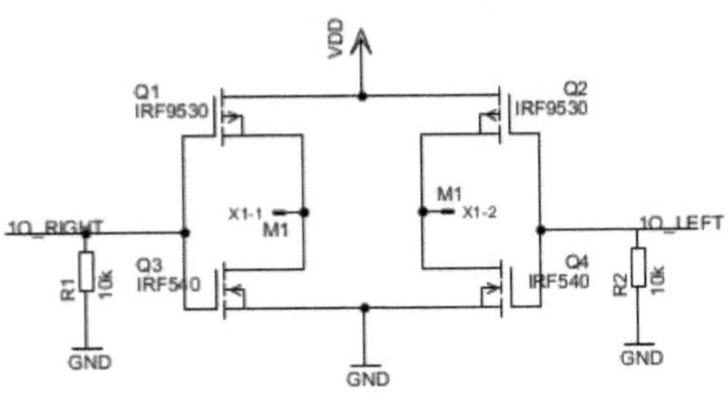

Fig. 8 Final stage amplifier – H bridge

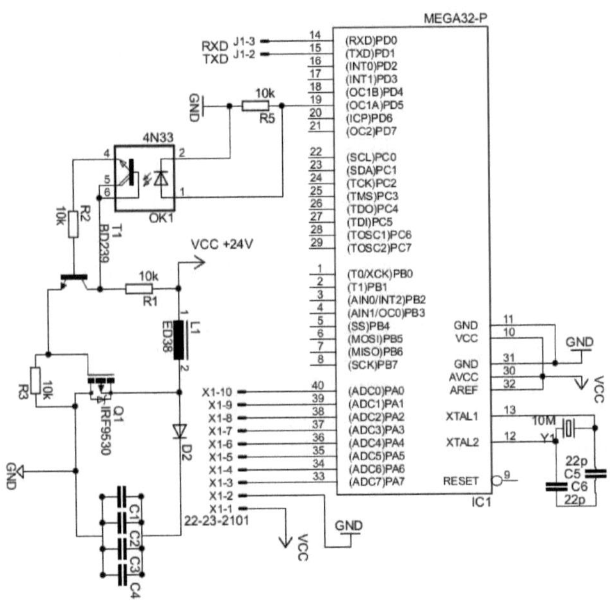

Fig. 9 ERF brake final stage amplifier and force controller

IV. Conclusions

Exoskeletons, in our days, used as rehabilitation systems are powerful systems that raise the rehabilitation process ton a high level of development. The microcontroller based control system becomes a necessity in order to control all the exoskeleton modules according with the exercises proposed by the therapist. Moreover this type of controlling system is flexible over a range of different users with different grades of disabilities. The communication with an external PC offers the possibility to load system parameters and acquired data into a database for further use and analysis.

The proposed innovative ERF braking system allows execution of active exercises with different variation functions and in respect with an imposed force.

Acknowledgment

Research supported by PCCA nr. 180/2012, A Hybrid FES-Exoskeleton System to Rehabilitate the Upper Limb in Disabled People (EXOSLIM).

Conflict of Interest

The authors declare that they have no conflict of interest.

References

1. Jonhson, M.J., et. all, (2006) Development of aADLER: The Activities of Daily Living Exerciser Robot, Proc. of the Int. Conference BIOROB, Rome.
2. Kazerooni, H., (2008) Exoskeletons for Human Performance Augmentation, Springer Handbook of Robotics, pp 773-793.
3. Noveanu S., Chetran B., Tătar O., Răducanu G., Mândru D. (2013), Structural Synthesis of the Upper Limb Modular Wearable Exerciser, Proc. of the 17th Int. Conference on System Theory, Control and Computing (ICSTCC-2013), Sinaia, pp. 693-697.
4. Chetran B., (2012) Studies And Researches Regarding Kinetoterapy Smart Systems, PhD Thesis, Technical University of Cluj-Napoca.
5. Graeve, O., (2007) Electrorheological Fluids and Magnetorheological Suspensions, World Scientific Publishing Co. Pte. Ltd., ISBN-10 981-277-119-0.
6. Schweizer K., (2010) DC and BLDC Motor Control Ics, http://www.atmel.com/images/ article_ac7_dc-and-bldc-motor-control-ics.pdf
7. Hauke B., (2014) Basic Calculation of a Boost Converter's Power Stage, Application Report SLVA372C, http://www.ti.com/lit/an/slva372c/slva372c.pdf

Author: Beniamin Chetran
Institute: Technical University of Cluj-Napoca
Street: 28 Memorandumului
City: Cluj-Napoca
Country: Romania
Email: Beniamin.Chetran@mdm.utcluj.ro

Neuromuscular Electrical Stimulation for Mobility Support of Elderly

W. Mayr[1], M. Krenn[1], M. Hendling[1], M. Haller[1], T. Nepomucky[1], E. Unger[1],
J. Cvečka[2], M. Sedliak[2], V. Tirpáková[2], D. Hamar[2], H. Fruhmann[3], S. Löfler[3], C. Hofer[3,4], and H. Kern[3,5]

[1] Center for Medical Physics and Biomedical Engineering, Medical University of Vienna, Vienna, Austria
[2] Faculty of Physical Education and Sports, Comenius University, Bratislava, Slovakia
[3] Ludwig Boltzmann Institute for Electrical Stimulation and Physical Rehabilitation, Vienna, Austria
[4] Otto Bock Healthcare Products GmbH, Vienna, Austria
[5] Department of Physical Medicine and Rehabilitation, Wilhelminenspital, Vienna, Austria

Abstract— **Ageing is associated with progressive degradation of physiological functionalities. Especially sarcopenia associated with loss of skeletal muscle mass, force and function strongly impairs mobility and autonomous living of senior citizens in their later years. Neuromuscular training based on non-invasive electrical stimulation could be a powerful and cost effective countermeasure capable of substantially delaying immobility and maintaining independent living.**

An electrical stimulation system was developed, with special focus on the requirements of safe and easy use by elderly persons, even if their cognitive abilities and fine motor skills appear diminished. The system is intended for neuromuscular training of the anterior thigh (quadriceps muscles).

The portable stimulation system consists of a control unit, providing an optimized user interface (simple and error-avoiding operation), and two stimulation modules, supplied and controlled via cable connections and carrying integrated electrodes and fixation means. Each stimulation module contains a microcontroller for data management and impulse generation, a power output stage for delivery of biphasic rectangular, charge balanced and voltage controlled impulses, and a measurement unit for recording of muscle twitch patterns (integrated accelerometer sensors) and electrode impedance (impulse current).

During operation an implemented compliance monitor permanently stores data on timing of stimulation, changes in parameter adjustments and recorded twitch and current values for later off-line analysis via a Visual Studio C# program, supporting guidance of training by supervising physicians.

In a validation study 5 subjects tested the system for observation periods of up to 10 weeks with 2 weekly training sessions of 3x6 minutes, in the first 2 weeks and sessions of 3x10 minutes duration in the remaining period.

The recorded data proved both failure free system operation and consequent use of the system in line with guidelines by all subjects, thus enabling valid correlation of training activity with physiological follow-up assessments on muscle function, morphology and molecular biology.

Keywords— **Neuromuscular electrical stimulation, muscle training, sarcopenia, mobility, elderly**

I. INTRODUCTION

The process of aging is associated with a variety of degenerative changes in the human organism. Especially the progressive loss of neuromuscular functionality, reduces and inhibits mobility of elderly persons, sooner or later reaches a disability threshold and in final consequence leads to loss of independent living.

Reduction of muscle mass and muscle function, generally described by the term "sarcopenia", are obvious macroscopic indications accompanying growing mobility deficits, can act as predictors for coming disabilities [1]. Studies report a decrease in isometric knee extension torque of in average 40% between 25 and 80 years old subjects [1]. Pronounced aging dependent degeneration is also depicted in the microscopic scale: Histological analyses show reduction of muscle fiber size and metabolic shift towards slow twitch type. Electron microscopy documents degeneration and loss of cellular excitation contraction coupling (ECM) units, reduction in mitochondrial density and structural disassembly of contractile protein structures [2].

Other studies show that active exercising can dramatically improve muscle strength and functional abilities of elder individuals [3,4]. An extensive review confirms strong evidence that neuromuscular electrical stimulation (NMS) is an efficient possibility for increasing muscle strength and maintaining muscle performance through periods of hypokinetic conditions [5].

The aim of our work was development of an efficient, safe, easy to handle and cost effective methodology and associated equipment for maintaining mobility of elderly persons and substantially delaying their reach of disability threshold. This method builds on neuromuscular electrical stimulation applied as regular home-based training under professional supervision and guidance on the basis of permanently recorded compliance data.

Special demands had to be considered on reduced cognitive and fine motoric ability of operating technical equipment autonomously in home environment. Further specific requirements were simple, robust and easily cleanable construction principles.

II. MATERIAL AND METHODS

The home based electrical stimulation training targets the anterior thigh muscles, quadriceps femora, which are

S. Vlad and R.V. Ciupa (eds.), *International Conference on Advancements of Medicine and Health Care through Technology*,
IFMBE Proceedings 44,
DOI: 10.1007/978-3-319-07653-9_3,

essential for safe and self-confident stand-up and sit-down maneuvers as well as walking on up- and downwards tracks and stair climbing. For safety reasons the training is exclusively applied in sitting position and knee extensions were performed unilaterally in alternating sequences of left and right leg (Fig. 1).

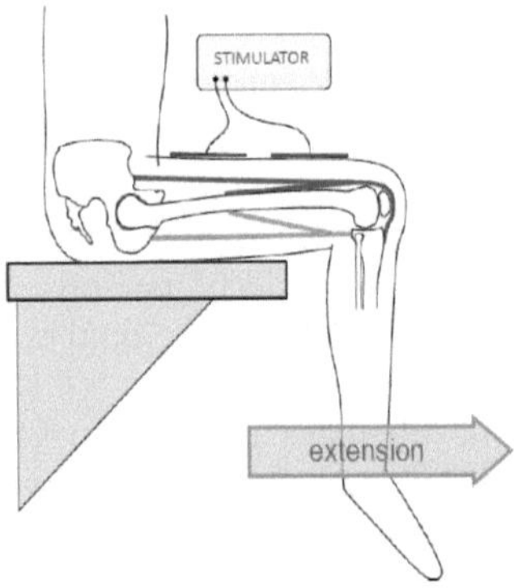

Fig. 1 Stimulation setup with subject in sitting position and alternating NMS supported voluntary knee extension of left and right leg

Training needed to remain restricted to minimal need of time and to avoid complicated handling and sensible discomfort to ensure regular application over longer time periods. Therefore, the NMS-training protocol was limited to 3x6 minutes, twice weekly, for an accommodation phase of two weeks and further on 3x10 minutes twice a week for 5 weeks and three times weekly for the remaining 4 weeks. Parameters were pre-evaluated with respect to sensibly well-accepted impulse width, frequency and burst shape. Accordingly biphasic rectangular impulses with 300 μs per phase were delivered at a frequency of 60 pps (pulses per second). Activation bursts had a length of 3.5 s including an initial amplitude ramp of 0.5 s and an inter-burst pause of 4.5 s. Voltage-controlled impulse delivery was chosen to avoid unpleasant sensations in case of partial conductivity loss at electrode skin contact surface respectively loosening of contact during operation. Adjustment of intensity levels was left to the subjects' discretion with the rule to go for the maximum intensity still perceived as comfortable and readjust any time if felt to be necessary. To improve motivation and add neuromuscular coordination tasks to the exercise design stimulated extension was combined with voluntary extension with the subjects instructed to perform full knee extension and add the necessary voluntary effort to the stimulated support.

Study: 5 subjects, 1 male, 4 female, were included in the validation study, the observation period was nine weeks. In the initial accommodation phase of two weeks, the subjects performed 2 weekly sessions with 3 times 6 minutes (45 contractions per leg) of continuous training and 5 minutes rest in-between. For the further period activity was increased to 3 weekly sessions with 3 times 10 minutes (75 contractions) separated by 5 minutes pause. The study had been approved by the Medical Ethics Committee of the City of Vienna (decision nr. EK-08-102-0608) and subjects gave their written informed consent before their inclusion.

Stimulation System: The developed stimulation system is the outcome of a series of prototype versions [6]. The actual model produced in a small series for the study is modular in design and relies on software based functionality. The user version consists of 3 modules: a central unit with 3 switches, graphical display, microcontroller with interface circuitry and rechargeable battery and 2 stimulation modules, each containing a coordinating microcontroller unit, stimulation end-stage including voltage step-up converter and direct current (DC) decoupling current sensing and a 3D accelerometer sensor unit. The stimulation modules are linked to the central unit via multipolar cables for power supply, control and data exchange. An USB-cable with medical grade galvanic separation can be used to connect the central unit safely to any external computer for programming and transfer of recorded compliance data (Fig. 2).

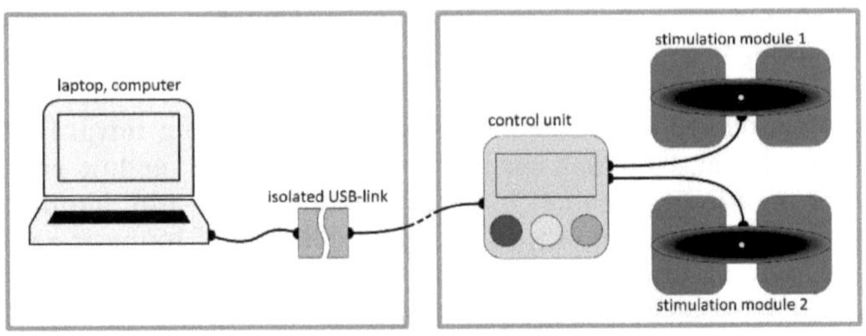

Fig. 2 Basic design of the stimulation unit (right) and notebook interface with medical grade galvanic separation in the USB line (left)

Details of the electronic circuitry of central unit and stimulation modules are shown in Fig. 3. The heart of the main control unit is a microcontroller PIC32MX795F512L (Microchip Technology Inc., Chandler AZ, USA) responsible for control of internal peripheral modules. Stimulation protocol and compliance data are stored on a secure-digital (SD) memory card with a capacity of 4 Giga Byte (GB). A real time clock is used to synchronize stored data especially in long-time home-based application. The unit contains a Lithium Polymer rechargeable battery with 3.7 V and 1500 mAh (milli Ampere hours) providing over 8 hours operation time. The battery is charged via Qi-certified wireless power link. The interactive user interface is reduced to a high contrast LC-Display, 2 multicolor status LEDs, 3 colored membrane pressure point trigger switches (diameter 20 mm) for command inputs and a 3D accelerometer sensor, which can trigger an emergency stop in case the user drops the unit and loses control.

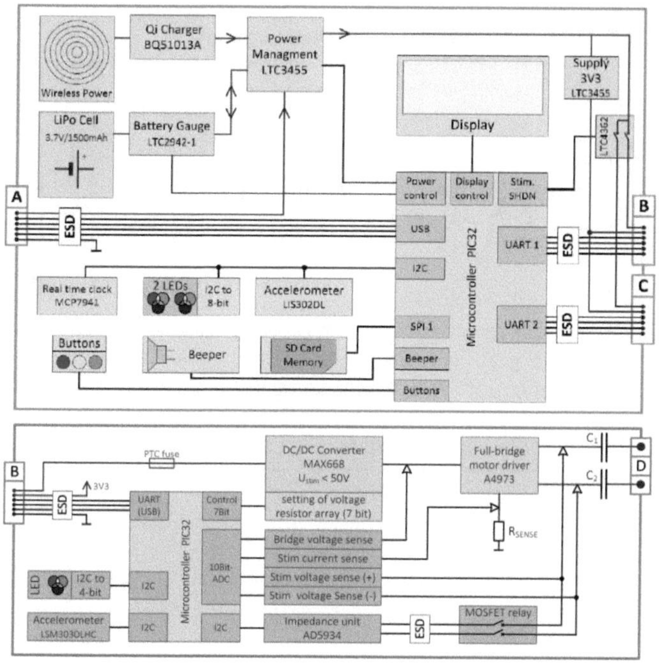

Fig. 3 Block diagrams of central unit (upper scheme) and one stimulator module (lower scheme) with all main functional elements. 2 stimulator units are connected with multipolar cables for power supply and data exchange.

Two multipolar cables for power supply and bidirectional data exchange are connected to the two stimulator units. In the lower scheme of Fig. 3 functional details of one stimulator unit are displayed. The modules contain their own microcontroller (PIC32MX250F128D, Microchip Technology, Chandler, AZ, USA) for management of stimulus delivery, data recording and communication. Further main elements are a step-up voltage converter transforming the battery voltage to adjustable levels of up to 45 V as needed for the H-bridge based stimulation end-stage. To ensure strict charge balance, capacitors decouple the electrode terminals to ensure blocking of direct current even in case of any thinkable technical failure. Output current is permanently monitored and allows indirect monitoring of electrode impedance. The integrated 3D-accelerometer-sensor has 3 functions: it (1) monitors muscle twitches via displacement movements of the muscle belly with attached stimulator, (2) monitors the position of the thigh to enable or block stimulation if subject is or is not sitting correctly and finally (3) detects mild shocks by strikes on the module case, which acts as an option for emergency shutdown. Current-, voltage- and accelerometer signals are permanently sampled and are part of the compliance data record. A centrally placed multi-color LED acts as a simple status indicator for operation or failure of the module. The stimulator units further carry 2 conductive rubber electrodes (9 x 14 cm, Schuhfried Medizintechnik, Vienna, Austria), touch protected by a non-conductive silicone insulation layer, and applied via water soaked foam sheet pockets and soft elastic bands with Velcro fixation.

The adjustment ranges for the most relevant parameters are defined in Table 1.

Table 1 Stimulation parameter ranges

	Parameter range		
Amplitude	3.0 V	to	+/-45 V
Impulse width	2 x 50 µs	to	2 x 1 ms
Pulse rate	0.01 pps	to	200 pps
Burst duration	5 ms	to	7200 s
Inter-burst pause	5 ms	to	7200 s

Compliance monitoring is an important extension in stimulator design, increasing motivation for accurate and regular application, as the subject is of course fully informed and aware of the data recording, and allows objective analysis of impact of a training strategy and thus an effective guidance by therapeutic supervisors. In order to be efficient, a compliance monitor needs to have sufficient sampling capacity for fast transients, like impulse current traces, and enough storage capacity for recording over weeks. It is further essential, that an interactive graphical user interface displays extracted key features and time courses of relevant activities and changes in a clear overview for fast interpretation by medical personnel.

In our stimulation device all actively applied protocols, adjustments of intensity and detailed shape of current impulses and sensed muscle twitches are protocolled over time. The sampling rate for time dependent curves is 83.3 kS/s (kilo-Samples per second), the available memory 4 GB (actual SD-card, expandable). As current data sampling per training session requires less than 1 MB (Mega Byte) of memory space there is room for theoretically more than 4000 sessions, no real limitation for any study. Timing is documented by storing time points read from the real-time clock. Data pre-reduction is achieved by real-time analysis and extraction and storage of just exemplary data. An example is handling of impulse bursts, where number of inherent impulses, mean-, maximum- and minimum-amplitude values and single representative impulses in full resolution sampling can be stored.

The evaluation software is programmed in Visual Studio C# (Microsoft, Redmond, WS, USA). It allows import of the stored data from the stimulator unit and analysis and visualization of recent training activities as a whole and in relevant details. This software tool is designed as a versatile and flexible tool with a preserved complete set of imported raw data and basic functionalities for automated feature extraction and time course visualizations that can be altered and extended freely at any time if necessary. Typical visualizations in the current version are, in addition to all preprogrammed protocol parameters and amount and distribution of activities, time course of intensity adjustments along the whole observation period or in single training sessions, time course of electrode impedance or special detail issues like charge per impulse in relation to externally recorded muscle reactions, as suggested in [7].

III. Results

The stimulation system has been autonomously applied by 5 subjects for observation periods of up to 10 weeks in home environment. The system was working without technical problems or user complains. Compliance data records were analyzed after the period individually and in intra-individual comparison. Only exemplary results of this validation study are presented here.

Table 2 shows mean values and standard deviations of recorded stimulation voltage and stimulation current intensities for each participant for the entire period of the NMS-training study. Intensity adjustments as well as reproducible electrode impedance are basic conditions for studies of this kind and their monitoring is essential for quality assurance. Of course this verification of valid experimental conditions is only complete, if the entire protocol was consequently followed without discontinuities, which would also be visible in the course of this data set as a whole.

Table 2 Average (avg.) voltage and current (standard deviation) of all training sessions for each subject.

subject no.	avg. voltage (V)	avg. current (mA)
A219	17.45 (2.22)	67.64 (4.24)
B028	19.05 (2.97)	61.61 (6.63)
B026	16.62 (3.76)	58.89 (5.02)
B029	20.22 (2.47)	62.80 (5.14)
B024	15.93 (2.83)	54.75 (4.74)
mean value (standard deviation)	18.81 (2.58)	57.33 (5.78)

These average data are extracted from more detailed individual records as shown in Figure 4. Mean values and standard deviation for each trainings series (3 series per trainings day) are plotted for voltage and current amplitude for the initial 6 protocol weeks of subject A219.

In further refinement of analysis of recorded data Figure 5 shows progressive voltage amplitude adjustments along the 10-minute training sequence of subject A219. After careful beginning with 12 V impulses a first level of 24 V is reached and maintained. After half of the sequence a further increase to a final plateau of 28 V is visible.

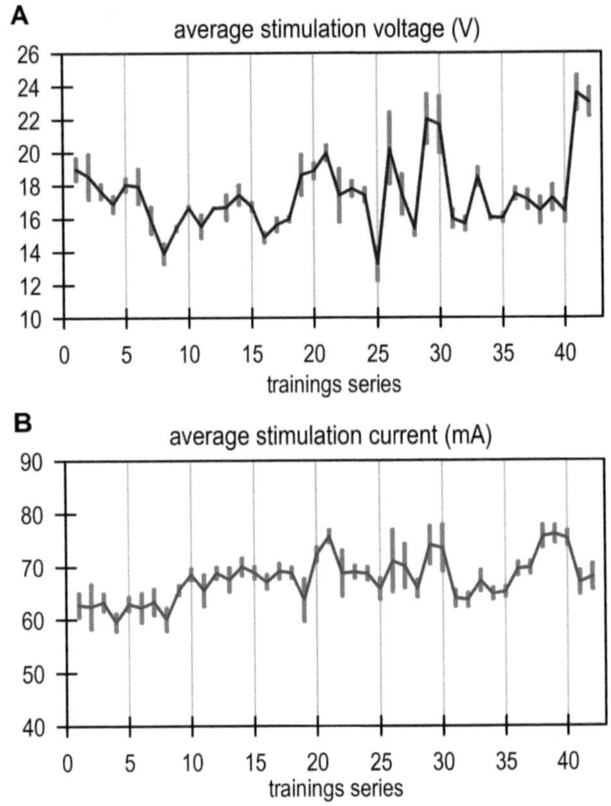

Fig. 4 Average stimulation voltage (A) and current amplitude (B) of a training series through the initial 6 weeks (14 training days, 42 stimulation sequences) for subject A219. The bars show the standard deviation.

Current traces are sampled with 83.3 kS/s, one representative impulse (after first half of burst duration) from each delivered burst (Figure 6) is stored in the compliance protocol in full resolution. Figure 6 shows an overlay of 3 voltage and current traces stored during the 10-minute stimulation sequence displayed in Figure 5.

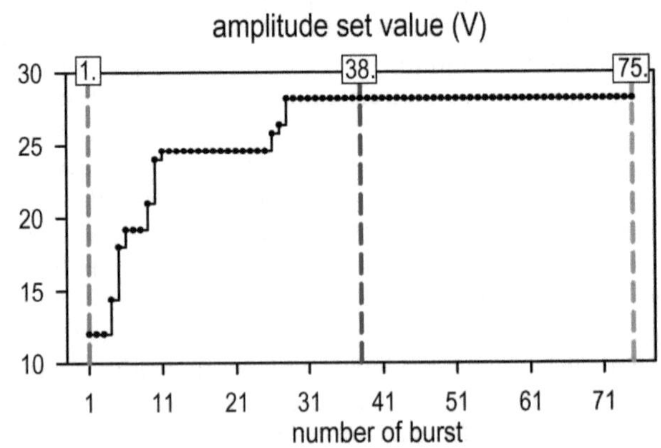

Fig. 5 Adjustments of voltage amplitude by subject A219 along its 10-minute stimulation sequence

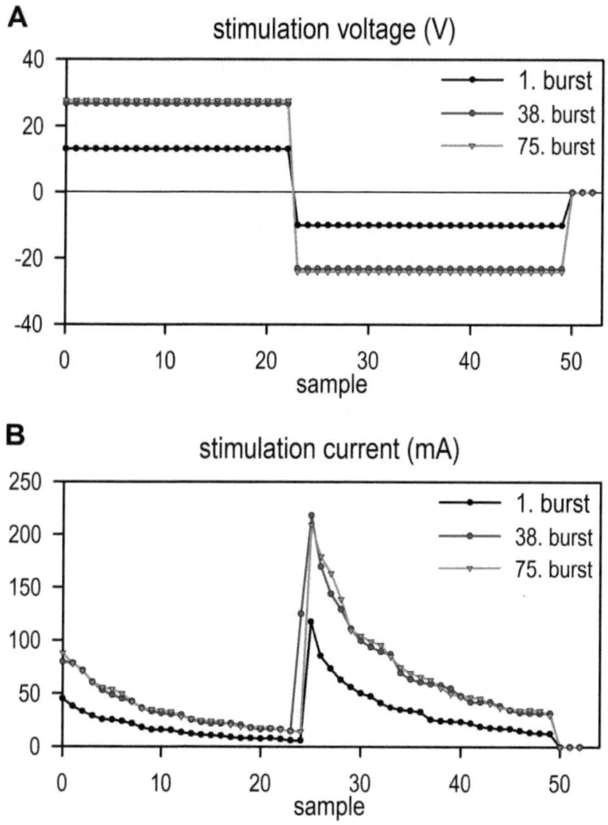

Fig. 6 Impulse samples of stimulation voltage (A) and current (B), sample rate 83.3 kS/s; single representative biphasic impulses (300 µs per phase) from 1st, 38th and 75th burst of the sequence in Figure 5 are plotted

IV. Discussion

NMS in combination of voluntary efforts in home-based application of our equipment and protocol leads to significant improvements in muscle cell physiology, voluntary knee extension torque and functional coordination tasks, as published elsewhere [8,9].

The technical equipment needs to consider special issues for safe, effective and motivated long-term use in home environment. A simple user interface can compensate mental and fine motoric deficits and reduced visual skills, automated safety monitoring with switch-off in case of improper conditions and easy cleaning are further important features.

An integrated compliance monitor system has turned out to be of essential added value and in some respects an indispensable prerequisite for safe and efficient home-based operation. As the system is able to trace all activities and most possible failures it supports guidance of training in self-responsibility and more deeply by qualified medical personnel from a supervising outpatient clinic. For scientific studies it provides at the same time a powerful tool for standardization and evaluation of validity of data.

Intensity adjustment is a very critical basic parameter in studies where it is based on individual decisions rather than measured feedback parameters. In our study subjects had to decide on sensible comfort/discomfort versus subjectively perceived strength of muscle contractions. The instruction to go for maximum achievable contractions just below pain threshold involves some systematic variance induced from individual sensitivity, placement and condition of electrodes, etc. Therefore monitoring of the whole course of individually adjusted intensity levels is of high value for later objective data interpretation.

The values in Table 2 show mean voltage levels, resulting current intensities and their fluctuation ranges for each participant and for the entire study group. These data per se allow judgment on constancy and inter-individual comparability of applied intensity and electrode setup. In addition to intensity adjustments electrode impedance, delivered current amplitude and impulse charge are important and most relevant evaluation parameters. Especially high-resolution sampling of current- and impedance-traces and charge per impulse allow accurate post-analysis of electrode stability, movement artefacts and electrolytic stress at the electrode-tissue interface.

In real time monitoring those can be observed in correlation with recorded muscle twitch traces provided from the integrated accelerometer sensors, which allows e. g. differentiation between losses in electrode contact versus muscle fatigue phenomena and automated instructions for corrective action to the user or emergency shut down if necessary. Similar automations can support safe and simplified start conditions in each training session with checking proper electrode conditions and recruitment of muscle twitches by plausible stimulus intensities.

Even so we have not yet implemented all mentioned functionalities in our system yet all necessary hardware features are already implemented and we were able to demonstrate stable and reliable sampling and collection of all necessary data sets. Finally the system is designed openly enough for future studies on further optimization of training effect versus amount of needed time.

Acknowledgment

The authors would like to acknowledge the support of the European Regional Development Fund: Cross Border Cooperation Program Slovakia – Austria 2007 - 2013 (Interreg IVA) for funding the project "Mobilität im Alter", MOBIL, N00033 (Partners: Ludwig Boltzmann Institute of Electrical Stimulation and Physical Rehabilitation, Austria, Center for Medical Physics and Biomedical Engineering, Medical

University of Vienna, Austria, and Faculty of Physical Education and Sports, Comenius University in Bratislava, Slovakia; Austrian national co-financing: Vienna Medical University, Austrian Ministry of Science and Research and Ludwig Boltzmann Society, Vienna, Austria).

Conflict of Interest

The authors declare that they have no conflict of interest.

References

1. Lauretani F, Russo CR, Bandinelli S et al (2003) Age-associated changes in skeletal muscles and their effect on mobility: an operational diagnosis of sarcopenia. *J Appl Physiol*, vol. 95, no. 5, pp. 1851-1860
2. Boncompagni S, d'Amelio L, Fulle S, Fanò G, Protasi F (2006) Progressive disorganization of the excitation-contraction coupling apparatus in aging human skeletal muscle as revealed by electron microscopy: a possible role in the decline of muscle performance. J Gerontol A Biol Sci Med Sci, 61:995–1008.
3. Ferri A, Narici M, Grassi B et al (2006) Neuromuscular recovery after a strength training session in elderly people. *Eur J Appl Physiol,* vol. 97, no. 3, pp. 272-279
4. Melov S., Tarnopolsky MA, Beckman K et al (2007) Resistance Exercise Reverses Aging in Human Skeletal Muscle. *PLoS One*, vol. 2, no. 5
5. Bax L, Staes F, Verhagen A (2005) Does neuromuscular electrical stimulation strengthen the quadriceps femoris? A systematic review of randomised controlled trials. *Sports medicine,* vol. 35, no. 3, pp. 191–212
6. Krenn M, Haller M, Bijak M, Unger E, Hofer C, Kern H, Mayr W (2011) Safe Neuromuscular Electrical Stimulator Designed for the Elderly. *Artificial Organs* vol. 35, no. 3, pp. 253–6
7. Chen CF, Chen WS, Chou LW, Chang YJ, Chen SC, Kuo TS, Lai JS (2012) Pulse energy as a reliable reference for twitch forces induced by transcutaneous neuromuscular electrical stimulation. *IEEE Transactions on neural systems and rehabilitation engineering,* vol. 20, no. 4, pp. 574–83
8. Kern H, Loefler S, Hofer C et al (2012) FES Training in Aging: interim results show statistically significant improvements in mobility and muscle fiber size. Eur J of Trans Myol - BAM, (1&2):61-67
9. Sarabon N, Loefler S, Cvecka J, Sedliak M, Kern H (2013) Strength training in elderly people improves static balance: a randomized controlled trial. Eur J of Trans Myol 23(3):85

Author: Winfried Mayr
Institute: Medical University of Vienna
Center for Medical Physics and Biomedical Engineering
Street: Waehringer Guertel 18-20, 4L
City: Vienna
Country: Austria
Email: winfried.mayr@meduniwien.ac.at

Towards Knowledge Extraction from Electronic Health Records – Automatic Negation Identification

I. Bărbănţan and R. Potolea

Computer Science Department, Technical University of Cluj-Napoca, Cluj-Napoca, Romania

Abstract— **Along with the adoption of the Electronic Health Records (EHRs) a step forward had been taken in the health care industry as it becomes easier and less time consuming to store and retrieve information. The EHRs are free text format documents, where although a certain structure may exist, the information is usually spread across the entire document, with no standard specific structure. Our current work represents a step in providing an accessible format to EHRs. While the ultimate goal for structuring EHRs is knowledge extraction for assisting the medical diagnosis, the correct identification of terms in documents is essential. In order to do this, the paper deals with negation identification. We consider negation representing disjoint sets of concepts as it can be expressed with explicit terms and prefixed terms. Most of the medical negation terms expressed using prefixes are not usually found in common dictionaries that could help in identifying their truth values. We compare our approach with the standard NegEx[1] on a dataset of 2132 sentences, and report better performance (with 27% improvement of recall, with the cost of less than 3% degradation of precision) in negation identification. We implemented a rule-based approach for identifying explicit negation and a vocabulary-based approach for the case when negation is expressed with prefixes. To the best of our knowledge, other works dealing with negation do not include an analysis negation expressed with prefixes, although in medical documents it represents an important trait in communicating information. In contrast to the baseline algorithm, NegEx, and other similar systems, our approach automatically identifies negated concepts and includes identification of negation expressed using prefixes.**

Keywords— **Text Mining, information extraction, prefix, negation, Electronic Health Records, vocabulary**

I. Introduction

Knowledge extraction from unstructured medical records is an important task in the development of medical decision support systems. In this attempt, structuring documents and identifying relevant items in free text is the first challenge which in turn faces, among others, the difficulty of detecting negated terms. We present a method that identifies negation in medical discharge summaries. The method is based on simple regular expressions that match negation identifiers and word parsers that split compound words into prefixes and root words. The use for such a tool improves the quality of the information extracted from documents and thus, the development of better applications for assisting medical decisions.

Extracting information and knowledge from narrative medical reports in free format has the advantage of both enhancing the current knowledge bases, provides the possibility of designing new applications for (semi)automated decision systems and improving the quality of existing medical systems.

The analysis of the medical textual data offers information like predicting adverse reactions by analyzing the interaction of drugs (when combined) or identifying comorbidity risks, forecasting possible conditions that may occur based on previous studies and cases, recommending investigations for a thorough diagnosis, suggesting diagnostic or follow up. The availability of large amounts of data may seem convenient, but diverts from focusing on the significant data. A clinical discharge document in raw format informs about document structuring into chapters containing grouped information regarding: Symptoms, Diseases, Diagnosis, patient's Historical information, Medical procedures [2], Medication [3], Investigations, Demographic data or Follow-up information [4].

Negation is part of the inter-human communication stating refusal, denial or changes opinions. Negation is used in mathematics, computer science or reasoning to change the truth value of sentences. In natural language negation has different connotations. The following two sentences generate subtle problems, because one of them states the complete absence of tiredness ("I'm not a bit tired."), whereas the other sentence describes a condition of exhaustion ("I'm not a little tired.") [5].

Negation can be formulated using specific words ("not"), prefixes ("non") or operators ("¬","!"). The process of information extraction from text is preceded by several text preprocessing tasks that include understanding and disambiguating the concepts in the text. For example, there are two interpretations in the analysis of the concept "fever" in the text "*The patient presented with no fever*". Depending on the focus of the analysis, the output could be "yes, the concept fever appears in the provided text" or "the concept fever is denied as the patient did not have a temperature of

S. Vlad and R.V. Ciupa (eds.), *International Conference on Advancements of Medicine and Health Care through Technology*, IFMBE Proceedings 44,
DOI: 10.1007/978-3-319-07653-9_4, © Springer International Publishing Switzerland 2014

over 35 degrees" when a semantically analysis of the concept is performed. Among other missions, disambiguation encompasses a negation analysis task where the goal is identifying and analyzing the influence of negation and how it spreads on the entire sentence ("The patient did not present with fever, headache or ocular pain.") and changes the meaning of the concepts. Some issues that may occur when performing text disambiguation by analyzing negation are that the negation identifiers may not be placed in the proximity of the term they negate; they can spread to other concepts and negate several terms and change the truth value of an entire sentence.

Free text documents like medical discharge summaries are usually saved in databases. By interrogating them to obtain documents containing similar clinical content like patients with comparable symptoms or diagnosis, poor information may be delivered when data is improper interrogated. When negation particles are not considered with their specific meaning, much of the generated outcome may be erroneous. Thus, even though the generated output contains a matching of the symptoms, a semantic approach would not consider these results.

The rest of the paper is organized as follows. In chapter II a description of similar systems dealing with EHRs is presented. Next, in chapter III the EHRs are briefly introduced along with the advantages and disadvantages of their adoption. Our solution is detailed in chapter IV with the dataset description, experiments performed, and the results we obtained. The last two chapters present the conclusion of our work, future enhancements we propose and the references.

II. Related work

Extracting information from health records is a problem that many researchers tackled. Some steps involved in the information extraction process, especially the preprocessing ones, are language dependent – like loading specific word dictionaries and the grammar processing. Most researchers focus on specific information contained in the medical document like symptom identification, diagnosis prognosis or coding [6], identification of follow-up information [7] or text disambiguation. Prediction of the disease from the content of a clinical discharge note is approached by Yang et all in [6]. Their goal is twofold: to identify explicit references to diseases in text and predict disease when their evidence is not stated. The mention of the explicit references to diseases is estimated using the NegEx algorithm. The sentences are annotated with yes, no or questionable based on the concepts that are negated in each sentence. A combination of dictionary look-up, rule-based and Machine Learning methods are included in the proposed approach. An analysis of 507 discharge summaries is performed and the authors report promising results.

The NegEx algorithm used in [6] is the most proeminent negation identification algorithms. Developed by Chapman et all. [1], the algorithm is based on regular expressions that identify the presence or absence of negation in medical documents. The authors report a specificity of 94.5 and a positive predictive value of 84.5% on 1000 sentences taken from discharge summaries. The regular expressions are written based on lists of negative expressions grouped into categories. The algorithm works by first specifying the medical term that must be identified. The stop words are not removed from the discharge summaries as these words may be included in the negative expressions provided by the negation lists.

From a medical report, information regarding medical conditions, symptoms and diseases can be extracted and used later for establishing relations and diagnosis for similar inputs. One approach of extracting medication information is presented in [8]. Using linguistic pattern matching and semantic rules the authors propose extracting medication relevant information like medication name, dosage, mode/route, frequency and duration. A set of 547 discharge summaries are used in the analysis and the performance is reported from the analysis of 251 manually annotated discharge summaries. The process consists in the following three steps: linguistic preprocessing that deals with sentence splitting and POS tagging followed by the dictionary interrogation and pattern matching. The medication names and identifiers like common affixes are detected using a dictionary of medication names. A second dictionary defining generic medication types is included in the system. The dictionaries are combined with the standard dictionary provided by UMLS. Also, a list of nouns, affixes and prepositions that are commonly found alongside medication names is generated.

In [9] the authors introduce the way negation is characterized in Natural Language and present an approach of automatically determining the scope and focus of negation. The frequency of the negation-bearing words in the corpus they use in their analysis leads to considering negation only the determiners *not* and *n't*. The scope of negation was identified with 66% accuracy. As future enhancement of their work, the authors propose including the negation prefixes in determining the scope and focus of negation. They suggest removing the prefix and determining whether the word without prefix is still valid. When dealing with polysemantic words, the authors suggest using a dictionary of antonyms.

III. Electronic health records

A. What Are EHRs?

As described in [10], the EHR "is a longitudinal electronic record of patient health information generated by one or more encounters in any care delivery setting." The EHR can also contain demographics, progress notes, problems, medications, vital signs, past medical history, immunizations, laboratory data and radiology reports. EHRs focus on all medical aspects of a patient and help find correlation between actual condition and previous investigations and conditions. [11]

Although EHRs increase the quality of the medical services and medical knowledge, there are also some aspects that make the adoption of EHRs more complicated. Some of the positive and negative aspects of EHRs are presented in the following.

B. Advantages and Disadvantages of EHRs

The EHRs are intended to keep track of the medical history and progress of a patient and also provide a legal document distinctive to each patient. The advantages of the EHRs exceed their disadvantages in terms of patient health care. Most of the disadvantages are related to the requirements of implementing, acquiring and maintaining the system.

a) Advantages

The time required investigating a patient's condition and establishing a diagnosis decreases and alongside the patient's suffering as the medical history of the patient is easily accessible. The current condition of the patient becomes easier to be handled as the EHRs are provided with templates where the information is stored in a structured fashion. Thanks to the electronic storing of the information, the medical tracks are harder to get lost and so are the electronic medical prescriptions. Due to easier access of the medical notes and the integration of medical resources, recent studies or treatments and more powerful information availability it the medical decisions are more accurate.

b) Disadvantages

The disadvantages of the EHRs include the costs of acquisition and maintenance of the system. [12] Some of the medical staff may be reluctant to the adoption of the new system as it represents a new technology that requires time and money spent in training and learning. One disadvantage that may affect the patient is the problem of privacy because of the availability of the medical records that can be accessed by many people, some of them not being authorized. Also, because of the repeated access to the medical records, information may be altered. [13]

IV. Proposed method

We present a method that identifies negation in medical discharge summaries. The method is based on simple regular expressions - that match negation identifiers - and word parsers - that split compound words into prefixes and root words.

We propose a two-step approach for identifying negation in medical documents. The algorithm uses as input data clinical discharge summaries, presented in more detail in the *Dataset* section. The method is focused on the main forms of negation: expressed using specific words and with prefixes.

The proposed algorithm analyzes negation using a combination of two approaches. In the rule-based approach the words that introduce negation are matched with the content of the discharge summaries. In this case regular expressions are constructed. The second approach deals with negation identification expressed with prefixes where a bag of words approach is included to obtain a list of words to represent the documents. A set of discharge summaries are used to generate an initial vocabulary of roots that are used as reference when searching for prefix negated words. We included this approach as we noticed that the negation words expressed with prefixes are not included in common dictionaries. The medical terms like *nontender*, *afebrile* or *nonfasting* do not have a definition in WordNet and become difficult to be interpreted by a non specialized person who reads a medical document.

A. Step1: Rule-Based Approach

In order to identify negation a list of words that introduce negation included in NegEx is used. The words are organized into six lists: Pseudo negation terms - phrases that look like negation terms but do not negate the clinical condition and are skipped when identified ("no increase", "not extend"), Pre-condition negation term that are placed before the term they negate ("absence of", "denies"), Pre-condition possibility terms ("rule out", "will be ruled out for"), Post-condition negation term placed after the term they are negating ("unlikely", "is ruled out"), Post-condition possibility terms ("did not rule out", "being ruled out") and Termination terms that indicate that the scope of the negation term should end ("but", "still").

By applying a stemming algorithm as preprocessing step the lists of negation determiners is reduced by 20%; thus reducing the size of the dictionary resulting in a faster matching algorithm. Also, it is likely that not all possible representations for each expression is contained in the lists. Defining lists with root forms increases the matching probability between the text and the expressions defined. The removed entities are nouns present both in their singular and plural forms ("cause of/causes of") together with different verbs occurring with several verbal tenses. For example these three entries from the PreConditionNegation list "was ruled out, is ruled out, are ruled out" are all set to their dictionary form "is rule out".

Our solution uses Gate's Annie tool [14] in order to implement the pattern matching part of our proposed method. Annie relies on finite state algorithms and the JAPE language. We defined lists for each negation list from NegEx and created a new jape processing resource where we added the rules for a grammar to identify occurrences of the expressions defined in the gazetteers in the provided text documents. By applying the pipeline on our corpus of medical documents we can estimate the performance of the system by analyzing the annotations generated.

B. Step2: Vocabulary-Based Approach

Using a Machine Learning approach for document filtering, we implemented a negation identification approach that recognizes whether the words are prefixed with negation prefixes. As we are dealing with medical documents, the use of the specific terms is large and we assume that the negated concept occurs in the same document and set of documents without the negation as well; thus, the pair <concept, prefix_negated_concept> is likely to appear; for example <bloody, nonbloody>. Starting from this assumption we propose creating a vocabulary using concepts obtained from a sample of discharge summaries. The vocabulary consists of unique occurrence of the words from the selected corpus of documents described in more detail in the *Dataset* section. The list of words is created by converting the corpus of documents into a bag of words. The steps involved in identifying the prefixed words are outlined in Figure 1. For each word in a new document it is verified whether it is a possible candidate to being prefixed. The possible prefixes are: out, anti, non, ir, a, un, dis, im. In Table 1 is briefly shown the meaning of each of these prefixes justifying the reason they were selected.

To avoid false positives, we created specialized rules for the prefixes, relying on the assumption that the length of a word without prefix should be greater than two characters. A new word is obtained by removing the prefix found in the beginning of the word. The word is then searched for in the vocabulary. If the word with no prefix is found in the bag of words, we consider that the word can exists in common language, so in this case we are dealing with a prefixed

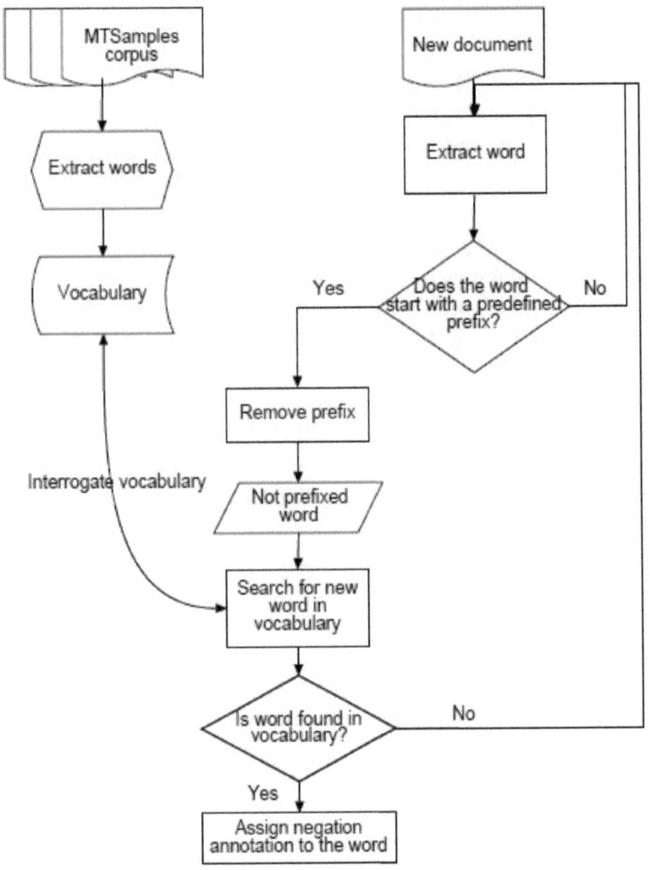

Fig. 1 Steps involved in the vocabulary-based approach

word. When the word cannot be found in the vocabulary we draw the conclusion that the word is not prefixed.

The two types of negations we tackle are disjoint sets and should be treated differently. The inclusion of prefixes in identifying negation is justified by the amount of negations expressed using prefixes which is significant in the medical domain. As presented in Table 3, almost 40% of all negations in the documents we analyzed are expressed using prefixes, so, handling prefixed negation in medical records makes sense.

Table 1 Negation prefixes and their meaning

Negation Prefix	Meaning
A, an	Not, without
Anti	Opposing, against
Dis	Negation, removal, expulsion
In, il, im, ir	Not, without
Non	Absence, negation
Un	Not, reversal, cancellation, deprived of

Table 2 Statistics of negation identifiers in documents

Average negations/doc	8.31
Average negation prefixes/doc	5.47
Average negation and negation prefixes/doc	13.78
Average words/doc	730.92
Average sentences/doc	59.22

Table 3 Negation in documents - Statistics

Word types	Explicit negation	Negation with prefixes
Number of words	1.14(%)	0.75(%)
Number of negations	60.28(%)	39.72(%)

A. Dataset

The dataset we used in our analysis consists of clinical discharge summaries, and we refer to it as the MTSamples dataset. The documents describe the evolution of a patient's status from the time they were hospitalized to the point of discharge with reference to past conditions. The documents were collected from [15] and are DE identified. We collected a total of 100 documents, 36 being used for evaluation and 64 in building a vocabulary. The documents used for evaluation were manually annotated for negation occurrences.

A statistic of the distribution of the words in the documents is presented in Table 2. The 2132 sentences provided for analysis contain a total of 26313 words, 299 being words negated using explicit terms and 197 words are expressing negation through prefixes. The average explicit negation words per document is 8 while the average prefix negation words is 5.

The performance of the baseline algorithm NegEx on our selected corpus of documents is presented Table 3 in column 2. Also, because the NegEx method does not include prefixes as negations, the recall in its case is unacceptably small. The evaluation of NegEx is performed on a dataset of 1000 sentences whereas our own evaluation includes more than 2000 annotated sentences making our analysis more reliable.

B. Experiments

The experiments we performed consist in analyzing the content of clinical discharge summaries. In order to evaluate negation in a document, we go through the content of the document and verify whether the words may represent a negation that can be expressed with explicit words or if they are prefixed with a negation inducing prefix. If the word represents an explicit negation we analyze it using a set of regular expressions. If the word is prefixed with a negation prefix we feed it to the vocabulary-based approach and determine whether the root of the word is a real word and annotate it with as negation in case the result is positive.

a) Evaluation of NegEx on the MTSamples Corpus

To obtain accurate results we evaluated the performance of NegEx on our annotated set of documents. The selected test documents are fed together with the identified negations to the NegEx tool. NegEx easily identifies the negated concepts determined by the words contained in the lists, but performs poorly in the case of prefix negation identification, as none of the negated words using prefixes is identified, thus resulting in a poor performance value for recall (46.63%), Table 4, second column.

b) Exp1: Initial Evaluation

The algorithm we proposed consists in a set of regular expressions used to identify explicit negation in texts and a vocabulary-based approach that is intended to identify negation expressed with prefixes. We evaluated the performance of the proposed algorithm on 2132 sentences. Due to the fact that we introduced the prefix identification method, an important increase in the recall (almost 20%) of the system is obtained when comparing to the performance of NegEx on the same corpus of documents. We noticed a small decrease in the precision of identifying negations (less than 1%). The results of the evaluation are presented in Table 4, third column.

c) Exp2: Evaluation on the Normalized MTSamples Dataset

For the second experiment we normalized the content of the documents by applying a stemmer to extract the root of the words. The results we report with respect to NegEx represent again a small degradation of precision, but an important increase in the recall of the system of almost 27%, as shown in Table 4 in the last column. As the recall of the system increases, in spite of the decrease of less than 3% of the precision, we report an improvement in the negation identification in medical documents compared to the baseline algorithm.

Table 4 Results

Method	NegEx	Exp1	Exp2
Precision (%)	100	99.39	97.84
Recall (%)	46.63	65.92	73.63

V. Conclusions and Future Work

We propose a system that automatically identifies negation expressed both with explicit terms and with prefixes in electronic health documents. We compare our approach with the standard NegEx[1] on a dataset of 2132 sentences, and report better performance (with 27% improvement of recall, with the cost of less than 3% assumed degradation of precision) in negation identification. Our proposed solution deals with negation identification using a rule-based matching algorithm and a vocabulary-based approach for identifying negated concepts expressed with prefixes using a generated vocabulary from the medical documents. To the best of our knowledge systems dealing with negation expressed using prefixes are not yet reported in literature. We found only that Blanco and Moldovan [9] consider a similar approach as a future enhancement in determining the scope and focus of negation.

The results of evaluating our solution are promising and as future work we propose testing our approach on documents from other domains. We want to extend the dictionary we created by using the WordNet dictionary and implement a semantic approach to the negation identification process using the definitions of the words.

ACKNOWLEDGMENT

This work is aligned with the COST Action IC1303 AAPELE.

CONFLICT OF INTEREST

The authors declare that they have no conflict of interest.

REFERENCES

1. Chapman, W. W., Bridewell, W., Hanbury, P., Cooper, G. F., & Buchanan, B. G. 2001. A Simple Algorithm for Identifying Negated Findings and Diseases in Discharge Summaries. Journal of Biomedical Informatics, 34(5), 301-310.
2. Long, W. 2005. Extracting Diagnoses from Discharge Summaries. AMIA 2005 Symposium Proceedings, 470-474.
3. Halgrim, S. R., Xia, F., Cadag, E., & Uzuner, Ö. 2011. A cascade of classifiers for extracting medication information from discharge summaries. Journal of Biomedical Semantics.
4. Rudd, K. L., Johnson, M. G., Liesinger, J. T., & Grafft, C. A. 2010. Automated detection of follow-up appointments using text mining of discharge records. International Journal for Quality in Health Care, 229–235.
5. Gindl, S. 2006. Negation Detection in Automated Medical Applications. A Survey. Vienna: Vienna University of Technology. http://publik.tuwien.ac.at/files/pub-inf_4604.pdf
6. Yang, H., Spasic, I., Keane, J.A., Nenadic, G., 2009. A Text Mining Approach to the Prediction of Disease Status from Clinical Discharge Summaries. J Am Med Informs Assoc. July 2009;16(4):596-600. Epub 2009 Apr 23.
7. Rudd, K. L., Johnson, M. G., Liesinger, J. T., & Grafft, C. A. 2010. Automated detection of follow-up appointments using text mining of discharge records. International Journal for Quality in Health Care, 229–235.
8. Spasic, I., Sarafraz, F., Keane, J. A., & Nenadic, G. 2010. Medication information extraction with linguistic pattern matching and semantic rules. J Am Med Inform Assoc, 532-535.
9. E. Blanco, D. Moldovan. “Some issues on detecting negation from text”. Proceedings of the Twenty-Fourth International Florida Artificial Intelligence Research Society Conference, 2011.
10. Electronic Health Records http://www.himss.org/library/ehr/ ?navItemNumber=13261
11. The Advantages of Electronic Health Records. American Psychological Association. May 2012, Vol 43, No. 5 http://www.apa.org/monitor/2012/05/electronic-records.aspx
12. Menachemi, N., Collum, T.H., Benefits and Drawbacks of Electronic Health Record Systems. Dovepress Journal, May 2011 Volume 2011:4, Pages 47 – 55.
13. Pharmica Consulting, Top Five Potential Drawbacks of Electronic Health Records, http://www.pharmicaconsulting.com/top -five-potential-drawbacks-of-electronic-health-records/
14. Cunningham, H., Maynard, D., Bontcheva, K., & Tablan, V. 2002. GATE: A Framework and Graphical Development Environment for Robust NLP Tools and Applications. Proceedings of the 40th Anniversary Meeting of the Association for Computational Linguistics (ACL'02). Philadelphia.
15. Transcribed Medical Transcription Sample Reports and Examples, http://www.mtsamples.com/ , accessed 23/10/2012.

Importance of Lateral Cephalogram in Treating Class III Patients

V. Țărmure*, O.C. Almășan*, D. Buhățel, A. Ilea, P. Jiman, M. Iancu, and A. Pop

Iuliu Hațieganu University of Medicine and Pharmacy, Cluj-Napoca, Romania
*Authors had the same contribution

Abstract— **Introduction: The need for an early identification and treatment of the skeletal Class III malocclusion is accepted worldwide. The treatment success in class III patients depends on the malocclusion type and the case individualization. The treatment choice is extremely difficult, and increases with involvement of the skeletal and occlusal structures. In certain situations, when growth pattern is unfavourable, combined surgical-orthodontic treatment needs to be applied. The aim of this paper is to discuss some aspects of the skeletal class III malocclusion. Subjects and methods: patients who addressed our Orthodontic Department, in Cluj-Napoca, Romania, during 2010-2013. Twenty-five subjects, diagnosed with class III malocclusion have been studied. The diagnosis has been established clinical and paraclinical. The treatment was individualized in each case based on patient's age and difficulty index of the malocclusion. Lateral cephalometry was used to assess skeletal pattern before and after treatment. Skeletal vertical and horizontal relationships were evaluated according to Tweed, Sassouni and Hasund/Segner. Statistical data processing was performed using the Statistica 7.0 software version for Windows, using the Principal Component Analysis (PCA) and the Varimax method. Results and discussion: There were encountered associated anomalies: mandible shift (20%), asymmetries (20%), crowding (40%), canine impaction (4%), open bite (4%), tooth transposition (4%). Nineteen patients (76%) were treated without extractions; 6 patients (24%) had tooth removal (bicuspids or first molars). Six patients (24%) were treated by orthodontic treatment and orthognathic surgery. Conclusion: A stepwise analysis influences the individual treatment of skeletal class III malocclusion, which predicts the treatment choice: orthodontic treatment or a multidisciplinary approach.**

Keywords— **class III malocclusion, lateral cephalogram, orthodontics, orthognathic surgery**

I. INTRODUCTION

The need for early identification and treatment of the skeletal Class III malocclusion is accepted worldwide. In class III patients the success of the treatment depends on the malocclusion type and the case's individualization [1]. The treatment choice is extremely difficult, and it increases with involvement of the skeletal and occlusal characteristics. In certain situations, when growth pattern is unfavourable, a combined surgical-orthodontic treatment has to be chosen [2]. The difficulty of the case increases when class III malocclusion is associated with open bite or mandible shift. The treatment needs to be individualized [3]. The treatment plan should include all the patient's symptoms. The treatment type is chosen depending on the patient's symptoms and on the analysis of the lateral cephalogram. Usually the orthodontic treatment precedes the surgical treatment, having the role to correct the jaw discrepancy and to obtain proper teeth alignment. The surgical approach involves commonly both, the maxilla and mandible, being in accordance to the skeletal and occlusal modifications of the malocclusion [4,5]. The maxilla is enlarged and jaw surgery is performed to establish occlusal harmony [6,7].

The aim of this paper is to discuss the management of skeletal class III malocclusion.

II. MATERIAL AND METHODS

Twenty five patients (14 females and 11 males, SD=4.89) with class III skeletal malocclusion (selected through a prospective method from patients who were referred to our orthodontic department, from Cluj-Napoca, Romania between 2010 and 2013 (treated by an orthodontist, VT) with ages between 6 and 23 were studied. Lateral cephalometry was used to establish skeletal pattern before and after treatment. Lateral cephalograms were performed directly with a 3D device (50–90 kV, 2–10 mA, exposure time 0.5-1.0 s). For ensuring the reliability of scanning, patients kept their teeth in centric occlusion during exposure, whilst using the cephalostat system. Skeletal vertical and horizontal relationships were evaluated according to the methods described by Tweed, Sassouni and Hasund/Segner. Following variables were evaluated: patient's age, the angles FMA, FMIA, IMPA, SNA, SNB, ANB, Z, PrAF, IdBM, Ii, NSL-ML, NSL-ML, Go (in degrees) and the distances AO-BO, HFA, HFP, OB, OJ (in mm). Statistical data processing was performed using the Statistica 7.0 software version for Windows, applying the Principal Component Analysis (PCA) and the Varimax method in order to determine the correlation between different variables. The cephalometric evaluation at the start of treatment showed the intermaxillary discrepancy in the antero-posterior and vertical dimension (Fig. 1). After orthodontic and surgical treatment, occlusal balancing and improvement of the intermaxillary relationships and of the esthetics of the face could be noted (Fig. 2). Six months after appliance removal, the overlapping of the lateral cephalograms shows no tendency to relapse and the maintenance of the results (Fig. 3).

S. Vlad and R.V. Ciupa (eds.), *International Conference on Advancements of Medicine and Health Care through Technology*,
IFMBE Proceedings 44,
DOI: 10.1007/978-3-319-07653-9_5, © Springer International Publishing Switzerland 2014

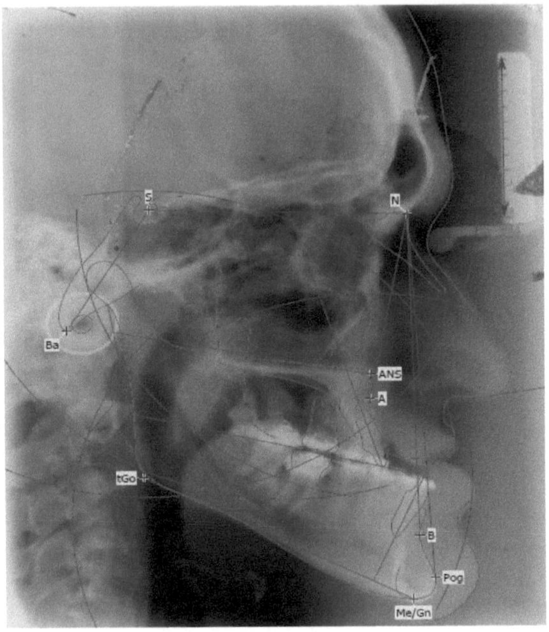

Fig. 1 Patient C.R., lateral cephalometric radiography, orthodontic stage, before treatment

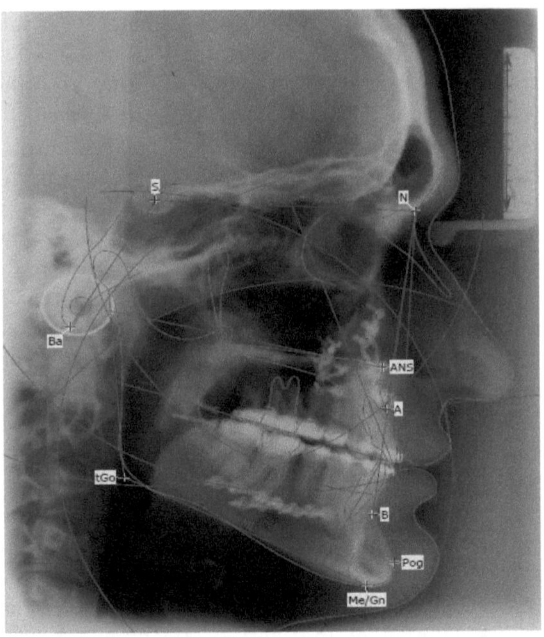

Fig. 2 Patient C.R., lateral cephalometric radiography, after orthodontic and surgical treatment

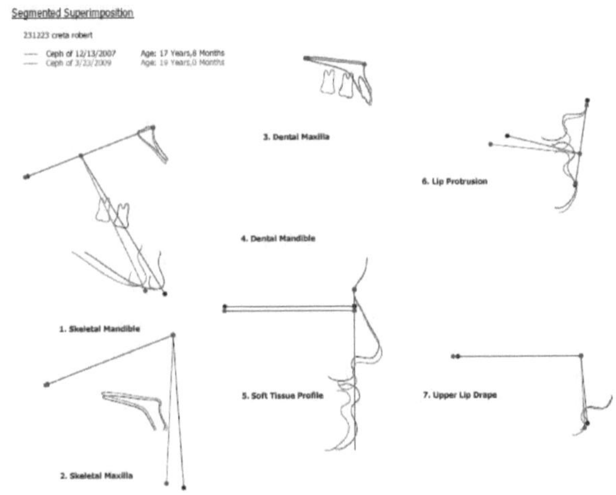

Fig. 3 Patient C.R.: Segmented superimposition before treatment, and after orthodontic and surgical treatment. An improvement of the occlusal relationships and esthetics can be observed.

III. Results and Discussion

Associated anomalies of the patients have also been diagnosed: mandible shift 20%, asymmetries 20%, crowding 40%, canine impaction 4%, open bite 4%, tooth transposition 4% (Fig. 4). When considering the type of space achievement, nineteen patients (76%) were treated without extractions; six patients (24%) have been treated by tooth removal (bicuspids or first molars). Regarding the treatment type, orthodontic or orthognathic treatment, six patients (24%) have been treated by orthodontics and orthognathic surgery, the other 19 patients (76%) being treated only through orthodontic methods.

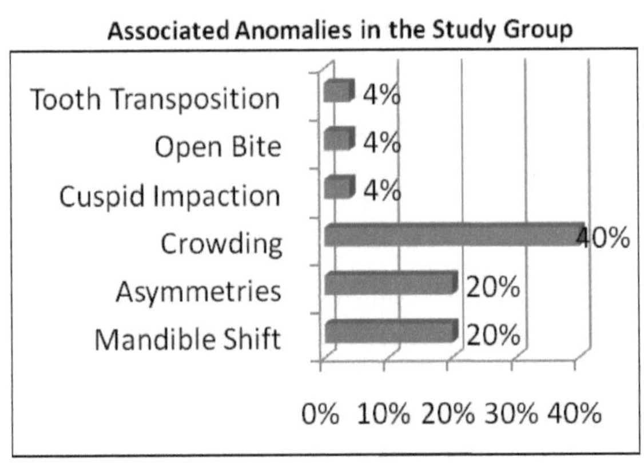

Fig. 4 Associated anomalies of the study group (SD=3.6)

Among the studied variables we aimed to identify the existence of certain groups of variables that were correlated to each other. The Principal Component Analysis (PCA) is a factorial analyzing method used in highlighting the association pattern between variables. The problem of determining the common pattern among certain variables was solved by applying numerical and geometrical methods. Thus, the variables have been represented through points on the unit sphere. From the analysis of the own values which measure the amount of variance due to each main component, there have been identified eight factors (principal components). In order to simplify the interpretation of the principal components, we used the Varimax method. This indicated as significant those components that had the correlation coefficient higher than 0.70, thus remaining only two principal components for analysis: Factor 1 and Factor 2. The optimal factorial solution is that with two extracted factors because they explained a maximal amount of variance. Proportion of variance explained by the first factor was 31.82%, the second explained 18.62%. Consequently, the cumulative percentage of variance accounted for by the first two factors was 50.44%. Figure 5 suggests that the factor rotation does not change the proportion of the total common variance explained by the first two factors.

The PCA method suggested that the anterior facial height, Wits' appraisal, SNA angle, anterior-posterior intermaxillary relationship (recorded by the ANB angle), IMPA angle, FMIA angle and overjet have varied to the contrary with the profile type (Sassouni) and the Z angle (Fig. 5.a). To the contrary, the SNB angle, the SNA angle and patient age have varied to the contrary with the lower face angulation (shown by the NSL-ML angle) (Fig. 5.b). On the other hand, FMA angle, NL-ML angle and the gonial angle (measured by the Ar-Go-Me angle) have varied to the contrary with the SNB angle (Fig. 5.c.).

Functional and esthetic disorders of patients with class III malocclusion can be observed even since the temporary dentition. These situations require the establishment of an early treatment plan, case monitoring and careful treatment planning of all treatment stages. Treatment choice is more provocative the higher the degree of the skeletal and dental involvement of the malocclusion. The orthodontic and combined orthognathic treatment is challenging, depending on the extent of the skeletal deformity, the degree of dental and soft tissue compensations and the patient's concern.

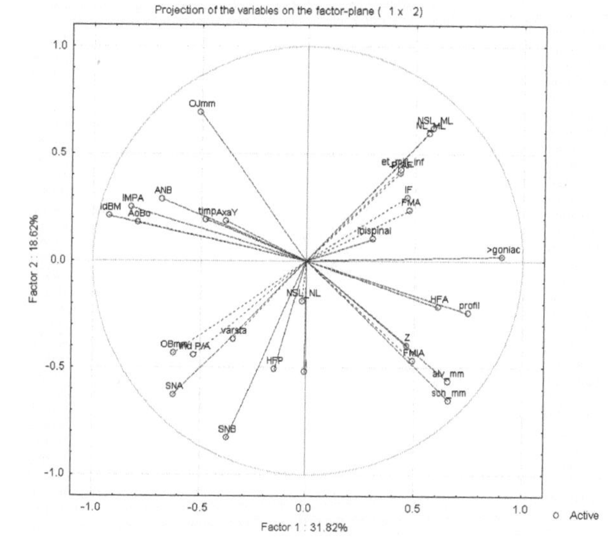

a.

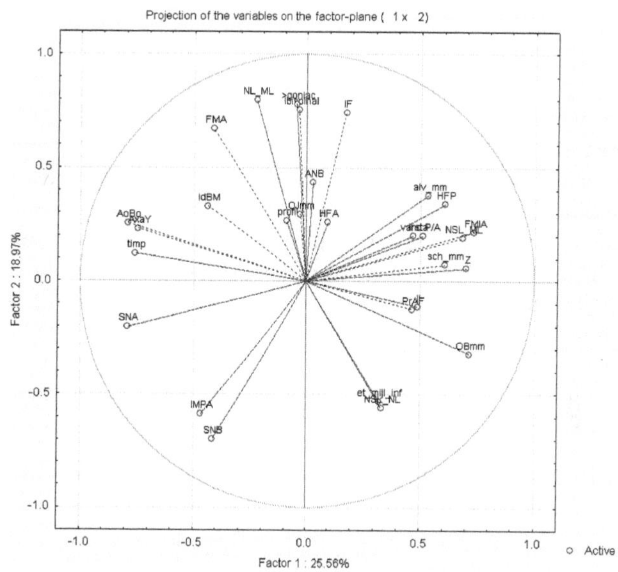

b.

Fig. 5. PCA method analyses

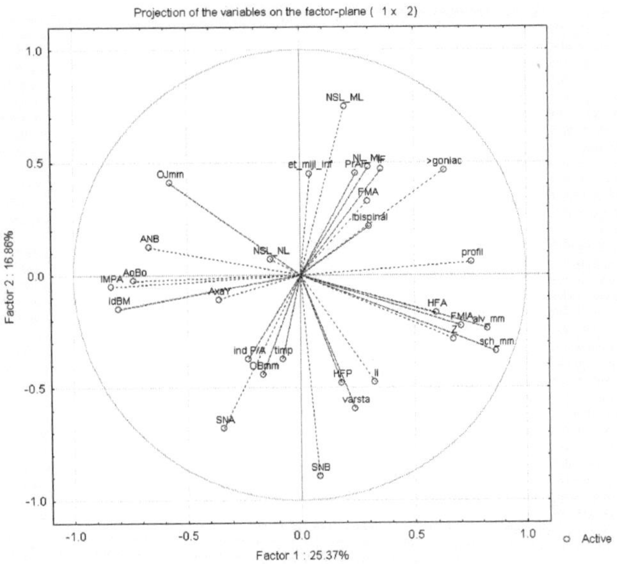

c.

Fig. 5 PCA method analyses

IV. Conclusions

A well planned analysis, step by step, of each case influences the individual treatment of the skeletal class III malocclusion, which predicts the option of an orthodontic or combined treatment: orthodontic and surgical. Early diagnosis is very important to control the evolution of the malocclusion, because otherwise the orthodontic treatment remains just a preliminary step of a multidisciplinary treatment.

Conflict of Interest

The authors declare that they have no conflict of interest.

References

1. Fang N, Duan Y, Huo N (2009) Camouflage treatment in skeletal Class III cases combined with severe crowding by extraction of four premolars. Orthod Waves 68:80-87
2. Troy BA, Shanker S, Fields HW, Vig K, Johnston W (2009) Comparison of incisor inclination in patients with Class III malocclusion treated with orthognathic surgery or orthodontic camouflage. Am J Orthod Dentofacial Orthop 135(2):146e1-9
3. León-Salazar V, Janson G, de Freitas MR, de Almeida RR, León-Salazar R (2009) Nonextraction treatment of a skeletal Class III malocclusion. Am J Orthod Dentofacial Orthop 136(5):736-745
4. Takeshita N, Ishida M, Watanabe H, Hashimoto T, Daimaruya T, Hasegawa M, Takano-Yamamoto T (2013) Improvement of asymmetric stomatognathic functions, unilateral crossbite, and facial esthetics in a patient with skeletal Class III malocclusion and mandibular asymmetry, treated with orthognathic surgery. Am J Orthod Dentofacial Orthop 144(3):441-454
5. de Haan IF, Ciesielski R, Nitsche T, Koos B (2013) Evaluation of relapse after orthodontic therapy combined with orthognathic surgery in the treatment of skeletal class III J Orofac Orthop. 74(5):362-369
6. Vieira BB, Sanguino AC, Moreira MR, Morizono EN, Matsumoto MA (2013) Surgical-orthodontic treatment of Class III malocclusion with agenesis of lateral incisor and unerupted canine. Dental Press J Orthod 18(3):94-100
7. Kim YJ, Lee Y, Chun YS, Kang N, Kim SJ, Kim M (2014) Condylar Positional Changes Up to 12 Months After Bimaxillary Surgery for Skeletal Class III Malocclusions. J Oral Maxillofac Surg 72(1):145-156.

Corresponding author:

Author: Tarmure Viorica, Almasan Oana
Institute: Iuliu Haţieganu University of Medicine and Pharmacy
Street: 33 Motilor
City: Cluj Napoca
Country: Romania
Email: tarmure@yahoo.com, oalmasan@ymail.com

The Use of Digital Imaging in the Evaluation of Perception in Facial Asymmetry Caused by Facial Nerve Disorders

A. Ilea[1], C. Vâjâean[1], L.C. Hurubeanu[2], B. Boşca[3], V. Ţărmure[4], V.E. Trombitaş[5], R.S. Câmpian[1], and S. Albu[5]

[1] "Iuliu Haţieganu" University of Medicine and Pharmacy Cluj-Napoca, Faculty of Dentistry, Department of Oral Rehabilitation, Oral Health and Dental Office Management, Romania
[2] "Iuliu Haţieganu" University of Medicine and Pharmacy Cluj-Napoca, Faculty of Dentistry, Department of Oral and Maxillo-Facial Surgery, Romania
[3] "Iuliu Haţieganu" University of Medicine and Pharmacy Cluj-Napoca, Faculty of Medicine, Department of Histology, Romania
[4] "Iuliu Haţieganu" University of Medicine and Pharmacy Cluj-Napoca, Faculty of Dentistry, Department of Orthodontics, Romania
[5] "Iuliu Haţieganu" University of Medicine and Pharmacy Cluj-Napoca, Faculty of Dentistry, Department of Cervicofacial and ENT Surgery, Romania

Abstract— **Facial asymmetry may be caused by facial nerve dysfunctions, as in the case of facial paralysis. The aim of this study is to evaluate the usefulness of manipulated digital images in facial paralysis diagnosis, to determine facial attractiveness, emotional perception and the level of knowledge among students of the Faculty of Dentistry. The results show that facial symmetry plays an important role in assessing facial attractiveness, and emotional perception is influenced by the presence of smile or smile mimicked by the asymmetrical pulling of the oral commissure. In conclusion, manipulated digital facial images facilitate the diagnosis of facial palsy or paralysis. On the other hand, these images are partially impersonal and cannot accurately convey the emotional experiences of the subjects.**

Keywords— **digital images, facial asymmetry, facial paralysis, facial palsy, perception**

I. INTRODUCTION

Facial asymmetry is present in both the face and the body starting with the intrauterine period. The two hemibodies apparently develop independently, so that the development of the human body is more often asymmetric than symmetric [1]. Usually, the right hemiface is wider than the left one, causing a slight deviation of the chin to the left [2]. The lower third of the face most frequently shows asymmetry compared to the other parts of the face [3].

The most obvious asymmetries are caused by the asymmetrical contraction of facial muscles [1]. Facial asymmetries can have multiple causes: they can be congenital, developmental and acquired after illnesses or traumas [4, 5, 6]. Among acquired facial asymmetries, we can mention facial palsy and paralysis. This is caused by peripheral or central damage to the facial nerve. Facial paralysis is characterized by static asymmetries due to hemifacial ptosis: the eyebrow is lowered, the eye is lagophthalmic, the tip of the nasal pyramid may be deviated towards the healthy part, the oral commissure is lowered and pulled towards the healthy side, hemifacial lines are effaced. These asymmetries become much more obvious during voluntary mimicry, when the paralyzed hemiface is immobile and pulled towards the healthy side, and the occlusion of the palpebral fissure is partial.

When we look at the facies of the person in front of us, we initially identify the person, and then we read the emotional state transmitted [7]. Facial emotion perception depends on the cultural psychology of a specific society [8].

The study undertaken by Eugene A. Chu et al. showed that in the first two seconds, the general population perceives asymmetries in the eyebrows and the perception threshold is 4 mm. If, however, the face viewing time is ten seconds, then eyebrow asymmetries and oral commissure asymmetries are simultaneously perceived. In this case, the perception threshold is 3 mm [9].

The aim of this study was to evaluate the utility of digital imaging and the level of the visual perception of facial asymmetry among fifth and sixth year students of the Faculty of Dental Medicine of Cluj-Napoca. The facial attractiveness and the emotions transmitted to students watching manipulated digital images, as well as the interventional attitude and the level of knowledge about the diagnosis of the pathological condition were assessed.

II. MATERIAL AND METHODS

The study was conducted through a questionnaire consisting of seven questions for fifth and sixth year students of the Faculty of Dental Medicine Cluj-Napoca, Romania, in the second week of the first semester of the 2012-2013 academic year. The students expressed their written consent to participate in the study. The forms were anonymous and contained: 6 questions, the grading scale and the serial number of the projected images. Question number 7 was related to the diagnosis of subjects with facial asymmetry. This question was projected on the screen at the end of the

S. Vlad and R.V. Ciupa (eds.), *International Conference on Advancements of Medicine and Health Care through Technology*, IFMBE Proceedings 44,
DOI: 10.1007/978-3-319-07653-9_6,

survey, and the students were asked to write the diagnosis on the form. Images of 12 subjects, 10 females and 2 males, previously created in Photoshop, were projected in Power Point. The images were manipulated so that clinical aspects of peripheral facial paralysis of different grades on the House-Brackmann scale were created (Fig. 1).

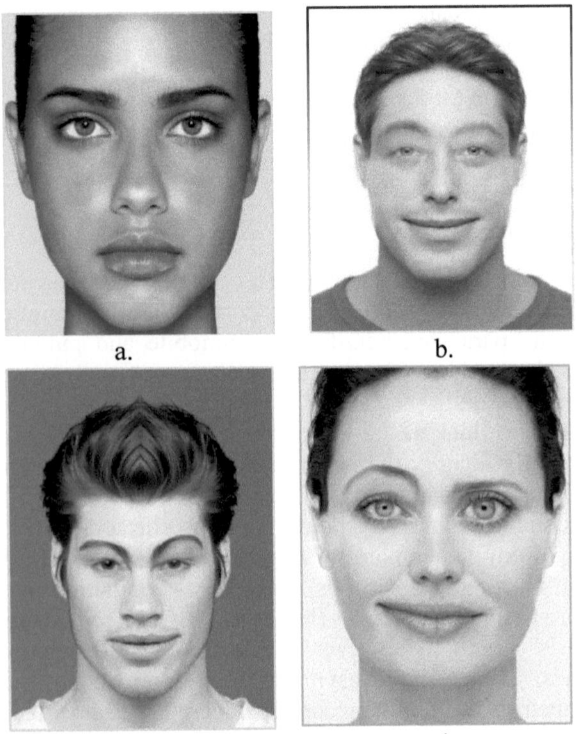

a. b. c. d.

Fig. 1 a. - Facial symmetry, b. - Grade II left peripheral facial palsy, c. - Grade IV right peripheral facial palsy, d. - Grade VI left peripheral facial paralysis

Among facies images with right and left facial paralysis, symmetrical facies images were randomly inserted. The watching time for each image was 2 minutes, followed by 1 minute, the time required for completing the questionnaire. Question number 7 was projected on the screen for 3 minutes after watching the 12 subjects, with the opportunity to answer in writing within this period.

The degree of facial paralysis was established according to the House-Brackmann scale [10]. For each 0.25 cm shift of the oral commissure towards the healthy side, one point was given. The maximum score was 4 points for a 1 cm shift of the oral commissure. In the same way, one point was given for each 0.25 cm eyebrow lowering, with a maximum of 1 cm. Six grades could be obtained by the summing up of the two parameters based on functional deficit; of the six grades, grade I was normal (Table 1).

Table 1 The House-Brackmann scale

Grade	Description	Score	Function %
I	Normal	8/8	100
II	Mild	7/8	76-99
III	Moderate	5/8 - 6/8	51-75
IV	Moderate-severe	3/8 – 4/8	26-50
V	Severe	1/8 – 2/8	1-25
VI	Total	0/8	0

The questionnaire with the 6 questions is shown in Table 2.

Table 2 Questionnaire

1. How do you assess the facial symmetry of the subject?	1= symmetric facies 2= slightly asymmetric facies 3= asymmetric facies 4= very asymmetric facies
2. How is the facial appearance of the subject ?	1=very unpleasant 2= unpleasant 3=neutral (neither pleasant, nor unpleasant) 4=pleasant 5=very pleasant
3. What state of mind does the subject's facies express?	1=a very negative state 2= a negative state 3= a neutral state 4= a positive state 5= a very positive state
4. How do you consider facial asymmetry in subjects with an asymmetric facies?	1=acceptable 2=unacceptable 0=no asymmetry was observed
5. Would you suggest surgery for the correction of the facial appearance?	1=yes 2=no
6. What feeling do you experience when you look at this facies?	1= sadness 2=anxiety 3=joy 4=pain 5=concern 6=optimism 7=fear 8=confusion

The results were statistically processed using SPSS and Microsoft Excel. To compare the mean ranks for two samples, the Mann-Whitney test was used (questions 1-3).

The χ^2 (square chi) test and the Fisher exact test for discrete variables (categorical, including dichotomous ones) were used (questions 4-7). The significance threshold for the tests used was $\alpha = 0.05$.

III. Results

The study involved 256 fifth and sixth year students. The participation rate was 54.7% for sixth year students and 62.9% for fifth year students. Incomplete questionnaires for questions 1-6 were excluded, so that 96 fifth year student questionnaires and 112 sixth year student questionnaires remained valid.

A. Perception of Facial Asymmetry

Facial symmetry was observed by most students (81%) of the two years of study when they watched symmetrical faces. Facial asymmetry in subjects with grade II facial palsy (who had one eyebrow 2.5 mm lower than the other) was observed by 74% of fifth year students and 78% of sixth year students. In contrast, in the case of subjects with grade III facial palsy (with both a 2.5 mm lowered eyebrow and a 2.5 mm contralateral shift of the oral commissure), facial asymmetry was detected by a lower percentage of students (66%). The number of students who detected facial asymmetry increased with the increasing grade of facial palsy: IV, V and VI. There were no statistically significant differences between students of the fifth and sixth year regarding the assessment of facial symmetry of the subjects. There were statistically significant differences in the perception of facial paralysis ($p < 0.001$) between grade I and the other House-Brackmann grades, between grades III and IV, and also between grades IV and V.

B. Facies Attractiveness

A proportion of about 75% of the students in the two years of study found symmetrical faces to be the most attractive. Although facial symmetry was present in both subjects 4 and 9, the face of subject no. 9 was seen by a greater number of students as more attractive than the face of subject no. 4. Although subjects with grade III facial palsy showed facial asymmetry, their faces were considered by more than half (53.6%) of the students as attractive. In the case of the subject with grade II facial palsy, although facial asymmetry was of only 2.5 mm, his face was considered attractive only by approximately 30% of the students. For grades IV, V and VI, with the increase of facial asymmetry, the proportion of students who considered the faces unattractive also increased. There were no statistically significant differences in the assessment of facial attractiveness between fifth and sixth year students.

C. Facies Expression

Symmetrical faces were considered by almost half of the students (48.5%) as being neutral, and only 38.2% of the students considered them as being positive facial expressions. Instead, the faces of subjects with grades II and III facial palsy were considered by 60% of the respondents as being positive facial expressions and by only less than 10% of the students as being negative facial expressions. The face of the subject with grade VI facial paralysis was found to express a positive state by more than one third (35.5%) of the students. In contrast, subjects with grade V facial palsy were assessed as having a positive facial expression by only 11.6% of the students. Statistically significant differences between fifth and sixth year students were obtained in the assessment of neutral ($p = 0.005$) and negative ($p = 0.002$) facial expressions.

D. Acceptability of Facial Asymmetry and Interventional Attitude

Facial asymmetry was considered acceptable for grades II and III facial palsy by approximately 80% of the fifth and sixth year students. More than half of the students (63.8%) assessed as acceptable the facial asymmetries of subjects with grade IV facial palsy, but approximately 80% of them assessed as unacceptable those of subjects with grade V, and the percentage of students increased to 90% in the case of grade VI facial paralysis. More than half of fifth and sixth year students would not indicate surgical correction of facial asymmetry caused by grade IV facial palsy.

E. Emotional Perception

Symmetrical faces and faces affected by grade V facial palsy mostly generated feelings of sadness among the students. Feelings showing indecision and allowing for interpretations such as anxiety, concern and confusion were mostly determined by subjects with grades IV, V and VI facial paralysis and with symmetrical faces. Positive feelings of joy and optimism were determined in the highest proportion by subjects with grades II and III facial palsy. There were statistically significant differences between fifth and sixth year students regarding the emotional perception of the subjects' expressions ($p < 0.001$).

F. Level of Knowledge related to the Diagnosis of the Pathological Condition

Sixth year students were able to establish the diagnosis of facial palsy or paralysis in subjects with facial asymmetry in a proportion of 63.6% compared to 23.2% of fifth year students. The proportion of students who gave no response was double among fifth year students compared to sixth year students.

IV. Discussions

The facial asymmetry perception threshold was 2.5 mm for three quarters of the fifth and sixth year students of the Faculty of Dental Medicine of Cluj-Napoca. This threshold is lower than the one determined by Chu EA et al. in general population observers. This difference is most likely due to the fact that the questionnaire was applied to a group of subjects trained to perceive and correct oral and facial asymmetries.

Facial symmetry was an important but not the only element in the assessment of facial attractiveness. For almost half of the students, the feelings transmitted by symmetrical faces were neutral. This shows that digital images processed in order to achieve a perfectly symmetrical face are artificial and do not meet our social and cultural norms. Instead, the slight facial asymmetry in grade III facial palsy that creates the illusion of balanced asymmetry (the lowered eyebrow on one side and the contralateral shift of the oral commissure) was considered by more than half of the students as being a positive facial expression. This shows that mild and moderate facial asymmetries produced by digital imaging processing are not perceived as pathological aspects with a negative impact on facial expressiveness. Facial asymmetries were considered unacceptable by the vast majority of students only when they caused severe asymmetry (grades V and VI).

The emotional perception was influenced by the presence of the smile or asymmetric smile mimicked by the slight or moderate pulling of the oral commissure.

Although the succession of asymmetric faces was at random, two thirds of the sixth year students were able to determine the cause of facial asymmetry. Poorer results were achieved by the fifth year students as their knowledge of facial nerve pathology was limited.

V. Conclusions

Manipulated digital facial images facilitate the diagnosis of facial palsy or paralysis. On the other hand, these images are partially impersonal and cannot accurately convey emotional feelings. A digital image is unable to replace human and social interaction.

Conflict of Interest

The authors declare that they have no conflict of interest.

References

1. van Gelder RS, Borod JC (1990) Neurobiological and cultural aspects of facial asymmetry. J Commun Disord 23(4-5):273-86
2. Haraguchi S, Iguchi Y, Takada K (2008) Asymmetry of the face in orthodontic patients. Angle Orthod 78:421-6
3. Severt TR, Proffit WR (1997) The prevalence of facial asymmetry in the dentofacial deformities population at the University of North Carolina. Int J Adult Orthodon Orthognath Surg 12:171-6
4. Hegtvedt AK (1993) Diagnosis and management of facial asymmetry. In: Peterson LJ, Indressano AT, Marciani RD, Roser SM, eds. Oral and Maxillofacial Surgery. Vol 3. Philadelphia: Lippincott, 1993, pp 1400-14
5. Cohen MM Jr (1995) Perspectives of craniofacial asymmetry. Part III. Common and/or well-known causes of asymmetry. Int J Oral Maxillofac Surg 24:127-33
6. Reyneke JP, Tsakiris P, Kienle F (1997) A simple classification for surgical planning of maxillomandibular asymmetry. Br J Oral Maxillofac Surg 35:349-51
7. Bruce V, Young A (1986) Understanding face recognition. Br J Psychol 77 (Pt 3):305-27
8. Pogosyan M, Engelmann JB (2011) Cultural differences in affect intensity perception in the context of advertising. Front Psychol 2:313. doi: 10.3389/fpsyg.2011.00313
9. Chu EA, Farrag TY, Ishii LE et al. (2011) Threshold of visual perception of facial asymmetry in a facial paralysis model. Arch Facial Plast Surg 13(1):14-9. doi: 10.1001/archfacial.2010.101.
10. House JW, Brackmann DE (1985) Facial nerve grading system. Otolaryngol Head Neck Surg 93:146–7.

Corresponding author: Ilea Aranka
Institute: "Iuliu Haţieganu" University of Medicine and Pharmacy Cluj-Napoca, Faculty of Dentistry, Department of Oral Rehabilitation, Oral Health and Dental Office Management
Street: Victor Babes
City: Cluj-Napoca
Country: Romania
Email: arankailea@yahoo.com, cseh.aranka@umfcluj.ro

Towards Assisting Medical Decisions by Using Rule Based Protocols and Semantic Resources

Radu Răzvan Slăvescu[1], Alin-Cristian Groşan[1], and Kinga Cristina Slăvescu[2]

[1] Technical University of Cluj-Napoca, Department of Computer Science, Cluj-Napoca, Romania
[2] "Iuliu Haţieganu" University of Medicine and Pharmacy, Cluj-Napoca, Romania

Abstract— **We present a rule based system aimed to assist the medical doctors in routine tasks. It suggests a diagnosis and recommends a treatment for patients based upon their medical history and current symptoms. The system employs free technologies which best match this purpose. The system relies on a set of CLIPS rules implementing the standard medical guidelines which the doctors follow in the process of diagnosing and prescribing drugs. Open Linked Data resources are used for recommending possible medication. The proposed architecture is open and expandable so other technologies can be linked to improve the results.**

Keywords— **rule based system, medical diagnosis, medical protocols, CLIPS, SPARQL**

I. INTRODUCTION

The need for a prompt and accurate medical diagnosis and treatment makes it necessary to offer the doctors the technology able to accomplish this. Recent advances in knowledge representation and reasoning offer solutions for implementing systems able to assist physicians in obtaining the relevant information and making the right decisions. Such systems might benefit from at least two recent developments in Romania. The first one is the introduction of the electronic medical record (EMR), which gives access to the whole medical history of one patient. The second is the implementation of the medical protocols, designed to guide the doctors in taking proper actions in their daily activity.

In order to help the practitioners improve their accuracy and promptitude in routine tasks, we created a system that assists them in collecting data from patients, recommending examinations, diagnosing the disease, deciding the treatment and informing the patients about its details. This paper reports on the decisions we have made when developing the aforementioned system [1].

The system is primarily intended to help the doctors perform routine tasks in an automatic way, from investigation to diagnosis and treatment. It was not our purpose to emulate the whole reasoning process performed by an expert in the field, but rather to "hard-wire" those decisions which are standardized in the existing protocols, thus saving time and effort from the practitioner.

The main contribution consists in the proposed design which makes use of the available technologies and solutions and the architecture to integrate them. For its functionality and data source, the system relies solely on open access tools and resources. In the same time, its structure allows easily importing data from another sources as well. Another contribution consists in defining the terms employed for describing the symptoms and reasoning upon them according to the protocol. We had to identify and standardize a set of terms used by the existing medical protocols and by the practitioners for describing the patient condition. The system also has to make use of the medical terms recently introduced in our country for reporting symptoms and investigation. The set of terms in the aligned vocabulary is offered to the system user via the system interface. This facilitates describing the patient data in a controlled way, thus allowing further processing based on standard guidelines. In the same time, the system should be able to exchange data with the national EHR, so its architecture was thought to accommodate this through the data format and the access points. The system is able to interrogate Open Linked Data resources like DrugBank (`www.drugbank.ca`) and present the doctor a set of drugs which could be recommended for curing the disease.

The rest of this paper is structured in the following manner. Section II details the system's components and their functionality. Section III presents a working example. Section IV discusses some limitations of the system, as well as the performance aspects and sketches possible optimizations. Section V compares our system to some similar approaches. Section VI is dedicated to conclusions and future work.

II. DETAILED SYSTEM STRUCTURE

The system is organized in several modules that cooperate to produce the desired results. The overall architecture diagram is given in Figure 1.

A database is used in order to store the user's personal information and medical history. The information from the

[1] A prototype of the system in form of a desktop application is available at http://cs-gw.utcluj.ro/~srazvan/prj/foc/FOC.tar.gz or upon request at srazvan@cs-gw.utcluj.ro

S. Vlad and R.V. Ciupa (eds.), *International Conference on Advancements of Medicine and Health Care through Technology*, IFMBE Proceedings 44,
DOI: 10.1007/978-3-319-07653-9_7,

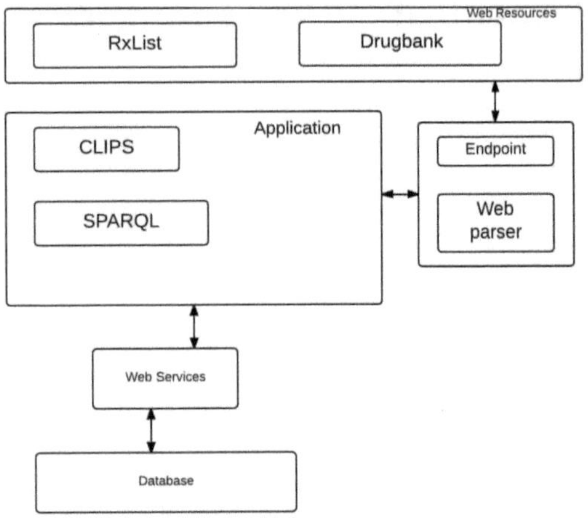

Fig. 1 System architecture

database is retrieved with a webservice which create the link between the database and the rest of the application. This allows importing data from other sources, perhaps from the national EHR. Another webservice is used for the CLIPS module which is responsible for reasoning using a set of rules written in the well known CLIPS language [1]. We chose the CLIPS language for protocol representation since it offers a flexible, declarative way for implementing rules. This makes it appropriate for implementing medical guidelines, which are known to be subject of a periodical review and update process by the medical community. Both webservices are implemented in C#. We use another webservice to bring the correct medication for the patient from an online free drugs database through SPARQL endpoint.

The front end of the application is structured in pages which replicate the layout of the medical file where the medical history of one patient is stored. A CLIPS rule based engine is integrated in this module. It uses a set of rules which actually implement the protocols. Based upon them, the rule based engine suggests the needed lab workups, the diagnosis and the treatment. Based on recommended treatment, the semantic web module selects the required medication for that patient from a series of drugs and also informs the patient about the side effects of the drug and the dosage required measured in tablets.

Once the doctor has filled in the fields of the form with the personal data received from the patient, this data is stored into a MySQL database via a C# webservice. The results of the lab workups are also saved in the same database.

These data are further used by a multi step CLIPS module, meaning that for the system to extract a valid diagnosis for a patient, multiple iterations might be needed. That is because usually the lab workups results help in ruling out one possible disease, but further investigation might be needed in order to reach a unique diagnosis. Therefore, the process of suggesting lab workups, receiving their results and drawing conclusions might iterate several times.

We are going to illustrate the system capabilities with the following scenario. One 11 years patient is brought to the hospital by his parents for abdominal pain. The doctor establishes the pain is situated in the upper abdominal area, namely in the right hypochondrium. The pain is permanent and localized. The patient also reports cough and vomiting. Then, the doctor proceeds to a physical examination and discovers the patient also has fever.

Based on the information he has just learned, the doctor would recommend a series of investigations for the patient. Once the lab results become available, some of the diseases are ruled out, but some more tests might be needed until one single diagnose is established. After that, the doctor recommends a treatment, typically in form of a medication, possibly combined with some sort of diet.

The doctor's behavior is guided by a set of guidelines based on studies and on medical consensus. An example of a rule from the abdominal pain protocol is given in Table 1. These protocols rules are translated into CLIPS rules so that the reasoning module could actually extract conclusions. The rules are developed in a format that is generic enough so that the system is scalable and offer the a degree of explicitness so that the CLIPS module is not mislead. An example of a CLIPS rule is presented in Listing 1 containing also some conditionally logic meaning that the rule will be triggered by any of the options from the "or" condition.

One issue we had to solve at this point was to deal with the differences existing between the set of terms used for describing the symptoms (one of them is presented in the first row of Table 1) and the terms used by the protocols (which are exemplified in the second row of Table 1). The terms in the first line belong to the set of Diagnosis Related Group (DRG), a system used for describing the hospital cases for health resources management which was recently adopted in our country (see [2] for details).

In the same time, the terms on which the existing medical protocols are grounded differ from those of the DRG, so an alignment issue had to be solved. The alignment was done manually and the corresponding sets of terms have been build. This is used in the system interface: the content of its drop-downs adapts dynamically, based on the prior selections and the content of those sets.

Table 1 A protocol excerpt

Step	Possible value
Get Pain Type	Upper abdominal pain
Localize pain	Right hypocondrium Left hypocondrium Epigastric
Get Pain Type	Local Spread
Establish Possible Diagnosis	Gastro-duodenal ulcer Gastritis Pancreatitis Cholecystitis Biliary Colic
Get associated symptoms	Nausea Vomiting Biliary vomiting Anorexia Haematemesis Diarrhea Constipation Haematochesia Dehydration Fever Sweating Cough Haematuria Disuria Polakiuria Weight loss
Order lab workups	White Blood Cell Hemoglobin Inflammatory Markers Liver Enzyme Blood Glucose Amylasemia Electrolytes Urinalysis Stool analysis Abdominal Ultrasound Upper/Lower gastrointestinal endoscopy Abdominal Radiography
Establish Diagnosis	Gastro-duodenal ulcer Gastritis Pancreatitis Cholecystitis Biliary Colic Urinary Tract Infection Dysmenorrhea Anal Fissure Appendicitis Twisted Ovarian Cyst Extrauterine Pregnancy

```
(defrule possible_diagnosis_DLPSA
 (pain (name upper abdominal pain))
 (or (localization
         (name rightHypocondrium))
     (localization
         (name leftHypocondrium))
     (localization
         (name Epigastric)))
=>
 (assert (pos-diagnosis
           (index 1)
           (name Gastro-duodenal_ulcer)))
 (assert (pos-diagnosis
           (index 1)
           (name Gastritis)))
 (assert (pos-diagnosis
           (index 1)
           (name Pancreatitis)))
 (assert (pos-diagnosis
           (index 1)
           (name Cholecystitis)))
 (assert (pos-diagnosis
           (index 1)
           (name Biliary_Colic))))
```

Listing 1 CLIPS rule example: possible causes for upper abdominal pain

Eventually, an exact diagnosis is generated and the doctor decides whether the patient needs to be admitted in the hospital or if he can follow the suggested treatment at home. Based on the established diagnosis, the system recommends a class of medication, e.g. antibiotics.

The name of the recommended treatment is entered in a SPARQL module, which uses JENA libraries to extract the needed information on that drug via a SPARQL endpoint. We chose the DrugBank database of drugs [3], which contains extensive data on the nomenclature, classification, action, or pharmaceutical properties of different drugs. We selected the following pieces of information: commercial name, description, indication, toxicity and a link for further information. The latter one provides the web address on `RxList` where information on the drug dose is published. The system uses a web parser to extract the dosage and the interaction information. Based on the interaction information, those drugs which cannot be prescribed to the patient for allergy/drug interaction reasons are filtered out, so only valid medication is presented to the doctor for selection.

On the application interface the doctor receives the recommended drug's name, his interaction with other drugs and the dosage based on the patient's weight.

III. A WORKING EXAMPLE

We conducted tests on different scenarios which might come across when the system is used in real world situations. This Section details the scenario in the prior Section in order to illustrate the system capabilities (see Fig. 2).

In Step 1 we introduced the first two entries in the system, pain and location of the pain. From the first item of the first line of the matrix we select the "Pain". In that field we selected "Upper abdominal pain". At his point, if we requested the system to reason and extract a diagnosis, the result was just the possible diagnosis and it requested more data; no precise diagnosis can be formulated. At a second step we added the information about the patients complains, age, the character of the pain, if it is intermittent or constant, and if the pain tends to spread or not. So, after selecting "Pain", on the same row in the next field we selected the localization of the pain. In that field we selected "Right hypocondrium". After we have selected the two options, the reasoning process is started. As an effect of that action the reasoning module returns us the possible diagnosis corresponding to the selected options. This were "Gastro-duodenal ulcer", "Gastritis", "Pancreatitis", "Cholecystitis", "Biliary Colic".

In the third step, we introduced the other symptoms. We selected the symptoms from the drop-down of checkboxes by checking the box near every symptom. From that entity we checked the boxes near "Fever", "Cough" and "Vomiting". In the fourth step we select the "Character" of the pain. In that field we selected "Constant" meaning the pain manifests itself all the time. In the fifth step we selected "No" for the "Spreading" field, meaning that the pain is localized in a small area rather than a larger part of the abdomen. After filling these data we repeated the reasoning process and the system replied with the lab workups the patient needs to undertake: "White Blood Cell", "Liver Enzyme" and "Electrolytes".

When the lab results become available, they indicate the "White Blood Cell" parameter was in the normal range, the "Liver Enzyme" value was "High" and the "Electrolytes" values were "Modified". Once they are introduced into the system, A third reasoning process ended up with suggesting the correct diagnosis for the patient, namely "Cholecystitis". The system also suggested a treatment for this diagnosis: a class of medications ("Antibiotics", in this particular case) and a specific diet ("Fat Free Diet"). It also recommends re-hidration of the patient due to the modified level of electrolytes. All these recommendations are made by a separate set of CLIPS rules which implement the corresponding knowledge.

Since the system knows the class of drugs needed for treatment, it will look up for the appropriate drugs. This is done by the SPARQL module, which queries the Open Linked Data endpoint about the drugs available in that class, adverse reaction it might have when combined with other drugs or his own side effects like headaches or fever. The system also calculates the dosage based on the patient's weight.

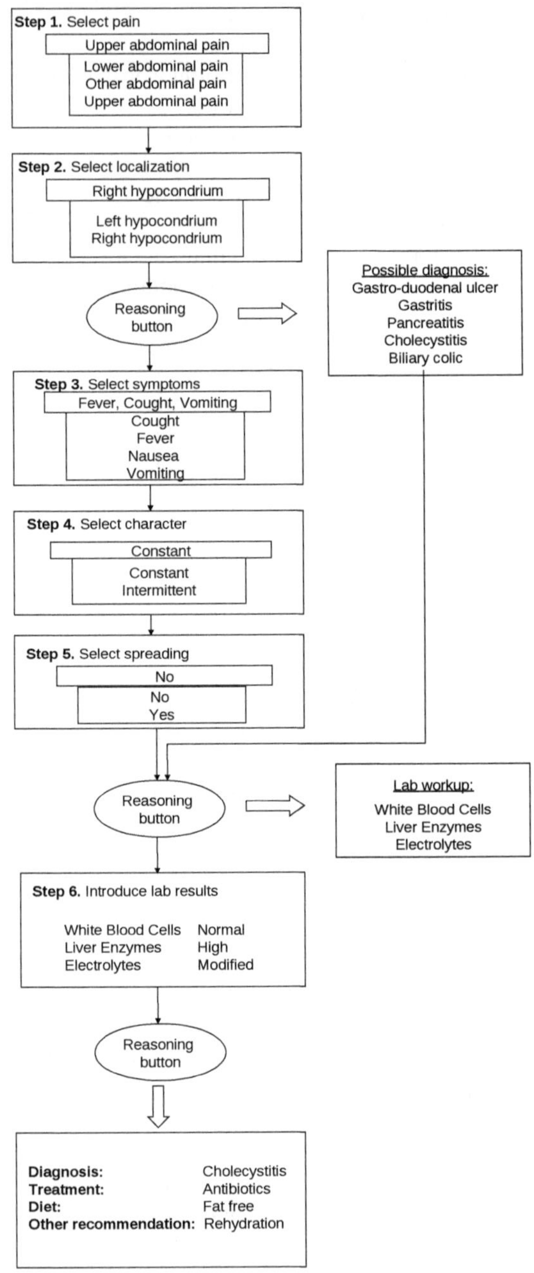

Fig. 2 Test scenario

```
Diagnosis = Cholecystitis
Treatment = Antibiotics
Recommended drug = Amoxicillin
Adverse drug effects:
 - Oxytetracycline and Amoxicillin:
   Possible antagonism of action
 - Demeclocycline and Amoxicillin
   Possible antagonism of action
 - Tetracycline and Amoxicillin
   Possible antagonism of action
 - Methotrexate and Amoxicillin
   The penicillin increases the effect
   and toxicity of methotrexate
 - Minocycline and Amoxicillin
   Possible antagonism of action
 - Methacycline and Amoxicillin
   Possible antagonism of action
Dosage = 25 mg/kg/day
```

From the displayed result we can observe the side effects that the recommended medicine in this case "Amoxicillin" has with various other drugs. The system also displays the drug dosage. This is calculated based on the weight of the patient and the pharmaco-cynetical properties of the drug (e.g. half life).

IV. DISCUSSION

Our system implements medical protocols used by the hospitals in our country. Its main purpose is to speed up the diagnose process by providing the doctor with suggestions regarding the most common, routine decisions involved in this process. All steps are consistent with the adopted terminology, as well as with the existing protocols. Also by using protocols we have a standardization of the information which makes it easier to further extend and update the system. The system is able to explain the reasoning line of the CLIPS module so the doctor can check its correctness. At each point, the doctor may overrule the system's suggestions by modifying them, deleting or adding information.

The system's interface is similar to the medical file and the doctors can associate very quickly the elements. We also reduced the human error factor in filling the forms by conditioning fields based on another set of protocols and by offering the opportunity of importing the previous personal data and medical history.

A strong point is speeding up the medication selection process, from detecting the available products to rejecting the incompatible ones to informing the patient, as bounded by the policies in our country, about the adverse reactions of a drug and the effects of it if combined with other drugs.

A good point of the system is that it uses nonproprietary technologies like CLIPS, C# or SPARQL, so a further development and deployment will raise no royalty issues.

A drawback of the system and in particular of the ontology that it uses for the extraction of the drugs is that without using efficient filters it will provide to the system information that is to broad for using it in real life situations. In the same time, the need of parsing large volume of data might have a negative impact over the execution time. Right now, this is kept at reasonable limits according to the doctors' (i.e., ultimate users) standards, but it remains a concern for us.

A limitation of the system is that its diagnoses are accurate for a large number of diseases but it cannot perform like an ideal doctor and have 100% accuracy with his diagnoses. The system assists the physician in their work and can give a strong and valid diagnosis for the diseases that are most likely to appear, but for more complicated investigations the doctor's assistance is mandatory.

The system assessment has been done manually and on a reduced set of scenarios. However, we intend to improve this by a systematic test involving more diagnoses and doctors scrutiny. Following the methodological line presented in [4], we also intend to test the system in a programmatic manner.

V. RELATED WORK

The medical diagnose systems such as EasyDiagnosis (`http://www.easydiagnosis.com/`) and Right Diagnosis (`http://www.rightdiagnosis.com/`) provide medical advise to a patient based on his complains. These systems seem to rely on symptoms frequency rather than on some standard protocols. The 5GL-Doctor Medical Diagnosis Software (`5glsoftware.webplus.net`) is similar to some point to our own. Both systems are based on matching rules on symptoms/signs/lab workups and generating short lists of possible diseases. 5GL-Doctor uses a large database into which information is brought from various web sources. The system's vast rulebase allows it to take into consideration the patient's geographical region and adjust the result accordingly. Right now, our system is focused on the protocols elaborated for our country.

The Kasimir system [5] uses Semantic Web technologies knowledge representation formalisms and open reasoning tools in order to assist decision making in oncology.

On the other hand, a number of guidelines [6] and/or protocols are collected and formalized in order to assist the doctor. Paper [7] provides a collection of such algorithms, based in part on extensive studies and in part on medical consensus, for the gastrointestinal area. The paper [8] presents a more comprehensive set of procedures and computation resources for a many medical applications.

In the area of medical ontologies, one significant research line is presented in [9], aiming to develop a large scale ontology for the medical field. Another progress factor comes from the efforts of developing standards for interoperability of health information technology (see `http://www.hl7.org/`) in order to establish standards for the emergent Electronic Medical Records. The Convergent Medical Terminology comprises a set of over 75,000 terms used internationally in order to offer a common lexicon to describe symptoms and diagnoses in a consistent manner. However, integrating the set of existing ontologies and data models remain a task for many researchers in the field. We can mention, for example, an openEHR archetypes-based approach for bridging the gap between the Health Level Seven (HL7) Virtual Medical Record standard and the ISO/CEN 13606 standard is presented [10].

VI. CONCLUSIONS AND FUTURE WORK

We presented the architecture and technologies used for building a rule based system designed to assist the doctors in their basic routine work. The system helps the practitioners when consulting a patient and provides them relevant information. It relies on free tools like CLIPS and on information and extracted from freely available Open Linked Data resources. The information extracted is the result of complex queries over various resources both local and over the web. One of the present paper's contributions consists of identifying the information resources and building the appropriated queries. This job required making use of the terms which are established in the medical practice and aligning them with the concepts employed by the resources mentioned.

As a future work, we intend to extend the system into more medical areas so it can diagnose a broader area of diseases and improve the work of cross area doctors. For now the system can extract diagnoses only for the gastroenterology area, but in the future we want to expand the system so it will be capable of offering assistance in other areas (e.g., neurology). In the same time, the system should exploit more information sources on drugs available on the web, which will required developments in the natural language processing part.

We also want to create a mobile version of the system with a more restricted functionality, mainly focused on interrogating the system about lab results, diagnosis justifying etc. For the mobile platform we want to create a system that can authenticate a patient and show to the doctor his medical history data by scanning a QR code on a bracelet. This way, the doctor could be more efficient in doing his job and not strictly linked to the work station.

CONFLICT OF INTEREST

The authors declare that they have no conflict of interest.

ACKNOWLEDGEMENTS

The authors thank Doru-Bogdan Terec for his contribution in implementing this system.

REFERENCES

1. Giarratano Joseph C., Riley Gary D.. *Expert Systems: Principles and Programming*. Pacific Grove, CA, USA: Brooks/Cole Publishing Co. 2005.
2. Mayes Rick. The Origins, Development, and Passage of Medicare's Revolutionary Prospective Payment System *Journal of the History of Medicine and Allied Sciences*. 2007;62:21-55.
3. Knox Craig, Law Vivian, Jewison Timothy, et al. DrugBank 3.0: a comprehensive resource for 'Omics' research on drugs *Nucleic Acids Research*. 2011;39:D1035-D1041.
4. Groot Perry, Hommersom Arjen, Lucas Peter J. F., et al. Using model checking for critiquing based on clinical guidelines *Artificial Intelligence in Medicine*. 2009;46:19-36.
5. d'Aquin Mathieu, Lieber Jean, Napoli Amedeo. Decentralized case-based reasoning and Semantic Web technologies applied to decision support in oncology *The Knowledge Engineering Review*. 2013;28:425–449.
6. Bickley L., Szilagyi P.G.. *Bates' Guide to Physical Examination and History-Taking*. Point (Lippincott Williams & Wilkins)Wolters Kluwer Health 2012.
7. Vandenplas Yvan, Gutierrez-Castrellon Pedro, Velasco-Benitez Carlos, et al. Practical algorithms for managing common gastrointestinal symptoms in infants *The International Journal of Applied and Basic Nutritional Sciences*. 2012.
8. Iyengar M. Sriram, Svirbely John R.. The Medical Algorithms Project *CoRR*. 2009;abs/0908.0932.
9. Rector Alan, Rogers Jeremy. Ontological and Practical Issues in Using a Description Logic to Represent Medical Concept Systems: Experience from GALEN in *IN REASONING WEB, SECOND INTERNATIONAL SUMMER SCHOOL, TUTORIAL LECTURES*:197–231 2006.
10. Gonzalez-Ferrer Arturo, Peleg Mor, Verhees Bert, Verlinden Jan-Marc, Marcos Carlos. Data Integration for Clinical Decision Support Based on openEHR Archetypes and HL7 Virtual Medical Record in *Process Support and Knowledge Representation in Health Care* (Lenz Richard, Miksch Silvia, Peleg Mor, Reichert Manfred, Riano David, Teije Annette. , eds.);7738 of *Lecture Notes in Computer Science*:71-84Springer Berlin Heidelberg 2013.

Preliminary Experiments on Using Subjective Logic for Reasoning on Diagnosis

Radu Răzvan Slăvescu[1] and Kinga Cristina Slăvescu[2]

[1] Technical University of Cluj-Napoca, Department of Computer Science, Cluj-Napoca, Romania
[2] "Iuliu Haţieganu" University of Medicine and Pharmacy, Cluj-Napoca, Romania

Abstract— **We present a system which implements a set of Subjective Logic operators, namely conjunction, abduction, deduction and fusion. The system's purpose was to investigate some patterns in the medical reasoning and to see whether they can be modeled using this subset of Subjective Logic. This approach would allow dealing seamlessly with rules of reasoning whose uncertainty level adjusts once more evidence becomes available. Our system allows assessing the rule confidence level in a programmatic way, based on the data stored in a database containing the previous patient examinations. It is also able to reason based on those rules and the input from the patient and to justify the conclusion.**

Keywords— **medical expert system, subjective logic, JESS, uncertainty models**

I. INTRODUCTION

The medical field raises a couple of challenges to the classical methods of reasoning, mainly because of the inherent uncertainty present in this area. The uncertainty comes from the lack of a comprehensive theory of the field, the difficulty of writing exceptionless rules for describing the causal relationships which exist between the entities and the practical impossibility of performing all the investigations required by a 100% guaranteed diagnosis [1].

The main shortcoming of the approach is the relatively high cost associated with such a study, which might limit the total body of knowledge which might be obtained. On the other hand, doctors are definitely developing their own "rules of thumb" once they accumulate enough experience. Such rules further guide them in the diagnosis process by providing valuable hints, even if they are not supported by a sound statistical survey. Building such rules and data to support them would be of interest for developing an expert system for the medical field. The rules might have associated a confidence level, but most of the time this level is indicated by the user rather than being computed based on prior evidence.

The main issue with the existing solutions is the probabilities they rely on are either expensive to find or are approximated, but no information on how the approximation's reliability itself is retained. The work presented in this paper aims to tackle this by employing Subjective Logic [2], which explicitly takes uncertainty into account. It deals with beliefs and operations on them in a manner similar to that of the Dempster-Shafer theory [3, 4].

The contributions made are the following. First, we identified a subset of the Subjective Logic operators we believe to be necessary for dealing with the reasoning patterns in the medical field. By employing this set of operators, we may seamlessly deal with both statistically validated rules and with those which are build from user observation and express their level of uncertainty accordingly. Then, we developed a system[1] which allows assessing the rule confidence level in a programmatic way, as well as building new rules and adding them to the system, together with the corresponding uncertainty. Last, the system have the possibility to justify the reasoning process which lead to a specific conclusion.

The rest of the paper is organized as follows. Section II introduces the basics of Subjective Logic. Section III presents the set of operators selected for the medical domain. Section IV shows the details of the implemented medical reasoner. Section V positions the work in the field, while Section VI concludes and sketches the intended future work.

II. SUBJECTIVE LOGIC FOR MEDICAL REASONING

Subjective logic (SL from now on) is a type of probabilistic logic that allows probability values to be expressed with degrees of uncertainty. The idea of probabilistic logic is to combine the strong points of logic and probability calculus. This means it has the binary logic's capacity to express structured argument models and the power of probabilities to add degrees of truth to those arguments. Subjective logic comes as an extension to probabilistic logic by adding the uncertainty dimensionality to the probability values making subjective logic suitable for reasoning in conditions of uncertainty or incomplete evidence.

The need for uncertainty comes from the subjective character of the world we live in. We have to take into consideration that whenever truths about propositions are assessed, they cannot be stated with absolute certainty (like in standard logic where fact are considered either true or false or in

[1]Prototype available on request at srazvan@cs-gw.utcluj.ro or for download at http://cs-gw.utcluj.ro/~srazvan/prj/slreasoner/SLReasoner.tar.gz

S. Vlad and R.V. Ciupa (eds.), *International Conference on Advancements of Medicine and Health Care through Technology*, IFMBE Proceedings 44,
DOI: 10.1007/978-3-319-07653-9_8,

probabilistic logic where to every fact a probabilistic value in the range [0,1] is attached). Also belief ownership must be taken into account because every assumption is made by an individual so it cannot represent a general, objective truth. As an example, one can consider two medical doctors who have significantly different degrees of working experience. Suppose both of them have to make an assumption regarding the possible connection between a disease D and a symptom S. Consider that the doctor with less experience has met in his career that from 10 cases of disease D 8 present symptom S while, on the other hand, the doctor with more experience has seen that from 100 cases of disease D, 80 present the symptom S. By using only probabilistic logic, one could infer in both cases that "80% cases of disease D present symptom S" which is correct in both cases, but what happens with the significantly greater experience of the second doctor? Shouldn't that count in some way? Shouldn't his opinion be more relevant to the assumption compared to the opinion of the less-experienced doctor? With the help of subjective logic we can model better this situation by assigning smaller value of uncertainty to the opinion of the more experienced doctor while the opinion of the less experienced doctor will receive a greater value of uncertainty.

As it can be seen, subjective logic can model more realistically real word situations and its conclusions reflect more adequately the ignorance and uncertainties that necessarily result from partially uncertain input arguments.

A. *Experience and Opinions*

SL argues that uncertainty involved in estimating the values of probabilities must be considered and assessed. The theory's basic block is the concept of *opinion* over a sentence. Given a proposition x, the opinion ω_x regarding the truth value of x is defined as a quadruple $\omega_x = (b_x, d_x, u_x, a_x)$. Its components represent the degree of belief (evidence supporting x), disbelief (evidence supporting $\neg x$) and uncertainty about the truth of x. By definition, they must sum up to 1. The atomicity a_x is a measure of the *prior* probability of the truth value of x. Within this paper, we will focus on a universe of discourse comprising only binomial, mutually exclusive sentences (x and $\neg x$ respectively), thus a_x defaults to 0.5.

For example, one can assign a value of 0.7 to the belief corresponding to the sentence "The patient has gastritis", 0.2 to the disbelief corresponding to the sentence "The patient does not have gastritis" and the remaining 0.1 to the uncertainty about the diagnosis. This one is due to the lack of perfect knowledge over the diagnosis and can be seen as second order probability (modeling uncertainty over a first-order probabilities). In this case, $\omega_x = (0.7, 0.2, 0.1, 0.5)$ means the agent issuing sentence x (i.e. the medical doctor) beliefs the sentence to a degree of 0.7; its negation $\neg x$ to a degree of 0.2 and has an uncertainty degree of 0.1 about it, possibly because of the lack of complete evidence. The value of a is 0.5 as, so far, we have considered only a binary universe of discourse for each sentence.

Given $\omega_x = (b_x, d_x, u_x, a_x)$, the corresponding probability expectation value (a generalization of a classical probability expectation), is defined by the formula below:

$$E(\omega_x) = b_x + a_x u_x \tag{1}$$

This definition corresponds to that of pignistic probability in [5] and is consistent with the principle of equally dividing frame belief among its singletons. The interpretation of a_x is the relative proportion of singletons of x.

As showed in [2], there exists a function mapping the evidence space for a sentence (i.e. prior observations over its truth) into opinion space. Based on this correspondence, sentence opinions can be synthesized out of sequences of observations over those sentences. Opinions are further combined according to specific operators to be defined later. The resulting algebra of opinions is equivalent, both from the point of view of semantics and expressiveness, with the distributions, but it has the advantage of being much more efficient from the computational perspective.

If for the sentence x, we have r experiences supporting x and s supporting $\neg x$, then the opinion's components b, d and u are computed in the following way:

$$\begin{cases} b = \frac{r}{r+s+2} \\ d = \frac{s}{r+s+2} \\ u = \frac{2}{r+s+2} \end{cases}$$

Some limit cases can be considered: $b = 1$ means logical $TRUE$ (probability 1), $d = 1$ means logical *FALSE* (probability 0), $u = 1$ means vacuous opinion (total uncertainty, absolute lack of experiences) and $b + d = 1$ gives the classical probability (no uncertainty). One should notice the latter case happens if the number of experiences is infinite. This property will be used further in this paper, when our extended formalism reduces to the original one when the number of experiences approaches ∞.

III. A Set of SL Operators for Medical Reasoning

This Section presents the SL operators employed for modelling the uncertain reasoning for the medical domain on which we have focused. Selecting them is one of the contributions made by this paper. There exist a large range of SL operations with the corresponding properties and applicability. To our best knowledge, this is the first attempt to build a subset of operations which are appropriate for modelling the reasoning in the medical field.

A. Conjunction

For $\omega_x = (b_x, d_x, u_x, a_x)$ and $\omega_y = (b_y, d_y, u_y, a_y)$, their conjunction $\omega_{x\wedge y}$, has the following components:

$$\begin{cases} b_{x\wedge y} = b_x b_y + \frac{(1-a_x)a_y b_x u_y + a_x(1-a_y)u_x b_y}{1-a_x a_y} \\ d_{x\wedge y} = d_x + d_y - d_x d_y \\ u_{x\wedge y} = u_x u_y + \frac{(1-a_y)b_x u_y + (1-a_x)u_x b_y}{1-a_x a_y} \\ a_{x\wedge y} = a_x a_y \end{cases}$$

Conjunction applies when the hypothesis of a rule is composed of more than one premises. In order to find the total opinion of the hypothesis we need to combine the premises' opinions. E.g. *IF bacteria has a spiral shape (first premise) AND Urease test is positive (second premise) THEN bacteria is Helicobacter Pylori (conclusion)*. In opinions we have $\omega_1 = (0.7, 0.2, 0.1, 0.5)$ and $\omega_2 = (0.6, 0.3, 0.1, 0.5)$ respectively, then their conjunction is $\omega_{hypothesis} = (0.4, 0.51, 0.09, 0.25)$.

The definition of the conjunction was first introduced in the paper [6], where is called normal binomial multiplication and is denoted by the operators $\cdot$. The operation is shown to be very good approximation of the analytically correct operators applied to the Beta probability density functions. Whilst the exact operations quickly become unmanageable, their SL counterparts preserve the simplicity thus allowing analyzing complex models [2]. The outcome, albeit approximate, will approach the exact results as the uncertainty decreases.

B. Abduction

In the medical field it is considered that every symptom attached to a disease is an effect of it. What our system tries to do is to discover the disease when knowing the symptoms, meaning that in our case we know the *consequent* and we try to find out the *antecedent*. The Subjective Logic Operator that reasons in this direction is called the Abduction Operator. The formula for this operator is omitted for brevity reasons; it can be found in [7].

Every rule in the system that matches a given symptom and asserts a new medical fact as a diagnose uses the Abduction operator. For example, for the rule `D_GA -> S_AP 2000 1000` (where 2000 represents the number of cases of Gastritis, while 1000 is the number of patients with Gastritis which presented Abdominal Pain) knowing that "Abdominal Pain(S_AP)" symptom is present, we compute the opinion of the diagnose "Gastritis(D_GA) with the Abductive Operator, taking into consideration

- ω_x the opinion related to the symptom x (i.e. Abdominal Pain)
- $\omega_{x|y}$ the opinion of the fact: "presence of symptom x in case of disease y (i.e. Gastritis)"
- $\omega_{x|\bar{y}}$ the opinion of the fact: "presence of symptom x when it is not the case of disease y"

in the formulas above.

For example, if the user chooses the *Abdominal Pain* symptom from the list, with the intensity of 0.74 out of 1, it means that an SL opinion for this medical fact will be generated with the values $\omega_x = (0.74, 0.26, 0.0, 0.5)$. By proceeding further, the rule engine will match the rule `D_GA -> S_AP 2000 1000` meaning that the aforementioned symptom is an effect of the *Gastritis* disease. This rule has requires three opinions in order to generate the opinion of the proposed diagnose through abduction:

- ω_x the opinion of the symptom
- $\omega_{x|y}$ the opinion of the fact:"symptom x is present in case of disease y"
- $\omega_{x|\bar{y}}$ the opinion of the fact:"symptom x is present in case of no disease y"

Having $\omega_x = (0.74\ \ 0.26\ \ 0.0\ \ 0.5)$, $\omega_{x|y} = (0.49\ \ 0.49\ \ 0.02\ \ 0.05)$ and $\omega_{x|\bar{y}} = (0.83\ \ 0.0\ \ 0.17\ \ 0.5)$ we obtain the opinion of the diagnose $\omega_{Gastritis} = (0.58\ \ 0.36\ \ 0.6\ \ 0.5)$. In other words, we "believe" that this is the correct diagnose with 58%, we "don't believe" this with 36% and we are "uncertain" with an amount of 6%.

C. Deduction

We use it if we have information about the *antecedent* and want to find out about *consequent*. For example, for the following medical rule:

```
IF the bacteria has a spiral shape
THEN the bacteria is Helicobacter Pylori
```

meaning that we use input data (symptoms and/or tests) to deduce the existence of another symptom and not a disease. Deduction has the same formula as in the case of Abduction but with the conditionals inverted [8]. We need three opinions in order to deduce the opinion of conclusion: ω_x (the opinion of the hypothesis), $\omega_{y|x}$ (the opinion of the fact that y is true when x is true) and $\omega_{y|\bar{x}}$ (the opinion of the fact that y is true when x is not true). A relevant numerical example would be to consider: $\omega_x = (0.1\ 0.8\ 0.1\ 0.5)$ (i.e. approximately 10% of the bacterias have spiral shape), $\omega_{y|x} = (0.3\ 0.65\ 0.05\ 0.5)$ (i.e. approximately 30% of the spiraled bacterias are

Helicobacter Pylori) and $\omega_{y|\bar{x}} = (0.2\ 0.7\ 0.1)$ (i.e. approximately 20% of bacterias that don't have spiral shape are Helicobacter Pylori). We deduce $\omega = (0.21\ 0.69\ 0.10\ 0.5)$.

D. Fusion

It can be the case that two rules can abduce the existence of the same disease. That means that in the working memory of the engine will exist two medical facts that correspond to the same disease but have different opinions. We need to "fuse" those facts into a single, final fact. The intuition is that a patient with 2 symptoms of a disease D is more likely to have it than a patient having only one of the symptoms. The opinions are merged using the Cumulative Fusion Operator [9].

For example, if the user chooses two symptoms from the list: *Abdominal Pain* and *Pirosis* with intensities 0.74 respectively 0.27, it will trigger two rules from the rule engine:*D_GA -> S_AP 2000 1000* and *D_GA -> S_PI 2000 600*. We observe that both rules propose the same *Gastritis* diagnose. It means that, by means of abduction, two facts corresponding to this diagnose will be generated: $\omega_1 = (0.58\ 0.36\ 0.6\ 0.5)$ and $\omega_2 = (0.25\ 0.74\ 0.1\ 0.5)$. With the help of the Fusion Operator, we combine these two intermediate results and we propose a final *Gastritis* diagnose with the opinion: $\omega_{Gastritis} = (0.26\ 0.73\ 0.1\ 0.5)$.

IV. Detailed System Structure

A. Objectives

Our objective was to develop an interactive rule-based expert system that will help in the medical diagnosis process. The system will use subjective logic to model the facts and the rules that form the knowledge base of the system and also adequate subjective operators will be used in the reasoning process.

Our intention is to extend the probabilistic logic reasoning by adding uncertainty values to rules and facts so we can model the degree of confidence we attach to each knowledge data.

Regarding the knowledge acquisition, the system will be able to model rules that are deduced from specialized medical studies, rules that come from doctors' own experience that are not yet validated by studies and also it will be able to build rules automatically by learning from medical patients databases.

The application flow will be as follows: the user will select symptoms from a list together with their intensity level as input and the system will display possible diagnoses as a result ranked by the degree of belief and the expectancy value for that diagnose. The user can select one of the results to receive justification and further explanations for it in a graphical manner. The system will provide also functionality for updating the rules that form the knowledge base.

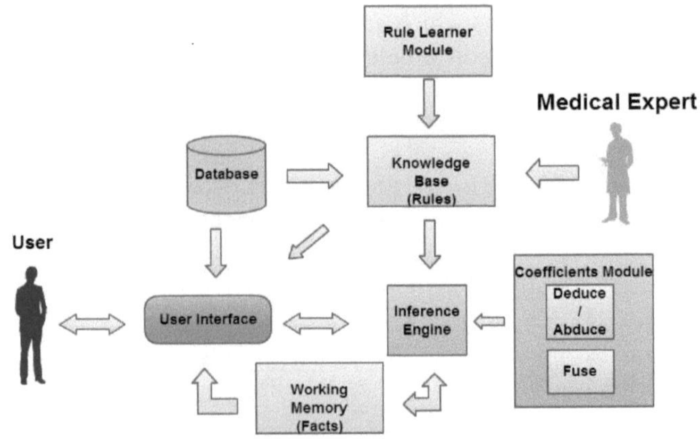

Fig. 1 Structure of the system

The system is organized into separate dedicated modules as presented in Figure 1.

The user interacts with the system via a user interface which allows him to select from a list of possible symptoms or medical tests (e.g. Abdominal Pain, Pirosis, Fever, Sour Taste, Biopsy Test, Amylase Test). Also for the input, the user selects the intensity level to which the symptom is present (i.e. a scroll bar with values from 0 - "no pain" to 100 - "excruciating pain") or the test has proved positive or negative. The output is presented initially as a list of possible diagnoses ordered by their belief degree and expectancy level. The user can select one of the diagnoses and ask for justification. The justification comes in form of a deduction graph tree that shows how the conclusion (i.e., the diagnose) was inferred given the input (i.e., the symptoms).

A set of rules have been written in JESS (Java Expert System Shell), an efficient forward chaining rule based system. The rules we have written implement on top of JESS a very simple inference engine which is able to represent Subjective Logic rules and facts (see Listing (see Listing 1 and 2) as JESS facts and to combine their respective opinions according to the Subjective Logic operators. The Coefficients Module computes, for every generated fact, its corresponding opinion. It is designed as a JESS script containing functions that manipulate JAVA objects representing the Subjective Logic operators of Deduction, Abduction and Fusion. Their justification will come later in this paper.

The knowledge base represents the set of all the rules the engine tries to reason with. These rules act as a model for the expertise provided by a doctor or a medical study. The rules in this form can be translated as follows: from 2000 cases of Gastritis(D_GA), 1000 subjects presented Abdominal Pain

(S_AP) or from 1000 cases of Pneumonia (D_PN), 950 of them presented symptoms of Fever(S_FV). This form is implemented as a JESS rule (see the sample Listing 1).

```
(defrule r1 "D_GA␣->␣S_AP␣2000␣1000"
  (medicalFact
    (description S_AP)
    (opinion ?b ?d ?u ?a)
    (index ?i))
  (parameter (rule r1)
  (params ?p1 ?p2 ?p3 ?p4 ?p5 ?p6 ?p7))
=>
  (bind ?list
    (computeResult ?b ?d ?u ?a
      ?p1 ?p2 ?p3 ?p4 ?p5 ?p6 ?p7))
  (bind ?newI (sym-cat r1 - ?i))
  (assert (medicalFact
            (name Gastritis)
            (description D_GA)
            (opinion (nth$ 1 ?list)
                     (nth$ 2 ?list)
                     (nth$ 3 ?list)
                     (nth$ 4 ?list))
            (rule r1)
            (symptoms ?i)
            (subsum 0)
            (index ?newI)
            (type D))))
```

Listing 1 A JESS rule implementing a reasoning step

Every rule tries to match a fact from the working memory representing a symptom. Each symptom has attached an opinion (belief, disbelief, uncertainty). Also every rule has a parameter fact that serves as a support for the Subjective Logic Operator that will be used in order to deduce a diagnose.

The working memory consists of two types of facts: ones that represent a medical fact that can be either a symptom or a diagnose and facts that serve as rule parameter base when computing the opinion values for the results.

```
(deftemplate medicalFact
 (multislot name)
 (slot description)
 (multislot opinion)
 (slot rule)
 (multislot symptoms)
 (slot subsum)
 (slot index)
 (slot type))
```

Listing 2 Medical Fact template

The database contains medical records describing patients' symptoms in a hospital and the corresponding diagnose. It can serve as an input for the Rule Learner Module or to update existing rules' parameters from the user interface. It is updated periodically as new patients are added.

In the diagnosis phase, the doctor first introduces the symptoms of the patient. They are converted into opinions with no uncertainty and a belief equal to the symptom's intensity selected on the interface. Then, the reasoning process is started and the results are presented the user Here, the results can be sorted by the Expectancy or Belief. Distinguishing between the two is possible within the framework of the Subjective Logic only. Belief could be interpreted as "reasons to support the diagnosis", while Expectancy is a combined value which incorporates both the supportive reasons for a diagnosis and the reasons due to the uncertainty component of the computation. It is up to the doctor to decide on which ground the final decision is made. The justification of the reasoning is available in form of a tree.

After the user checks the presence of a symptom and selects its intensity, the opinion for the fact that is generated in the working memory is computed as follows:

$$\begin{cases} b = \textit{the scroll value from the interface} \\ d = 1 - b \\ u = 0 \\ a = 0.5 \end{cases}$$

V. Related Work

Dealing with uncertainty in the area of Expert Systems could be traced back to MYCIN [10] and PATHFINDER [11]. Mycin was an early expert system that used rules endowed with certainty factors to identify bacteria causing severe infections and to recommend antibiotics, with the dosage adjusted for the patient's body weight. The rule for combining the evidence had some difficulties and was changed over time. Our system will differ from the MYCIN-like medical system on two important aspects. First, rather than using human obtained assessments of the certainty factors for rules and diagnoses, our systems offers the opportunity not only to express probabilities, but also to express how accurate the probability estimations actually are. Second, our system is able both to learn new rules from patients' records and to adjust the rules parameters to match the newly acquired data.

One approach for dealing with uncertainty is the based on graphs whose nodes model diseases and symptoms, while the weighted arcs show their mutual dependence. The doctor search for evidence able to discriminate among some mutually exclusive potential diagnoses. The lack of explicit uncertainty might lead to counter-intuitive results because the lack of evidence for some disease might be interpreted as support for another one. Our system allows the user to rank the potential diagnoses either based on expected values or belief levels. The former gives results consistent with the probabilities, while the latter could be interpreted as how much support we have for a specific diagnosis, but without artificially interpreting the lack of support for one disease as a support for the opposite.

Paper [12] presents the rule-based automated induction reasoning method based on rough sets, including exhaustive search, post-processing procedure, estimation for statistic test and the bootstrap and re-sampling methods. For the time being, we do not induce rules, but stick with the existing one and only update their opinions.

VI. Conclusions and Future Work

We identified a set of reasoning patterns used by the specialists in the medical field and showed how they can be emulated using the Subjective Logic operators of conjunction, abduction, deduction and fusion. We presented a system which implements the operators and performed preliminary experiments on the field. Our system allows assessing the rule confidence level in a programmatic way, based on the data stored in a database of previous patient examinations and to justify the reasoning process which lead to a specific conclusion. By employing this set of operators, we may seamlessly deal with both statistically validated rules as well as those which are build from user observation and express their level of uncertainty accordingly.

As a future work, we first intend to conduct comprehensive experiments for comparing the diagnosis accuracy versus the human expert's. So far, only a preliminary set of tests, on a limited number of use cases, have been done. Then, we foresee testing it on a more comprehensive patient database in order to identify the reasoning chain which might appear and to test whether in this situation the conclusions of the system match those of the medical experts. Automatically generating new rules and adding them to the system, together with the corresponding opinions should also be explored.

Conflict of Interest

The authors declare that they have no conflict of interest.

Acknowledgements

The first author wants to thank Alexandru Marchiş for his contribution in the system implementation.

References

1. Russell Stuart, Norvig Peter. *Artificial Intelligence: A Modern Approach*. Prentice Hallsecond ed. 2003.
2. Jøsang Audun. *Subjective Logic*. Draft book 2013.
3. Dempster A. P.. Upper and lower probabilities induced by a multivalued mapping *The Annals of Mathematical Statistics*. 1967;38:325–339.
4. Shafer Glenn. *A Mathematical Theory of Evidence*. Princeton: Princeton University Press 1976.
5. Smets Philip, Kennes R.. The transferable belief model *Artificial Intelligence*. 1994:191–234.
6. Jøsang Audun, McAnally David. Multiplication and Comultiplication of Beliefs *International Journal of Approximate Reasoning*. 2004;38:19–51.
7. Jøsang Audun. Abductive Reasoning with Uncertainty in *Proceedings of the 12th International Conference on Information Processing and Management of Uncertainty (IPMU2008)*(Malaga, Spain) 2008.
8. Jøsang Audun, Pope Simon, Daniel Milan. Conditional deduction under uncertainty in *Proceedings of the 8th European conference on Symbolic and Quantitative Approaches to Reasoning with Uncertainty*(Berlin, Heidelberg):824–835Springer-Verlag 2005.
9. Jøsang Audun, Diaz Javier, Rifqi Maria. Cumulative and averaging fusion of beliefs *Information Fusion*. 2010;11:192–200.
10. Shortliffe Edward H., Buchanan Bruce G.. A model of inexact reasoning in medicine *Mathematical biosciences*. 1975;23:351–379.
11. Heckerman D.E., Horvitz E.J., Nathwani B.N.. The Pathfinder project report ksl-90-08Medical Computer Science Group, Section on Medical Informatics, Stanford UniversityStanford, CA 1990.
12. Ai-Ping LI, Yan Jia, Quan-Yuan WU. On Rule Induction Method Based Rough Sets in Diagnostic Expert System in *Proceedings of the 2006 International Conference on Hybrid Information Technology - Volume 01*ICHIT '06(Washington, DC, USA):392–398IEEE Computer Society 2006.

Design of a Multi-site Electrical Stimulation System for Transcutaneous Lumbar Posterior Roots Stimulation

M. Krenn[1], S.M. Danner[1,2], A. Schweiger[1], U.S. Hofstoetter[1], K. Minassian[1], and W. Mayr[1]

[1] Center for Medical Physics and Biomedical Engineering, Medical University of Vienna, Vienna, Austria
[2] Institute for Analysis and Scientific Computing, Vienna University of Technology, Vienna, Austria

Abstract— **Lumbar posterior roots in humans can be activated by transcutaneous electrical spinal cord stimulation (tSCS). This method employs paravertebral stimulation and can be used to control spasticity and modify gait patterns in people with upper motor neuron dysfunctions. Furthermore, when single stimuli are applied reflexes are elicited in all lower limb muscle groups simultaneously, posterior root-muscle reflexes, which can be used for electrophysiological studies. It is important to control stimulation settings and site. Here, a novel multi-site stimulation system is presented. The stimulation module is based on a microcontroller and delivers biphasic, voltage-controlled pulses with amplitudes up to +/-45 V. The stimulator is controlled and powered by a computer using the Universal Serial Bus (USB) data link. Software-controlled stimulation allows flexible parameter settings. The stimulator integrates a measurement unit, which records pulse shape and electrode impedance. An electrode array, based on a flexible printed circuit board with 8 gold coated square electrode contacts (1x1cm^2) in a row on a flexible polymer base foil. These foil strips provide access lines and mechanical fixation means to assemble 2-dimensional array configurations. A 3x8 contact configuration was tested for delivery of impulses to the skin surface above the rosto-caudal spinal cord in combination with an abdominally placed 200cm^2 reference electrode.**

Selectivity in eliciting reflex activity in lower extremity muscle groups could be demonstrated with potential advantages in automated stimulation site adjustment and multi-site test procedures.

Keywords— **posterior root muscle reflex, voltage-controlled stimulator, electrode array**

I. Introduction

Electrical stimulation of the human lumbosacral spinal cord via transcutaneous electrodes can elicit muscle twitches in multiple lower limb muscles [1]. These responses result from synchronous depolarization of Ia afferent fibers within the posterior roots and the subsequent monosynaptic activation of motor fibers innervating the lower limb muscles [2]. Furthermore, it has been shown that epidural spinal cord stimulation can elicit functional movements, locomotor-like activity and extension of the lower limbs, in motor complete spinal cord injured individuals [3, 4]. Transcutaneous spinal cord stimulation is used for a noninvasive investigation of neural circuits of the lumbar spinal cord in human [3] and is a promising method for neuromodulation applications, like reduction of spasticity and modification of gait [5]. Currently, the stimulation technique is based on a simple setup. Usually, two small (5 cm diameter) stimulation electrodes are placed paravertebrally between T11-12 and a large indifferent electrode over the abdomen [1]. However, due to anatomical differences between patients the positioning of the paraspinal electrodes can be a very time consuming procedure. Furthermore, when the body position (supine, prone and standing) is changed a rearranging of the electrode position becomes necessary.

The aim of this project was to develop a flexible stimulation system consisting of an USB-powered stimulator that is controlled by a computer, and an electrode array for focused delivery of stimuli.

The requirements on the system were as follows: The computer application must enable the user to adjust amplitude, pulse width and frequency of the applied pulses. Power consumption of the output stage should not exceed 500 mA in order to enable USB powering. Furthermore, simultaneous recording of stimulation voltage and current should be implemented, that allows monitoring of load impedance. The multi-electrode array has to be made from flexible material, since it has to adapt perfectly to the shape of the subject's body surface. Moreover, each electrode pad of the array should be activated independently.

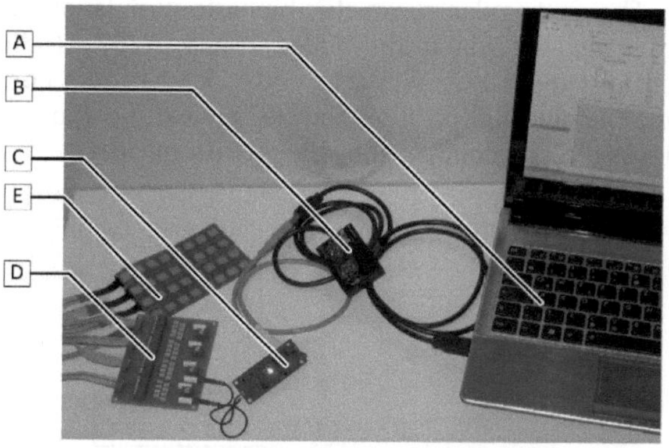

Fig. 1 Stimulation system: A computer controls the stimulator (A), medical graded USB insulation (B), one channel electrical stimulator (C), adapter board (D) and electrode array (E)

S. Vlad and R.V. Ciupa (eds.), *International Conference on Advancements of Medicine and Health Care through Technology*, IFMBE Proceedings 44,
DOI: 10.1007/978-3-319-07653-9_9, © Springer International Publishing Switzerland 2014

II. Stimulation Sytem

The electrical stimulator is powered and controlled by a computer (Fig. 1) whereas a galvanic isolation ensures basic safety for the subject. Every pad of the electrode array can be switched on independently via an adapter board.

Controller. The stimulator is controlled using a 32-bit microcontroller PIC32 (PIC32MX250F128D, Microchip Technology Inc., Chandler, AZ, USA) that operates at a clock frequency of 32 MHz. The supply voltage of the microcontroller is in the range of 2.3 V to 3.6 V. The used peripheral features of the microcontroller include an I2C module, a 10-bit analog digital convert (ADC) and a USB 2.0-compliant module. The stimulation pulse timing was derived from a 32-bit timer with a resolution of 1 µs. Therefore, the PIC32 controlled two main functions, first the generation of the pulses to stimulate the neural system and second to manage the communication with the computer.

Power Supply. The stimulation module is USB-powered and therefore supplied with a voltage range from 4.75 V to 5.25 V [6]. According to the specification the USB port can deliver up to 500 mA. The USB-port is protected using reset-able fuses with a switch-off threshold of 500mA (13.2 V, 0.15 Ω) in the power line. Microcontroller and other integrated circuits (IC) were supplied with 3.3 V, using a positive voltage regulator (TPS73133, Texas Instruments Inc., Dallas, TX, USA). For human safety the USB-data-link and power path were galvanically isolated from the PC using an USB-port isolator ADuM4160 (Analog Devices, Norwood, MA, USA) and a DC/DC converter ISQ0505 (XP Power Limited, Singapore, SG).

Generation of stimulation pulses. A boost converter (LM3488, Texas Instruments Inc.) was used to generate the stimulation voltage level. The output voltage was set using a resistor array (Table 1) connected to the feedback input, which allowed a digital control of the step-up converter. The linear increment of the output voltage was around 360 mV. The rectangular, symmetric biphasic stimulation pulses were generated via a full-bridge driver A4973 (Allegro MicroSystems, LLC, Worcester, MA, USA). This component generated the positive and negative stimulation pulse and was directly controlled by the microcontroller.

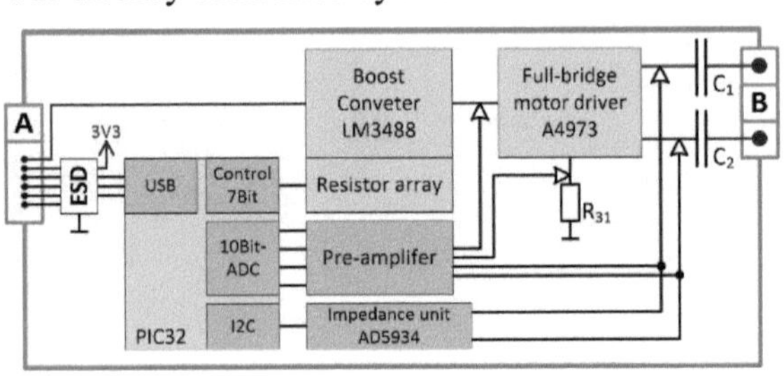

Fig. 2 Basic stimulator design consisting of a microcontroller, an output stage and peripherals for data acquisition

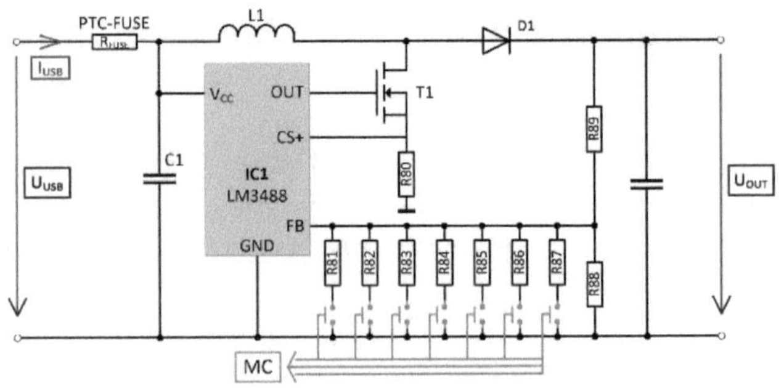

Fig. 3 Schematic of the boost converter. L1 = 100µH; IC1 = LM3488, T1 = FDMS86103L (Fairchild Semiconductor), D1 = STPS3150 (STMicroelectronics), R80 = 50mΩ, RFUSE = MF-NSMF050-2 (Bourns Inc.), values of R81 to R89 (see Table 1)

Electrode array. The electrode array with 3 x 8 contact pads was made from a flexible printed circuit board (Fig. 6). The material of the base foil is polyimid, the contact pads (10x10 mm) are gold coated copper layers. The indifferent reference electrode was positioned on the abdominal skin surface using two 8 x 13 cm electrodes (STIMEX, Schwa-Medico GmbH, Ehringshausen, Germany). To increase application flexibility each electrode pad is contacted separately from the interface board. The interface integrated switching ports allowed activating or deactivating of each stimulation array contacts independently. Joining arbitrary pads to form one cumulative electrode allowed modulation the induced electrical field configuration.

Table 1 Output voltage (U_{out}) of the step-up converter, R_{RES} is the resulting value of the parallel resistor array of R81 to R88. According to a desired U_{out} the open drain outputs of the microcontroller are open "0" or closed "1". R88 was 560 kΩ and R89 was 18 kΩ.

R81 1 kΩ	R82 2 kΩ	R83 4 kΩ	R84 8 kΩ	R85 16 kΩ	R86 32 kΩ	R87 64.9 kΩ	R_{RES} (kΩ)	U_{OUT} (V)
0	0	0	0	0	0	0	560	1.34(1)
⋮	⋮	⋮	⋮	⋮	⋮	⋮		⋮
0	1	0	1	0	1	0	1.523	16.02
0	1	0	1	0	1	1	1.488	16.38
⋮	⋮	⋮	⋮	⋮	⋮	⋮		⋮
1	1	1	1	1	1	1	0.507	45.65

(1) minimum output voltage is equal to U_{USB}, i.e. 5 V

III. Material and Methods

Electrode array. The electrode array with 3 x 8 contact pads was made from a flexible printed circuit board (Fig. 4). The material of the base foil is polyimid, the contact pads (10x10 mm) are gold coated copper layers. The indifferent reference electrode was positioned on the abdominal skin surface using two 8 x 13 cm electrodes (STIMEX, Schwa-Medico GmbH, Ehringshausen, Germany). To increase application flexibility each electrode pad is contacted

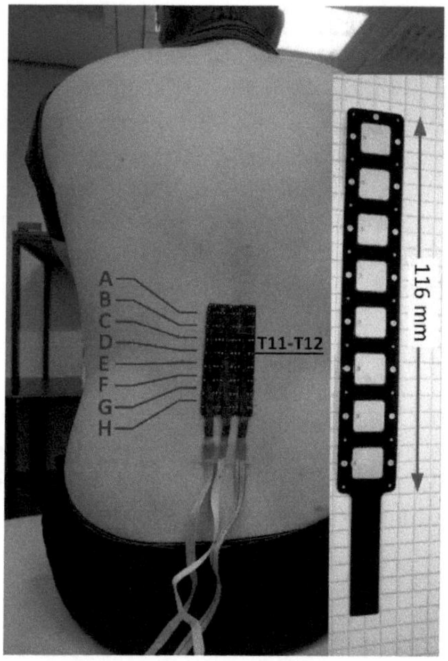

Fig. 4 Electrode array which was placed on the back with self-adhesive hydrogel layer. Level D of the electrode array was in-line with the interspinous space T11-T12.

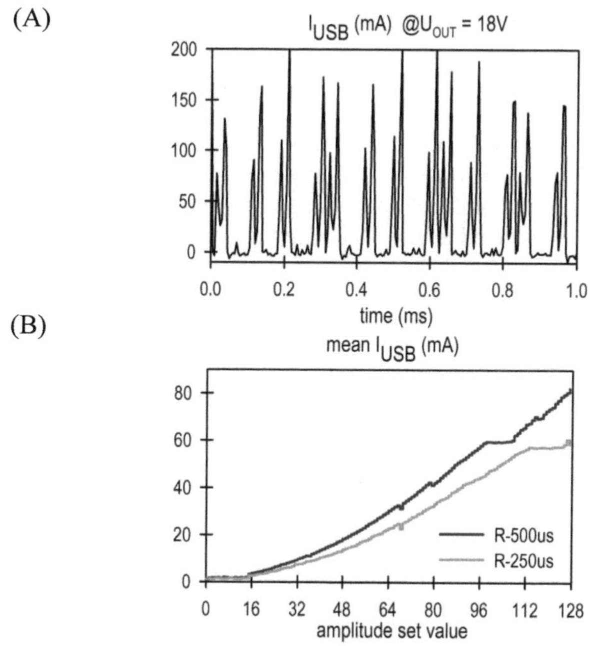

Fig. 5 Current consumption of the stimulation module. The time signal current intake of the boost converter (A). Mean current consumption for increasing output voltage – amplitude set value (B).

separately from the interface board. The interface integrated switching ports allowed activating or deactivating of each stimulation array contacts independently. Joining arbitrary pads to form one cumulative electrode allowed modulation the induced electrical field configuration.

Testing of stimulation module. An ohmic load resistor of 500 Ω was used to verify the generate stimulation pulses and current consumption to the module. Stimulation parameters were either 2x250 µs or 2x 500 µs at a stimulation rate of 50 pulses per second. The amplitude was increased in steps of 300 mV up to the maximum intensity.

Verification of the stimulation system. The system was verified in a preliminary measurement performing lumbar spinal cord stimulation in a subject (male, 28years) with intact nervous system. The study was approved by the Ethics Committee of the City of Vienna, Austria. The stimulation set-up (Fig. 4) consisted of an electrode array at the back with 8 levels and two large reference electrodes (8x13 cm, STIMEX, Schwa-Medico GmbH, GER) over the abdomen. Each level of the array consisted of three electrodes strips and spanned 8 cm caudal and 4 cm rostral, centered to the interspinous space T11-T12 [7]. Every level was separately addressed for stimulation. The stimulation parameters were kept constant during the whole trial. Biphasic, rectangular and charge-balanced stimulation pulses with a width of 2 x 1 ms were delivered. Electromyographic activities were recorded in quadriceps (QM), and soleus (TS) bilaterally. At each level four responses were collected.

IV. Results

The boost converter (LM3488) reached the maximum output voltage when all resistors (R81 to R87) were switched on, i.e. the microcontroller set value was 127. In that case, the measured output voltage of the boost converter was 45 V with a duty cycle of 90 % of the boost converter. The current intake was around 80 mA at the load configuration 1. The current consumption over the whole output voltage range and the output voltage of the stimulator was measured for different loads (Fig. 5).

A verification measurement of the posterior-root muscle reflexes is presented in graphs Fig. 6. The responses of quadriceps and triceps surae were compared at two different stimulation levels (A and H of Fig. 6). The evoked muscle activation shows dependency to rostro-caudal changes of the stimulation site. Quadriceps reflexes were larger when stimulation was applied at the rostral site (A). The converse was the case for reflexes in triceps surae. At the time 0 ms the stimulation artifact is visible which can be identified in all muscle groups.

V. Discussion and conclusion

Even though the distribution of the generated electrical field with transcutaneous electrodes is dispersed in relation to the target structures selective stimulation is possible to some degree [2].

The presented stimulation system allows flexible stimulation of posterior roots respectively spinal root structures. The computerized control, which was programmed in Visual C# 2012, allows the user to control the stimulation amplitude, pulse width and pulse frequency and enables the generation of various stimulation patterns. Additionally, the hardware is capable of measuring the stimulation voltage and current as well as the load's impedance, which provides valuable feedback during the stimulation [8]. The stimulation system also detect and record application errors.

Under real test conditions the current consumption of the output stage was acceptably low, which allows USB-port supply. The interface board enabled a fast relocation and change of the size and position of the cumulative electrode, even during stimulation patterns, eliminating the need to remove and reposition electrodes through optimization periods. Furthermore, the design allows every attached array-segment to be supplied with a distinct signal. The electrode array combined with the self-adhesive hydrogel pads is easy to apply and, due to its flexible material, conforms well to the shape of the subject's body surface. The modular design of the arrays allows it to be expanded and placed as needed, maximizing the flexibility of the system. It has been shown that a single activated pad induces a focused electrical field, with only little crosstalk to surrounding tissue.

Future steps include the improvement of the stimulator's hardware to enable delivery of higher stimulation voltages amplitudes and further refinement of the array design and selectivity of stimulation. Moreover, the adapter PCB's mechanical switches will be replaced by electrically controlled ones in order to enable software induced activation and deactivation and real-time access to fields modulation.

The presented stimulation system allows for fast positioning of the applied stimulation and enables novel neuromodulatory approaches by allowing complex stimulation patterns and electrical field configurations.

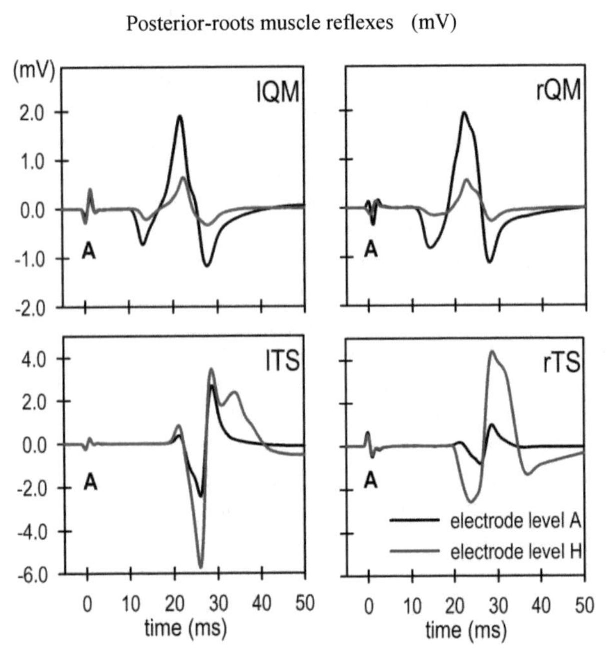

Fig. 6 Compound muscle action potential (CMAP) of the left (l) and right (r) muscle groups QM and TS. The stimulation intensity was 60 mA for level A and 45 mA for level H. The stimulation artifact (A) was present in all recordings.

Acknowledgment

We would like to acknowledge the support of Wings for life spinal cord research foundation, Salzburg, Austria; Project: WFL-AT-007/11 and of the Vienna science and technology fund, Vienna, Austria; Project: LS11-057.

Conflict of Interest

The authors declare that they have no conflict of interest'.

References

1. Minassian K, Persy I, Rattay F, Pinter MM, Kern H, Dimitrijevic MR (2007) Human lumbar cord circuitries can be activated by extrinsic tonic input to generate locomotor-like activity. Hum Mov Sci 26:275–95.
2. Danner SM, Hofstoetter US, Ladenbauer J, Rattay F, Minassian K (2011) Can the human lumbar posterior columns be stimulated by transcutaneous spinal cord stimulation? Artif Organs 35:257–62.
3. Dimitrijevic MR, Gerasimenko Y, Pinter MM (1998) Evidence for a spinal central pattern generator in humans. Ann N Y Acad Sci 860:360–376.
4. Jilge B, Minassian K, Rattay F, Dimitrijevic MR (2004) Frequency-dependent selection of alternative spinal pathways with common periodic sensory input. Biol Cybern 91:359–376.
5. Hofstoetter US, McKay WB, Tansey KE, Mayr W, Kern H, Minassian K (2014) Modification of spasticity by transcutaneous spinal cord stimulation in individuals with incomplete spinal cord injury. J Spinal Cord Med 37:202–11.
6. Kollman R, Betten J (2002) Powering electronics from the USB port (slyt118). Analog Appl J 2Q:28–35.
7. Krenn M, Toth A, Danner SM, Hofstoetter US, Minassian K, Mayr W (2013) Selectivity of transcutaneous stimulation of lumbar posterior roots at different spinal levels in humans. Biomed Tech (Berl) 58:1–2.
8. Hendling M, Krenn M, Haller MA, Loefler S, Kern H, Mayr W (2013) Compliance monitoring of home based electrical stimulation training of elderly subjects. Biomed Tech (Berl) 58:1–2.

Author: Matthias Krenn
Institute: Medical University of Vienna
Center for Medical Physics and Biomedical Engineering
Street: Waehringer Guertel 18-20, AKH 4L
City: Vienna
Country: Austria
Email: matthias.krenn@meduniwien.ac.at

Imaging Techniques in the Assessment of Liver Tumoral Vascularization

I. Grigorescu[1], Z. Sparchez[2], R. Badea[2], M. Dragoteanu[2], M. Thelen[3], S.L. Popa[1], and D.L. Dumitrascu[1]

[1] 2nd Medical Department, "I.Hatieganu" University of Medicine and Pharmacology Cluj-Napoca, Romania
[2] "Octavian Fodor" Regional Institute for Gastroenterology and Hepatology Cluj-Napoca, Romania
[3] Radiological Clinic, "J.Gutenberg" University Mainz, Germany

Abstract— **Several imaging methods may describe the vascular pattern of a solid tumor and assess through this its benign/malignant character. Gray-scale ultrasound (US) represents the first method of detecting a liver tumor. Doppler US helps further in establishing the vascularization of the tumors and their architectural pattern. The detectability rate of intratumoral vessels is higher in Power Doppler comparative to B-flow, especially in deep seated lesions. Malignancy is suggested at contrast-enhanced US (CEUS) by hypoenhancing areas (in late phases) and washout (portal-venous phase), but benign tumors with high-shunt flow, atypical focal nodular hyperplasias (FNH) and adenomas should not be excluded. Classical scintigraphy used alone had not specific images in FNH, adenomas, abscesses, cysts, hepatocarcinomas and pseudotumors; colloidal and in vivo labeled SPECT are important in diagnosing hemangiomas>2cm. There exists a correlation at liver angioscintigraphy (LAS) between increased hepatic perfusion index (HPI) values and large tumoral volumes ($r=0.313$, $p<0.001$) in benign tumors, although it is known that arterialisation usually correlates with malignancy. Lack of detection of the central scar in 60% cases of FNH at MR appears because of the large tumoral volume and/or underlying steatosis. Resovist administration enhances the diagnostic specificity in FNH and malignant transformed nodules. Dynamic imaging methods using contrast agents, always interpreted in the patient's clinical and biological context, are important methods of investigation, used in order to enable positive and differential diagnosis in tumor masses of the liver.**

Keywords— **contrast-enhanced imaging methods, liver tumor, tumor vascularization**

I. Introduction

Imaging techniques have increased importance in the assessment of any tumoral nodule, especially if this is located on chronic liver disease. Corroborating clinical imaging data and the comparison with pathological examination through different criteria and algorithms for prediction of malignant or benign etiology aims to establish a positive diagnosis. There are several noninvasive imaging methods of investigation, which can assess the vascularization in case of tumor masses of the liver.

II. Material and Methods

Our study including 348 patients with suspected benign liver tumors (35 of them having several masses at the same time), were investigated ultrasonographically (gray-scale ultrasound (US) and Doppler US with Logiq 7 (GE, USA) and Sonoline Si2000 (Siemens) devices, 46 of them were investigated also at Power-Doppler and B-flow, 38 underwent also contrast-enhanced US (CEUS) with Sonovue. 261 of these tumors were evaluated scintigraphically by the tomographic scintillation camera SPECT Orbiter Siemens with parallel colimator of high resolution and low energy (203 with radiocolloid, 188 with *in vivo* labeled RBC), 109 by contrast-enhanced CT (CT Somatom Plus-4-Spiral-CT-Scanner (Siemens, Germany), and 29 by contrast-enhanced MR (*Gd*-chelate; Resovist; and Primovist) with a device of 1,0 T (Gyroscan Intera Philips, Netherland). If diagnosis could not be established only by US methods, following a diagnostic algorithm, scintigraphy, CT or MR, or even invasive techniques were used in order to have a positive diagnosis. Histological examination was considered the gold standard. The control group consisted in 60 patients with malignant liver tumors. The studies on US, scintigraphy and MR were performed by us at the „O.Fodor"Regional Institute for Gastroenterology and Hepatology Cluj-Napoca and on CT at the Radiological Clinic of Mainz, Germany. In order to assess the statistical significance for quantitative variables we used the Mann-Whitney, Kruskal-Wallis tests and Spearman correlation coefficient; association between qualitative variables was tested by Pearson Chi Square or Fisher Freeman-Halton tests and Phi and Cramer correlation coefficient.

III. Results

A. Abdominal Ultrasound (US)

The final diagnosis in our 348 patients-group, after corroborating imaging with invasive techniques (with final histological examination), included: 270 hemangiomas, 18 focal nodular hyperplasias (FNH), 7 adenomas, 7 abscesses, 1 angiomyolipoma, 25 biliary and 11 hydatid cysts, 6 polycystic liver diseases, 13 fatty free areas, 5 focal

S. Vlad and R.V. Ciupa (eds.), *International Conference on Advancements of Medicine and Health Care through Technology*, IFMBE Proceedings 44,
DOI: 10.1007/978-3-319-07653-9_10,

steatosis, 2 post-surgical scars, 1 neuroendocrine tumor, 1 hematoma, 12 regenerative and 2 dysplastic nodules, 2 portal cavernomas, 1 hepatocarcinoma (HCC), 1 cholangiocarcinoma, and in 2 cases there co-existed hemangiomas with HCC and gastric carcinoid. The highest sensitivity (94.81%), and specificity (99.16%) rates of US in solid tumors were obtained in hemangiomas and FNH. The classical criteria of hyperechoic, well delimited tumor without vascular signal was found in 81.85% hemangiomas (Fig.1). Histological examination was needed in 7/18 patients with FNH, where imaging methods could not establish the diagnosis. Nonspecific patterns were found in adenomas and angiomyolipomas. Reconstruction in order to help the surgen's technique of removing a liver tumor is possible by means of 3D-US (Fig.2).

A group of 46 patients with liver tumors (14 benign and 32 malignant) were evaluated both by Power Doppler (Fig.3) and B-flow (Fig.4). Overall, both methods had an important role in detecting, describing the type and traiectory of intratumoral vessels, high specificity (93.33%) and moderate sensitivity (71.43%) rate in establishing the benign etiology. There was a high linear correlation between the number of vessels detected by the 2 methods ($r=0.95$, $p<0.0001$). Irregular, tortuous vessels are typical for malignancy, but can be found also in atypical hemangiomas or FNH.

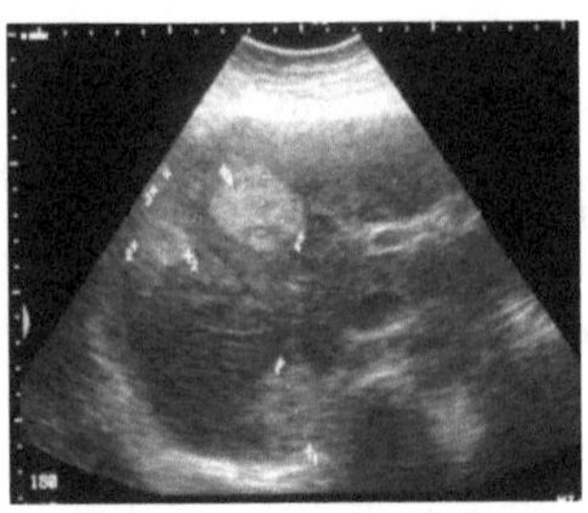

Fig. 1 Gray-scale US: hemangioma

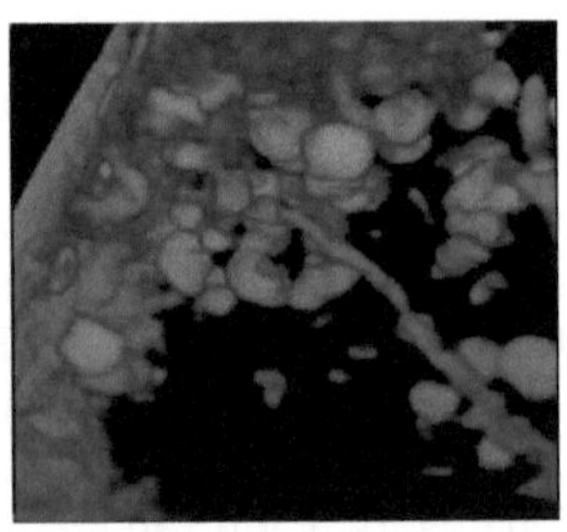

Fig. 2 3D-US: liver metastases

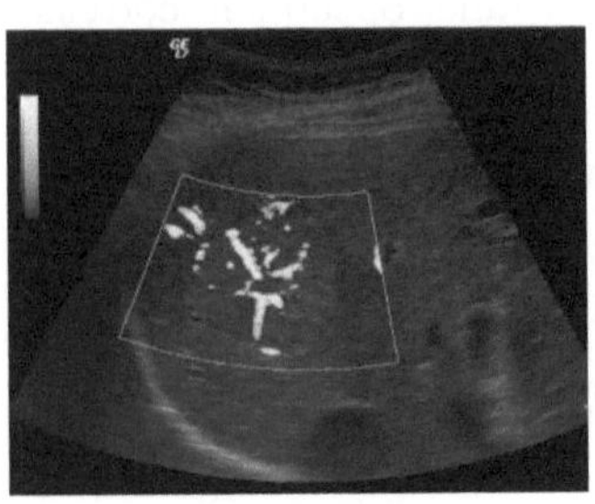

Fig. 3 Power-Doppler: FNH

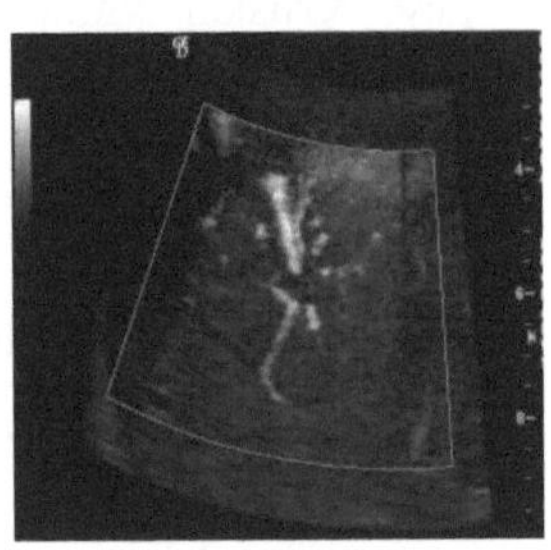

Fig. 4 B-flow: FNH

Contrast enhanced ultrasonography (CEUS) had high sensitivity and sensibility rates (92.00 and 92.30%) in the 38 patients investigated with Sonovue, according to the EFSUMB guidelines, especially in the small lesions and the ones grafted on chronic liver diseases in our study. Centripetal and centrifugal filling of the tumors was encountered in 87.5% cases of hemangiomas and 60% of FNH.

B. Liver Scintigraphy

Liver scintigraphy is another technique used in differentiating liver tumors, providing functional information that is inaccessible through morphological imaging methods. In exploring liver tumors, scintigraphic radio colloid (Fig.5), is used in conjunction with liver angioscintigraphy and red blood cell scintigraphy.

In our study classical scintigraphy used alone was considered not specific in FNH, adenomas, abscesses, cysts, HCC and pseudotumors; the classical SPECT aspect of blood stasis was found in 95/117 (81.19%) of our cases (Fig.6).

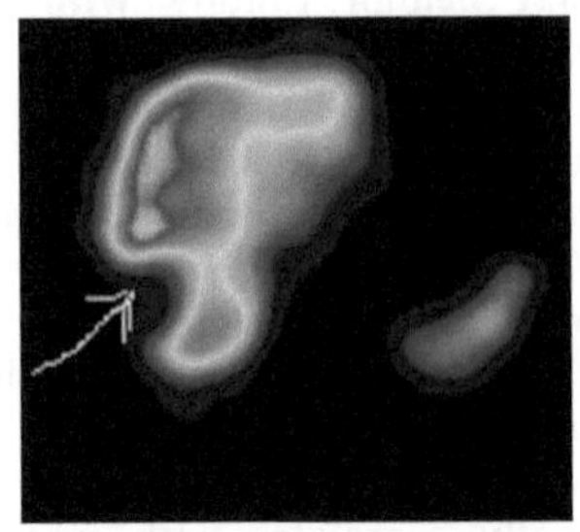

Fig. 5 SPECT with ^{99m}Tc – phytate: hemangioma

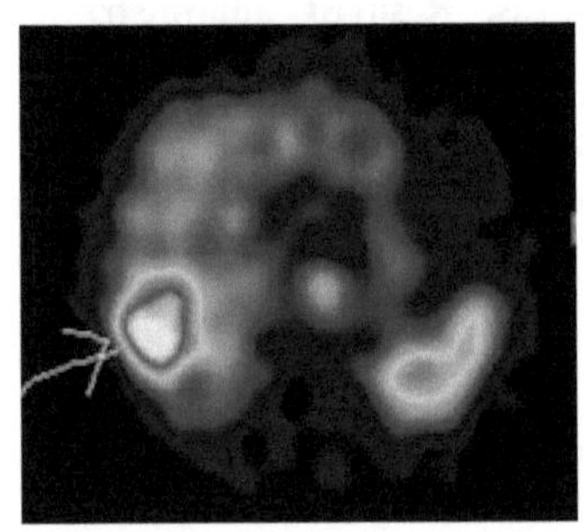

Fig. 6 SPECT with in vivo RBC: hemangioma

Liver angioscintigraphy (LAS) allows the assessment of the arterialization of liver perfusion in neoplasia, by means of calculating the hepatic perfusion index (HPI). Tumoral masses were investigated by LAS in 149 patients, using the arterio-portal perfusion ratio in order to evaluate their benign/malignant character. We obtained a correlation between increased HPI values and large tumoral volumes ($r=0.313$, $p<0.001$) in benign tumors.

C. Computed Tomography (CT)

CT is an imaging technique produces a cross - sectional image of the patient using X-ray in a non-conventional manner.

Our contrast enhanced CT- study on 109 patients with presumtive diagnosis of benign liver tumors, showed a high sensitivity (82.35%), but a lower specificity rate (41.67%). Most hemangiomas (28/41) showed the "Iris phenomena"(Fig.7), the rest had an atypical dynamic behaviour, especially those grafted on chronic liver diseases. Small FNH grafted on steatosis had atypical features in dynamics. The sensitivity of 100% was found in small cysts grafted on chronic liver diseases.

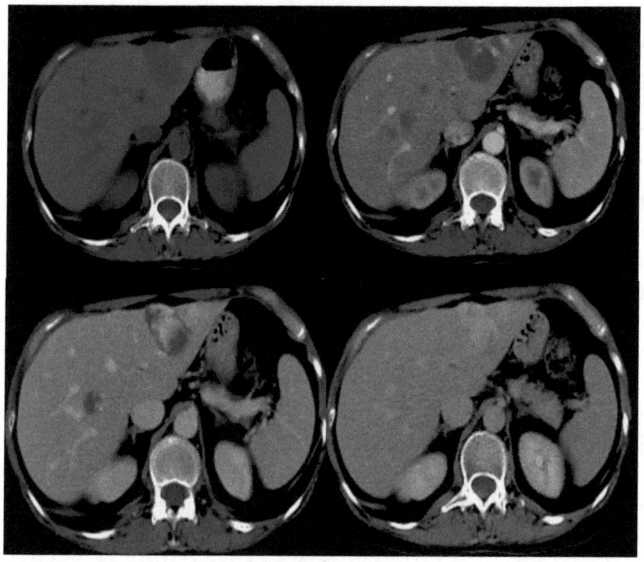

Fig. 7 MDCT: hemangioma (native, arterial, portal and late phases)

D. Nuclear Magnetic Resonance (MR)

Patients with problems of differential diagnosis in other imaging methods (n=29) were evaluated by contrast enhanced MR (*Gd*-chelate; Resovist; and Primovist) with a device of 1,0 T (Gyroscan Intera Philips, Netherland); hemangioma diagnosis was established in all cases in our study because of the typical T2-hypersignal image and centripetal filling.

IV. Discussion

Abdominal ultrasound (US) is a diagnostic method in "real time", accurate, inexpensive, non-irradiating, with broad accessibility. Other advantages are: possibility of guiding interventional maneuvers (for diagnostic and therapeutic purposes). Limitations of the method are, however: impossibility of exact differentiation between benign- malignant, artifacts, obesity, noncooperation of patient, impossibility of characterization air containing organs (lungs) and bone, subjectivity and dependence on the examiner.

Gray-scale US is the first step in the detection and classification of tumor in a particular category. If transabdominal examination of liver tumors is done, we use low frequency transducers (2.25 - 3.5MHz) and for the operatory use high frequencies (5-7.5- 10MHz) [1]. *3D-US* enables reconstruction plans in a region of interest and the ability of the 3D representation of surfaces of organs [2].

Contrast enhanced ultrasonography (CEUS). The use of microbubble contrast agents such as Levovist® (Schering AG) or SonoVue® (Bracco) allows a better characterization of liver tumors; persistence of the contrast in the portal venous and late phase suggests benignity and malignancy is suspected if washout of micro bubbles is present [3]. CEUS is not perfectly superimposable over contrast enhanced CT/MRI, because contrast agents that are used in US remain in intravascular space. Hypoenhancing areas (in late phases) at CEUS and washout (portal-venous phase) are highly suggestive for malignancy, but benign tumors with high-shunt flow, atypical FNH or even adenomas should not be excluded.

Laparoscopic US has a double role, in diagnosis and treatment, identifying and locating small not palpable (deep) lesions, or those masked by cirrhosis, representing a useful method in the detection of metastases during surgery for cancers, puncture, US-guided biopsy/ethanol injection in liver tumors (HCC<3cm), and drainage of intra/per hepatic leakage. If hydatid cysts are found, the information brought by this method allows reliable detection of multiple lesions, avoiding surgery if there is increased risk of vascular injury or biliary - cystic fistula [4].

Doppler exploration of tumors is done by *color Doppler* (shows the presence of blood and direction of blood circulation) and *spectral Doppler* (reveals character, speed of flow and peripheral resistance), establishing the pattern of tumor vascularization and the permeability of liver vessels. The limits of the method are the difficulty of: evaluation of blood supply of small nodules or deep seated lesions/located near the heart, detecting arterial-venous shunts and low speed flows. Usually, malignant tumors are characterized by elevated systolic speed, flow rate and increased speed in the hepatic artery, arterial flow type, while the vascularization of benign tumors show variable configurations. In case of malignant tumors, Doppler US can detect relatively high speed because of the increasing blood flow or the presence of arterial-venous fistulas. *Power Doppler* detects movement of the erythrocytes, having an increased sensitivity to slow flows, but without being able to specify their direction. Doppler US can calculate hepatic perfusion index [5], determining the arterial and portal blood flow in the hepatic hilum and calculating the relative arterial ratio to the total perfusion. *B–flow US*, a non-Doppler technique in gray scale (GE Medical Systems) allows the direct real-time visualization of the blood echo, similar to that obtained after IV injection of the contrast agent [6]. Its images are less influenced by breathing or cardiac cycle, being considered to be a suitable method in order to assess better hyper vascular tumors using contrast agents [7]. The detectability rate of intratumoral vessels was higher in Power Doppler comparative to B-flow, especially in deep seeated lesions.

Liver scintigraphy with radio labeled colloid (^{99m}Tc - phytate, 13mCi for planar scintigraphy, 10-15mCi for SPECT), uses ^{99m}Tc – phytate, which is injected IV and then removed from circulation by Kupffer cells; liver viewing is possible by gamma radiation emitted by the tracer. In the case of benign or malignant tumor, areas without Kupffer cells are highlighted with an accuracy of 60 % (planar scintigraphy) or 87 % (SPECT tomoscintigraphy). False-positive images without colloid caption (areas of fibrosis, atrophy, sclerosis) may occur in cirrhosis. SPECT scintigraphy method delectability limit is 1.5-2cm. In exploring liver tumors, scintigraphic radio colloid is used in conjunction with liver angioscintigraphy and red blood cell scintigraphy.

Liver scintigraphy with "in vivo " labeled red blood cells (RBC), is especially important in the diagnosis of hepatic hemangiomas, having as principle the accumulation in the hemangiomatous dilatations of these tumors. It is performed by IV injection 10 - 15mg of stannous agent (Medrone or pyrophosphate) which is fixed on the surface of RBC followed (after 30 minutes) by injecting IV 20mCi 15 ^{99m}Tc - pertechnetate (radioactive tracer), which binds instantly the erythrocyte membrane, marking the entire volume of circulating blood. Typical image shows up as "positive" RBC stagnation in the areas highlighted as areas without colloid caption on the colloid scintigraphy. False-negative results may occur with sclerotic, thromboses, or small (< 2cm) hemangiomas. SPECT with labeled RBC have a sensitivity of 85% for hemangiomas 1.5-3cm and 95-100 % in the >3cm (values comparable to those offered by MRI) [8] but a lower sensitivity and specificity compared to MRI tumors < 2cm [9].

Liver angioscintigraphy (LAS) uses the same colloidal tracers injected for subsequent planar imaging. It allows the assessment of the arterialization of liver perfusion in neoplasia. Hepatic perfusion index (HPI) represents the ratio between arterial perfusion and the portal-venous pressure, calculated after Sarper [10] by dividing the amplitude of the arterial segment to the summation of arterial and venous segments. Normal values of HPI are below the percentage of 40 %; HPI indicator is suggestive of cancer (more than 50 % in up to 90 % of the cases, in a non-cirrhotic liver), in contrast to benign tumors that present a normal HPI [11]; changes of the flow arterial-portal ratio appear in some benign masses (abscesses) or overlays on chronic liver disease [12]. Limitations of the method are: overlapping tumors with cirrhosis (compensatory growth of hepatic arterial flow), the presence of anatomical variations of the arterial pedicle (the impossibility of calculating HPI correctly), liver intra-arterial catheters (for chemotherapy in HCC) and liver tumors invading the liver by contiguity (normal HPI), altered circulatory dynamics (congestive heart failure), failure of bolus injection (inaccessible or sclerotic veins). Compared to other imaging methods (US, CT, planar scintigraphy), CT and LAS proved to have the highest sensitivity by detecting 90% of metastases from colorectal neoplasm [13]. LAS sensitivity in the detection of occult metastasis of the digestive carcinomas is 92-97% [14]. Classical scintigraphy used alone had not specific images in FNH, adenomas, abscesses, cysts, hepatocarcinomas and pseudotumors; colloidal and *in vivo* labeled SPECT are important in diagnosing hemangiomas>2cm. We noticed a correlation at LAS between increased HPI values and large tumoral volumes ($r=0.313$, $p<0.001$) in benign tumors, although it is known that arterialisation usually correlates with malignancy.

Computed tomography (CT) measures the absorbed X-rays by the various structures of the body through the detector. Slices may range from 0.5- 10mm.

2D images obtained from computerized reconstruction of multiple projections at different angles are called sections/slices, each image corresponds to a certain tissue thickness (2mm→1-1.5cm). CT values (HU - Hounsfield units) are displayed on the display as gray-scale images, the latter being represented by an matrix made up of a variable number of elements (pixels), each pixel in the image having a certain shade of gray. This HU scale (-1024 HU: air→4000 HU: bone) tissue attenuation values are reported to the water's value (0HU), with positive values for bone and soft tissue structures, and negative for air or fat tissue. Thus, analyzing the various pathological processes, we can distinguish their different densities relative to neighboring regions: identical (iso dense), lower (hypo dense), or high (hyper dense). From the clinical point of view, we can emphasize the advantages of the CT method, consisting of: increased spatial resolution, ability to determine the differences between structures with different densities, guiding interventional maneuvers (biopsies), and 3D visualization of the anatomy. On the other hand, CT has also some disadvantages and limits: the high price, poor accessibility, radiation dose, potential contrast allergenic substances, and impossibility of investigating during pregnancy, renal or severe cardiac failure, millimeter lesions, and intestinal mucosal lesions.

Multi-detector CT (MDCT) allows detection of millimeter masses by scanning of anatomical regions in a single apnea. There are scanners that manage to aquire 4, 8, 16 and 64 sections simultaneously. MDCT technique transformed an axial cross-sectional imaging technique in a 3D one. The use of contrast agents (iodine, e.g. Ultravist ®) increases the contrast between adjacent tissues and allows the assessment of vascularization of any lesion; depending on its behavior one can classify a finding having a specific etiology (inflammatory, benign/malignant), it also enables the description of masses, which were iso-dense and undetectable at native CT. There are several ways of contrast administration: intravenous (IV), orally, in enema. Main contraindications are: renal insufficiency, increased serum creatinine (> 1.5mg/dl), hyperthyroidism, allergy to contrast agents. Multiplanar reconstruction of CT has led to "perfusion maps" that assesses liver tumor angiogenesis and vascularization of the tumor by the tumor and regional volume flow measurement. Images made by overlapping two imaging methods PET and CT have a higher resolution.

Nuclear magnetic resonance (MR) imaging uses the hydrogen nuclei (^{1}H) of the tissue structure in order to obtain the MR image. Images or base sequences are called T1 (relaxation in the parallel plane to the magnetic field of the device) or T2 (transverse relaxation). The contrast of the images is given by the density of protons in a tissue and times T1 and T2. Slice thickness to examine liver is 4-5 or 5 -7mm. Protocol for focal liver lesion detection, used also in our patients, involves: T1 and T2 sequences (preferably suppression technique) and three phases dynamic images with gadolinium (*Gd*).

This diagnostic method is assigned an important role in detecting iso dense masses (CT) as small HCC (small hyper intense lesions) within a regenerative nodule (hypo intense). It uses 3 types of contrast agents: hepatic-biliary, gadolinium -based compounds (extracellular) and those taken up by the reticulo-endothelial system (super paramagnetic). Contrast agents having as target the reticulo-endothelial system (Resovist) consisting of super paramagnetic iron oxide particles (SPIO), produce distortion of the local magnetic field; Kupffer cells play an important role in capturing these particles. This type of contrast agents allow differential diagnosis between benign -malignant liver masses, being known that a malignant lesion does not change its intensity signal in T2 sequences after administration of SPIO. Some limitations of this method include: the presence of motion artifacts; presence of pace-makers or metallic materials (prosthetic valves or joints, metallic foreign bodies) are absolute contraindications. Among the relative contraindications are: claustrophobia, pregnancy, difficult collaboration. Although Magnevist is considered to be useful in atypical FNH, we could not detect the central scar in 60% cases of FNH, most probable because of the large tumoral volume and/or underlying steatosis. Resovist administration enhances the diagnostic specificity in FNH and malignant transformed nodules, the latter being indicated by the nonenhancing areas inside the dysplastic nodules.

Positron emmision tomography (PET) with 18 - FDG (fluoro - deoxy - glucose) in malignant tumors, is the most sensitive method to detect metastases with different origin (colorectal, stomach, esophagus). It is performed especially when somatostatin receptor scintigraphy is negative, but suspicion of metastasis of a gastrinoma or poorly differentiated carcinoid tumor persists. Unfortunately, however, examination costs are very high.

Liver angiography allows the assessment of the hepatic artery and hepatic portal flow with particular importance for the surgeon in pre-operative assessment. The contrast agent is inserted through a catheter (Seldinger technique) or puncture (spleno-portography). Hypervascularized small (< 1cm) metastases do not allow highlighting their nutritional artery, capillary phase allowing the view of heavily vascularized areas around the tumor. Angiography is considered more efficient than labeled colloid scintigraphy for the hyper vascular metastases, but CT is preferred in the less vascularized ones.

V. Conclusion

Dynamic imaging methods using contrast agents, always interpreted in the patient's clinical and biological context, are important noninvasive methods of investigation, used in order to enable positive and differential diagnosis in tumor masses of the liver.

Conflict of Interest

The authors declare that they have no conflict of interest and there is no disagreement in this new approach of imaging assessment of liver tumors.

Statement of human rights

The procedures were in accordance with the ethical standards of the responsible local and national committee on human experimentation and with Helsinki Declaration of 2000.

References

1. Dudea SM.Elemente tehnice ale aparatelor de diagnostic ultrasonografic. In: Badea R, Mircea PA, Dudea S, Stamatian F. Tratat de ultrasonografie clinică- vol.I Principii, abdomen, obstetrică şi ginecologie. Ed. Medicală Bucureşti, 2000; 39-44
2. Dudea SM, Badea R. Tehnologii noi în ultrasonografie. In: Badea R, Mircea PA, Dudea S, Stamatian F. Tratat de ultrasonografie clinică-vol.I. Ed. Medicală Bucureşti, 2000; 45-55
3. Albrecht T, Blomley M, Bolondi L et al. EFSUMB Study Group. Guidelines for the Use of Contrast Agents in Ultrasound. Ultraschall in Med 2004; 25: 249-256
4. Vlad L. Ecografia intraoperatorie a ficatului. In: Vlad L. Chirurgie hepato-biliară. Curs de specializare. Tipogr.UMF Cluj. 1999: 43-48
5. Leen E, Anderson JR, Robertson J et al. Doppler index perfusion in the detection of hepatic metastases secondary to gastric carcinoma. The American Journal of Surgery 1997; 173: 99-102
6. Wachsberg RH. B-flow, a non-Doppler technology for flow mapping: early experience in the abdomen. Ultrasound Quarterly 2003; 19: 114-122
7. Furuse J, Maru Y, Mera K et al. Visualisation of blood flow in hepatic vessels and hepatocellular carcinoma using B-flow sonography. J Clin Ultrasound 2001; 29(1): 1-6
8. Zerib E. Radionuclide imaging and diagnosis of benign tumours of the liver. Medicine Nucleaire (Elsevier Paris) 1966; 20: 324-329
9. Birnbaum BA, Weinreb JC, Megibow AJ et al. Definitive diagnosis of hepatic hemangiomas: MR imaging versus Tc-99m-labeled red blood cell SPECT. Radiology. 1990 Jul; 176(1): 95-101
10. Sarper RV, Fajman E, Rypins J. A non-invasive method for measuring portal venous/total hepatic blood flow, by hepatosplenic radionuclide angiography. Radiology 1981; 141: 179-184
11. Dragoteanu M, Marin M, Căinap C et al. Angioscintigrafia hepatică versus ecografia în detecţia tumorilor hepatice. Rom J Gastr 2002;11:134-5
12. Dragoteanu M, Cotul SO, Pîgleşan C, Tamaş St. Liver angio - scintigraphy: clinical applications. Rom J Gastroenterol 2004;13: 55-63
13. Hemingway DM et al. Clinical correlation of high activity dynamic hepatic scintigraphy in patients with colorectal cancer. Br J Cancer 1992; 65(5): 781-2
14. Carter R, Hemingway D, Cooke TG et al. A prospective study of six methods for detection of hepatic colorectal metastases. Ann R Coll Surg Engl 1996; 78(1): 27-30

Author's address:
Author: Ioana Grigorescu
Institute: 2nd Medical Department, „Iuliu Hatieganu" University of Medicine and Pharmacology Cluj-Napoca, Romania
Street: Clinicilor Str. 2-4
City: Cluj-Napoca
Country: Romania
E-mail: ioanaducagrigorescu@gmail.com

The Use of Breath Test for the Assessment of Gastric Emptying Rate in Clinical Practice

T. Surdea-Blaga, L. David, and D.L. Dumitrascu

2nd Medical Department, "Iuliu Hatieganu" University of Medicine and Pharmacy, Cluj-Napoca, Romania

Abstract— **Dyspeptic symptoms such as early satiation, postprandial fullness, and nausea or epigastric pain are very common in the general population. These symptoms are classically attributed to gastrointestinal dismotility, and are commonly seen in functional dyspepsia and in diabetes. In a subset of patients the pathogenesis of dyspeptic symptoms is attributed to a delayed gastric emptying rate. There are several techniques used to assess the gastric emptying rate. In this paper we presented our experience in the assessment of gastric emptying rate using a non-invasive and non-radioactive method, the 13C labeled-octanoic acid breath test. First we described the technique and the parameters returned by the system. In the end we discussed several cases of symptomatic patients, with diabetes mellitus and functional dyspepsia. The dyspeptic symptoms are not very specific, and gastric emptying proves to be normal quite often, suggesting that other mechanisms are involved in the pathogenesis of the symptoms. Gastric emptying tests should be performed before initiating treatment with prokinetics. In this context, the breath test is an easy method to assess the gastric emptying rate.**

Keywords— **gastric emptying, breath test, functional dyspepsia, diabetes mellitus**

I. INTRODUCTION

Dyspeptic symptoms such as early satiation, postprandial fullness, and nausea or epigastric pain are very common in the general population, and are commonly seen in functional (FD) and organic dyspepsia, as well as in diabetes mellitus. These symptoms are classically attributed to gastrointestinal dismotility [1]. In a subset of patients with FD (up to 50%), gastric emptying (GE) is delayed compared with healthy controls [2]. However, the relationship between delayed GE and symptoms is not yet very clear [3,4]. In addition, the term gastrointestinal motility is rather general and includes also impaired gastric accommodation and changes in postprandial antral motility [1] Forty % of patients with FD were found to have an impaired gastric accommodation of the proximal stomach to a meal, and this motility change was associated with early satiety [5]. The prevalence of delayed GE in longstanding type 2 diabetes was observed in 30% of cases, but upper gastrointestinal symptoms seem to be a poor predictor of delayed GE in unselected diabetic patients [6]. Gastroparesis is a complication of diabetes mellitus (consequence of intrinsic and extrinsic neuropathy) and the typical symptoms, observed in more than 2/3 of cases are early satiety, bloating, nausea, vomiting and abdominal pain [7].

At least in a subgroup of patients with FD and diabetes, symptoms like early satiety, bloating, nausea, vomiting or postprandial fullness, are associated with alterations in the GE rate. The gold standard for the assessment of GE is scintigraphy. This method is expensive and not widely available. Since its first use in 1993, there is a constant and growing interest in measuring the GE using breath tests (BT) with stable isotopes 13C or 14C. Twenty years ago, using octanoic acid 13C BT Ghoos et al showed that scintigraphic parameters (scintigraphic half-emptying time, and lag phase) had strong correlations with parameters of GE determined using the BT (GEBT) [8]. GEBT was found to be as reproducible as scintigraphy, and had a good sensitivity (93%) to identify accelerated GE, or delayed GE (89%) [9]. 13C acetic acid or acids labeled with 14C, as well as 13Cspirulina platensis BT can also be used.

Nowadays, the measurement of GE using BT is considered to be a simple, non-invasive and non-radioactive method to assess the GE rate. For clinical use, there are available some systems that measure GE in a real-time fashion, using continuous measuring of exhaled CO_2, and providing reliable and reasonably accurate data for GE rate estimate [10]. One of these systems is BreathID® (Exalenz Bioscience Ltd., Israel). We would like to present the experience of our department in using 13C octanoic acid GEBT, a continuous BT in symptomatic patients.

II. MATERIALS AND METHODS

GE rate was analyzed by a continuous BT in real time using the BreathID® system. All patients were tested in the morning, after fasting overnight for at least 8 hours. After a 10 minutes baseline collection of the patient's breath, a standard solid labeled meal EXPIROGer® (Sofar S.p.A. Milano, Italy) was administered and 250 mL of water. The patients were requested to consume the meal in 5 minutes. The standard meal had 378kcal (5.8% proteins, 60,8% carbohydrates and 33,3% lipids), and contained 13C labeled octanoic acid. After the administration of the meal, the patients were asked to remain seated for 4 hours, close to

S. Vlad and R.V. Ciupa (eds.), *International Conference on Advancements of Medicine and Health Care through Technology*, IFMBE Proceedings 44,
DOI: 10.1007/978-3-319-07653-9_11, © Springer International Publishing Switzerland 2014

the machine, with a nasal breathing cannula fixed all the time. The patients were connected to the device via nasal cannula. Octanoic acid is retained in the solid phase of the test meal as long as the test meal is mixed and grinded, followed by rapid disintegration of food in the duodenum, the subsequent absorption of the octanoic acid in portal venous system. Octanoic acid is oxidized in the hepatic mitochondria, with release of the 13CO2 in the blood, which is expired [11]. The BreathID® system continuously and non-invasively collected breath samples, and measured the changes in the isotopic ratio 13CO2/12CO2 in the exhaled air, using molecular correlation spectroscopy. The ratio is normalized for patient weight, height and 13C substrate and dose. The device provides percentage dose recovery (PDR) [proportion of the administered dose excreted per unit time %/hour] and cumulative percentage dose recovery (CPDR). It then calculates T1/2 (the time needed to discharge 50% of the labeled meal), tlag (the analog to the scintigraphy lag time for 10% emptying of the labeled meal) and gastric emptying coefficient (GEC) based on analysis according to a non-linear model to obtain tlag, T1/2 and GEC as described by Ghoos et al. [8].

Previous papers using a similar system, defined normal ranges of GE parameters based on earlier studies of Ghoos et al. and Maes et al. [8,12]. We used the 5 and 95 percentiles (in order to be able to detect patients even with slightly impaired motility and not just those with significant impaired motility) of Maes et al. [12] to define normal ranges of GE parameters, as follows: T1/2 41-109 min, tlag 3-69 min and GEC 2.75–3.88 (delayed emptying <2.75).

III. Results

So far we tested 28 patients (11 males). Two patients vomited during the test, so we considered the final result as being inaccurate, and they were excluded. One patient was retested after treatment. All tested patients were symptomatic, and the majority had either FD or diabetes mellitus with dyspeptic symptoms such as epigastric pain, early satiation, postprandial fullness, nausea, or vomiting. As we did not have all clinical data about all the patients, only several cases are mentioned. T1/2 ranged from 17.1 min to 219,3 min, tlag ranged from 14.5 min to 142.1 min and GEC from 1.8 to 7.0.

The use of octanoic breath test in patients with functional dyspepsia

We tested nine patients with FD. Four of them had postprandial distress syndrome (PDS), 3 had epigastric pain syndrome (EPS) and two had mixed FD (symptoms from both syndromes). Five patients had abnormal GE coefficients (at least one parameter). Three patients had a delayed T1/2 (> 109min), one of them having EPS, and the other mixed FD. Another patient with FD had a GEC< 2.75. Thus, four patients with FD had a delayed GEBT. One patient with FD had a very rapid GE, with T1/2 = 17 min.

Seven patients also completed a 9 item questionnaire - Patient Health Questionnaire (PHQ-9), developed to identify very rapidly symptoms of depression [13]. All these patients had signs of depression – 1 patient minimal depression, 4 patients mild, 1 moderate and 1 severe depression.

Case history 1. A 21-year-old woman was referred to a gastroenterologist by her primary care physician (PCP) because of nausea and epigastric pain that has been present during the last six months. The epigastric pain was related with the ingestion of meals, but the patient perceived pain as continuous and not intermittent. The pain was not influenced by antacids or antisecretory drugs. The symptoms were present daily, and rated as very severe (4 points on a Likert scale from 0 – absent to 4 – very severe). She also accused moderate bloating (scored as 2 on the same Likert scale), more than 3 days/week. Only occasionally she accused postprandial fullness and early satiety (less than once a week, and moderate as severity). Her medical history was negative for other conditions that could explain the pain. Physical examination was normal, blood tests, upper gastrointestinal (GI) endoscopy (including duodenal biopsies) were normal. The patient did not take non-steroidal-anti-inflammatory drugs (NSAIDs), was a nonsmoker, and did not use alcohol. Her family history was negative for GI disease. A diagnosis of FD - EPS was made. We evaluated the presence of depression in this patient using PHQ-9, and the final score was 10, suggesting moderate symptoms of depression. The GEBT revealed a much delayed GE (T1/2 = 219 min, tlag = 92 min, GEC = 2.01) (figure 1). She was given a prokinetic agent – domperidone 10mg, 3 times daily for 4 weeks. After 2 weeks she reported an improvement in symptoms severity (epigastric pain was rated as moderate, and nausea was rated as mild), she still had pain every day, but nausea was less frequent (1-3 days/week). After 4 weeks from the first GEBT, we repeated the GEBT, and we noted that T1/2 decreased by 20% (from 219 min to 175 min), with tlag = 84.3, and GEC = 2.18. However, at this time, her symptoms were rated as very severe, and were present daily.

Case history 2. A 39-year old male was referred to a gastroenterologist by her PCP because of epigastric pain, early satiation, postprandial fullness and vomiting, that has been present during the last 12 months, and were present at least 3-4 times a week. The patient rated the symptoms as moderate in intensity. The personal history, blood tests, upper GI endoscopy, abdominal ultrasound, could not reveal other conditions that could explain the symptoms. A diagnosis of mixed FD was made. We performed a GEBT which revealed a very rapid GE of the solid meal, with T1/2 = 17.1 min, tlag = 14.5 min, GEC = 7.0 (figure 2).

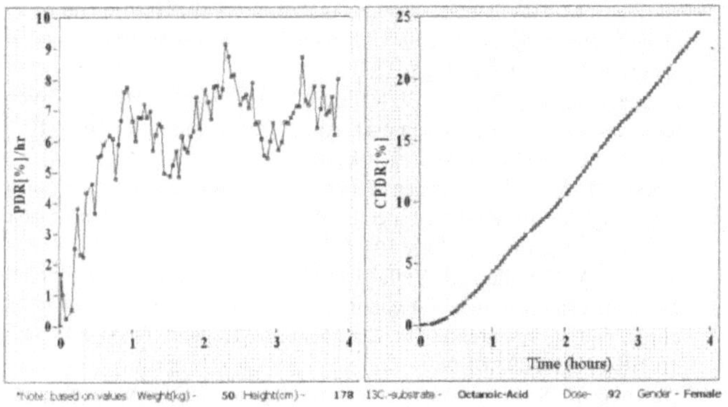

Fig. 1 Delayed gastric emptying time in a patient with functional dyspepsia – epigastric pain syndrome

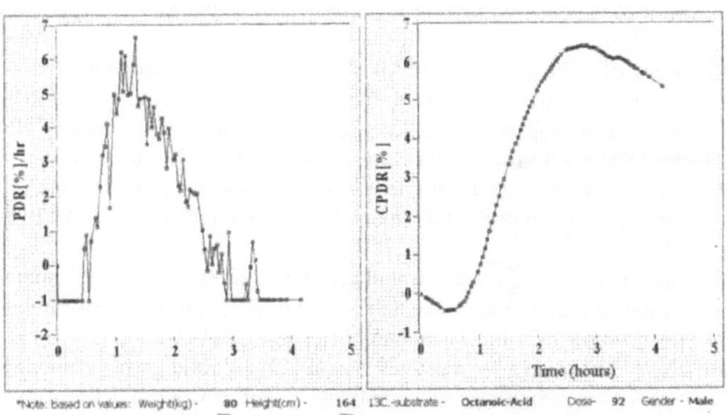

Fig. 2 Rapid gastric emptying time in a patient with mixed functional dyspepsia

The use of octanoic breath test in patients with diabetes mellitus

Case history 3. A 70-year-old male, with type 2 non-insulin-dependent diabetes, was referred to gastroenterologist for nausea, bloating and pain in the upper abdomen. The symptoms have been present in the last 6 months. Blood tests, abdominal ultrasound, upper GI endoscopy were negative for other conditions that could explain the symptoms. The symptoms were suggestive of gastroparesis and we performed a GEBT, which revealed a delayed GE with T1/2 = 183 min, Tlag = 142 min, and GEC = 1.8 (figure 3).

Case history 4. A 53-year-old patient with type 2 non-insulin-dependent diabetes consulted for nausea and epigastric pain. The symptoms have been present in the last 2 months. Blood tests, abdominal ultrasound, upper GI endoscopy were negative for other conditions that could explain the symptoms. We performed a GEBT, but the GE was rather rapid, with T1/2 = 39 min.

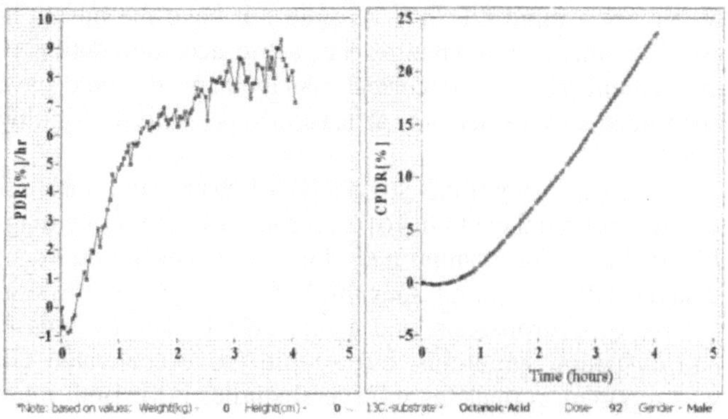

Fig. 3 Delayed gastric emptying time in a patient with diabetes

IV. Discussions

Since they were first described a lot of studies aimed to validate GEBT. Currently, this technique is considered to have a good accuracy when compared with scintigraphy [10,14]. BreathID® system has the advantage that evaluates continuously the GE, and immediately provides the results. GEBT is rapid, and easy to use in a clinical setting and compared with scintigraphy has some advantages: is safer than scintigraphy, particularly if repeated assessments are required, can be performed in pregnant or breast feeding women and in children.

The dyspeptic symptoms are not specific enough to predict the GE rate. That's why, not all patients with postprandial fullness benefit from prokinetic agents. In addition, as observed in case 1, even in patients with delayed GE, prokinetics do not always improve symptoms. Probably, our patient associated other gastric motility changes that generated the symptoms, and that would have required other drugs. The relationship between delayed GE and symptoms is still debated [3,4]. There are studies showing that delayed GE of solids was associated with postprandial fullness and vomiting, and delayed GE of liquids was associated both with postprandial fullness and early satiety [3]. Other studies found no correlation between symptoms and T1/2 [4]. Not only delayed GE can determine symptoms, but also does accelerated GE at 1 h, and impaired gastric accommodation. Studies reported the presence of each of these pathogenic mechanisms in more than 1/3 of cases [15]. The second case was the case of a patient with mixed FD and a rapid GE. There are some hypotheses that rapid GE also plays a role in FD. Kusano et al., found a significant correspondence between FD-PDS and accelerated GE in the early postprandial period, and suggested that the duodenum and the duodeno-gastric interaction could have an important role in the pathophysiology of FD [16]. In addition, impaired gastric accommodation induces a high luminal pressure, and secondary a rapid GE [17]. We did not have the means to assess if there were changes in gastric accommodation in this patient, but for the correct management, it would have been necessary to perform at least a hyper caloric drinking test.

Not always symptoms suggestive of gastroparesis are associated with delayed GE [6]. Gastroparesis cannot be diagnosed based on symptoms alone and confirmation of delayed GE is required. Our third case had symptoms suggestive of gastroparesis, and a delayed GE. The forth case, had dyspeptic symptoms, but a rapid GE. Accelerated GE was reported in diabetes in several studies [18]. Both insulin-induced hypoglycemia [19] and elevated plasma ghrelin levels [20] accelerate GE in diabetes.

In conclusion, symptoms as early satiation, postprandial fullness, and nausea or epigastric pain are not always a sign of delayed GE. GE tests should be performed before initiating treatment with prokinetics. In this context, GEBT is an easy method to assess GE rate, response to treatment, and can be repeated without safety concerns.

Conflict of Interest

The authors declare that they have no conflict of interest.

Statement of human rights

The procedures were in accordance with the ethical standards of the responsible local and national committee on human experimentation and with Helsinki Declaration of 2000

References

1. Tack J, Talley NJ, Camilleri M, Holtman G, Hu P, Malagelada JR , et al. Functional Gastroduodenal Disorders. In Drossman DA, Corazziari E, Delvaux M, Spiller RC, Talley NJ, Thompson WG, Whitehead WE, editors: Rome III - The functional gastrointestinal disorders (3rd edition). McLean (VA): Degnon Associates Inc; 2006, p. 419–488
2. Haag S, Talley NJ, Holtmann G (2004) Symptom patterns in functional dyspepsia and irritable bowel syndrome: relationship to disturbances in gastric emptying and response to a nutrient challenge in consulters and non-consulters. Gut 53:1445-1451 DOI: 10.1136/gut.2003.030049;
3. Sarnelli G, Caenepeel P, Geypens B et al (2003) Symptoms associated with impaired gastric emptying of solids and liquids in functional dyspepsia. Am J Gastroenterol 98:783-788 DOI 10.1111/j.1572-0241.2003.07389.x
4. Wilmer A, Van Cutsem E, Andrioli A et al (1998) Ambulatory gastrojejunal manometry in severe motility-like dyspepsia: lack of correlation between dysmotility, symptoms, and gastric emptying. Gut 42:235-242 DOI 10.1136/gut.42.2.235
5. Tack J, Piessevaux H, Coulie B et al (1998) Role of impaired gastric accommodation to a meal in functional dyspepsia. Gastroenterology 115:1346-52
6. Horowitz M, Harding PE, Maddox AF et al (1989) Gastric and oesophageal emptying in patients with type 2 (non-insulin dependent) diabetes mellitus. Diabetologia 32:151–159
7. Hoogerwerf WA, Pasricha PJ, Kalloo AN et al (1999) Pain: the overlooked symptom in gastroparesis. Am J Gastroenterol 94:1029–1033 DOI 10.1111/j.1572-0241.1999.01008.x
8. Ghoos YF, Maes BD, Geypens BJ et al (1993) Measurement of gastric emptying rate of solids by means of a carbon-labeled octanoic acid breath test. Gastroenterology 104:1640–1647
9. Szarka LA, Camilleri M, Vella A et al (2008) A stable isotope breath test with a standard meal for abnormal gastric emptying of solids in the clinic and in research. Clin Gastroenterol Hepatol 6:635-643 DOI 10.1016/j.cgh.2008.01.009
10. Dickman R, Steinmetz A, Bernnstine H et al (2011) A novel continuous breath test versus scintigraphy for gastric emptying rate measurement. J Clin Gastroenterol 45:22-25 DOI 10.1097/MCG.0b013e3181dadb23
11. Van V, Schoonjans RS, Struijk DG et al (2002) Influence of dialysate on gastric emptying time in peritoneal dialysis patients. Perit Dial Int 22:32-38
12. Maes BD, Ghoos YF, Hiele MI et al (1997) Gastric emptying rate of solids in patients with nonulcer dyspepsia. Dig Dis Sci 42:1158–1162
13. Kroenke K, Spitzer RL, Williams JB (2001) The PHQ-9: validity of a brief depression severity measure. J Gen Intern Med 16:606–613
14. Szarka, Delbende B, Perri F et al (2000) 13C-octanoic acid breath test for gastric emptying measurement. Eur J Gastroenterol Hepatol 12:85-91
15. Bredenoord AJ, Chial HJ, Camilleri M et al (2003) Gastric accommodation and emptying in evaluation of patients with upper gastrointestinal symptoms. Clin Gastroenterol Hepatol 1:264–272
16. Kusano M, Zai H, Shimoyama Y et al (2011) Rapid gastric emptying, rather than delayed gastric emptying, might provoke functional dyspepsia. J Gastroenterol Hepatol 26 Suppl 3:75-78 DOI 10.1111/j.1440-1746.2011.06627.x
17. Lunding JA, Tefera S, Gilja OH et al (2006) Rapid initial gastric emptying and hypersensitivity to gastric filling in functional dyspepsia: effects of duodenal lipids. Scand J Gastroenterol 41:1028–1036 DOI 10.1080/00365520600590513
18. Nowak TV, Johnson CP, Kalbfleisch JH, et al (1995) Highly variable gastric emptying in patients with insulin dependent diabetes mellitus. Gut 37:23-29
19. Russo A, Stevens JE, Chen R, et al (2005) Insulin-induced hypoglycemia accelerates gastric emptying of solids and liquids in long-standing type 1 diabetes. J Clin Endocrinol Metab 90:4489-4495 DOI 10.1210/jc.2005-0513
20. Ariga H, Imai K, Chen C et al (2008) Does ghrelin explain accelerated gastric emptying in the early stages of diabetes mellitus? Am J Physiol Regul Integr Comp Physiol 294:R1807-1812 DOI 10.1152/ajpregu.00785.2007

Author: Teodora Surdea-Blaga
Institute: 2nd Medical Department, „Iuliu Hatieganu" University of Medicine and Pharmacy Cluj-Napoca, Romania
Street: 2-4 Clinicilor Str.
City: Cluj-Napoca
Country: Romania
Email: teodora@gastroterra.com

Artificial Intelligence Applied in Diagnostic and Treatment of Dukes C Colorectal Cancer

B. Micu[1], C. Micu[2], A. Andercou[3], and N. Constantea[1]

[1] "Iuliu Hateganu" University of Medicine and Pharmacy, 5th Surgical Department, Cluj-Napoca, Romania
[2] "Iuliu Hateganu" University of Medicine and Pharmacy, Department of Anatomy and Embryology, Cluj-Napoca, Romania
[3] "Iuliu Hateganu" University of Medicine and Pharmacy, 2nd Surgical Department, Cluj-Napoca, Romania

Abstract — **One of the most common causes of morbidity and mortality from malignant tumors of the gastrointestinal tract is colorectal cancer. The paper presents a case analysis of Dukes C colorectal cancer patients who underwent radical surgery at the County Clinic Hospital, Cluj-Napoca, Romania. In order to predict the survival rate of colorectal cancer patients an artificial intelligence neural network has been implemented by the authors based on obtained statistical data.**

Keywords— **malignant tumors, colorectal cancer patients, survival rate prediction, artificial intelligence, neural networks**

I. Introduction

The prevalence of colorectal cancer is increasing worldwide and this becomes a problem of public health. We must improve efforts to find mechanism for optimize cancer care through accurate staging and appropriate treatments [1].

Within TNM staging, N stage describes the number of lymph nodes invaded by the tumor. There are studies showing that the total number of invaded lymph nodes does not allow accurate staging of colorectal cancer [2,3]. Lymph node ratio (LNR) is defined as the ratio of the number of metastatic lymph nodes over the total number of resected lymph nodes. Many studies confirm the influence of LNR on survival in breast cancer [4], bladder cancer [5], pancreatic cancer [6], gastric and lung cancer [7,8].

The paper aims to highlight the role and impact of LNR on survival of patients with stage III colorectal cancer, who underwent radical surgery, and to develop a postoperative survival rate prediction system according to patient's cancer staging parameters including LNR.

II. Case Study

An evaluation of the patients with Dukes C colorectal cancer who underwent radical surgery, at the County Clinic Hospital, Cluj-Napoca, 5th Surgical Clinic, between January 2005 and December 2008. Patients with histopathological type of cancer other than adenocarcinoma, those who were operated in emergency and those with incomplete or lost data were excluded from the study. The data analyzed were represented by: age, gender, tumor location, TNM Dukes C stage (IIIA, IIIB, IIIC), T stage, N stage, number of excised lymph nodes, number of invaded lymph nodes, lymph node ratio. LNR was calculated by dividing the number of metastatic lymph nodes to the total number of excised lymph nodes. Based on this criterion, patients were divided into 5 groups, the cut-off points where set at <0.10, 0.11-0.21, 0.22-0.36, 0.37-0.6, and >0.61 respectively, this classification of LNR has been already applied in several previous studies [8]. Patients were evaluated during a postoperative follow-up period of 5 years, at every 6 months in the first two years and at 1 year over the next three years.

The study has been approved by the medical ethical commission of the County Clinic Hospital, Cluj-Napoca.

Table 1 Sample of collected patient's cancer stage parameters

No.	TNMStage	Stage T	Stage N	LNR	Survival [Months]
1	IIIC	T3	N2	0.44	50
14	IIIB	T3	N1	0.125	44
23	IIIA	T2	N1	0.2	≥60
36	IIIB	T4	N1	0.3	≥60
43	IIIC	T3	N2	0.5	18
58	IIIB	T3	N1	0.083	≥60

III. Statistical Data Analysis

Fifty-eight patients met the inclusion criteria in the study. Of these, 23 (39.7%) were women and 35 (60.3%) men. 31.4% (18 cases) were aged under 60 and 69% (40 cases) were aged over 60, see figure 1.

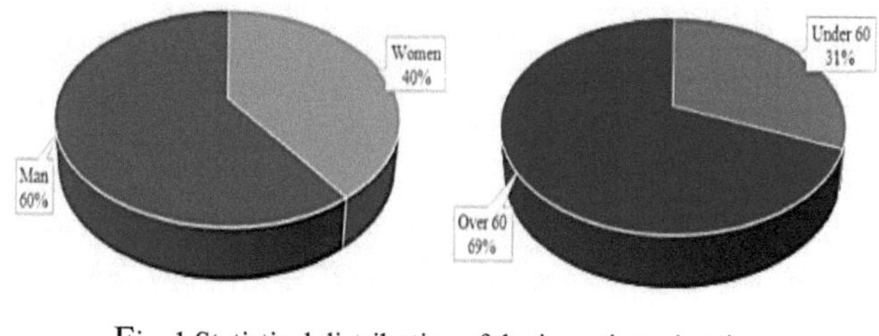

Fig. 1 Statistical distribution of the investigated patients

S. Vlad and R.V. Ciupa (eds.), *International Conference on Advancements of Medicine and Health Care through Technology*, IFMBE Proceedings 44,
DOI: 10.1007/978-3-319-07653-9_12, © Springer International Publishing Switzerland 2014

In terms of topography, 15 cases were located in the right colon, 18 in the left colon and 25 in the rectum. The number of lymph nodes excised during surgery for cancer of the right colon was significantly higher. The number of excised lymph nodes was not statistically significant based on tumor location.

The comparison of the relationship between the number of excised lymph nodes and the number of invaded lymph nodes reveals a positive trend.

The five-year survival by stage was higher in stage IIIA, 13 cases, (75%), than in stage IIIB, 22 cases, (55%), and superior to stage IIIC, 23 cases (10.71%), ($p<0.006$).

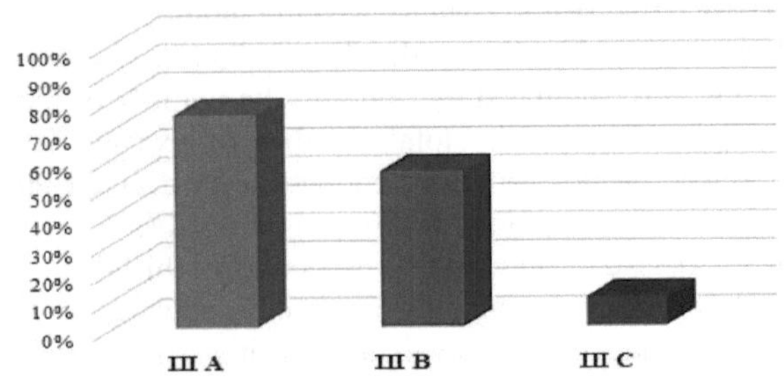

Fig. 2 Patients five-year survival rate according to TNM stage

The increase in T stage determines a decrease in survival. Survival in T2 group (15 cases with 66.67% five-year survival rate) compared to T3 (38 cases with 33.82% five-year survival rate) and T4 (5 cases with 33.3% five-year survival rate) groups reveals a higher value.

The analysis of N stage shows that 35 patients (60.31%) were in N1 stage and the remaining 23 (39.7%) were in N2 stage. The five-year survival rate in N1 group was 64.62% compared to the N2 group, where it was 8.57% ($p<0.001$).

The lymph node ratio (LNR) groups consisted of 8 cases (13.8%) in LNR1 group (<0.1), five-year survival rate 100%, 10 cases, in LNR2 group (0.11-0.21), five-year survival rate 83.33%, 13 cases, in LNR3 group (0.22-0.36), five-year survival rate 37.5%, 20 cases, in LNR4 group (0.37-0.60), survival rate 0%, and LNR5 group, 7 cases, (>0.6), survival rate 0%. (see figure 3)

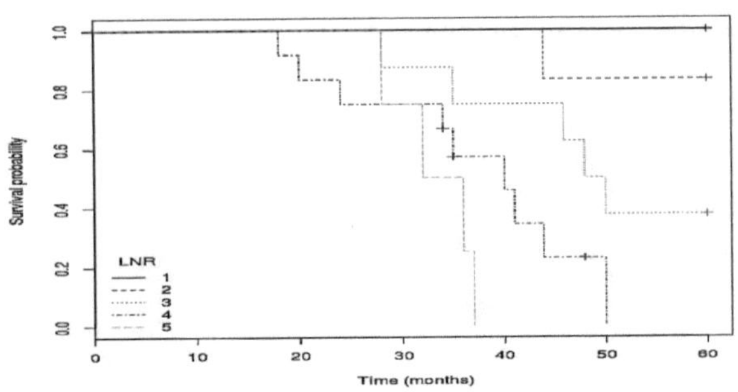

Fig. 3 Kaplan-Meier survival curve by LNR groups

LNR is associated with N stage. In patients staged N1 (LNR 1- 8 cases, LNR2-10 cases, LNR3-8 cases, LNR4-7 cases, LNR5-2 cases) or N2 (LNR 1- 0 cases, LNR2-0 cases, LNR3-5 cases, LNR4-13 cases, LNR5-5 cases) and divided in subgroups using LNR, five-years survival rates was different between N1 and N2 stage.

IV. Artificial Intelligence Approach

In order to predict the survival rate of colorectal cancer patients who underwent radical surgery according to different cancer stages the authors prose a neural network based artificial intelligence technique.

Artificial Neural Networks (ANN) belong to a special group of data analysis techniques that do not resemble with other classical techniques. ANN are learning about the chosen subject from the information provided to them, by detecting relationships between input and desired output data, rather than being defined by user [9].

A. The Structure of an Artificial Neural Network

The design of artificial neural networks has been inspired from the structure of human brain the most complex neural network from nature.

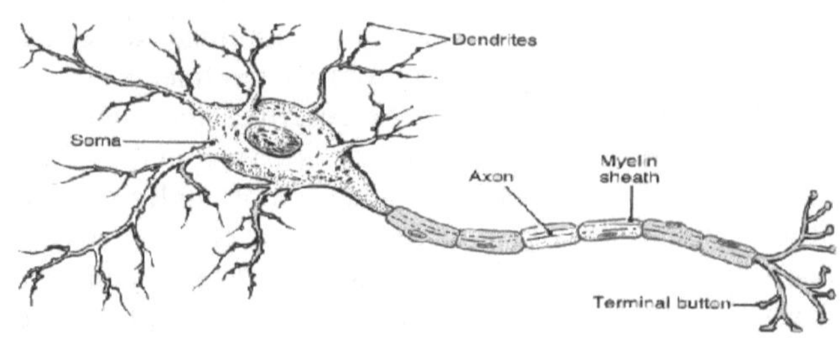

Fig. 4 Structure of a biological neuron [10]

Therefore, the building bloc of an ANN, the artificial neuron (figure 5) like the biological one (figure 4) is a system with a variable number of inputs u_k, $k=1..m$ (dendrites) and only one output y (axon).

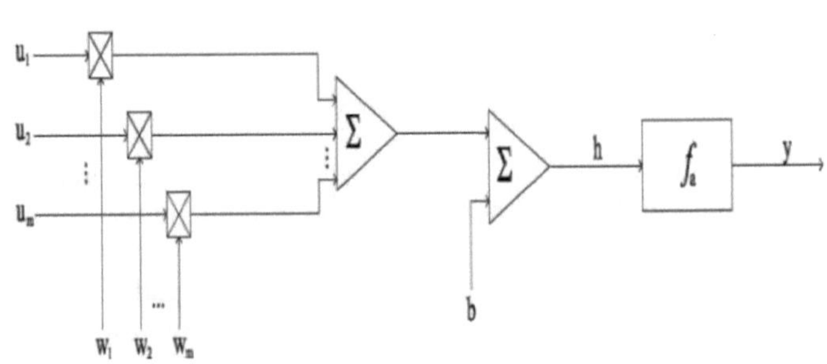

Fig. 5 Structure of an artificial neuron [11]

The inputs are multiplied by some w_k weighs and added to the bias b. And finally, the so obtained sum is sent as an argument to a transfer function that produces the output of the artificial neuron [11]:

$$y = f_a\left(\sum_{k=1}^{m}(u_k \cdot w_k) + b\right) \quad (1)$$

A group of artificial neurons, which work in parallel, form a layer. The layer gathering the neurons which provide the ANN output is called *output layer*, while the layers which contain the neurons interposed between the global inputs and the inputs of the output layer neurons are called hidden layers. Usually, in prediction or forecasting applications there are used feed-forward ANN which contain a hidden layer and an output layer.

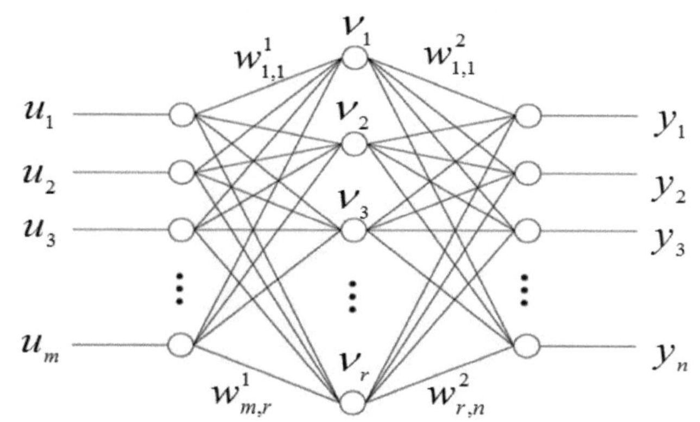

Fig. 6 Feed-forward neural network

Figure 6 presents the simplified block diagram of a two layer feed-forward neural network. From this block diagram, the relation which defines the output values of a feed-forward ANN, when u_k input values are known, could be deduced:

$$y_i = f_{a2}\left(\sum_{j=1}^{r}(v_j \cdot w_{i,j}^2) + b_i^2\right) \quad (2)$$

where:

$$v_j = f_{a1}\left(\sum_{k=1}^{m}(u_k \cdot w_{k,j}^1) + b_j^1\right) \quad (3)$$

B. Training an Artificial Neural Network

The training of a neural network is the process in which it is taught to provide the desired output values. Figure 7 shows the basic principle of the training process. According to this the weights and bias values of each neuron are adjusted depending on the error between the actual ANN outputs and the desired ones, evaluated numerically by a *performance function* (usually a mean square error function) [12].

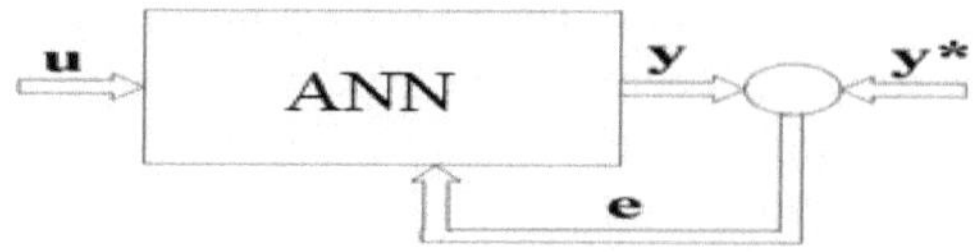

Fig. 7 Working principal of the ANN training process

C. Proposed survival rate prediction system

The proposed neural network prediction system for colorectal cancer patients survival rate evaluation, has the following input parameters:

- *TNM_Stage*, an integer value between 1 and 3 (1 for stage IIIA, 2 for stage IIIB and respectively 3 for stage IIIC);
- *Stage_N*, equal to 1 or 2 according to stage N1 and respectively stage N2;
- *Stage_T*, an integer value between 1 and 4 according to stage T1, T2, T3 and respectively stage T4;
- *LNR_Group*, an integer value between 1 and 5, which describes the lymph node ratio (1 if *LNR* is less then 0.1, 2 if *LNR* is between 0.1 and 0.21, 3 if *LNR* is between 0.21 and 0.36, 4 if *LNR* is between 0.36 and 0.6, and respectively 5 if *LNR* has a higher value than 0.61).

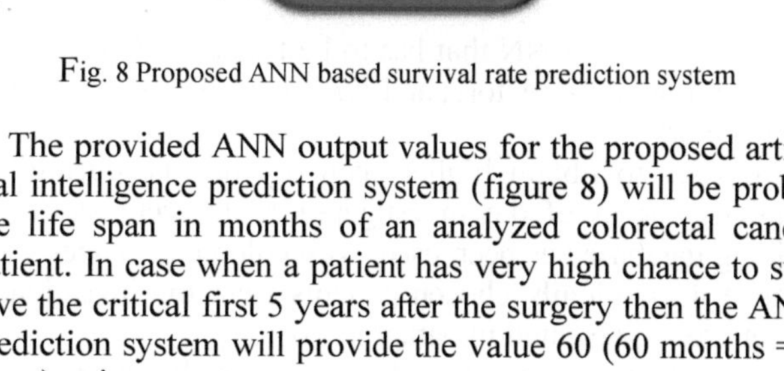

Fig. 8 Proposed ANN based survival rate prediction system

The provided ANN output values for the proposed artificial intelligence prediction system (figure 8) will be probable life span in months of an analyzed colorectal cancer patient. In case when a patient has very high chance to survive the critical first 5 years after the surgery then the ANN prediction system will provide the value 60 (60 months = 5 years) at its output.

V. Prediction System Implementation

In order to implement the proposed artificial intelligence based prediction system the *Neural Networks* toolbox of the *MatLab* software package was used [13].

To determine the optimal structure of the proposed ANN, at first different feed-forward architectures with one hidden layer and one output layer have been tested. The number of neurons on the hidden layer was varied between 5 and 30 with a step of 5 neurons. The transfer function of the hidden layer neurons has been set the hyperbolic tangent sigmoid function (*tansig*) while the output layer neurons transfer function was chosen one by one from the hyperbolic tangent tansig, the linear *purelin*, and respectively the logarithmic sigmoid *logsig* functions [12]:

$$\mathrm{tansig}(x) = \frac{1-e^{-2x}}{1+e^{-2x}} \tag{4}$$

$$\mathrm{purelin}(x) = x \tag{5}$$

$$\mathrm{logsig}(x) = \frac{1}{1+e^{-x}} \tag{6}$$

Therefore, almost 20 different feed-forward ANN with a single hidden layer have been investigated, using a custom *MatLab* function developed by the authors. To create a feed-forward network the following predefined *MatLab* function has been used:

$$net = \mathrm{newff}(Vin,\ Vtrg,\ LS,\ TF) \tag{7}$$

where: *Vin* represents the input data vectors; *Vtrg* represents the desired (target) output data vectors; *LS* represents the hidden layer structure (number of neurons in each layer); and respectively *TF* represents the transfer function used for each ANN layer.

To provide the desired output data, once an ANN is created, it is submitted to a training process using the Levenberg-Marquard training method combined with a descendent gradient with momentum weight backpropagation learning rule:

$$net = \mathrm{train}(net,\ Vin,\ Vtrg) \tag{8}$$

where: *net* is the ANN that has to be trained; *Vin* is a set of training input data vectors; and *Vtrg* represents output target data vectors.

In order to obtain higher accuracy results, during the training process of the investigated ANN architectures, a training database has been used, with colorectal cancer stage data of 43 randomly chosen patients from the investigated target group presented in paragraph II.

To compare the output values provided by each one of the investigated ANN architectures and to identify the optimal ANN configuration a performance function, was applied equation (9). This function is based on the average evaluation error applied for both the training data sets and for a testing database formed by the remaining 15 patients data that were not provided to the implemented ANN structures during the training process.

$$Perf = \frac{1}{n}\cdot\left(\sum_{i=1}^{n}\frac{\left(y_i^* - y_i\right)}{y_i^*}[\%]\right) \tag{9}$$

where: y^* represent the desired output values, y represents the provided output values, and n represents the number of input/desired output values.

Comparing the performance result for each of the investigated ANN structures the best configuration with one hidden layer and one output layer has been identified to be an ANN with 30 neurons on the hidden layer and with the *logsig* function for the output layer neurons. In this case the average evaluation error for the training data sets was 8.15% and respectively 14.13% for the testing data sets. Figure 9 presents the evaluation error distribution on accuracy classes for both training and testing data sets:

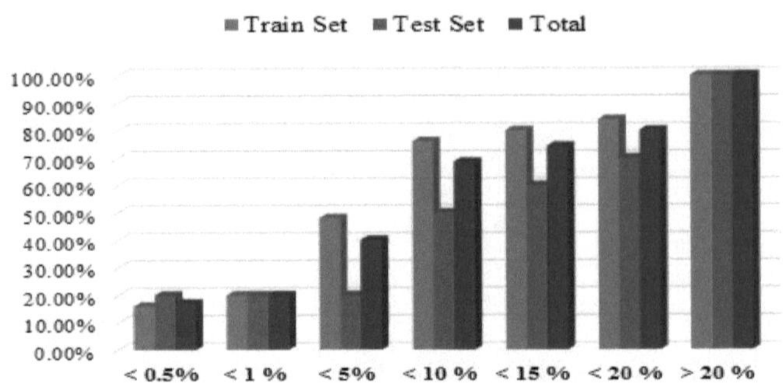

Fig. 9 Evaluation error distribution for the best single hidden layer ANN based survival rate prediction system

From figure 9 results that for 40% of the all testing and training data sets the evaluation error of the predicted patient life span is less than 5%, while 74% of the data sets fit in the 15% evaluation error limit.

In order to determine the proper post-surgery cancer care and treatment techniques for the colorectal cancer patients the based on the predicted life span the absolute accuracy of the implemented ANN has to be known. Therefore, in table 2 result provided for each training and testing data sets are classified in 6 accuracy classes:

Table 2 Absolut accuracy for the best single hidden layer ANN

Accuracy	Training Sets	Test Sets	All Sets
1 Month	44%	20%	37%
2 Months	44%	20%	37%
4 Months	56%	50%	54%
6 Months	76%	50%	69%
12 Months	84%	70%	80%
18 Months	96%	80%	91%

Analyzing the data presented in the above table we observe that only for 37% of all the training and testing data sets we get a 1 Month absolute prediction accuracy while only 54% of all data sets provide a 4 Months prediction accuracy.

Therefore, to prove the efficiency of the proposed ANN survival rate prediction system in the following a more complex feed-forward architecture has been considered, with two hidden layers and one output layer. To identify the optimal ANN configuration the neurons on the hidden layers have been varied between 5 and 30 with a step of 5 neurons. Considering the experience gained from implementing and testing the different ANN structures with one single hidden layer the transfer function for the hidden layers has been set to *tansig*, while the transfer function of the output layer neurons have been set to *logsig*.

Therefore, more than 30 different feed-forward ANN structures with two hidden layers have been investigated. Comparing the results provided by each one of them the optimal ANN configuration was identified to be a feed-forward ANN with 15 neurons on each hidden layer. In this case the average evaluation error for the training data sets was 6.41% and respectively 9.92% for the testing data sets.

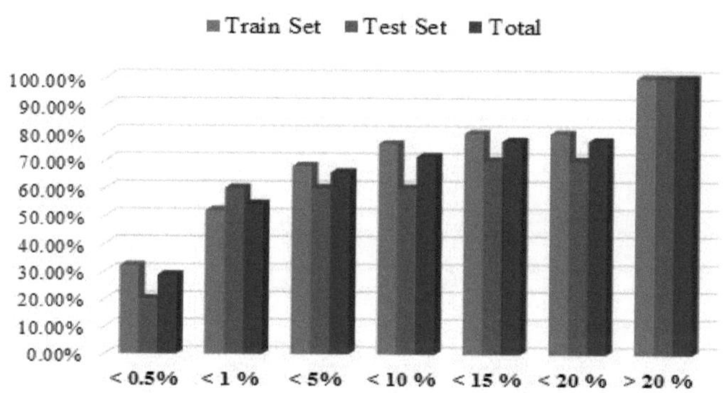

Fig. 10 Evaluation error distribution for the best two hidden layer ANN based survival rate prediction system

Figure 10 presents the evaluation error distribution on accuracy classes for both training and testing data sets. It can be observed that for this two hidden ANN configuration more than 50% of all training and testing data sets present an evaluation error less than 1%, while for more than 70% the evaluation error is less than 10%.

Analyzing the absolute accuracy for each of the testing and training data sets (table 3), the implemented optimal two hidden layer ANN prediction system provides result with 1 Month accuracy for 60% of the patients and a 6 Month prediction accuracy for 71% of the investigated patients.

Table 3 Absolute accuracy of the best two hidden layer ANN

Accuracy	Training Sets	Test Sets	All Sets
1 Month	60%	60%	60%
2 Months	64%	60%	63%
4 Months	72%	60%	69%
6 Months	76%	60%	71%
12 Months	80%	70%	77%
18 Months	96%	100%	97%

VI. Conclusions

An evaluation of the patients with Dukes C colorectal cancer who underwent radical surgery, between January 2005 and December 2008 at the County Clinic Hospital, Cluj-Napoca (Romania) has been made.

In the presented the authors established the cut-off points of the LNR at <0.1; 0.21; 0.36; 0.6; >0.61, and divided the patients in five groups (1 to 5) based on cut-off interval and shown a statistically significant proportionality in the relationship between the five-year survival rates and the five LNR groups.

According to the results of this study, when the patients in N1 and N2 stage were divided by LNR, respectively, the five-year survival rates were different by LNR in patients in the N1 and N2 stage. This data shows that the patients divided by N staging based on the absolute number of metastatic lymph nodes are not distributed consistently and the use of LNR, along with the current TNM staging, can give a better prognosis.

Therefore, an artificial intelligence based prediction system for the post-surgery five-year survival rate (life span) of the colorectal cancer patients according to their cancer stage parameters (TNM stage, stage N, stage T and LNR group) has been proposed. The implemented feed-forward ANN (best two hidden layer configuration) has a 1 Month prediction accuracy for 60% of the test cases.

The proposed ANN survival rate (life span) prediction system could be used to determine subgroups of patient at risk of relapse or death that could benefit from new therapeutic options, especially personalized cancer treatments for each patient.

As future development of the proposed survival rate prediction system could be an implementation with more input parameters like patient age or gender, and an investigation of a three hidden layer ANN configuration influence on the accuracy of the provided output values.

Conflict of Interest

The authors declare that they have no conflict of interest.

References

1. Parson H.M., Tuttle T.M., Kuntz K.M., Begun J.W., McGovern P.M., Virgin B.A. (2011) Association between lymph node evaluation for colon cancer and node positivity over the past 20 years. The Journal of the American Medical Association, vol. 306, no. 10, pp 1089-1097.
2. Sobin L.H., Wittekind C. (2002) TNM classification of malignant tumors. International Union Against Cancer 6th Edition, ed. Wiley, NewYork, USA.
3. Wang J., Kulaylat M., Rockette H., Hassett J., Rajput A, Dunn K.B., Dayton M. (2009) Should total number of lymph nodes be used as a quality of care measure for stage III colon cancer? Annals of Surgery, vol. 249, pp. 559-563.
4. Truong P.T., Vinh-Hung V., Cserni G., Woodward W.A., Tai P., Vlastos G. (2008) The number of positive nodes and the ratio of positive to excised nodes are significant predictors of survival in women with micrometastatic node-positive breast cancer. European Journal of Cancer, vol. 44, pp. 1670-1677.
5. Herr H.W. (2003) Superiority of ratio based lymph node staging for bladder cancer. Journal of Urology, vol. 169, pp. 943-945.
6. Pawlik T.M., Gleisner A.L., Cameron J.L., Winter J.M., Assumpcao L., Lillemoe K.D., Wolfgang C., Hruban R.H., Schulick R.D., Yeo C.J., Choti M.A. (2007) Prognostic relevance of lymph node ratio following pancreaticoduodenectomy for pancreatic cancer. Surgery vol. 141, pp. 610-618.
7. Marchet A., Mocellin S., Ambrosi A., Morgagni P., Garcea D., Marrelli D., Roviello F., de Manzoni G., Minicozzi A., Natalini G., De Santis F, Baiocchi L., Coniglio A., Nitti D. (2007) The ratio between metastatic and examined lymph nodes is an independent prognostic factor in gastric cancer regardless of the type of lymphadenectomy: results from an Italian multicentre study in 1853 patients. Annals of Surgery, vol. 245, pp. 543-552.
8. Gajra A., Newman N., Gamble G.P., Kohman L.J., Graziano S.L. (2003) Effect of number of lymph nodes sampled on outcome in patients with stage I non-small-cell lung cancer. Journal of Clinical Oncology, vol. 21, pp. 1029-1034.
9. Micu D.D., Czumbil L., Christoforidis G.C., Ceclan A.: (2011) Layer Recurrent Neural Network Solution for an Electromagnetic Interference Problem. IEEE Transaction on Magnetics, vol. 47, no. 5, pp. 1410-1413.
10. Carlson, N.A. (1992) Foundations of Physiological Psychology. ed. Simon & Schuster, pp. 36, Massachusetts, USA.
11. Czumbil L., Micu D.D., Ceclan A. (2009) Artificial Intelligence Techniques Applied to Electromagnetic Interference Problems. International Conference on Advancements of Medicicne and Health Care Throught Technology, IFMBE Proceedings, vol. 26, pp.339-344.
12. Micu D.D., Czumbil L., Christoforidis C., Simion E. (2012) Neural Networks Applied in Electromagnetic Interference Problems. Revue Roumain des Sciences Techniques – Serie Electromagnetique et Energetique, vol. 57, no. 2, pp. 162-171.
13. Demuth H, Beale H (1998) Neural Networks Toolbox. Users's Guide, ver. 3.0, The MATHWORKS Inc., 1998

Glaucoma Risk – Correlations between Measurements from Optical Coherence Tomography and Ocular Response Analyzer

H. Demea[1], S. Demea[1], R. Holonec[2], and G. Lupu[2]

[1] Ophthalmological Center – Review, Cluj-Napoca, Romania
[2] Technical University, Electrical Engineering Faculty, Cluj-Napoca, Romania

Abstract— **Glaucoma can lead to blindness if it is not diagnosed in time. To detect it in a patient, a complex assessment is necessary, including: intraocular pressure (IOP) measurements and detection of its influence upon the optic nerve. Our work is based on the hypothesis that retinal nerve fiber layers (RNFL) are influenced by IOP and corneal properties. First, investigations were made with the Reichert Ocular Response Analyzer (ORA) for the intraocular pressure (Goldman- correlated Intraocular Pressure: IOPg, Compensated Intraocular Pressure: IOPc) and corneal properties (Corneal Hysteresis: CH, specific damping capacity: φ). Then patients were measured with Optical Coherence Tomography (OCT) for retinal nerve fiber layers thickness: average and superior, inferior, temporal, nasal quadrants. The unified database comprises all these data collected from 4343 eyes and its construction was based on a text extraction method that uses image processing, optical character recognition (OCR) and virtual instrumentation techniques. Appropriate technical data (ORA, OCT) collected, properly computed and judged are very useful in glaucoma diagnosis and management, which is demonstrated in one of the largest databases studied (more than 4,000 eyes measured).**

Keywords— **intraocular pressure, ocular response analyzer, optical coherence tomography, retinal nerve fiber layer, optical character recognition**

I. INTRODUCTION

From the early 1880's until the last quarter of the 20th century, glaucoma was defined as "pressure within the eye higher than the statistical normal of the population." It was believed that this elevated intraocular pressure (IOP) would cause a certain type of damage to the optic nerve, which would eventually cause blindness if left untreated.

The American Academy of Ophthalmology now defines glaucoma as "a group of diseases with certain features including an intraocular pressure that is too high for the continued health of the eye." Glaucoma can be regarded as a group of diseases that have as a common end-point a characteristic optic nerve damage which is determined by both structural change and functional deficit [1].

In order to quantify in a patient the risk of glaucoma, first it's necessary to measure at least two important parameters: intraocular pressure and optic nerve characteristics (structure and function), and then integrate the collected data with the rest of the clinical data.

II. WORK HYPOTHESIS

Glaucoma is a leading cause of irreversible blindness throughout the world. The common denominator of the glaucoma is a characteristic optic neuropathy, which derives from various risk factors including Intraocular Pressure (IOP). Although elevated IOP is clearly the most frequent causative risk factor for glaucomatous optic nerve atrophy, it is not the only factor, and attempts to define glaucoma on the basis of ocular tension are no longer advised.

It has been demonstrated that corneal biomechanical properties influence the results and outcomes of various ocular measurements and procedures, and may hold clues to diagnosing and managing ocular diseases [2].

It's crucially important, therefore, to quantify in some way the influence of the mentioned factors upon the optic nerve.

The correlation between the most important factors in diagnosis and evaluating a glaucoma suspect patient were studied: *Intraocular Pressure* (IOP) - as a risk factor, *corneal biomechanical properties* - as modulating factors upon IOP's influence on the optic nerve and *retinal nerve fiber layers* (RNFL) - as a measure of the optic nerve damage in glaucoma suspects patients.

III. METHODS

A database was built, where the measured parameters from 4383 eyes were collected. Only 4343 of them, with valid data, were used in the statistical research. The investigations took place during the years 2006-2012. Every patient carried out the following investigations: intraocular pressure and corneal properties with Reichert Ocular Response Analyzer (ORA), retinal nerve fiber layers with Optical Coherence Tomography (OCT).

S. Vlad and R.V. Ciupa (eds.), *International Conference on Advancements of Medicine and Health Care through Technology*, IFMBE Proceedings 44,
DOI: 10.1007/978-3-319-07653-9_13, © Springer International Publishing Switzerland 2014

A. Ocular Response Analyzer Data

The Reichert Ocular Response Analyzer utilizes a dynamic bi-directional applanation process to measure the biomechanical properties of the cornea and the intraocular pressure of the eye. The basic output of the measurement process is a Goldman - correlated intraocular pressure measurement (IOPg), and a measure of corneal tissue properties called Corneal Hysteresis (CH), which is the result of viscous damping in the corneal tissue. The CH measurement also provides a basis for a new additional parameter: Corneal Compensated Intraocular Pressure (IOPcc), frequent different from IOPg. IOPcc is an Intraocular Pressure measurement that is less affected by corneal properties than other methods of tonometry, such as Goldman. Human corneal tissue is a complex *viscous-elastic* structure. The CH measurement is an indication of viscous damping in the cornea. The subjects whose corneas exhibit low CH, which can be thought of in simple terms as a “soft” cornea, are probable candidates for a variety of ocular diseases [3]. The specific corneal damping capacity (φ) is calculated using relation (1).

$$\varphi=\frac{D}{U}=\frac{CH}{2\cdot IOPg} \tag{1}$$

The specific damping capacity (φ) is defined as the energy loss per cycle (D) divided by the peak energy stored (U), which for the being considered spring mass system is the energy stored in the spring at maximum deflection [4].

B. Optical Coherence Tomography Data

Optical Coherence Tomography (OCT) performs high-resolution, micron-scale, cross-sectional, or tomography imaging of the eye internal microstructure. OCT enables real-time in situ imaging of tissue structure with resolution of 3 to 15 microns, which are 10 times to 100 times higher than conventional clinical imaging technologies such as ultrasound, magnetic resonance or computer tomography. OCT measurement beam is in the infrared, no ionizing radiation, so imaging is well tolerated by patients [5].

To search for optic nerve damage in a patient a structural eye parameter was used in this study: Retinal Nerve Fiber Layers (RNFL) that was measured with Stratus 3000 - Carl Zeiss Optical Coherence Tomography (OCT). To measure RNFL: circular scans were obtained with a diameter of 3.4 mm centered on the optic disk [6]. The scan was initiated at clock dial 9:00 and proceeded clockwise (Figure 1). The mean RNFL thickness values were automatically calculated globally and separately for the superior, inferior, temporal, and nasal quadrants (90 degrees each) using OCT software version A5 (Humphrey-Zeiss Medical Systems).

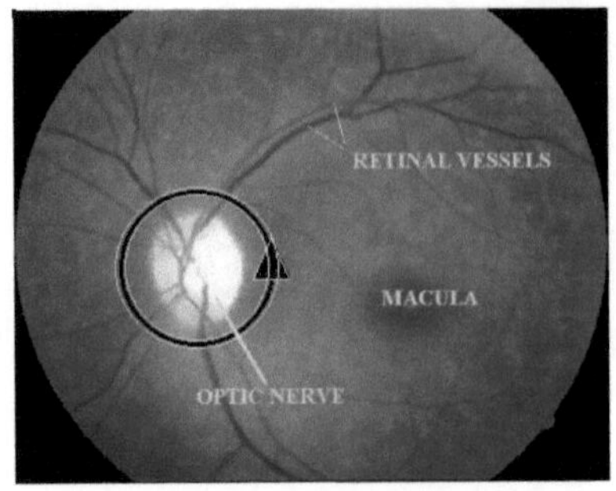

Fig. 1 RNFL circumpapillary scan type (black arrow - around optic nerve head) represented on an ocular fundus image (with macula, optic nerve and retinal vessels marked)

Two different parameters were collected from the "pdf" file with the scan results (OCT printout - in Figure 2). The first was the mean RNFL thickness of the entire circumference of the optic disk, labeled as "fiber avg" in database. The second parameter was quadrant thickness of RNFL, labeled as "fiber S", "fiber I", "fiber T" and "fiber N" - for superior, inferior, temporal respectively nasal quadrants.

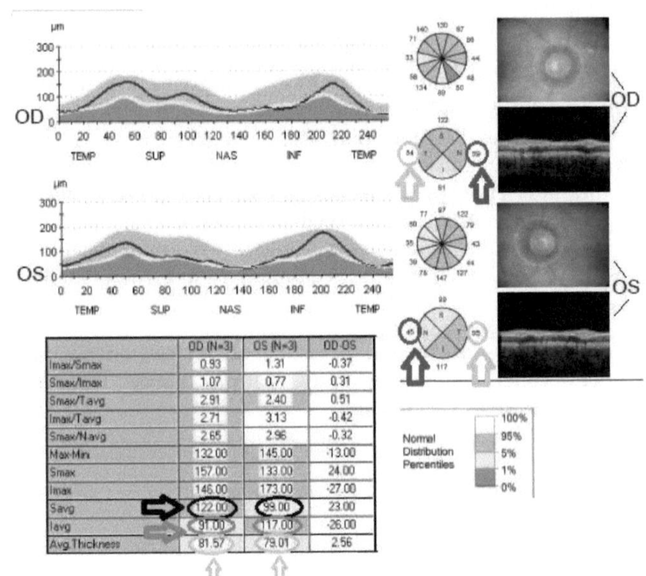

	OD (N=3)	OS (N=3)	OD-OS
Imax/Smax	0.93	1.31	-0.37
Smax/Imax	1.07	0.77	0.31
Smax/Tavg	2.91	2.40	0.51
Imax/Tavg	2.71	3.13	-0.42
Smax/Navg	2.65	2.96	-0.32
Max-Min	132.00	145.00	-13.00
Smax	157.00	133.00	24.00
Imax	146.00	173.00	-27.00
Savg	122.00	99.00	23.00
Iavg	91.00	117.00	-26.00
Avg.Thickness	81.57	79.01	2.56

Fig. 2 OCT printout –PDF file

OCT printout reveals the appearance of RNFL scan and automated analysis for both eyes (right eye and left eye, labeled as OD/OS). The collected data from the OCT printout, that are integrated in the final database, are marked with circles and arrows of different colors for different quadrants, as in Fig2: light blue for temporal quadrants (labeled as "fiber T"), indigo for nasal quadrants (labeled as "fiber N"), black for superior quadrants ("fiber S"), brown for inferior quadrants ("fiber I"), pink for average thickness of RNFL ("fiber avg"). Each eye from a patient was considered and analyzed separately in the database, because of various differences between right and left eye regarding IOP, corneal properties and possibility in a patient to have optic nerve damage / secondary glaucoma only in one eye.

C. Building the Integrated Database

In order to achieve clinical a research goal in ophthalmologists practice the extraction of the relevant information from different types of documents become one of the most important. Biomedical information exists in form like: text, journal articles, databases or electronic health records [7]. The OCT device from Review Ophthalmological Center gives the patients results in "pdf" documents and ORA device gives the results in "csv" files. In order to extract the necessary information and to build an integrated database a set of virtual instruments (vi) in Labview (National Instruments) were implemented.

For required OCT data, the "pdf" files (Figure 2) were converted in "tiff" files. By using the NI Vision Assistant and NI Vision Development Module an optical character recognition (OCR) based application was implemented (Figure 3) [8].

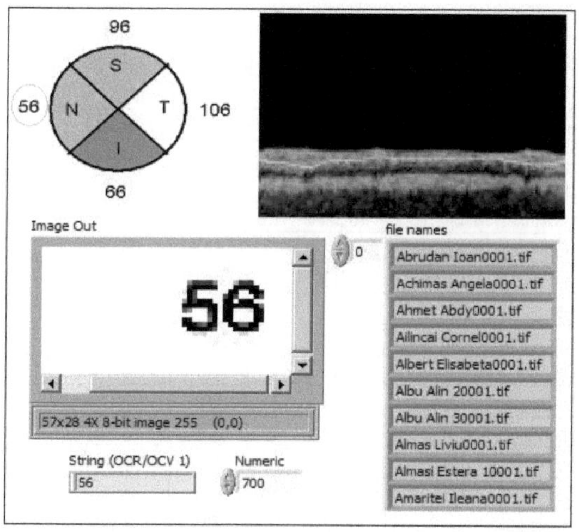

Fig. 3 The application for ORA data retrieval-The vi. front panel

For each feature the values were determined after some image enhancement algorithms: low pass filter for smoothing, Look Up Table (LUT) –exponential for contrast or masking for select the region of interest (ROI). Finally, after the OCR session the characters set were read.

The collected data from ORA and OCT were put together and exported in an "excel" file, wherefrom 4343 eyes values were available to be statistically computed.

The built integrated database that is used finally for the statistical analysis contains for each eye the next features: The gender and the age of the patient, Goldman - correlated Intraocular Pressure (IOPg), Compensated Intraocular Pressure (IOPcc), Corneal Hysteresis (CH), Corneal Resistance Factor (CRF), computed specific damping capacity (φ), retinal nerve fiber layers thickness - as a mean ("fiber avg") and the average measurements for each of the four quadrants ("fiber S, I, T and N") around the optic nerve (Figure 2).

For statistical analyze of data SPSS version 13.0.1 was used, with descriptive statistics, bivariate correlation, linear regression and multiple stepwise regression statistics procedures.

Database from the "excel" file was imported as a "sav" file in SPSS to be studied. First an overview was made and the main features of the collected data were analyzed. The correlation indices (Pearson and Spearman) were computed, to see the *strength* of association between variables. Multiple stepwise regression analysis was used to *quantify* different associations. This study was made because all previous studies show that IOP (for example) produces a RNFL thickness decreasing [1], [5], [14], and the goal is to know which variables or association are more related with this RNFL loss.

IV. EXPERIMENTAL RESULTS

The 4343 studied eyes are coming from a group of patients with ages are distributed between 8 and 95 years, with a mean of 53.17 years old and a standard deviation of 17.46 years old (Figure 4). The gender distribution was: 1572 male and 2771 female.

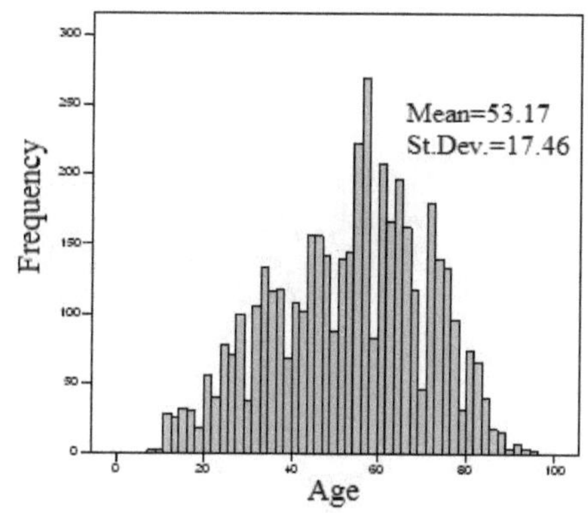

Fig. 4 The frequency of studied patients (4343) grouped according to age

Descriptive statistics on our database revealed: Goldman - correlated Intraocular Pressure (IOPg) between 4.1 and 65.9 mmHg, Compensated Intraocular Pressure (IOPcc) between 6.2 and 70.7 mmHg, Corneal Hysteresis (CH)

between 0 and 26.6 , Corneal Resistance Factor (CRF) with values between 3.4 and 27, computed specific damping corneal capacity (φ) between 0 and 1.195, retinal nerve fiber layers thickness - as an average around the optic nerve (fiber avg) between 23.96 - 150.20 microns and the measurements for each of the four quadrants around the optic nerve (fiber S, N, T, I) respectively 9 - 191, 10 - 174, 15-175, 1-199 microns as minimum - maximum measurements (Table 1).

Table 1 Descriptive statistic of the database in study

	N	Minimum	Maximum	Mean	Std. Deviation
Fiber-S	4343	9	191	124.06	22.972
Fiber-N	4343	10	174	79.96	19.154
Fiber-T	4343	15	175	70.84	14.854
Fiber-I	4343	1	199	124.29	22.653
Fiber -Avg	4343	23.96	150.20	99.804	15.060
IOPg	4343	4.1	65.9	18.356	5.0162
IOPc	4343	6.2	70.7	18.974	5.3419
CRF	4343	3.4	27.5	10.851	2.0794
CH	4343	.0	26.6	9.913	2.1272
φ	4343	.000	1.195	.291	.1022
Valid N (listwise)	4343				

Correlations between age and RNFL thickness (average and the four quadrants) with the other measured parameters: IOP, corneal properties and φ were computed (Table 2).

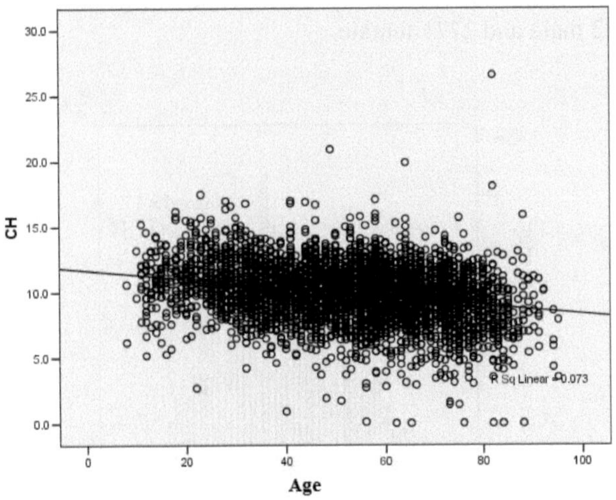

Fig. 5 Regression scatterplot for CH dependence on age

The regression scatterplot for CH negative linear relation by age is illustrated in Fig. 5: CH is decreasing with the increasing age (r = - 0.271). The regression constant (point at which the regression line would hit the vertical axis of the graph) is 11.67 (CH value for age 0); Regression unstandardized coefficient is -0.033. It is therefore a possibility to predict CH by knowing the age by using the relation (2)

$$CH = 11.67 - 0.033 \times age \qquad (2)$$

Statistically significant correlations for all studied variables were found with the exception of those between temporal RNFL and IOPg and CRF; some of them are positive (RNFL is decreasing when the studied parameter - CH, CRF, φ - is decreasing) and others are negative (RNFL is decreasing when the studied parameter - IOPg and IOPc - are increasing). In Table 2 the most significant correlations between age and the measured or computed parameters are included; they are sorted in decreasing order by statistical relevance; RNFL thickness and corneal parameters decrease with the age (negative correlations); IOPg and especially IOPc increase with the age.

Table 2 Pearson and Spearman correlation coefficients (ordered decreasing by clinical relevance) and their statistical significance for the most significant correlations detected between age, RNFL ("fiber" avg, I, S, N, T), intraocular pressure (IOPg, IOPc), corneal parameters (CH, CRF and φ)

Studied Variables		Pearson correl. coeff.	Statistic. signific. (p)	Spearman correl. coeff.	Statistic. signific. (p)
age	fiber avg	-0.322	0.000	-0.331	0.000
age	fiber S	-0.313	0.000	-0.324	0.000
age	CH	-0.271	0.000	-0.261	0.000
age	fiber I	-0.244	0.000	-0.236	0.000
age	φ	-0.204	0.000	-0.224	0.000
age	IOPc	0.203	0.000	0.098	0.000
age	fiber T	-0.191	0.000	-0.204	0.000
age	fiber N	-0.188	0.000	-0.206	0.000
age	CRF	-0.167	0.000	-0.150	0.000
fiber avg	CH	0.165	0.000	0.136	0.000
fiber avg	IOPc	-0.162	0.000	-0.130	0.000
fiber I	IOPc	-0.160	0.000	-0.127	0.000
fiber I	CH	0.157	0.000	0.129	0.000
fiber avg	φ	0.150	0.000	0.141	0.000
fiber S	CH	0.150	0.000	0.0123	0.000
fiber I	φ	0.148	0.000	0.137	0.000
fiber S	IOPc	-0.139	0.000	-0.139	0.000
fiber S	φ	0.125	0.000	0.115	0.000
fiber I	IOPg	-0.114	0.000	-0.084	0.000
fiber avg	IOPg	-0.112	0.000	-0.084	0.000
fiber N	φ	0.104	0.000	0.115	0.000

Multiple stepwise regressions revealed the influence of different associations between the collected parameters, and show which of these associations are better to predict RNFL loss in glaucoma suspect patients. (Table 3)

The best predictors, with negative correlation, are associations: age + IOPc, age+ CH, Age+ φ (Beta = -0.3, multiple R= 0.11), but they still only account for 11% of RNFL variability. Considering different association for age, IOP, CH correlation coefficients are increasing significant (Beta = -0.34 for IOPg+IOPc, -0.39 for IOPg+IOPc+CH comparative with -0.322 for age) so their increase is a better predictor for RNFL loss, than any other studied parameter considered alone.

Table 3 Multiple regression stepwise, with different predicting variable association, considering "Fiber avg" as Dependent variable (the most significant correlations are highlighted)

Dependent Variable: Fiber -Avg		Unstandardized coefficients		Standardized Coefficients		
Variable	R^2	B	standard error b	Beta	t	Signif. of t
IOPg	0.013	-0.33	0.045	-0.112	-7.426	0.000
IOPg,	0.033	0.59	0.106	0.198	5.594	0.000
IOPc		-0.96	0.100	-0.342	-9.655	0.000
IOPg,	0.033	0.71	1.825	0.238	0.392	0.695
IOPc,		-1.10	2.114	-0.391	-0.522	0.602
CH		-0.15	2.295	-0.021	-0.066	0.947
IOPg,	0.115	-0.17	1.790	-0.056	-0.095	0.925
IOPc,		-0.16	2.057	-0.057	-0.078	0.938
CH,		0.51	2.261	0.072	0.225	0.822
φ,		-7.80	5.421	-0.053	-1.439	0.150
age		-0.26	0.013	-0.297	-19.97	0.000
Age	0.104	-0.28	0.012	-0.322	-22.41	0.000
Age, φ	0,111	-0.26	0.013	-0.304	-20.81	0.000
		12.95	2.153	0.088	6.013	0.000
Age,	0.110	-0.26	0.013	-0.299	-20.12	0.000
CH		0.60	0.105	0.084	5.651	0.000
Age,	0.115	-0.26	0.013	-0.297	-19.96	0.000
CH,		0.50	0.107	0.070	4.600	0.000
IOPg		-0.20	0.044	-0.067	-4.594	0.000
Age,	0.114	-0.26	0.013	-0.302	-20.71	0.000
IOPc		-0.29	0.041	-0.103	-7.062	0.000

V. Discussions

There are many parameters to look for when we try to distinguish between a normal and a glaucomatous patient. The variability between individuals and within an individual over a lifetime make difficult to appreciate the situation of a patient at one moment. Biomechanical properties of the eye structures, measured by ORA are very important to assess a glaucoma suspect, and there are many studies focused on these properties [9]. By now nearly everyone recognizes that the current gold standard for measuring IOP, the Goldmann tonometer, has considerable flaws. The IOP measure is affected by corneal properties including rigidity, thickness, structure, hydration curvature and perhaps other factors not yet identified. ORA is capable to provide pressure measurements that are less affected by corneal properties, and give us additional information. All of these were taken into account and they determine us to make a step on ward to introduce these data into our daily medical practice.

Recent studies [10] shows that IOP induce a certain amount of stress and strain at the optic nerve head and lead to apoptosis of he ganglion cells; process depend on biomechanical properties of sclera and lamina cribrosa. Our study sustains these findings: computed "R square" is 0.01 for IOPg considered alone as RNFL predictor and triple, 0.03, for IOPg+CH as associated predictors for RNFL loss.

Multiple stepwise regression revealed that RNFL thickness (fiber avg) is much better predicted by age, or associations age + IOPc, age+ CH, Age+ φ (R square is 0.11) than by IOP g, or IOPc, IOPc+ CH (R square is 0.01 respectively 0.03), thus the older definition of glaucoma - that elevated intraocular pressure (IOP) would cause a certain type of damage to the optic nerve - is no longer sustained. As we can see in Table 2, for IOPg considered alone, R square is only 0.013, thus it can explain only 1% RNFL variability, while association age+CH+IOPg account 11% of RNFL variability (ten times more).

Statistics in other studies show also a higher correlation for (in order) superior, inferior quadrants and average thickness of RNFL with IOP [5], [14], [15]. Present work (with a studied sample far greater than other studies) shows also significant statistical correlations between IOP and RNFL thickness, as follows: average, inferior, superior, nasal and temporal (ordered decreasing by relevance). Considering these we improved our daily medical practice, with an appropriate technical and engineering support; uncovering the measure of correlation between IOP and RNFL loss, we also search for other possible RNFL loss causative factors, just as mentioned in other studies [16].

VI. Conclusions

Glaucoma risk or its clinical diagnosis in a patient requires a lot of work and attention between his clinical and paraclinical measured data. Technical support to integrate, compute and judge all patient's collected data offer a better approach of clinical cases.

RNFL thickness is one of the most important parameter used to categorize a patient as healthy, borderline (glaucoma risk) or ill (glaucomatous) and is known to be influenced by elevated IOP in the presence of certain properties of the cornea [13],[14]. Different considered associations between the mentioned parameters - as predictors for RNFL loss - increases the accuracy in categorize a patient. Present work sustain these, showing a good statistical correlation between

RNFL and ORA measured parameters (IOP, corneal properties), as well as with computed corneal specific damping capacity (φ).

The best correlations we found are between age and RNFL thickness (in order: medium, superior, inferior, temporal, nasal, with "r" respectively -0.32, -0.31, -0.24, -0.19,- 0.18 , for all p< 0.001); correlations between RNFL thickness (medium and inferior) with IOPc, CH and φ (r = -0.15 /-0.16, p<0.001) are better than between RNFL (superior and nasal) and IOPc, CH and φ (r =-0.14/-0.10, p<0.001); there is a very low positive correlation between RNFL (medium, inferior, superior, temporal) and CRF (r=0.06 / 0.02, p<0.001).

The best predictors for RNFL damage are associations: age + IOPc, age+ CH, Age+ φ (R square is 0.11), but they still only justify a rate of 11% for RNFL variability (loss).

Though, low/medium values of the correlation coefficients (Pearson' r and Spearman not greater than 0.33) show that the studied parameters are not enough for a complete and complex assessment of a glaucoma suspect patient; RNFL thickness decrease is certainly demonstrated now, determined by a more complex combination of factors than IOP and corneal properties [16].

The best predictors for RNFL loss (measure for the optic nerve *structure)* are associations: age + IOPc, age+ CH, Age+ φ, age+CH+IOPg (R square is 0.11), but they still only justify a rate of 11% for RNFL variability (loss).

Future studies with additional collected data about patients (for example: visual field as a measure for the optic nerve *function,* or ocular blood perfusion pressure responsible for optic nerve *nutrition*) are needed to improve rate of prediction for RNFL loss in glaucoma suspects.

Machine Learning Classifiers are also in our focus to increase the speed and accuracy of framing a glaucoma suspect patient, in daily clinical ophthalmological practice.

Conflict of Interest

The authors declare that they have no conflict of interest.

Statement of human rights

The procedures followed were in accordance with the ethical standards of the responsible committee on human experimentation (institutional and national) and with the Helsinki Declaration of 1975, as revised in 2000 and 2008.

References

1. American Academy of Ophthalmology, Basic and Clinical Science Course, Section 10, Glaucoma - *The Eye MD Association*, San Francisco, CA, 2007-2008, p 15-32
2. H. Demea, S. Demea, R. Holonec, A Corneal effort mapping system for glaucoma risk based on ocular response analyzer; *IEEE International Conference on Automation, Quality and Testing, Robotics; AQTR,* Cluj-Napoca, Vol.1,2008, p 333-336,
3. Luce D, Taylor D. Reichert Ocular Response Analyzer measures corneal biomechanical properties and IOP: provides new indicators for corneal specialties and glaucoma management. *Ocular Response Analyzer White Paper.* March 2009
4. B.J. Stone, A summary of basic vibration theory. *The University of Western Australia*, Crawley, Australia, 2007
5. Schuman JS, Puliafito CA, Fujimoto JG. Optical coherence tomography of ocular diseases. *Slack Inc. Thorofare, USA*, 2005:26-35
6. Schuman JS, Pedut-Kloizman T, Hertzmark E, et al. Reproducibility of nerve fiber layer thickness measurements using optical coherence tomography. *Ophthalmology,* 1996 103(11):1889 –1898
7. D. Ghai and N. Jain, Text Extraction from Document Images- A Review. *International Journal of Computer Applications* 84(3):40-48, 2013, Foundation of Computer Science, New York, USA.
8. S.P. Rasal. Bio-Medical Science with Optical Character, *International Journal of New Trends in Electronics and Communication (IJNTEC),* Vol.1, Issue. 2, Sep. 2013.
9. Wang M, Lu AT, Varma R, Schuman JS, Greenfield DS, Huang D (2014) Advanced Imaging for Glaucoma Study Group. Combining information from 3 anatomic regions in the diagnosis of glaucoma with time-domain optical coherence tomography. *J Glaucoma.* 23(3):129-135.
10. D. Howit, D Cramer *Introducere in SPSS pentru psihologie, Third edition,* Ed. Polirom, 2006, p 75-83, 198-205
11. M. Harris and G Taylor, *Medical Statistics made easy, 2nd edition,* Scion Publishing Ltd, 2008, p 48-57
12. C. F. Burgoyne, J. C. Downs, A. J. Bellezza, J.K. Suh and R. T. Hart, The optic nerve head as a biomechanical structure: a new paradigm for understanding the role of IOP-related stress and strain in the pathophysiology of glaucomatous optic nerve head damage , *Prog Retin Eye Research*, 2005, 24 (1), pp 39-73
13. Miki A, Medeiros FA, Weinreb RN, Jain S, He F, Sharpsten L, Khachatryan N, Hammel N, Liebmann JM, Girkin CA, Sample PA, Zangwill LM. Rates of Retinal Nerve Fiber Layer Thinning in Glaucoma Suspect Eyes, *Ophthalmology*, 2014 S0161-6420(14)00048-7.
14. Xu G, Weinreb RN, Leung CK. Retinal nerve fiber layer progression in glaucoma: a comparison between retinal nerve fiber layer thickness and retardance. *Ophthalmology,* 2013 Dec;120(12):2493-500.
15. McGlynn MM, Ehrlich JR, Marlow ED, Chee RI, Silva FQ, Van Tassel SH, Radcliffe NM. Association of blood and ocular perfusion pressure with structural glaucomatous progression by flicker chronoscopy. *British Journal of Ophthalmology.* 2013 Dec; 97(12):1569-1573

Author: Sorina Demea
Institute: Ophthalmological Center – Review
Street: 9th Moților St., ap. 8
City: Cluj-Napoca
Country: Romania
Email: sdemea@yahoo.com

Age-Specific Basal Rate Profile Characteristics at Initiation of Insulin Pump Therapy

G. Ghimpeteanu[1], G. Roman[1,2], D. Ciobanu[1], and A. Alionescu[2]

[1] University of Medicine and Pharmacy "Iuliu Hatieganu", Cluj-Napoca, Romania
[2] Clinical Center of Diabetes, Cluj-Napoca, Romania

Abstract— **The use of insulin pumps in the treatment of type 1 diabetes mellitus increased tremendously in the developed countries during recent years. In order to successfully switch patients previously treated with multiple daily insulin injections to insulin pump therapy, a proper distribution of total daily insulin is required. An important step is to determine the daily basal rate, and to tailor the basal rate pattern according to the 24-hourly basal insulin need. The aim of our study was to identify the age-dependent characteristics of basal rate profiles at the initiation of insulin pump therapy during hospital admission; 70 patients who met the criteria of the national program for insulin pumps were included; they were divided into 4 age-groups (Group 1: 6 to < 12 years; Group 2: 12 to < 18 years; Group 3: 18 to < 25years; Group 4: >25 years), and the daily basal rate requirement and hourly distribution of the basal rate were investigated. A significant difference between basal insulin requirements was observed among the four groups (Group 1-0.36±0.14; Group 2 -0.64±0.21; Group 3 -0.64±0.19; Group 4-0.57±0.20; p<0.001), and a bimodal distribution of basal insulin need was observed for all age-groups, but with variable age-dependent amplitudes. Identification of the optimal proportion of insulin and the 24-hourly basal insulin distribution for different age groups can help easily initiate and implement the right pattern right from the beginning of insulin pump therapy.**

Keywords— **type 1 diabetes, insulin pump, CSII, insulin dose**

I. Introduction

Since the discovery of insulin in the 1920s, type 1 diabetes (T1DM) disease course changed dramatically, from a slowly fatal condition treated by starvation, to a lifelong, insulin-controllable disease. Continuous efforts have been made during the past 30 years in order to achieve the best glycaemic control by mimicking nondiabetic insulin secretion patterns: a slow, basal delivery throughout 24h with boosts at meal times. Two treatment options are available to achieve this target: multiple daily insulin injections (MDI) or continuous subcutaneous insulin infusion (CSII) by insulin pumps. Insulin pumps are small, electromechanical devices which infuse rapid-acting insulin via a subcutaneously inserted cannula, providing an hourly programmed basal insulin delivery and patient-activated prandial boluses[1].

Insulin pump use has considerably increased in pediatric diabetes care during the past decade in developed countries, especially in preschool children [2, 3]. The main indications of CSII therapy are in T1DM in children, pregnancy, disabling hypoglycaemia with MDI and T1DM uncontrolled on MDI [4]. Several studies have shown better glycaemic control, less severe hypoglycaemia, improved quality of life, treatment satisfaction and blood glucose variability with CSII versus MDI [5-8], but with the downsides of higher treatment costs, complexity and reduced access in developing countries, due to budgetary constraints in healthcare systems.

When switching patients from MDI to CSII, a decrease by 10-20% of total daily insulin dose is expected, due to pharmacokinetic differences between the modalities [9]. An important step in starting CSII is to determine the basal insulin dose requirement, usually representing 30-50% of the total pump-adjusted daily insulin dose [3, 10].

The objective of our research was to identify the characteristics of the optimal basal insulin profile according to age groupings, in order to improve the insulin pump initiation process. While different basal rate profile recommendations have been made for adolescents and adults by diabetes care settings across different geographies, there is no current consensus on how to start CSII in different age groups.

II. Patients and Methods

Case records from 70 type 1 diabetes patients aged 6 to 40 years who were switched from MDI to CSII from 2002 until 2011 at the Clinical Center of Diabetes, Nutrition and Metabolic diseases in Cluj-Napoca, were examined. Patients who met the inclusion criteria to be part of the National Diabetes Program for free insulin pumps[11], were referred to the above mentioned clinic from different diabetes care settings across Transilvania.

Informed consent was obtained either from the participants or from their parents. The study was conducted in accordance with the ethical standards of the local ethics committee and with the ethical principles for medical research involving human subjects stated in the revised Helsinki Declaration.

S. Vlad and R.V. Ciupa (eds.), *International Conference on Advancements of Medicine and Health Care through Technology*, IFMBE Proceedings 44,
DOI: 10.1007/978-3-319-07653-9_14, © Springer International Publishing Switzerland 2014

All pumps were started on rapid-acting insulin analog during hospital admission. The total daily insulin dose (TDD) on MDI was used to calculate the pump start doses. TDD was decreased by at least 20%. The basal rate was divided into 5 blocks: 12:00 AM-3:00 AM, 3:00 AM-7:00 AM, 7:00 AM-12:00 PM, 12:00 PM-6:00 PM and 6:00PM-12:00AM. Nighttime hourly basal rate from 12:00 AM to 3:00 AM was 0,1U/h lower or higher than 3:00 AM-7:00 AM, depending on individual tendencies for nighttime hypoglycaemia. Also, daytime hypoglycemia-prone time intervals were covered by 0,1U/h lower insulin doses. Basal rate adjustments were made based on 6 h fasting tests performed on successive time intervals on consecutive days during hospital admission.

Patients were divided into 4 age groups: prepubertal 6 to < 12 years (n=14), adolescent 12 to < 18 years (n=20), young adult 18 to <25years (n=18) and adult >25years (n=18). For all statistical analyses SPSSv.22 was used.

III. Results

Study group mean age was 19.1±8.9 years, mean duration of diabetes at pump start 11.4±8 years, 60% female and 88.5% from urban area. Mean duration of MDI treatment before pump initiation was 7.7±5.7 years. The proportion of patients on pre-pump basal insulin analog and rapid-acting analog was 92.8% and 88.5% respectively. Pump patient basic characteristics and insulin requirement are presented in Table1.

Table 1 Pump patient characteristics by age group

	Group 1 6 to <12 years	Group 2 12 to <18 years	Group 3 18 to <25 years	Group 4 >25 years
N	14	20	18	18
Age (years)	9.3±2.1	13.6±1.6	19.9±1.6	32.2±4.5
Male (%)	21.4	35.7	28.6	14.3
Weight (Kg)	33.8±14.1	51.7±11.8	61.8±5.1	65.8±15.4
Height (m)	1.39±0.11	1.60±0.08	1.68±0.06	1.69±0.10
BMI (kg/m^2)	17.1±5.6	19.8±3.5	21.8±1.8	22.6±3.1
HbA1c at pump initiation (%)	8.2±1.2	8.7±1.7	8.3±1.4	8.5±1.2
Diabetes duration (years)	5,6±3,0	8,3±3,3	9,8±5,9	21,1±8,0
Total daily insulin pump dose (U/day)	23.8±9.6	37.5±7.1	36.5±7.6	34.3±7.0
Total daily basal rate need (U/day)	8.8±3.4	15.5±5.1	15.4±4.6	13.8±2.6
Basal rate percent (%)	37.8	41.2	42.1	40.7
Total insulin need U/kg/day	0.99±0.40	1.56±0.29	1.52±0.31	1.43±0.29
Basal rate need U/kg/day	0.36±0.14	0.64±0.21	0.64±0.19	0.57±0.20

Mean HbA1c at the initiation of insulin pump therapy was 8.4±1.4%, with no significant differences between groups (p>0.05). Mean total pump daily insulin requirement was 33.7±9.1 U/day, with significantly lower doses in the prepubertal group. The lowest basal insulin requirement was in the prepubertal group (P<0.05), with no significant differences between the other groups. The mean total daily insulin/kg was the highest in the pubertal group, and the lowest in the prepubertal group; the mean basal requirement/kg/day was the highest in the adolescent and young adult groups. The lowest basal rate requirement as percent of daily totals was in the 6-<12years group. Overall, as percentage of the daily total insulin, the mean basal rate was around 40%. The hourly basal rate distributions according to age groups are represented in Figure1, as percent of mean total 24h basal need.

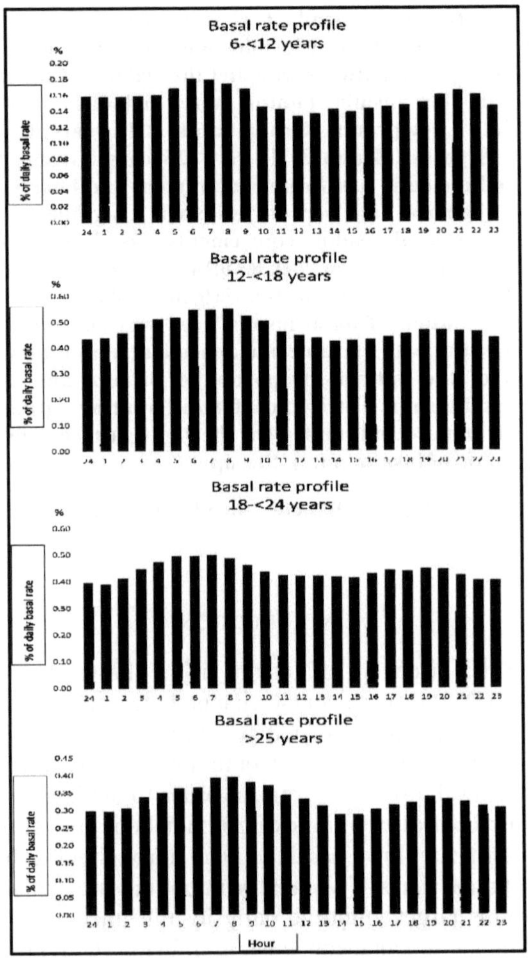

Fig. 1 Insulin pump hourly basal rate profiles in different age groups

The bimodal distribution of daily basal rate across all age-groups is of immediate practical importance, with a lower basal need between 11:00 and 15:00, indicating a higher insulin sensitivity around midday. In prepubertal children, the highest basal insulin need was between 5:00-9:00, with the second lower peak between 19:00-22:00. The other three groups revealed the highest basal insulin need between 3:00-10:00, and a lower peak between 17:00-21:00. Among the last three groups, the lowest basal insulin requirement and highest insulin sensitivity respectively was observed in the group aged > 25 years between 13:00-16:00.

IV. Discussion and conclusions

Clinical trial data of CSII in different T1DM subpopulations shows clear benefits [12-14]: achievement of good/better glycemic control with much lesser injections than MDI, less severe hypoglycemia, more flexibility and a clear patient preference for insulin pump therapy and better perception of general and mental health status[5]. In order to achieve all these benefits, a rigorous patient selection is required. Most people with T1DM can achieve acceptable glycemic control with MDI, when this option is applied sufficiently rigorously. It is better to reserve the CSII option for the ones in which the most robust clinical evidence exists. Guidelines draw clear criteria in this respect, the pediatric population being considered one in which MDI is inappropriate or inacceptable. In adolescents, non-adherence, insulin resistance, changing activity and sleep patterns can lead to treatment failure, both with CSII and MDI, but though, they are often better managed with an insulin pump [3]. Moreover, studies have shown that teenagers are more likely to have high glycated hemoglobin levels on CSII, leading even to pump treatment discontinuation and switch back to MDI [15].

Considering that insulin requirements vary across age-groups[16], knowing the age-related basal rate profile characteristics can help establish an optimal insulin profile from the beginning of CSII, the greatest variability being found in the pediatric age-group. According to certain authors, basal rate should be ~ 50% of daily totals[17], but others recommend it as 40% of daily totals[18]. Our study group adhere to the least recommendation, with even lower basal rate requirements below the age of 12 years. The recommendations for basal rate distribution patterns vary widely across geographies, as some clinics prefer to start with the same hourly rate, others with four different daily basal rates, and others with sliding ruler scales developed according to body weight and age[19]. In our analysis, the biphasic daily basal rate profile observed across all age-groups might be attributed to the differences in counter-regulating hormones in different age-groups, as the dusk phenomenon decreases amplitude > 12 years and the dawn phenomenon marks the highest basal need interval.

The findings of our research can be used to easier successfully initiate future patients in our setting in insulin pump therapy, knowing what sort of profile to expect, optimizing and tailoring the basal rate accordingly.

Conflict of Interest

The authors declare that they have no conflict of interest.

References

1. Pickup, J C (2012) Management of diabetes mellitus: is the pump mightier than the pen? Nat Rev Endocrinol 8: 425-433 DOI 10.1038/nrendo.2012.28
2. Berghaeuser, M A, Kapellen, T, Heidtmann, B, et al. (2008) Continuous subcutaneous insulin infusion in toddlers starting at diagnosis of type 1 diabetes mellitus. A multicenter analysis of 104 patients from 63 centres in Germany and Austria. Pediatr Diabetes 9: 590-595 DOI 10.1111/j.1399-5448.2008.00416.x
3. Phillip, M, Battelino, T, Rodriguez, H, et al. (2007) Use of insulin pump therapy in the pediatric age-group: consensus statement from the European Society for Paediatric Endocrinology, the Lawson Wilkins Pediatric Endocrine Society, and the International Society for Pediatric and Adolescent Diabetes, endorsed by the American Diabetes Association and the European Association for the Study of Diabetes. Diabetes Care 30: 1653-1662 DOI 10.2337/dc07-9922
4. Pickup, J C (2012) Insulin-pump therapy for type 1 diabetes mellitus. N Engl J Med 366: 1616-1624 DOI 10.1056/NEJMct1113948
5. Misso, M L, Egberts, K J, Page, M, et al. (2010) Continuous subcutaneous insulin infusion (CSII) versus multiple insulin injections for type 1 diabetes mellitus. Cochrane Database Syst Rev CD005103 DOI 10.1002/14651858.CD005103.pub2
6. Schreiver, C, Jacoby, U, Watzer, B, et al. (2013) Glycaemic variability in paediatric patients with type 1 diabetes on continuous subcutaneous insulin infusion (CSII) or multiple daily injections (MDI): a cross-sectional cohort study. Clin Endocrinol (Oxf) 79: 641-647 DOI 10.1111/cen.12093
7. Bode, B W, Tamborlane, W V, and Davidson, P C (2002) Insulin pump therapy in the 21st century. Strategies for successful use in adults, adolescents, and children with diabetes. Postgrad Med 111: 69-77; quiz 27
8. Danne, T, Battelino, T, Kordonouri, O, et al. (2005) A cross-sectional international survey of continuous subcutaneous insulin infusion in 377 children and adolescents with type 1 diabetes mellitus from 10 countries. Pediatr Diabetes 6: 193-198 DOI 10.1111/j.1399-543X.2005.00131.x
9. Lauritzen, T, Pramming, S, Deckert, T, and Binder, C (1983) Pharmacokinetics of continuous subcutaneous insulin infusion. Diabetologia 24: 326-329
10. Pankowska, E, Szypowska, A, and Lipka, M (2008) Basal insulin and total daily insulin dose in children with type 1 diabetes using insulin pumps. Pediatr Diabetes 9: 208-213 DOI 10.1111/j.1399-5448.2008.00375.x
11. http://www.ms.ro/?pag=133
12. Kordonouri, O, Hartmann, R, and Danne, T (2011) Treatment of type 1 diabetes in children and adolescents using modern insulin pumps. Diabetes Res Clin Pract 93 Suppl 1: S118-124 DOI 10.1016/S0168-8227(11)70027-4

13. Gonzalez-Romero, S, Gonzalez-Molero, I, Fernandez-Abellan, M, et al. (2010) Continuous subcutaneous insulin infusion versus multiple daily injections in pregnant women with type 1 diabetes. Diabetes Technol Ther 12: 263-269 DOI 10.1089/dia.2009.0140
14. Pickup, J C, and Sutton, A J (2008) Severe hypoglycaemia and glycaemic control in Type 1 diabetes: meta-analysis of multiple daily insulin injections compared with continuous subcutaneous insulin infusion. Diabet Med 25: 765-774 DOI 10.1111/j.1464-5491.2008.02486.x
15. Hofer, S E, Heidtmann, B, Raile, K, et al. (2010) Discontinuation of insulin pump treatment in children, adolescents, and young adults. A multicenter analysis based on the DPV database in Germany and Austria. Pediatr Diabetes 11: 116-121 DOI 10.1111/j.1399-5448.2009.00546.x
16. Cemeroglu, A P, Thomas, J P, Zande, L T, et al. (2013) Basal and bolus insulin requirements in children, adolescents, and young adults with type 1 diabetes mellitus on continuous subcutaneous insulin infusion (CSII): effects of age and puberty. Endocr Pract 19: 805-811 DOI 10.4158/EP13099.OR
17. Scheiner, G, and Boyer, B A (2005) Characteristics of basal insulin requirements by age and gender in Type-1 diabetes patients using insulin pump therapy. Diabetes Res Clin Pract 69: 14-21 DOI 10.1016/j.diabres.2004.11.005
18. King, A B (2010) How much do I give? Reevaluation of insulin dosing estimation formulas using continuous glucose monitoring. Endocr Pract 16: 428-432 DOI 10.4158/EP09308.OR
19. Klinkert, C, Bachran, R, Heidtmann, B, et al. (2008) Age-specific characteristics of the basal insulin-rate for pediatric patients on CSII. Exp Clin Endocrinol Diabetes 116: 118-122 DOI 10.1055/s-2007-990296

Author: Gabriela Ghimpeteanu
Institute: University of Medicine and Pharmacy "Iuliu Hatieganu"
Street: 8, Victor Babes Street
City: Cluj-Napoca, Romania
Country: Romania
Email:gabrielagrossu@gmail.com

The Informatised Follow Up of the Therapeutics Effects of Levonorgestrel Releasing Intrauterine Device – Mirena®

D. Muresan[1], I. Rotar[2], and S. Mirel[3]

[1] University of Medicine and Pharmacy "Iuliu Hatieganu", Faculty of Medicine, IIIrd Ginecology Department, Cluj-Napoca, Romania
[2] University of Medicine and Pharmacy "Iuliu Hatieganu", Faculty of Medicine, I[st] Ginecology, Cluj-Napoca, Romania
[3] University of Medicine and Pharmacy "Iuliu Hatieganu", Faculty of Pharmacy, Medical Devices Department, Cluj-Napoca, Romania

Abstract— **The levonorgestrel intrauterine system (LNG-IUS) offers a new therapeutic concept that combines a highly efficient contraceptive effect. The device is also used in the therapy of idiopathic menorrhagia. Our study analyses the therapeutically efficiency of an intrauterine medical device (Mirena) used by patients with idiopathic menorrhagia for one year. 20 woman patients were supervised based on a trimestrial questionnaire, sent by the patient to their gynecologist. At the beginning and at end of the study all the patients have submitted a clinical and ultrasound evaluation. Also usual hematological examinations have been performed. The results showed a significant decrease in duration and quantity of menstrual bleeding (p<0.05). The correlation between the electronic data and clinical data was very good (p<0.05), and the acceptance of monitoring system used was excellent. We can conclude that the Mirena treatment is efficient, well tolerated and is suitable for internet medical follow-up.**

Keywords— **intrauterine devices, monitoring, clinical data, electronic data**

I. Introduction

Hormonal intrauterine devices were introduced 30 years ago in order to improve the contraceptive action and to reduce the side-effects of other contraceptive methods [1, 2]. The researches suggested that the addition of a progestogen to a non-medicated contraceptive device improved its contraceptive efficacy. The device provides fertility control, complete reversibility and convenience, and has an excellent tolerability [3]. Furthermore, these devices have proven to be effective in treatment of heavy menstrual blood losses. Affecting 20% of women, menorrhagia is defined as total menstrual blood loss of more than 80 ml per menstrual cycle [4].

Traditional medical management of menorrhagia consists of oral medications (nonsteroidal anti-inflammatory drugs, oral progestins or oral contraceptives). Surgical options include invasive methods such as endometrial resection or ablation and even hysterectomy.

The levonorgestrel intrauterine system (LNG-IUS) offers a new therapeutic concept that combines the contraceptive efficacy with a treatment that reduces menstrual blood loss in both normal women and those with menorrhagia.

The clinic studies reported that levonorgestrel - IUS is more effective than nonsteroidal anti-inflammatory drugs and is as effective as oral norethisterone in menorrhagia management. The treatment compliance is significantly higher in the case of LNG-IUS. After 3 months of treatment, women using the LNG-IUS have 82% reduction in menstrual blood loss—twice that observed with tranexamic acid and 4 times the reduction seen with flurbiprofen [5] After 3 months, the levonorgestrel intrauterine system reduces menstrual blood loss by an average of 94%, comparable to the 87% reduction in oral norethisterone users [6, 7]. After 12 months of treatment, the women in the LNG-IUS group registered an average 96% reduction in blood loss compared to pretreatment levels.

The device also compares favorably with less-invasive surgical treatments for menorrhagia, including endometrial resection and ablation [8, 9]. Reduction of excessive blood loss is seen as soon as the first menstruation after insertion and at 1 year the reduction is more than 90%. The therapeutic effect is maintained for more than 5 years after first placement of the LNG IUS in the uterine cavity [10].

The recent studies concluded that menorrhagia treatment with the LNG-IUS is advantageous for women who wish to preserve fertility [2]. The levonorgestrel-releasing IUS is equally effective and well- accepted option in all age groups [11] and the bodyweight of the user is not associated with failure of the method. [11, 12]. The complications and side effects are rare; the invasive procedures are avoided and the fertility is preserved [3, 13].

II. Materials

A. Devices Materials, Properties and Design

Constructed of polyethylene, the levonorgestrel IUS is a T-shaped device with a steroid reservoir around the vertical stem (Fig. 1). Mirena is an intrauterine contraceptive device (IUCD). It consists of a small T-shaped frame made of polyethylene. The arms of the T are approx. 3 cm in length. The vertical arm is surrounded by a cylindrical reservoir

S. Vlad and R.V. Ciupa (eds.), *International Conference on Advancements of Medicine and Health Care through Technology*, IFMBE Proceedings 44,
DOI: 10.1007/978-3-319-07653-9_15, © Springer International Publishing Switzerland 2014

containing levonorgestrel. Two fine plastic threads are attached to the tip of the vertical arm (which are used for removal of the system and to check its presence once it is in place). The polyethylene removal threads attached to the T-frame are pigmented with black iron oxide. The T-frame contains barium sulphate, which makes it visible in X-ray examinations.

The unfilled polymer is the polydimethylsiloxane (PDMS) polymer after peroxide catalysis, which is mixed in an equal ratio with levonorgestrel, to form the levonorgestrel releasing reservoir. The unfilled polymer is also mixed with inert colloidal silica to form the membrane tubing, which covers the levonorgestrel reservoir in order to control the release rate of levonorgestrel [14].

The active ingredient of the system is levonorgestrel, which is a progestogen usually present in contraceptive products. Levonorgestrel is a nortestosterone derivative with potent progestogenic effects. Its chemical name is 13-ethyl-17-hydroxy-18,19-dinor-17a-pregn-4-en-20-yn-3-one with following structural formula (Fig.2)

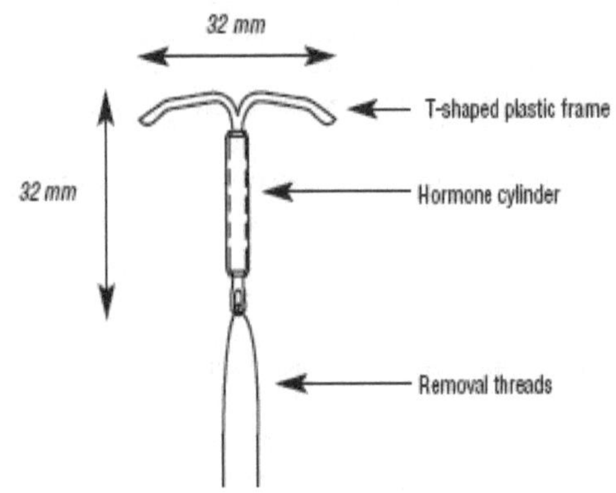

Fig. 1 The LNG-IUS construction (Mirena -IUCD)

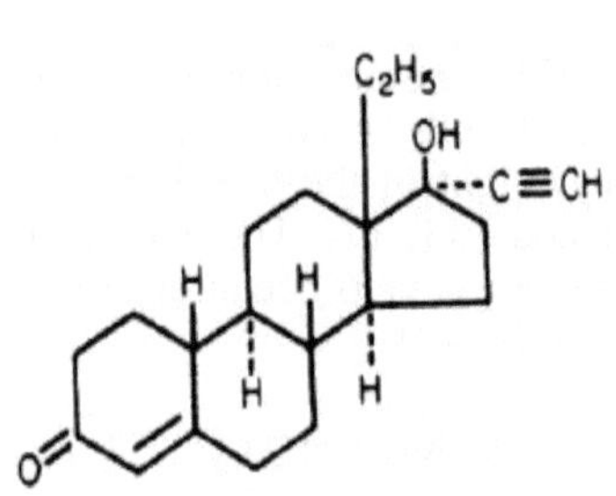

Fig. 2 Levonorgestrel structure

B. Mechanism of Action

This intrauterine delivery system has mainly local progestogenic effects exerts by a low doses of levonorgestrel in the uterine cavity.

The use of the levonorgestrel-releasing intrauterine system is associated with a strong reduction in duration and quantity of menstrual bleeding. This effect is based on the local action of LNG - IUS on the endometrium and could be explained by the substantial morphologic effects at this level. The local release of levonorgestrel into the uterine cavity results in a strong suppression of the endometrial epithelium as the epithelium becomes insensitive to estradiol released from the ovaries. This accounts for the reduction in menstrual blood loss [12, 16]. Reduction of menstrual blood loss results in improvement of the body iron balance and in an increase in hemoglobin concentration [10]. The significant reduction of MBL and the increase in hemoglobin and serum ferritin levels in the treatment of menorrhagia with the LNG-IUS has great implications for women's reproductive health [17]

III. EXPERIMENTHAL

A. Method

This study analyses the possibility and the efficiency of distant monitoring (via email) of the LNG-IUS intrauterine system's therapeutically effects, used in therapeutically purposes at woman patients with idiopathic menorrhagia.

We have designed a longitudinal, descriptive and analytic study. The patient after the insertion of LNG-IUS send email to their gynecologist via email concerning the duration of the menstrual bleeding, the amount of blood loss or the occurrence of any side effects such as amenorrhea, spotting. This information was resent to our team by email each 3 month. At the end of the study every patient had a clinical and ultrasound examination. Usual hematological (hemoglobin, hematocrit, erythrocyte blood count, seric iron level) parameter were taken at day 0 and at 12 months.

The Mirena device was used as conservative treatment of women suffering from idiopathic menorrhagia and secondary ferriprive anemia, in the absence of a severe gynecological pathology that would require an immediately surgical treatment.

The study protocol was approved by the local ethical committee (University of Medicine and Pharmacy "Iuliu Hatieganu" Cluj-Napoca, Romania) and is in accordance with guidelines set out in the Helsinki Declaration of human rights. The informed consent was obtained for every patient.

The study had many steps. At the entrance of the patient in the study a complete gynecological and pelvic ultrasound examination were performed. Complementary hematological examination was asked in order to asses the impact of the blood loss (hemoglobin, hematocrit, erythrocyte blood count, seric iron level).

The inclusion criteria are represented by:

- idiopathic menorrhagia (clinical and ultrasound parameters in the normal range)
- mild chronic ferriprive secondary anemia (hemoglobin values ranging between 8-12.5 g %)
- body mass index between 18-30
- the acceptance of the contraception for the whole duration of the study.

The exclusion criteria are represented by:

- the existence of associated disease that represent an absolute contraindication for the use of LNG – IUS (breast cancer, cervical cancer, ectopic pregnancy, hepatic disease) or relative contraindications (acquired immunodeficiency syndrome, anticoagulant therapy, bradychardia, cardiac disease, cerebrovascular disease, coagulopathy)

- women that have at least one child (after vaginal delivery or cesarean section).

An electronic form has been send to every patient regarding the quality of life after the insertion of LNG-IUS.

The recruitment of the woman patients took 6 moths. Afterwards, the patients were monitorised by an electronic questionnaire sent by email every 3 moths for one year. At the end of the study a clinical, ultrasound and hematological exam was done in order to verify the therapeutically results and the concordance of the 4 questionnaires completed by each patient with objective medical data. 23 patients took part in the study, 20 of them being monitorised until the end of the study and 3 of them haven't sent back all the 4 questionnaires, being eliminated.

During the study the patients have sent the results by email, by filling the questionnaire with quantitative results. They also have sent details about any given adverse reaction that might appear.

The electronic form was design using Microsoft Excel with the following fields:

- monthly bleeding pattern – the number of days of monthly bleeding
- for each day a quantification of the vaginal blood flow:
  - none
  - spotting
  - light bleeding
  - normal bleeding
  - heavy bleeding
- the concomitant medication
- adverse reactions
- laboratory analyses made at the beginning and at the end of the study
- the level of satisfaction of the patient concerning the device and it's effect on bleeding
- the level of satisfaction of the patient concerning the informative communication method.

At 12 months all the patients have been reexamined using clinical and ultrasound parameters. Also a blood drawn has been performed in order to evaluate the level of the anemia.

The data has been analyzed in order to find if there is any concordance between the data offered by patients during the monitoring period and the clinical results. The effectiveness of the use of LNG-IUS was analyzed taking into consideration the duration and the amount of the menstrual flow and its impact upon the hematological parameters.

The impact of LNG-IUS upon the endometrium was measured using 2D and 3D ultrasound technique. Using 2D the thickness of the endometrium was measured on a longitudinal section between miometrium-endometrium limit anterior and posterior, identified by an echogenicity difference (Fig. 3).

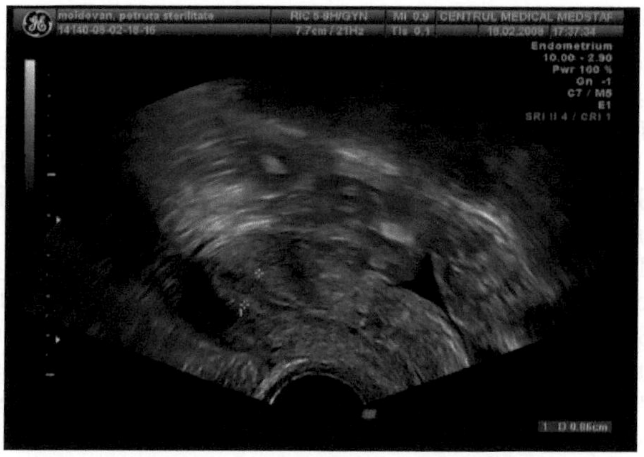

Fig. 2 Impact of LNG-IUS upon the endometrium using 2D ultrasound technique

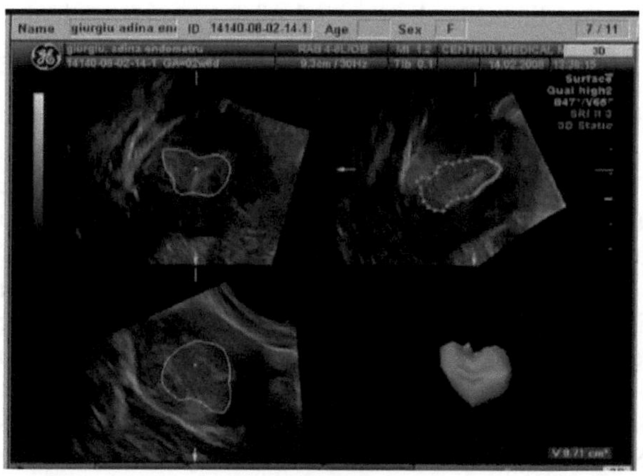

Fig. 2 The evaluation of the endometrial volume using 3D ultrasound technique

The measurement of the endometrial volume has been performed using a Voluson 730 Expert system equipped with a volumetric probe. The volume acquisition has been made using rendering mode and static 3D. For the image acquisition a median longitudinal uterine section using a volumetric acquisitioning angle of 65°.

The calculation of the volume have been made using VOCAL 2 (VIRTUAL ORGAN COMPUTER-AIDED ANALYSIS) software using the rotational technique, with a 15° step and with the manual drawing of the endometrial lining at each step (Fig. 4). The evaluation of the endometrial volume have been performed before inserting LNG-IUS and after 12 months.

The acceptability of the IUD and the comfort of the patient have been evaluated using a numeric scale ranging from 1 to 5 (1- unacceptable, 5 – no discomfort at all).

B. Results

The total number of the study participants was 20. They have sent all the 4 questionnaires by email and have been present at the final control.

There haven't been any important adverse reactions that could harm patient's health. The acceptance of the LNG-IUS system was very good, none of the patients having abandoned because of unpleasant secondary effects.

The minor secondary effects consisted of a prolonged bleeding in the first three month after the insertion of LNG-IUS in 4 cases (20%) that has remitted starting with the fourth month, mastodynia of reduced intensity in 3 cases (15%) and disturbance of the vaginal flora with the appearance of anaerobic bacteria in 3 cases (15%). The appearance of these minor secondary effects was notified to the examinator by electronic questionnaires filled each trimester by email, and also by this way the therapeutically method of resolving these has been immediately indicated.

The medium bleeding period of the woman patients has been reduced significantly from 7.8 days at the beginning of the study to 2.4 days at the end of the study ($p<0.05$). This decrease was gradual, being more significantly after the second questionnaire (6 months).

The amount of blood loss during a cycle has decreased from a high bleeding at the beginning of the study to a much reduced bleeding (16 patients) or the absence (4 patients) at the end of the study. Because of these changes the patient's satisfaction level concerning the LNG-IUS device progressively increased, from a media of 2.4 points to a media of 4.8 points at the end of one's year time. A high satisfaction score made all the patients to continue the use of the LNG-IUS device even after the end of the study.

The confirmation of the healing of idiopathic menorrhagia with Mirena has been made using 2D and 3D ultrasound examination and by the measurement of the hemoglobin level. The threshold value bigger than 12.5 g% has been considered to signify the hematological healing.

The average hemoglobin value was 9.6 g% at the beginning of the study, and it reached 12.7 g% at the end of the study ($p<0.05$). This study proves the correction of the anemia by the use of LNG-IUS.

The dimensions and the volume of the endometrium after one year of using LNG-IUS have decreased after 12 months of treatment. The hemoglobin level has increased. These parameters have been analyzed using Student test. A statistic significant modification has been observed ($p<0.01$) between the initial and final values of the endometrial thickness and volume and also of the values of hemoglobin (table I). These results indicate the therapeutic efficiency of the LNG-IUS system upon the endometrial hyperplasia and the correction of the anemia of the patients.

The calculation of the endometrial volume was more significant than the measurement of the endometrial thickness (volume p < thickness p) for the evaluation of LNG-IUS effect.

An inverse correlation has been found using the "r" Pearson correlation index when comparing the values of the endometrial thickness and the initial level of the hemoglobin ($r = -0.22088$) and between the initial endometrial volume and the initial hemoglobin level ($r = -0.32266$). This inverse correlation was stronger for the endometrial volume which can give a better prediction of the anemia degree (table II).

Table 1 Statistical parameters

	Initial thick-ness (mm)	Initial volume (cm^3)	Initial Hb g% ml	Final thick-ness (mm)	Final volume (cm^3)	Final Hb g%ml
Medium value and std dev	11,85 +/-1.88	10,80 +/-1.82	9,61 +/- 1.31	3,71 +/- 0.98	2,80 +/- 0.41	12,69 +/- 1.03
"p" initial - final				2,3461 E-12	1,8732 E-13	1,2588 E-06

Table 2 Pearson correlation

	Endometrial thickness	Endometrial volume	Hb	Correlation index Pearson "r"
Initial values	+		+	- 0.22088
Initial values		+	+	- 0.32266
Final values	+		+	- 0.17590
Final values		+	+	- 0.3888

At the end of the treatment period the endometrial volume was better correlated with the hemoglobin level (r = - 0.3888) than the endometrial thickness (r = - 0.17590).

The volumetric and dimensional modification of the endometrium confirms the efficiency of the LNG-IUS system, and it is in according with the degree of anemia correction of the patients. From the parameters that we have used, the calculation of the endometrial volume using 3D ultrasound, even if it requires complex ultrasound machines and experience represent a more sensitive method for the detection of the endometrial modifications.

The analysis of the concordance between the subjective data and the objective ones at the end of the study has showed a concordance of 96% between the subjective appreciation for the bleeding period and the hematological healing, and a concordance of 92% between the monthly blood loss and the values of hemoglobin at the end o the study.

At the beginning of the study the concordance between lost blood quantity appreciated by the patient and the hemoglobin level was only of 74%, value probably due to more difficult quantification of the massive bleeding of the patient and their different biological terrain.

The level of patient satisfaction for the e-mail communication was of 4.7 point on a scale between 1 to 5.

C. Discussions

The use of Mirena device with permanently liberation of levonorgestrel represents a modern method, noninvasive appropriate for the treatment of idiopathic menorrhagia [17, 18]. LNG-IUS has some advantages when compared with other therapies used for the treatment of this condition such as: easy application, maintaince of the integrity of the female genital and of a very small incidence of systematic secondary effects [19]. This system represents an efficient alternative to the hysterectomy for the perimenaupausal women [20]

The prolonged bleeding pattern found after the insertion of the LNG-IUS system is a transient phenomenon, which is not accompanied by increased blood loss and it disappeared spontaneously in the first 2 to 4 months of treatment. These finding has been confirmed by many multicentric studies [4, 21]. The actual studies confirm the value of the calculation of the endometrial volume by 3D ultrasound, with a good reproducibility and repetability. The determination of the endometrial volume using 3D technique can be applied in the diagnosis of the disorders that involve and excess of the endometrial volume (endometrial cancer or endometrial hyperplasia in idiopathic menorrhagia) and in the follow-up of their treatments [22, 23].

The calculation of the endometrial volume seems to be better correlated with the initial degree of anemia of the patients than the endometrial thickness. Also the endometrial volume sees to be better correlate with the final values of the hemoglobin, representing a more sensitive method for the evaluation of the therapeutically efficiency.

A better correlation of the volumetric data can be explained by the fact that the endometrium thickness represents an incomplete parameter, it is measured at a single level and it is not taking into consideration the aspect and the dimensions of the uterine cavity, while the volume measuring is analyzing the whole cavity.

The measurement of the endometrial volume can represent a new standard in the future for the evaluation of the conditions that involves endometrial changes [24].

The use of electronic questionnaires for evaluating the efficiency of the Mirena device represents a modern, easy and efficient way of controlling the treatment at distance. This method has reached a high satisfaction level from the patients and at final analysis of the study it presented a very good concordance with the medical objective data. This method of e-mail monitoring has allowed the avoidance of some useless walks for the patients, an efficient communication between the doctor and his patient, it allowed the continuously gathering of medical information and the decrease of some repeatable medical consultations.

The email based follow-up of the effects and the results can also be applied for other diseases, taking into consideration their particularities. In order to obtain correct medical results with statistic significance the questionnaire has to be extremely well design and it should include numeric and well defined qualitative parameters.

IV. Conclusions

LNG-IU represents an effective therapeutically method for the treatment of hormonal menorrhagia in 30 to 45 years old women. The method is easily accepted by patients and it often allows the avoidance of some aggressive chirurgical interventions, preserving the integrity of the genital organs.

This method fulfils the requirements of the minimal invasive techniques so valued in nowadays because of its local impact with almost no secondary side effects due to the systemic passage of the hormones (13). The key for the success of this device is represented by an attentive selection of the patient with idiopathic menorrhagia, with the exclusion of cases with other endometrial conditions.

The follow-up realized at distance by email represents an effective personal efficient surveillance, easy to realize at persons with different illness, located in isolated area with access difficulties. The data obtained by this method allow also the real time update of the treatment if necessary.

The results obtained through electronic monitoring are in a statistical significant concordance with the clinic and paraclinic data. The distance follow-up ca is considered an efficient method of surveillance of the therapeutic effect.

V. Conflict of Interest

The authors declare that they have no conflict of interest.

References

1. Rybo G, Anderson K, Odlind V (1993) Hormonal intrauterine devices. Ann Med., 25 (2): 143-147
2. Crosignani PG (2008) Intrauterine devices and intrauterine systems. Human Reproduction Update, 14(3):197–208, DOI 10.1093/humupd/dmn003
3. Sturridge F, Guillebaud J (1996) A risk-benefit assessment of the levonorgestrel-releasing intrauterine system. Drug Safety, 15 (6): 430-440
4. Lethaby A.E, Cooke I, Rees M (2005) Progesterone or progestogen-releasing intrauterine systems for heavy menstrual bleeding. Cochrane Database Syst. Rev, 19 (4), CD002126
5. Milsom I , Andersson K, Andersch B (1991) A comparision of flurbiprofen, tranexamic acid and a levonorgestrel- releasing intrauterine contraceptive device in the treatment of idiopapathic menorrhagia. Am J Obstet Gynecol, 164: 879-883
6. Irvine GA, Campbell-Brown M.B, Lumsden MA (1998) Randomised comparative trial of the levonorgestrel intrauterine system and norethisterone for treatment of idiopapathic menorrhagia. Brit J Obstet Gynaec, 10:. 592-598
7. Lethaby AE, Cooke I., Rees M (2000) Progesterone/progestogen releasing intrauterine systems versus either placebo or any other medication for heavy menstrual bleeding. Cochrane Database Syst Rev., vol 2, CD002126
8. Crosignani PG et al (1997) Levonorgestrel-releasing intrauterine device versus hysteroscopic endometrial resection in the treatment of dysfunctional uterine bleeding", Obstet Gynecol, 90: 257-263
9. Istre O, Trolle B (2001) Treatment of menorrhagian with the levonorgestrel intrauterine system versus endometrial resection, Fertil Steril, 76: 304-309
10. Luukkainen T (2000) The levonorgestrel intrauterine system: therapeutic aspects. Steroids, 65 (10-11): 699-702
11. Luukkainen T (1992) Contraception after thirty-five. Acta Obstet Gyn Scan 71 (3): 169-74
12. Backman T (2004) Benefit-risk assessment of the levonorgestrel intrauterine system in contraception. Drug Safety 27 (15): 1185-204
13. Kriplani A, Singh B M., Las S, Agarwal N. (2007) Efficacy, acceptability and side effects of the levonorgestrel intrauterine system for menorrhagia. Int. J. Gynecol Obstet 97 (3):190-194
14. www.rxlist.com/cg/generic/mirena/htm
15. Wildemeersch D, Rowe P (2004) Assessment of menstrual blood loss in women with ideopathic menorrhagia using the frameless levonorgestrel-releasing intrauterine system. Contraception, 70(2):165-168
16. Cameron IT (2001) The levonorgestrel intrauterine system: the benefits of reduced bleeding. Eur J. Contracept Reprod Health Care, 6 (1):27-32
17. Xiao B. et al (2003) Therapeutic effects of the levonorgestrel-releasing intrauterine system in the treatment of idiopathic menorrhagia. Fertil Steril, 79 (4): 963-969
18. Shaw R.W, Symonds IM, Tamisian Oet al. (2007). Randomised comparative trial of thermal balloon ablation and levonorgestrel intrauterine system in patients with idiopathic menorrhagia. Aust N Z J Obstet Gynecol 47(4):335-340
19. Mansour D (2007) Modern management of abnormal uterine bleeding - the levonorgestrel intra-uterine system. Best Pract Res Clin Obstet Gynecol, 21(6):1007-10021
20. Milson I (2007) The levonorgestrel-releasing intrauterine system as an alternative to hysterectomy in peri-menopausal women. Contraception, 75(6) :S152-154
21. Yazbeck C at al. (2006) Levonorgestrel-releasing intrauterine system in the treatment of dysfunctional uterine bleeding: A French multicenter study. Gynecol Obstet Fertil 34(10): 906-913
22. Martins W.P et al. (2007) Reliability and validity of tissue volume measurement by three-dimensional ultrasound: an experimental model. Ultrasound Obst Gyn, 29(2): 210-214
23. N. Raine-Fenning, B. Campbell, J. Collier, M. Brincat, I. Johnson (2002) The reproducibility of endometrial volume acquisition and measurement with the VOCAL-imaging program. Ultrasound Obst Gyn, 19(1):69-75
24. Odeh M et al. (2007) Three-dimensional endometrial volume and 3-dimensional power Doppler analysis in predicting endometrial carcinoma and hyperplasia. Gynecol Oncol, 106 (2): 348-353

Address of the corresponding author:

Author: D. Muresan
Institute: University of Medicine and Pharmacy "Iuliu Hatieganu"
Street: V. Babes 8
City: Cluj-Napoca
Country: Romania
Email: muresandaniel01@yahoo.com

Evaluation of Self-Measurements for Two Blood Pressure Devices

S. Mirel[1], A.T. Lup[1], L. Colobatiu[1], D. Pop Vornicescu[2], T. Pop[2], V. Mirel[3], and S. Pop[2]

[1] University of Medicine and Pharmacy "Iuliu Hatieganu", Faculty of Pharmacy, Cluj-Napoca, Romania
[2] University of Medicine and Pharmacy "Iuliu Hatieganu", Faculty of Medicine, Cluj-Napoca, Romania
[3] National Institute for Research and Development of Isotopic and Molecular Technologies, Cluj-Napoca

Abstract— **The study is aimed to evaluate and to compare the performance of two different types of blood pressure devices (the wrist and the upper arm monitors) – two models which are more accessible for patients due to their low price. 33 subjects aged 20 to 22 years were included (82% women). Our principal outcome was the mean relative difference for systolic and diastolic blood pressure values (SBP and DBP) measured with the selected monitors: *Flaem Nuova* and *AFK BDM-5B*. Both blood pressure monitors tested were found to be suitable for measuring at home, their performance being acceptable according to the European Society of Hypertension guidelines (considering mean differences of more than 5 mm Hg to be clinically significant). In addition, we investigated the accuracy of measurements in correlation with user's knowledge offered by specific training. The users must be properly instructed in the self-measurement technique.**

Keywords— **blood pressure devices, accuracy, self-measurement, users training**

I. Introduction

Hypertension (HTA) is an important problem of public-health, therefore the prevention, detection, treatment and control of this condition should take priority. The prevalence of hypertension was reported to be around 30–45% of the general population[1] and was predicted to increase by 60% in 2025 [2] - with no significant differences between developed and developing countries [3], but with a steep increase with ageing [4]. 45% of Romanian adult population has HTA 40%, and 75% of them have more than 65 years old [5].

An adequate control of blood pressure (BP) values can predict future cardiovascular events and decreased the risk of mortality due to cardiovascular disease. The blood pressure measurements made in the physician's office have been the standard for diagnosis of hypertension and determination of the efficacy of antihypertensive treatement [6]. Furthermore, the long-term monitoring of a patient with hypertension requires frequent blood pressure controls. In this context, the self-measurement and ambulatory monitoring are complementary to conventional office measurement [7, 8]. Self-measurement of BP may increase compliance with specific therapy and reduce the number of visits required for long term-monitoring, being a less expensive method of monitoring blood [6, 9] Morever, the SMBP allowed identification of patients with white-coat hypertension [8]. According to the European Society of Hypertension - European Society of Cardiology (ESH/ESC) guidelines for the Management of Hypertension, the blood pressure self-measurement (PBSM) at home is known to be a useful clinical tool [1] and is considered a valid method for providing the best-practice recommendations for obtaining the measurements. In this context, valid measurements of blood pressure must be reliable and accurate not only at clinicals and community settings, but also in home environments.

The availability of the home medical devices for blood pressure has considerably increased over the past decade. The home monitors (most of them automated oscillometric BP monitors) are easier to use compared with clinical sphygmomanometers, but it is important to establish their reliability. All devices should be validated according to standardized protocols and requirements concerning the effectiveness, accuracy and safety (for both patients and healthcare professionals). The new international standards [10] describe the requirements for the essential performance of automated non-invasive devices, in addition to recommendations for BP measurement. The upper arm BP devices (fully automated or semi-automated) are preferred over wrist- or finger devices which are currently not well recommended [11]. Moreover, the Internet commerce with this health products increases dramatically, but the sites don't offer a real support for consumer in purchasing a validated automated home blood pressure monitoring [12]. Furthermore, the self-measurement of BP requires appropriate training under medical supervision [13].

II. Experimental

A. Materials and Methods

We examined two blood pressure devices used for self-measurement of blood pressure: an upper arm automatic device (by Flaem Nuova, Italy) and a wrist blood pressure monitor (BDM-5B, AFK, Germany).

33 subjects were recruited from the students of Faculty of Pharmacy UMF Cluj-Napoca (second year of studies), which consent to participate in the study. All subjects had not previously self-measured their blood pressure and had no previously knowledge about devices and measurements

S. Vlad and R.V. Ciupa (eds.), *International Conference on Advancements of Medicine and Health Care through Technology*,
IFMBE Proceedings 44,
DOI: 10.1007/978-3-319-07653-9_16, © Springer International Publishing Switzerland 2014

techniques. Blood pressure was measured - used both self-monitoring devices (upper arm and wrist) – alternatively, in two protocols.

Initially (into the first protocol), the subjects measured their blood pressure following the user's manuals. All subject had 10 minutes to read the manufacturer's instructions.

In the second protocol, the self-measurement of blood pressure was performed after the subjects were trained concerning the correct measurement. All subject had 30 minutes training about preparation, technique and specific equipment (pharmacist) and a practical demonstration (with a practitioner).

In both protocol the measurement was performed under the supervision of the practitioner (medicine) and an observer (pharmacist).

In each case, the blood pressure was measured twice with two -three minutes of difference between each measurement including the time required to move between devices. BP was measured in sitting position (on a chair-supporting their backs and arms), with the legs uncrossed, after a five-minute rest. The left arm and wrist were used for all the measurements and a special attention was given to the position of the monitors - at the level of the heart The measurement points were 8 cm above the elbow joint and 4 cm above the wrist joint [1, 8].

The results were registered, compared and analyzed.

The study protocol has been approved by the Ethical Committee of University of Medicine and Pharmacy "Iuliu Hatieganu", Cluj-Napoca, Romania. The informed consents were obtained from all participants in the study.

Statistical Analysis

Statistical analysis were performed using SPSS software, version 16.0. The values are expressed as mean (SD). Group differences (calculated for systolic and diastolic blood pressure) were assessed with paired Student's t test.

B. Results

We had compared the SBP and BP values registered by two blood pressure devices which are more accessible for patients due to their low price. We had chosen two automated monitors designed for home use: an upper arm monitor (Flaem Nuova, Italy) and a wrist blood pressure monitor (BDM-5B, AFK Germany). Both of them used the oscillometric measurement technique and - according to their manufacturers - both of them are accurate, simple to use: (the one-touch button) and easy to read (large display). The principal characteristics of each device are summarized in table 1.

33 young subjects (mean age 20.2 years, 82% women), untreated by antihypertensive medication were included in our study. Table 2 presents the patients characteristics.

A total of 264 BP measurements (8 measurements per patient and 132 measurements per device) were performed.

Table 3 presents the obtained descriptive data.

The results showed that the average values were similar for SBP, but different for DBP. Thus, the averages of SBP measured by using the upper arm (*Flaem)* and the wrist *(AFK BDM-5B)* devices were similar: 117.5 mmHg (SD 12.8), respectively 116.7 mmHg (SD 10.2). The averages of DBP measured with the *Flaem* upper arm devices were significantly higher than those measured by *AFK BDM-5B* wrist devices: 69.5 mmHg (SD 13.9) respectively 63.6 mmHg (SD 11.4). Also, the averages of pulse values registered with the *Flaem* upper arm devices were higher than those measured by *AFK BDM-5B* wrist devices: 69.5 mmHg (SD 13.9) respectively 63.6 mmHg (SD 11.4).

Table 1 The characteristics of BP devices

Parameters	Devices	
	Flaem Nuova	AFK BDM-5B
Method	oscillometric	oscillometric
Measurements localization	upper arm	wrist
Measurements range	40 to250 mmHg	0 to 299 mmHg
Pressuure sensor	semi conductor	semi conductor
Validated	clinically validated AAMI	no data available
Accuracy	+/-3 mmHg	+/-3 mmHg
Memory function	2 channels with 60 memories for each	3 channels with 33 memories for each
Technology	Real Fuzzy	No data available
Display	LCD digital very large	LCD digital large
Weight	410 g	125 g
Cuff inflation	automatic	automatic
Batteries	4 * 1,5V AA	2* 1,5V AAA
Connection to PC	No	No

Table 2 Patients characteristics

Parameters	Mean
Gender: men: 6 women: 27	
Age (years)	20,2
Arm circumference (mm)	256
Wrist circumfer-ence (mm)	148
SBP (mmHg)	117,1
DBP (mmHg)	67,6

Table 3 The mean systolic and diastolic BP in two protocols

Devices	Parameters	Without training	After training
Flaem Nuova upper-arm	SBP (mmHg)	117.2 (SD 11.7)	118 (SD 13.5)
	DBP (mmHg)	66.2 (SD 14.4)	72.8 (SD 9.8)
AFK BDM-5B wrist	SBP (mmHg)	116.3 mmHg (SD 10.2)	117.1 mmHg (SD 11.5)
	DBP (mmHg)	64.4 mmHg (SD 9.4)	66.8 mmHg (SD 10.8)

On the other hand, it was seen that there are differences regarding the recorded values in the two proposed protocols. Thus, the systolic and diastolic blood pressure obtained in the first protocol (without training) and the second protocol (after training) were similar for wrist devices: 116.3 mmHg (SD 10.2)/ 64.4 mmHg (SD 9.4), respectively and 117.1 mmHg (SD 11.5) / 68.8 mmHg (SD 10.8).

Regarding the *Flaem* upper-arm monitor, there was no significant difference in SBP values (average of 117.5 mmHg (SD 12.8). But the diastolic blood pressure measured in the first protocol was on average lower (5 mmHg) than measurements taken after the specific training.

C. Discusion

It is known that individual blood pressure can vary due to the multiple factors, but when we analyzed the inconsistencies in the measuring of the various blood pressures using different type of home devices, usually we can speak about two factors: device performance (equipment accuracy) and users skills (knowledge and abilities, inadequate performance of measurement technique).

The selection of a blood pressure measuring device may be influenced by many factors (as price), but the most important requirement must be that it gives accurate measurements. First of all, it should be recommended to use only the devices that have been properly validated (even if their price is higher). In our study we used two home BP devices: an upper arm device sold usually in the community pharmacies (50 euro cost) and a wrist device (10 euro cost) bought from supermarket (non-medical field). Both devices used oscillometric method - which is considered to be the standard for automated blood pressure measurements. The method is based on the assumption that the maximal oscillation in the cuff-air pressure detected during deflation corresponds to the mean arterial pressure. Then, the BP values are computed through a specific algorithm, specific for each models and manufacturer [14]. Both devices include an electronic monitor with a pressure sensor, a digital display and an upper arm cuff. An electrically-driven pump raises the pressure in the cuff. We could not establish a relation between the type of device (concerning the localization measurement or commercial price) and the results of self measurements. It must be mentioned that blood pressure level at the wrist is influenced by many factors (angle between hand and fore-arm, hydrostatic pressure [15] which can affect our results. Although, the cheaper wrist-device tested - is not validated using the most widely used protocols (the British Hypertension Society (BHS) protocol and the standard protocols of the US Association for the Advancement of Medical Instrumentation (AAMI), the results was similar with the validated upper arm device (clinically validated AAMI). The small difference between the registered values could be explained by different algorithms use of the two manufacturers.

However, the compliance of users was higher than for upper arm device (the wrist-devices are considered to be much easier to handle). Generally, we assumed that the choice of the devices is often made by the patients and the price and the compliance aspects influence their decision.

Instead, we observe a relation between the correct use of device and the results of self measurements. The measures must be performed according to the conditions recommended by European Society of Hypertension guidelines [1]. The positioning of arm or wrist at heart level during measurement is the most important for the accuracy of BP values.

The inaccuracy in measurements often could occur as a result of human error and can be minimized through a good practice. The users should be instructed on the correct measure of their blood pressure by using the selected devices (how to prepare the measurements and how to operate the device). A short training course should preferably be given in order to obtain an accurate and reproducible result.

A limitation of our study was the fact that no reference sphygmomanometer was used in order to established which device is closest to the real value.

III. Conclusions

Valid measurements of blood pressure, both at clinical and in home environments, are essential for monitoring of hypertensive patients. The blood pressure devices used are available in various types and models, with different technical characteristics (concerning fast measurement, memory, sized cuffs). Our outcome was the mean relative difference for blood pressure values (SBP and DBP) measured with two type of self-monitoring devices. We considered mean differences of more than 5 mm Hg to be clinically significant.

It could be concluded that different devices can give different values. Further research must investigate the accuracy of home blood pressure measurements and the devices that are usually used. The users must be properly instructed in the measurement technique. The choice of devices and the education of patients are important for population monitoring and screening of blood pressure.

Conflict of Interest

The authors declare that they have no conflict of interest.

References

1. Mancia et al. (2013) Guidelines for the management of arterial hypertension: The Task Force for the management of arterial hypertension of the European Society of Hypertension and of the European Society of Cardiology J Hypertension 31:1281–1357 DOI:10.1097/01.hjh.0000431740.32696.cc
2. Kearney PM, Whelton M, Reynolds K, Muntner P, Whelton PK, He J. (2005) Global burden of hypertension: analysis of worldwide data. Lancet 365(9455):217-23
3. Pereira M, Lunet N, Azevedo A, Barros H. (2009) Differences in prevalence, awareness, treatment and control of hypertension between developing and developed countries. J Hypertens. 27(5): 963-75
4. Lewington S, Clarke R, Qizilbash N, Peto R, Collins R. (2002) Prospective studies collaboration. Age-specific relevance of usual blood pressure to vascular mortality: a meta-analysis of individual data for one million adults in 61 prospective studies. Lancet 360:1903-13
5. Dorobanţu M, Darabont R. O., Bădilă E. et al. (2006) Studiu de Prevalenţă a Hipertensiunii Arteriale şi evaluare a riscului cardiovascular în România. (2006) Rev. Rom. Cardiol., 2006; vol. XXI; 30-95
6. Staessen JA, Den Hond E, Celis H, et al. (2004) Antihypertensive treatment based on blood pressure measurement at home or in the physician's office: a randomized controlled trial. JAMA 291(8):955-64
7. Wagner S, Toftegaard T S, Bertelsen O W (2012) Challenges in Blood Pressure Self-Measurement, Int J Telemed Appl. 437350: DOI:10.1155/2012/437350
8. Celis H, Den Hond E, Staessen J A (2005), Self-Measurement of Blood Pressure at Home in the Management of Hypertension, Clinical Medicine Research. 3, 1: 19-26
9. Appel LJ, Stason WB (1993) Ambulatory blood pressure monitoring and blood pressure self-measurement in the diagnosis and management of hypertension. Ann Intern Med. 1, 118 (11):867-882
10. http://www.aami.org/publications/homehealthcare/articles/BehindTech.BPstandard.pdf
11. Lopez LM, Taylor JR.(2004), Home blood pressure monitoring: point-of-care testing. Ann Pharmacother 38(5):868-73
12. Graves JW (2005) A survey of validated automated home blood pressure monitors available for the Internet shopper, Blood Press Monit. 10 (2):103-7. at http://www.ncbi.nlm.nih.gov/pubmed/15812259
13. Campbell NR, Milkovich L, Burgess E, McKay DW (2001) Self-measurement of blood pressure: accuracy, patient preparation for readings, technique and equipment. Blood Press Monit. 6 (3):133-8
14. Braam RL, Th. Thien (2003) Home blood pressure measurement with oscillometric upper-arm devices. Neth J Med 61(10):307-312
15. Braam RL, Aslan B, Thien Th (2003) Oscillometric wrist blood pressure measuring devices, Neth J Med 61(10):313-317

Author: Mirel Simona
Institute: UMF Cluj-Napoca
Street: N. Pascaly 9
City: Cluj Napoca
Country: Romania
Email: smirel@umfcluj.ro

Real-Time System for Continuous and Remote Monitoring of Respiration during Sleep Using Wireless Sensors Networks

C. Rotariu[1], H. Costin[1,2], R. Ciobotariu[3], Al. Păsărică[1], and C. Cristea[1]

[1] Grigore T. Popa University of Medicine and Pharmacy, Faculty of Medical Bioengineering, Iasi, Romania
[2] The Institute of Computer Science, Romanian Academy – Iasi Branch, Romania
[3] Gheorghe Asachi Technical University of Iasi, Faculty of Electrical Engineering, Iasi, Romania

Abstract— **Sleep represents a dynamic physiological process having an important role in the restoration of the central nervous system. Nowadays, because a significant part of the population suffers of sleep disorders, the dynamic long time continuous monitoring of human respiration has an important role in diagnosis and treatment. This paper proposes a flexible, scalable and cost-effective integrated system for respiration frequency monitoring during sleep. The described system may be used to monitor especially patients suffering from obstructive sleep apnea episodes, within healthcare institutes or their homes, with a degree of accuracy similar to the most expansive commercial systems. Usually the long time continuous monitoring requires the use of sensors attached by wires to the medical devices, but they are very uncomfortable for patient during sleep. As an alternative, the patient's respiration frequency is continuously measured by using wireless sensor nodes and then transferred to a central monitoring station via a wireless sensor network. The sensor nodes use devices based on the impedance pneumography technique to measure the patient respiration frequency connected to wireless modules. On the central monitoring station a software application receives the patient's respiration frequency from wireless sensors network, displays it on its graphical user interface and activates the alerts in interface when obstructive sleep apnea episodes are detected. A prototype of the described system has been developed, implemented and tested.**

Keywords— **impedance pneumography, remote monitoring system, sleep disorders, wireless sensor networks**

I. INTRODUCTION

According to American Academy of Sleep Medicine approximately 20% of the population in modern societies suffers from sleep disorders. In these conditions the continuous long time monitoring of human respiration plays an important role in diagnosis and treatment for a number of medical conditions requiring circadian rhythm analysis, sleep related breathing disorder, or sudden death syndrome.

Usually the sleep monitoring represents a method widely used in the diagnosis of obstructive sleep apnea (OSA). OSA is a sleep related breathing disorder characterized by pauses in breathing, longer than 10 seconds, due to collapse of the upper airway, and with a prevalence of approximately 5% in the adult population. Due to increasing occurrence of OSA, there is a need to provide long time continuous patient monitoring services. The monitoring of human respiration may be performed at a variety of environments, within healthcare institutions or their home, during overnight with many electrodes and sensors attached to patient that collect a number of physiological signals including brain and heart signals, patient motion, respiratory frequency, or blood oxygen saturation.

Respiratory frequency (RF) is a vital physiological parameter, along with heart rate, oxygen saturation, blood pressure, and temperature. It is widely used in sleep monitoring systems because allows an assessment of the condition of OSA, the respiratory frequency and its fluctuations can be recorded promptly, and pauses in respiration can be easily detected.

Traditionally, the most used sleep monitoring systems include devices for respiratory frequency measurements having sensors attached to the patient by electrical wires. For example, some monitoring methods of the respiratory activity use thermistor based sensors [1], others use piezoelectric elastic bands connected across the thorax [2], microwave radars [3], or respiratory inductive plethysmography [4]. Other methods detect the respiratory signal from the low frequency variations of ECG waveform [5]. All these situations, although acceptable for shorter periods of time, involve sensors attached on patient, connected by unwieldy wires to monitoring devices that are not very comfortable for patient. In order to avoid this situation, we decided to use wireless devices.

II. MATERIALS AND METHODS

An overall view of the proposed continuous remote monitoring system (Fig.1) for sleep disorders consists of the following components: a) a wireless sensor network (WSN) used to measure RF from the patient during sleep; each Sensor Node is a wireless device attached on patient's chest; b) several repeater nodes distributed in WSN at fixed location; c) a central monitoring station running a patient RF patient monitor application.

S. Vlad and R.V. Ciupa (eds.), *International Conference on Advancements of Medicine and Health Care through Technology*, IFMBE Proceedings 44,
DOI: 10.1007/978-3-319-07653-9_17, © Springer International Publishing Switzerland 2014

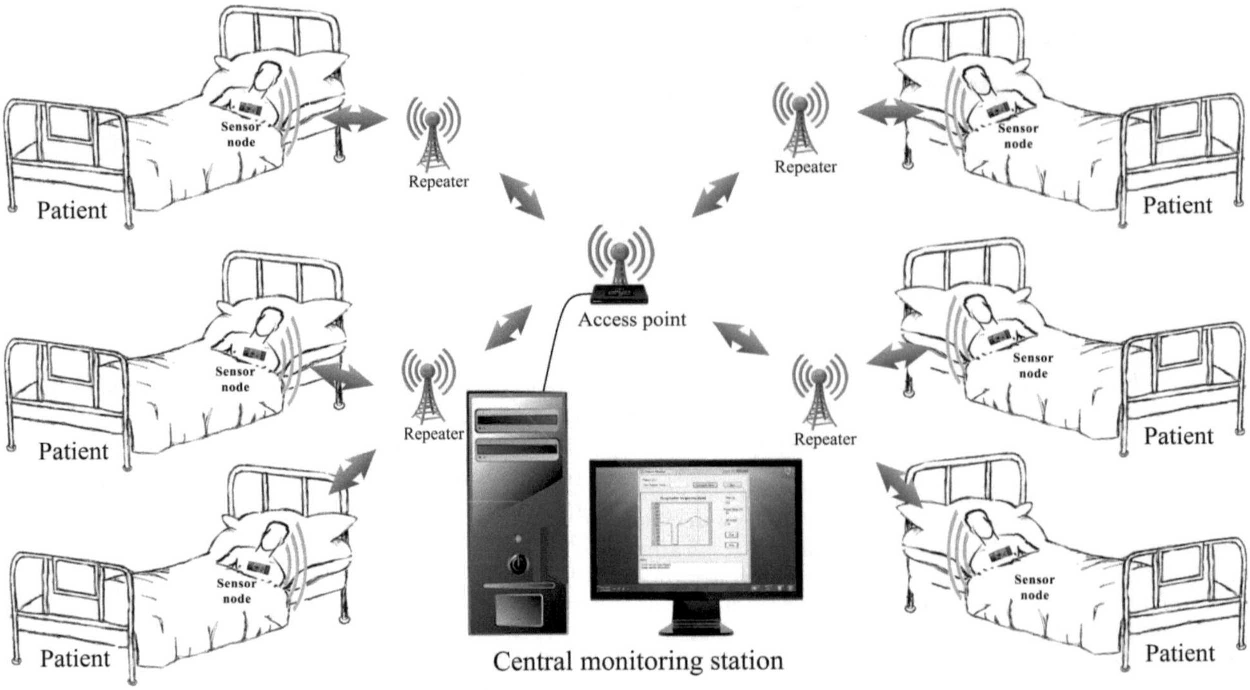

Fig. 1 Real-time continuous remote monitoring system for sleep disorders – network architecture

Each sensor node (Fig. 2) contains a custom developed acquisition board based on AD5933 Impedance Converter (Analog Devices) connected to an eZ430RF2500 module (Texas Instruments).

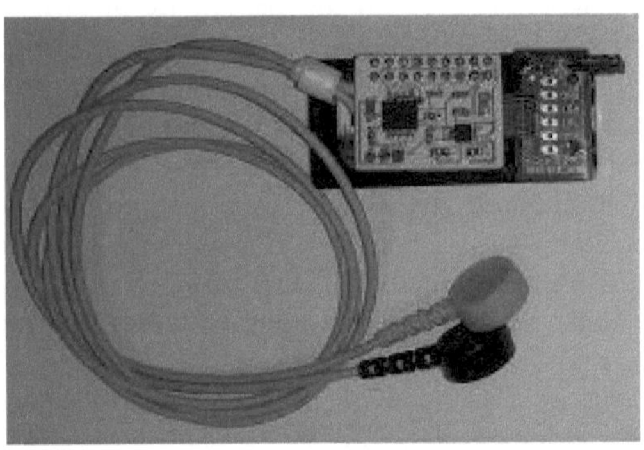

Fig. 2 Sensor Node - prototype

The eZ430RF2500 module is a small wireless radio development kit (Texas Instruments) based on the MSP430F2274 microcontroller and CC2500 wireless transceiver. It provides all the necessary hardware and software tools to evaluate the MSP430F2274 microcontroller and CC2500 2.4 GHz wireless transceiver. The applications can be easily developed using IAR Embedded Workbench Integrated Development Environment or Code Composer Essentials. The eZ430RF2500 module has a limited indoor/outdoor communication range (10/50 m line-of-sight for reliable data transfer) and for this reason necessitates repeaters to send the result of measurement to the central monitoring station.

The power consumption of each Sensor Nodes is an important characteristic of the WSNs having battery powered nodes [6]. For this reason we carefully chose for the proposed solution, low power circuits.

The AD5933 is used to measure variations in the electrical impedance of the patient's thorax caused by respiration. Impedance pneumography is a commonly used technique to measure a patient's respiration frequency by means of either two electrodes (as we used – Fig. 3) or four electrodes.

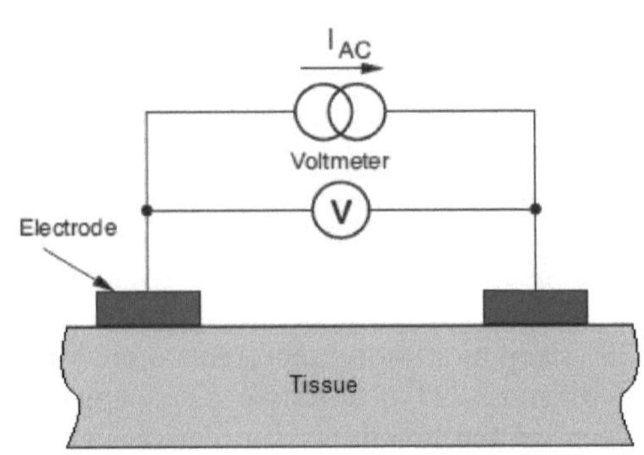

Fig. 3 Impedance pneumography using two electrodes

The AD5933 is a high precision impedance converter that can accurately measure a range of impedance values with an error rate less than 0.5%, measured with a 12-bit resolution and sampled with 1 MSPS. The AD5933 is connected to the MSP430F2274 using the standard I2C lines, as it is represented in Fig. 4.

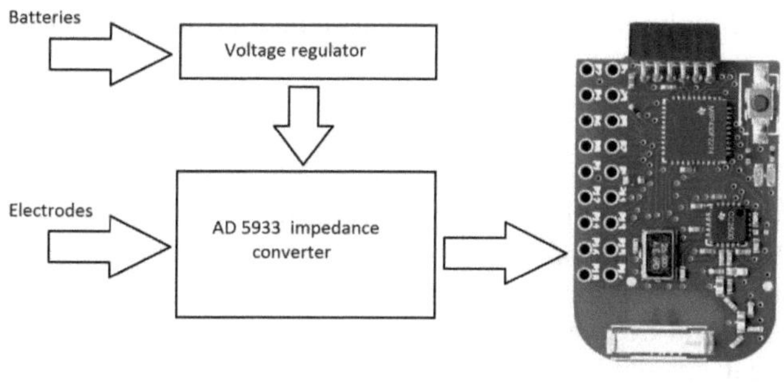

Fig. 4 Sensor Node - schematic

The AD5933 is powered at 3.3 V through a voltage regulator, implemented with TPS60240 (Texas Instruments). The TPS60240 is a switched capacitor voltage converter used for input supply voltage range of 1.8V up to 5.5V.

For the applications running on central monitoring station a very user-friendly Graphical User Interface (GUI) was developed by means of LabWindows/CVI programming environment (National Instruments – Fig. 5).

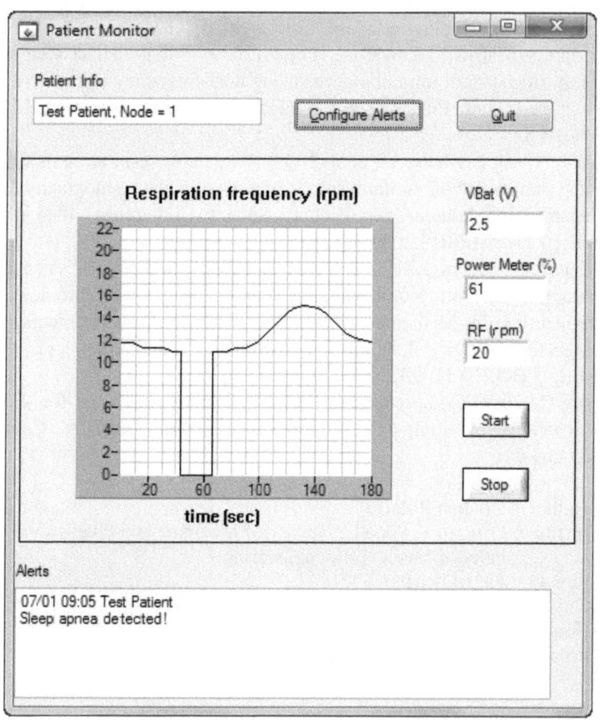

Fig. 5 Central monitoring station GUI

It is used to display the temporal waveform of the respiration frequency (RF) for monitored patient and several other status parameters of the Sensor Node (the battery voltage and the received signal strength indication, measured on the power present in the received radio signal, RSSI).

III. Results

The prototype of the continuous remote respiration system for sleep monitoring, as it was described above, has been implemented and tested.

The accuracy of measurements for RF test was performed by using the PNEUMOTRACE respiration transducer connected to a similar eZ430RF2500 wireless module, as it is represented in Fig. 6. The PNEUMOTRACE is a sturdy piezo-electric respiration transducer that generates a substantial, linear signal in response to changes in thoracic circumference associated with respiration.

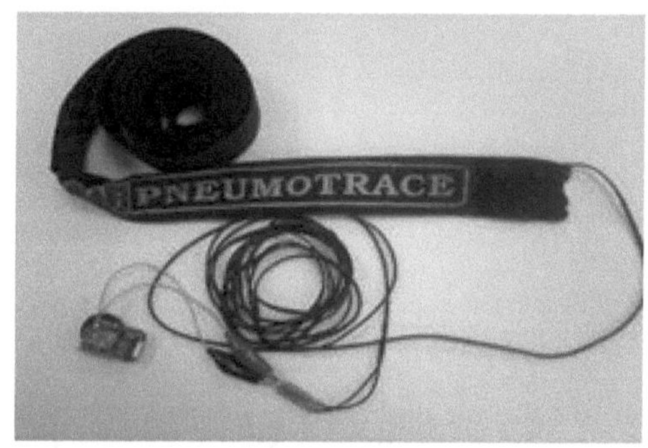

Fig. 6 PNEUMOTRACE chest belt connected to eZ430RF2500

The respiratory signal acquired using impedance pneumography is similar to the signal acquired using a standard respiration transducer, as it is presented in Fig. 7. The RF was computed by first filtering the raw respiratory signal with a moving average window of 21 samples and then applying an adaptive threshold based detection method. We tested the impedance transducer on 10 patients during sleep and the results show that the obtained accuracy of the RF, expressed by the formula

$$Acc = (TP + TN) / (TP + FP + TN + FN) \quad (1)$$

varied between 93.7% (subject no. 3) and 96.3% (subject no. 4), with respect to measurements made by means of PNEUMOTRACE chest belt took as reference. In (1) TP, TN, FP and FN mean true positive, true negative, false positive and false negative measurements, respectively. The recordings of the respiration signal lasted 10 minutes each.

We used the SimpliciTi protocol (Texas Instruments) to forward data from Sensor Node to central monitoring station through WSN. SimpliciTI is a small wireless protocol and has as features low memory needs, advanced network control, sleeping modes support. The sampling frequency of the respiratory signal was 10 Hz and data transmission rate between the ED and AP through RE was set at one transmission per second.

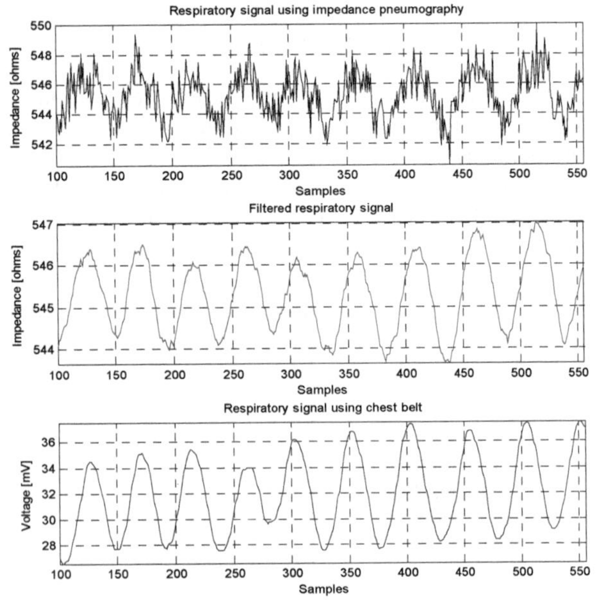

Fig. 7 Respiratory signals - impedance pneumography vs. PNEUMOTRACE respiration transducer (chest belt)

In order to compute and analyze the average current consumption profile of the Sensor Node, we used a simple hardware configuration. The current profile was acquired across a 5 Ω resistor, and then the integral of the voltage curve on it was computed. In this way we obtained an average current of 17 mA. To calculate the battery life expectancy of the Sensor Node we assumed that batteries still maintain their voltage ideally until their capacity (1250 mAh) is exhausted, and we obtained a value of 73.5 hours.

IV. Conclusions

A prototype of a flexible, scalable and cost-effective medical remote monitoring system for the detection of sleep-related disorders has been developed, implemented and tested.

The system is suitable for continuous long-time monitoring of human respiration for a number of medical conditions requiring analysis of respiratory rhythm, sleep-related respiration disorder, especially obstructive sleep apnea.

The described continuous remote respiration system for sleep monitoring allows persons with respiration diseases or elderly people to be monitored within their homes, as an alternative to medical supervision in healthcare institutions.

Conflict of Interest

The authors declare that they have no conflict of interest.

Statement of Human Rights

The proposed respiration sensors are absolutely safe for human being, as maximum working voltages do not exceed 5 V, applied on skin. Also, the informed consent has been obtained from the used subjects. Moreover, the prototype design and experimental set up were in accordance with the ethical standards of the responsible committee on human experimentation (institutional and national) and with the Helsinki Declaration of 1975, as revised in 2000 and 2008.

References

1. Jovanov E, Raskovic D, Hormigo R (2001) Thermistor-based breathing sensor for circadian rhythm evaluation, Proc. of the 38th Annual Rocky Mountain Bioengineering Symp., RMBS 2001, Copper Mountain Conference.
2. Ciobotariu R, Rotariu C, Adochiei F, and Costin H (2011) Wireless breathing system for long term telemonitoring of respiratory activity, Proc. of the 7th Int. Symp. on Advanced Topics in Electrical Engineering, University "Politehnica" of Bucharest, 635-638
3. Suzuki S, Matsui T, Kawahara H et.al (2009) A non-contact vital sign monitoring system for ambulances using dual-frequency microwave radars, Med. Biol. Eng. Comput. 47(1):101–105, DOI:10.1007/s11517-008-0408-x
4. Wu D, Wang L, Zhang YT et.al (2009) A wearable respiration monitoring system based on digital respiratory inductive plethysmography, Engineering in Medicine and Biology Society Conference, 4844–4847 DOI:10.1109/IEMBS.2009.5332665
5. Cerutti S, Bianchi AM, and Reiter H (2006) Analysis of sleep and stress profiles from biomedical signal processing in wearable devices, Engineering in Medicine and Biology Society 2006 Conference - EMBS'06. 28th Annual International Conference of the IEEE, DOI:10.1109/IEMBS.2006.260885
6. Tang C (2014) Comprehensive Energy Efficient Algorithm for WSN, International Journal of Computers, Communications & Control 9(2):209-216

Author: Cristian Rotariu
Institute: Grigore T. Popa University of Medicine and Pharmacy, Faculty of Medical Bioengineering
Street: Kogalniceanu 9-13
City: Iasi,
Country: Romania
Email: cristian.rotariu@bioinginerie.ro

Didactic Application for Monitoring Biomedical Parameters and Data Transfer over the Network Using Virtual Instrumentation

R. Munteanu jr.[1], C. Mureşan[1], D. Iudean[1], M. Munteanu[1], and B. Amza[2]

[1] Faculty of Electric Engineering, Technical University of Cluj-Napoca, Cluj-Napoca, Romania
[2] "Iuliu Haţieganu" University of Medicine and Pharmacy, Cluj-Napoca, Romania

Abstract— **Telemedicine is used on a large scale for monitoring the state of a patient and permits the real-time contact between the doctor and the patient. The software applications and the TCP/IP protocols, combined with the data acquisition techniques, allow the doctors and engineers to cooperate towards reliable medical equipment and solutions.**

This paper presents an application for monitoring two patients by a doctor, in laboratory conditions. The doctor is sending a request to connect to the server application, and selects the patient he wants to monitor. All the application was developed in LabVIEW. As future perspective, the application can be developed quite easily for monitoring the biological parameters as a didactic platform used by students in laboratory condition.

Keywords— **Telemedicine, client-server, TCP/IP, LabVIEW**

I. INTRODUCTION

Nowadays, medical engineering brings more useful technological solutions towards the health of the people. Telemedicine is used on a large scale for monitoring the state of a patient and permits the real-time contact between the doctor and the patient. At the same time, the real-time monitoring of a patient offers better chances to get immediate specialized medical care.

The software applications and the TCP/IP protocols, combined with the data acquisition techniques, allow the doctors and engineers to cooperate towards reliable medical equipment and solutions. These solutions could be used simultaneously in clinics and at home, in order to assure a better surveillance of the patient and a quicker response and act time of the doctor. Thus, by laboratory application, the students could be easily familiarized with such techniques.

Modern medical equipment uses communication networks based on TCP/IP suite of network and transport protocols, elements which are used in the present application.[4]

Transmission Control Protocol and Internet Protocol are at level 4 and level 3, respectively, on the Open Systems Interconnection reference model. As mentioned above, the present application is using only the TCP/IP model, and not the OSI model. Figure 1 shows the differences between the two reference models used in data communication [1],[5].

Internet protocol (IP) is a level 3 network protocol (OSI model) and at internet level in TCP/IP model. It is responsible with addressing information (data packages) between terminals and manages the information fragmentation and reassembly, respectively.

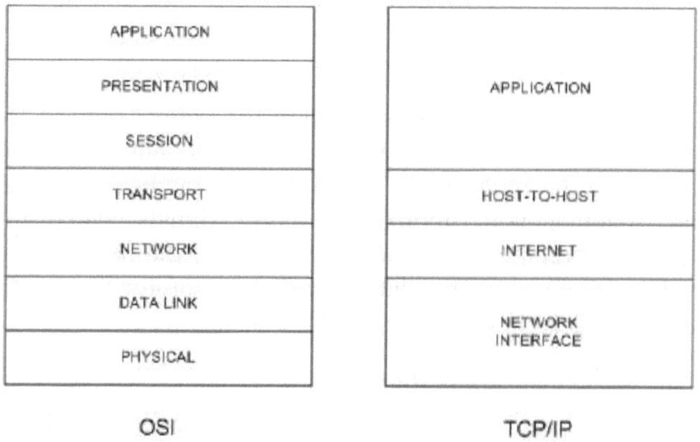

Fig. 1 Reference models used in data communication

Transmission Control Protocol (TCP) corresponds to level Transport, both in OSI and TCP/IP reference models. It provides to the higher levels and to applications a considerable number of transport and control services regarding the information transfer errors.

II. EXPERIMENTAL APPLICATION

The application presented in the paper is didactical and simulates the monitoring of two patients by a "lab doctor". The application is developed in laboratory conditions.

A server application runs on the patient's computer (the same computer for both patients), and a client application runs on the doctor's computer. The doctor is sending a request to connect to the server application, and selects the patient he wants to monitor. All the application was developed in LabVIEW (simulation of medical signals from the server, data transmission) [6],[8].

S. Vlad and R.V. Ciupa (eds.), *International Conference on Advancements of Medicine and Health Care through Technology*, IFMBE Proceedings 44,
DOI: 10.1007/978-3-319-07653-9_18, © Springer International Publishing Switzerland 2014

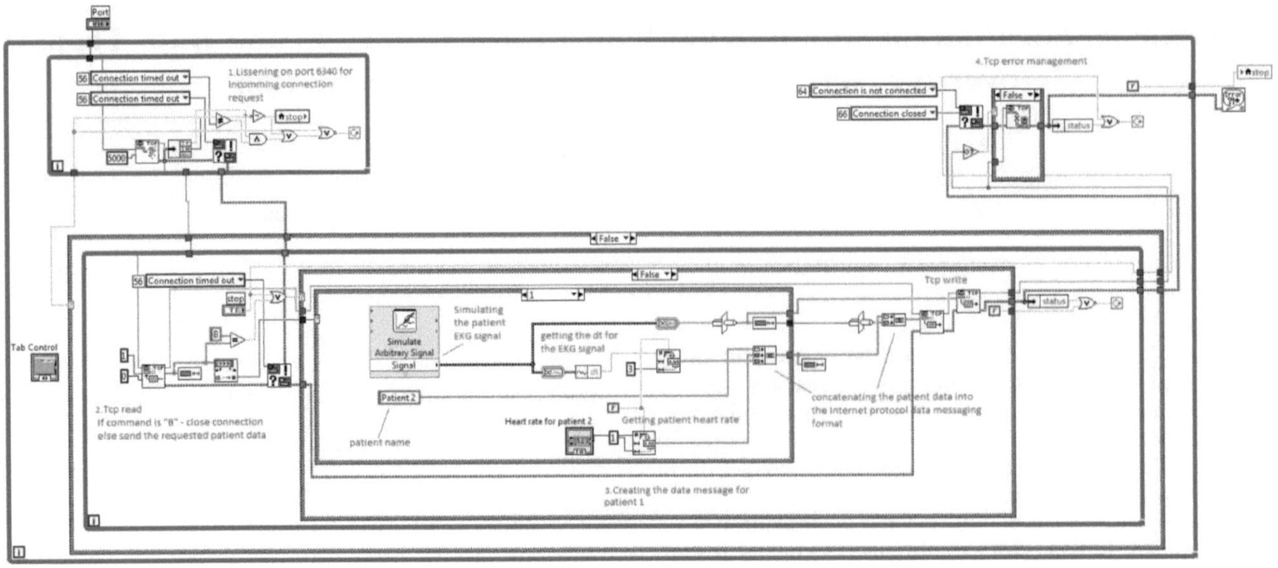

Fig. 2 The server's application LabVIEW Diagram

The server application is listening for a client request for monitoring patient number 1 or patient number 2, is processing the request and is sending the medical information, together with appropriate alarm signals, when the biological parameters of the patient exceed the normal limits. In such manner, the "lab doctor" can monitor the condition of the patient at any moment it considers.

A. Server-Client Application

The applications were realized in LabVIEW and are based on the TCP/IP reference model. The server's application LabVIEW Diagram and the client's application LabVIEW diagram are shown in Figure 2 and Figure 4, respectively. The block diagram of the applications is shown in Figure 3. The applications have the server-client form. The client is initiating the communication, and the server is providing the data [2],[3].

The server uses the TCP Listen subVI from LabVIEW in order to receive any TCP/IP connection request. The port 6340 is used for identifying the request at the transport protocol level (TCP). When the client application sends a connection request on the IP address of the server application (10.128.3.1), a client-server connection between the two terminals is established.

This consists of:

1. The "listening" structure for connection requests on port 6340 and for connection establishment with the client application.
2. The structure for receiving the data inquiry command regarding a certain patient, or the command to interrupt the connection.
3. The structure responsible for creating the message and for transmitting it.
4. Error management structure.

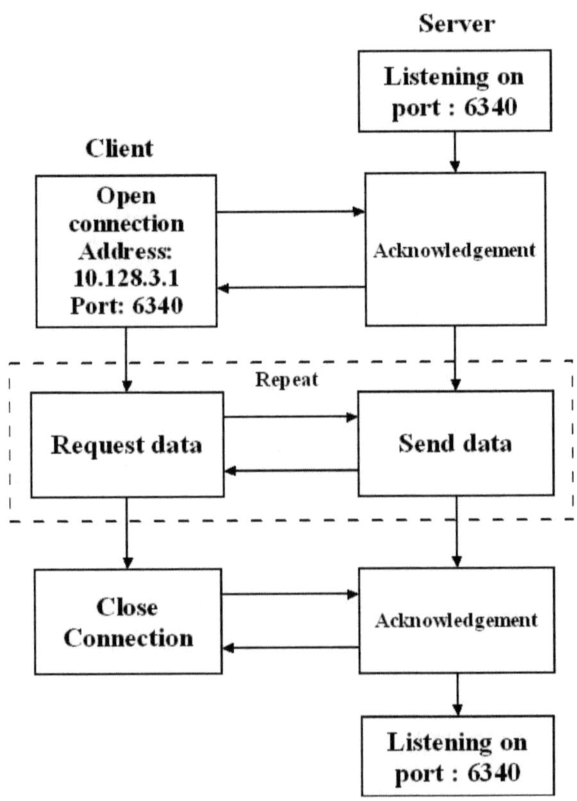

Fig. 3 Block diagram of the client-server applications

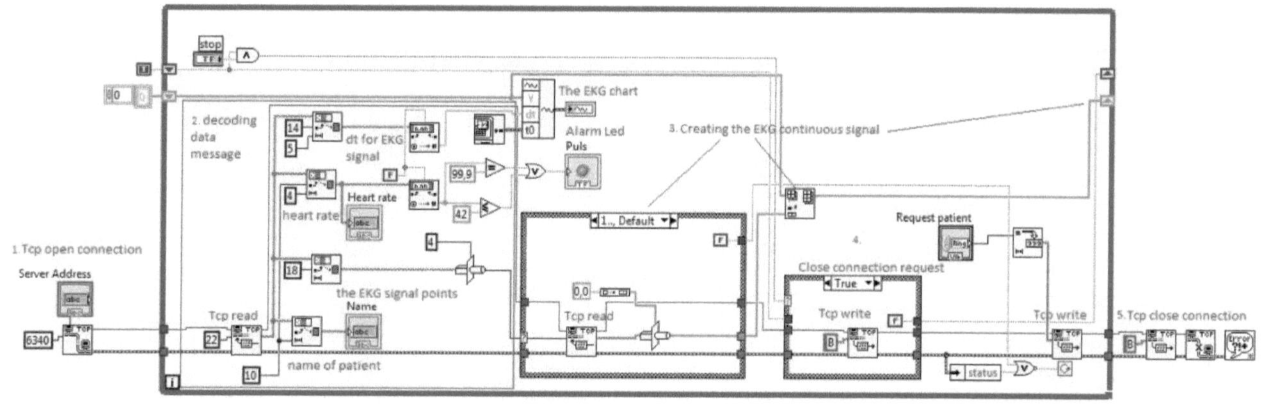

Fig. 4 The client's application LabVIEW diagram

	Time	Source	Destination	Protocol	Length	Info	
1	0.00000000	192.168.120.6	10.128.3.1	TCP	66	49380 > 6340 [SYN] Seq=0 Win=8192 Len=0 MSS=1460 WS=4 SACK_PERM=1	1. open connection ip:10.128.3.1 (sent SYN bit)
2	0.00387100	10.128.3.1	192.168.120.6	TCP	66	6340 > 49380 [SYN, ACK] Seq=0 Ack=1 Win=8192 Len=0 MSS=1460 WS=256 SACK_PERM=1	2. Aknowledgement received (SYN bit received)
3	0.00396700	192.168.120.6	10.128.3.1	TCP	54	49380 > 6340 [ACK] Seq=1 Ack=1 Win=65700 Len=0	3. Aknowledgement sent , Ok for push data
4	0.00687500	10.128.3.1	192.168.120.6	TCP	76	6340 > 49380 [PSH, ACK] Seq=1 Ack=1 Win=65536 Len=22	4. Patient data received
5	0.20947600	192.168.120.6	10.128.3.1	TCP	54	49380 > 6340 [ACK] Seq=1 Ack=23 Win=65676 Len=0	5. Aknowledgement for patient data sent
6	0.21064800	10.128.3.1	192.168.120.6	TCP	662	6340 > 49380 [PSH, ACK] Seq=23 Ack=1 Win=65536 Len=608	6. Patient data received
7	0.21099100	192.168.120.6	10.128.3.1	TCP	55	49380 > 6340 [PSH, ACK] Seq=1 Ack=631 Win=65068 Len=1	7. Aknowledgement for patient data sent , and request for patient 2 data sent
8	0.21651200	10.128.3.1	192.168.120.6	TCP	76	6340 > 49380 [PSH, ACK] Seq=631 Ack=2 Win=65536 Len=22	8. Patient 2 data received

Fig. 5 The TCP/IP messages transmitted in the client-server connection

The next step is the data transfer: the server application processes a request and provides the data, due to the client request. The data request and receiving will be presented in detail in the next paragraph.

This consist of:

1. TCP open connection – the subVI which sends the open connection request.
2. The message decoding sequence. In this structure, the message is decoded in order to display the data for the desired patient.
3. The structure for recomposing the EKG signal.
4. The structure where the connection interruption request is generated, and also the request for information regarding a certain patient.
5. TCP close connection – the subVI which closes the connection.

To close the connection, the client application sends a request, and the server application sends a confirmation, then enters in „listening" mode – waiting for a new connection request. The interrupt request connection is realized using the *TCP Close Connection* subVI.

The TCP/IP messages transmitted in the client-server connection are presented in Figure 5.

1. The client application sends a connection request to the server application.
2. The server application sends the confirmation for the connection request, and the connection between the two applications is established.
3. The client sends the confirmations message and sends a message stating that data transmission can be started.
4. The patient data is received.
5. The client transmits the confirmation message.
6. The patient data is received.
7. The client confirms receiving the data and makes a request for transmitting the data for the second patient.
8. Data for the second patient are received.

B. Data Transfer

Data transfer is realized as shown in the block diagram from Figure 6 [3]. The client application uses the *TCP write* subVI, transmitting the requested patient id number, and the server application reads and processes these data, using the *TCP read* subVI. The server application provides the requested data to the client application using again the *TCP write* subVI.

The EKG signal was simulated and saved in a file, using a LabVIEW subVI. The server application reads the EKG signal from file using the *Simulate Arbitrary Signal* subVI and is transmitted to the client application. The reading is continuous and cyclic [7],[9].

Transmission is done in two sequences. The first transmission stage (sequence 1) contains data regarding the patient name, heart rate and two pieces of information regarding the EKG signal's structure – the signal's *"dt"* and signal's samples data type (byte, word, double word).

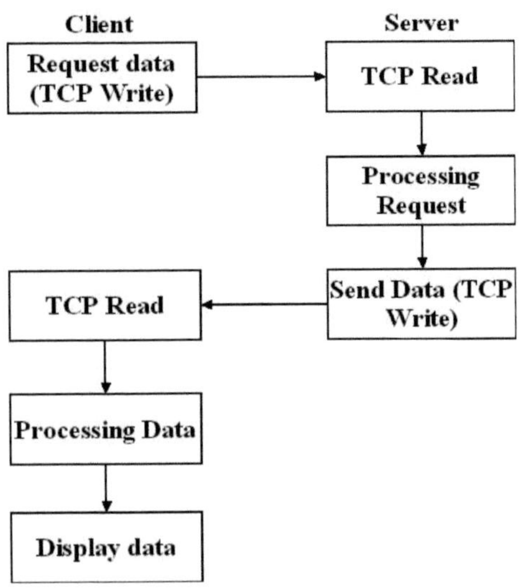

Fig. 6 Block diagram of the data transfer

The type for the data transmitted with TCP/IP must be *string,* hence the heart rate, *dt*, and data type must be converted from a numeric format in a string format using the "fraction number to string" subVI. Afterwards, these four pieces of information in string format are concatenated in a single string, using the "concatenate string" function, following to be transmitted further in *sequence 1.*

The second transmission stage contains only the EKG signal's samples. The data has to be converted in string format as well, and are transmitted afterwards to the client application in *sequence 2.*

Figure 7 shows the block diagram for the message to be sent.

The client application receives the data using the *TCP read* subVI and processes in order to display these information and to activate alarms on critically conditions, respectively. The received data and the alarms are displayed on the front panel of the client application.

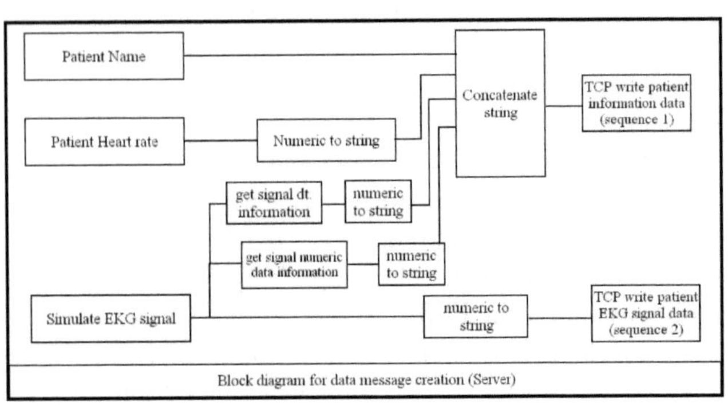

Fig. 7 The block diagram for the message to be sent

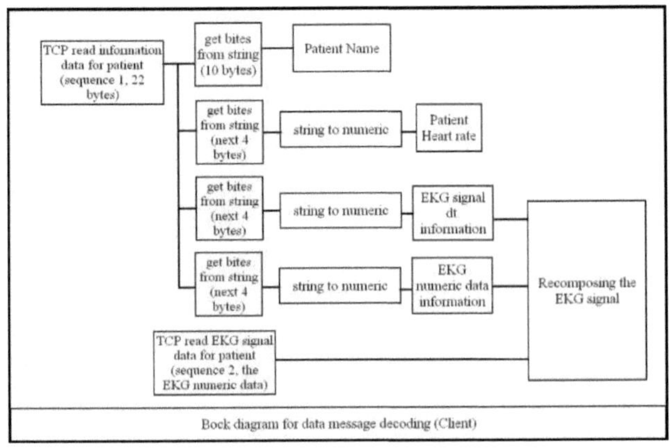

Fig. 8 The block diagram for the message decoding in the client application

The received data message is decoded in the client application in order to be displayed. In the first sequence, the data string (22 bytes) is received, which contains the patient's name (10 bytes), the patient's heart rate (4 bytes), the EKG signal's *dt* (4 bytes) and the information regarding the EKG signal's samples data type (4 byte). These pieces of information are extracted from the received message using the "get substring from string" VI. Afterwards, the heart rate, *dt* and data type are transformed in numeric format using the "string to fraction number" VI.

The block diagram for the message decoding in the client application is shown in Figure 8.

C. Displaying Results

The results provided by the server application displayed in the front panel of the client application are the EKG and the heart-rate of the patients. The heart-rate of each patient is simulated in the server application by numerical controls [7],[8].

The front panel of the client application displays the following information:

- menu for selecting the patient the "lab doctor" wants to monitor;
- patient's name;
- EKG and heart-rate of the patient;
- color indicator about the patient's condition – green if the monitored biological parameters are inside the normal limits or red if these parameters are outside the normal limits, signalizing a critical condition;
- IP address corresponding to server application's terminal (10.128.3.1);
- STOP button for closing the connection to server application.

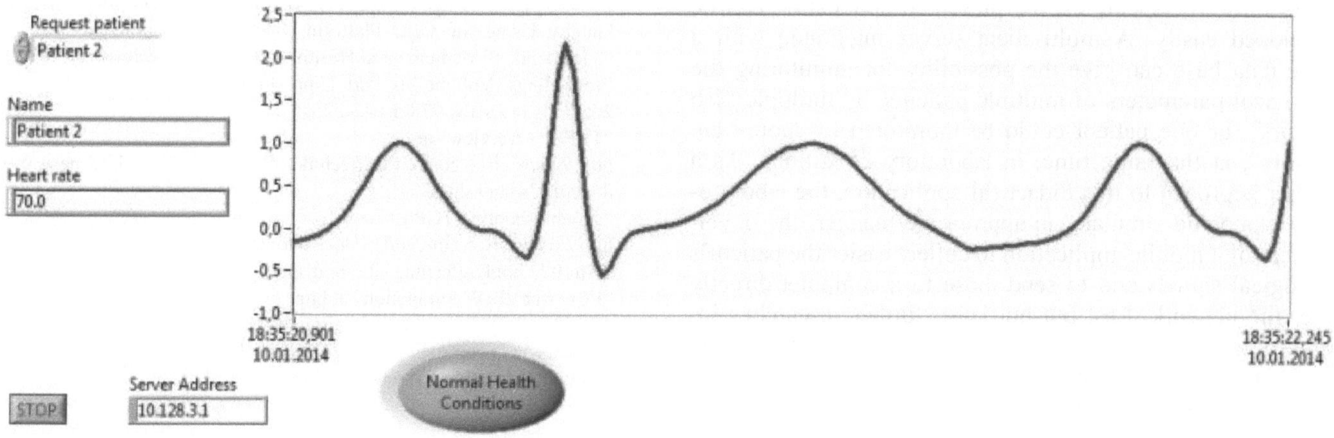

Fig. 9 Monitoring a patient in normal condition

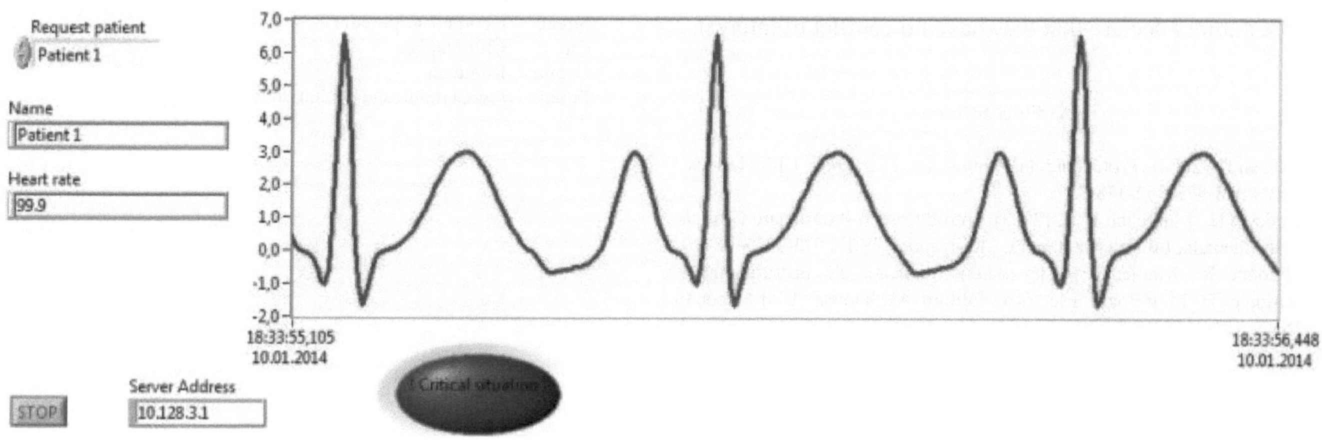

Fig. 10 Monitoring a patient in critical condition

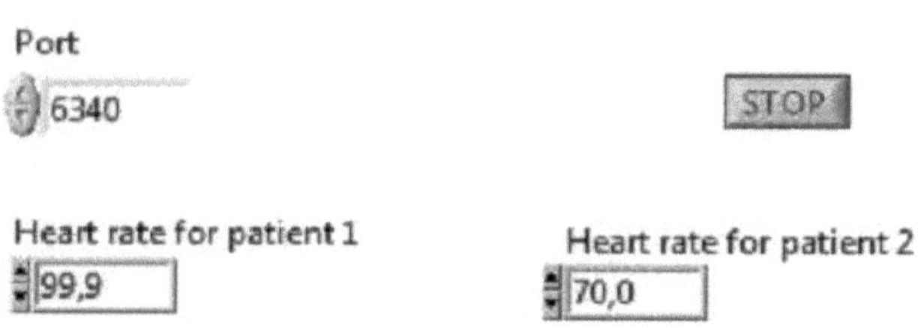

Fig. 11 Front panel of the server application

Figure 9 illustrates the case of monitoring a patient in normal condition, while Figure 10 shows the case of a patient in critical condition (accelerate heart-rate).

For the laboratory application, the front panel of the server application displays both heart rates of the two patients, the "listening" port for a connection request (6340) and a STOP button.

Figure 11 shows the front panel of the server application.

III. Conclusions

The paper presents a laboratory application for monitoring two patients (situated at the same location) by a "lab doctor". The data transmission is of type client-server and is based on the TCP/IP reference model. The applications were realized in LabVIEW, which brings the advantages of virtual instrumentation and gives an increased flexibility and reconfigurability to the application. In such manner, the "lab doctor" can monitor his patients, providing them a better response and act time, thus a better medical care. The application is a good example for the students, in order to get familiarized with real-time events.

The virtual instrumentation combined with the reliability of the internet data transmission give the possibility of the specialized medical personnel to be a discrete presence in the life of the patient, without interfering more than necessarily. At the same time, the patient could be more relaxed, knowing that his condition is under specialized control.

As future perspectives, the presented application can be developed easily. A multi-client server integrated with a large data base can give the possibility for monitoring the biological parameters of multiple patients, by multiple "lab doctors", or one patient could be monitored by more "lab doctors", at the same time, in laboratory conditions. As a further approach to this didactical application, the laboratory works could simulate, in appropriate manner, the development of a mobile application to collect easier the patient's biological signals and to send those to a computer/directly over the network. Last but not least, further researches intend to determine specific monitoring and data transmission applications, depending on specific biological parameters and medical demands, suitable for students.

Conflict of Interest

The authors declare that they have no conflict of interest.

References

1. Dragan F. (2008)- Protocoale de comunicatie, U.T. Press, Cluj-Napoca, ISBN 978-973-662-378-3.
2. Hedeşiu H., Munteanu R. jr. (2003) –Introducere în Programare Grafică Instrumentală, Editura Mediamira, Cluj-Napoca, ISBN 973-9357-48-2.
3. Holonec R., Munteanu R. jr. (2003)– Aplicaţii ale Instrumentaţiei Virtuale în Metrologie Electrică, Editura Mediamira, Cluj-Napoca, ISBN 973-9357-31-8.
4. Zaharia V.D., Drăgan F.,(2011) Monitoring System for a Medical Facility Using the OPC Platform; International Conference on Advancements of Medicine and Health Care through Technology, IFMBE Proceedings, Volume 36, Part 1, pp. 44-47, DOI: 10.1007/978-3-642-22586-4_11 ISBN: 978-3-642-22585-7
5. "TCP/IP Overview" at http://www.cisco.com/en/US/tech/tk365/technologies_white_paper09186a008014f8a9.shtml
6. "Troubleshooting TCP/IP" at http://www.cisco.com/en/US/docs/internetworking/troubleshooting/guide/tr1907.html?referring_site=bodynav
7. "ECG LabVIEW Simulation" at http://www.ni.com/example/31189/en/
8. "Basic TCP/IP Communication in LabVIEW" at http://www.ni.com/white-paper/2710/en/
9. National Instruments at www.ni.com

Author: Radu MUNTEANU jr.
Institute: Faculty of Electric Engineering, Technical University of Cluj-Napoca
Street: George Bariţiu 26
City: Cluj-Napoca
Country: Romania
Email: radu.a.munteanu@ethm.utcluj.ro

Low-Cost Platform for Remote Health Monitoring and Home Environment Analysis

V. Tompa, D. Hurgoiu, and C. Neamțu

Technical University of Cluj-Napoca, Design Engineering and Robotics Department, Cluj-Napoca, Romania

Abstract— **This paper aims to purpose an open, low-cost alternative to the existing health monitoring devices, without compromising key aspects such as accuracy, portability or communication features. Initial testing showed that it is possible to adapt the same features of a dedicated device, while keeping the versatility of a dedicated prototyping platform. Furthermore, the advantages introduced by the third generation LEGO EV3 platform will improve the results, especially for time sensitive measurements like EKG or NIBP.**

Keywords— **telemedicine, biosensors, low-cost platform**

I. Introduction

As the population ages, more medical resources are required for expanding the healthcare in hospitals, homecare, and community care. Furthermore, the low fertility rate in most European countries has resulted in insufficient human resources, so there were introduced various wireless technologies and established healthcare systems to reduce the workload on existing medical personnel [1].

This paper aims to purpose an open, low-cost alternative to existing telemedicine health monitoring devices, without compromising key aspects such as accuracy, portability or communication features. Also, the described platform can be reconfigured with minimum effort to analyze home environmental factors such as temperature and indoor oxygen levels.

Based on the most widely used educational platform, it will provide students a relatively inexpensive, reusable, robust and reconfigurable solution for telemedicine applications development, optimization and testing [2].

II. The hardware platforma

A. Lego Mindstorms NXT

LEGO® Mindstorms NXT 2.0 is a set of interconnecting bricks that provides a flexible low-cost alternative to dedicated Rapid Prototyping solutions. This multi-purpose kit contains inter-connectable bricks, sensors, motors and a microprocessor controller unit called the NXT Intelligent Brick (Figure 1). Its versatility enables students and educators to develop and test various applications and provide a quick proof of concept [3].

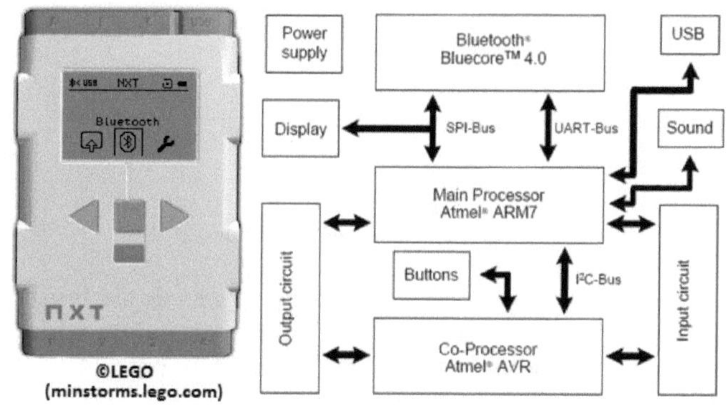

Fig. 1 NXT Intelligent Brick Hardware Architecture

One of the key features of the Mindstorms NXT platform is the ability to provide wireless communication via Bluetooth® technology through the Serial Port Profile (SPP). This means that it is able to connect to various devices (PCs, smartphones, tablets or routers) regardless of system architecture (x86-x64, RISC) or operating system (Windows, Windows Mobile, Android, iOS, Macintosh etc.)

B. Analog Input

In order to connect analog sensors that are not LEGO interfaced it is necessary to build a simple adapter that requires a 10kΩ resistor as the main component.

The internal 10 bit Analogue-to-Digital Converter scales the sensor input voltage to what are called *raw* units:

$$Raw = \frac{1024}{5}V \tag{1}$$

where 1024 is the highest number that can be expressed on a 10 bit resolution. The raw value is sampled every 3 milliseconds, thus resulting a maximum sampling rate of 333 Hz for each input channel [4].

The following equation calculates the sensor signal voltage (*Sig*) based on the measured raw input value [4]:

$$Sig[mV] = \frac{10000 \cdot Raw}{1024} - 5000mV \tag{2}$$

The diagram included in Figure 2 presents the circuit used for ±5V range analog signal input. Most Vernier analog sensors require a 5V DC source and provide a 0 – 5 volt raw signal [5].

S. Vlad and R.V. Ciupa (eds.), *International Conference on Advancements of Medicine and Health Care through Technology*, IFMBE Proceedings 44,
DOI: 10.1007/978-3-319-07653-9_19, © Springer International Publishing Switzerland 2014

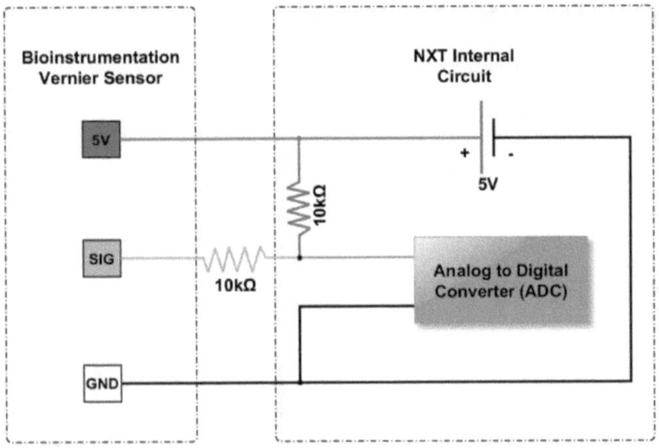

Fig. 2 Analog input circuit for ±5V range

As illustrated in Figure 2, the green wire feeds the sensor by connecting it to the NXT 5V DC power supply which has a total current limit of 180 mA for all input ports [4].

C. Vernier Biosensors

Vernier, a leading sensors and Transducers Company provides several biomedical engineering sensors that can be used by educators to teach students various biomedical engineering concepts [5]. The Vernier Bioinstrumentation kit includes the sensors presented in Figure 3:

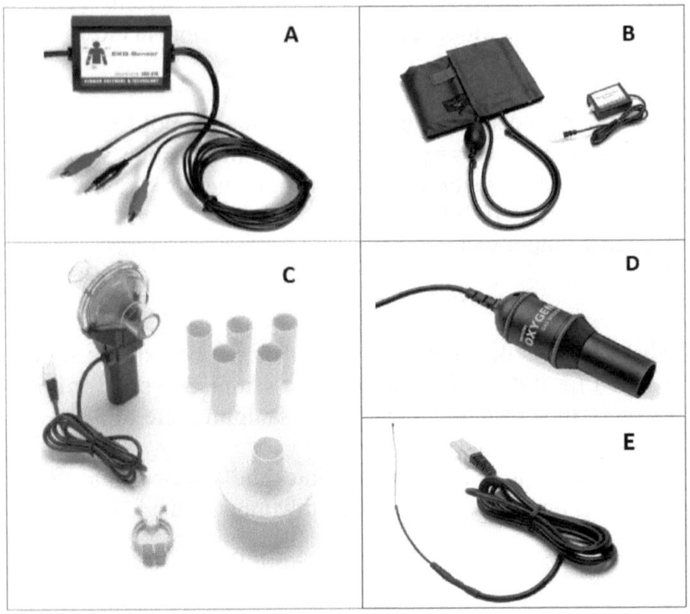

Fig. 3 Vernier Biosensors: A) EKG Sensor; B) Non-invasive Blood Pressure sensor (NIBP); C) Spirometer; D) O2 Gas Sensor; E) Surface Temperature Sensor

III. Data Acquisition

A. EKG

An electrocardiogram or EKG (Figure 4) is a graphical recording of the electrical events occurring within the heart. A typical EKG tracing consists of five identifiable deflections. Each deflection is noted by one of the letters P, Q, R, S, or T. The P wave is the first waveform in a tracing and represents the depolarization of the heart's atria. The QRS complex represents the depolarization of the heart's ventricles. The deflection that represents the repolarization of the atria is usually undetectable because of the intensity of the QRS waveform. The final waveform is the T wave and it represents the repolarization of the ventricles [6].

Table 1 EKG Sensor Specifications

Offset:	1.00 V (±0.3 V)
Gain:	1 mV body potential / 1 V sensor output
Isoelectric line:	1 V
DC output voltage:	[0…5] V range

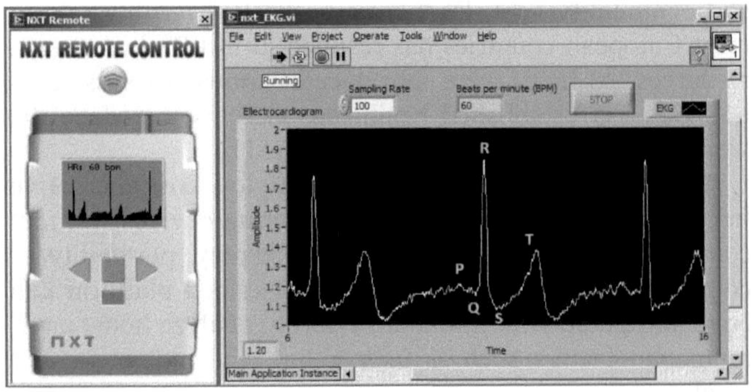

Fig. 4 Real Time EKG Data visible on NXT display (left) and PC (right)

The subject's heart rate is expressed in beats per minute and it is calculated by measuring the time between successive QRS complexes. If the intervals between QRS complexes (R-R intervals) are consistent, ventricular rhythm is regular. If intervals between P waves (P-P intervals) are consistent, the atrial rhythm is regular [7].

The EKG waveform cannot be interpreted accurately by reading the NXT display due to the screen's low resolution (100x64). Therefore, the data is transmitted via the USB port or Bluetooth connection to a higher screen resolution machine (like a PC, smartphone, tablet or even a smart router). The additional device also provides internet access and database connectivity, features that LEGO Mindstorms NXT lacks.

The NXT unit was programmed using LabVIEW, a visual development environment from National Instruments. Access to low-level resources is provided via the functions introduced by Lego Toolkit for LabVIEW. The Block Diagram of the EKG VI is presented in the Figure below.

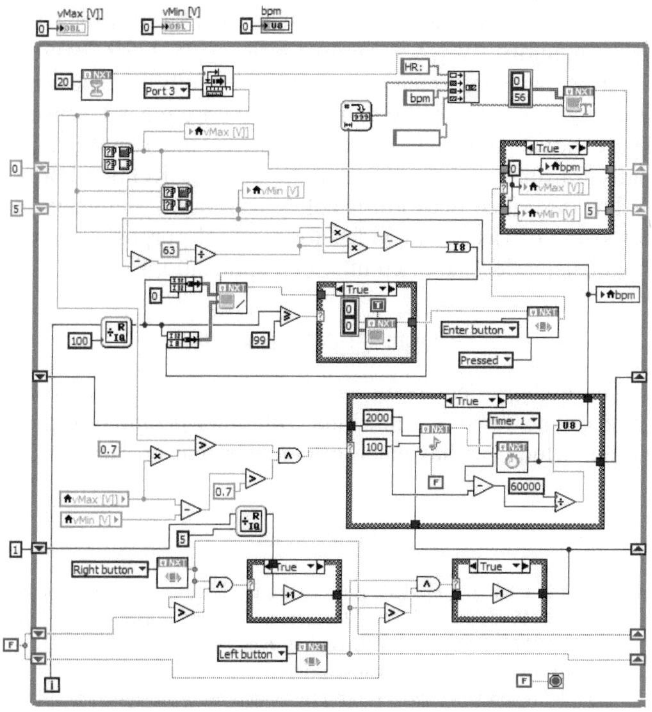

Fig. 5 NXT Targeted VI (EKG application)

The Mindstorms platform uses the cross-compilation concept: the application is created and compiled by using another machine (PC) and the executable program (containing byte code instructions) is transferred and deployed into the NXT memory.

B. Blood Pressure

The Vernier Blood Pressure Sensor (Figure 3B) is used to non-invasively measure mean arterial blood pressure and calculate both the systolic and diastolic blood pressure by using the oscillometric method [8].

Table 2 NIBP Sensor Specifications [8]

Sensing element:	SenSym SDX05D4
Pressure range:	0 mm Hg to 250 mm Hg
Typical accuracy:	±3mm Hg
Response time:	100 microseconds
Calibration:	slope = 56.11 (mm Hg/V); intercept = 0 (mm Hg)

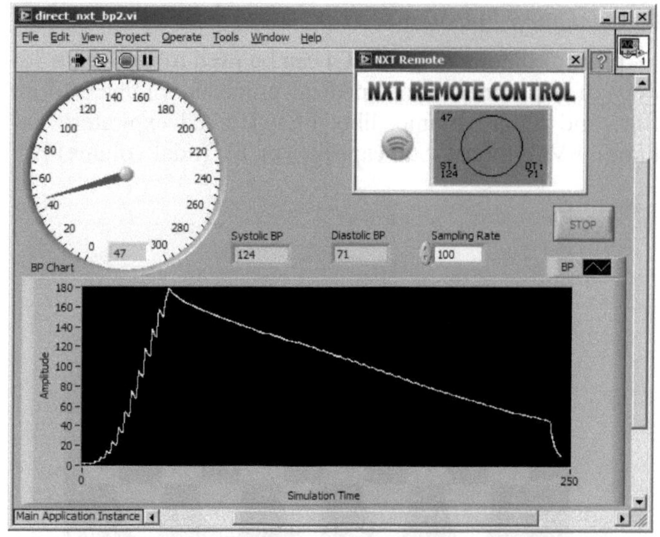

Fig. 6 Blood Pressure NXT and PC User Interface

The oscillometric method is based on the principle that blood pumped through the arteries by the heart causes the arterial walls to flex. When a cuff (placed around the upper arm to occlude the brachial artery) is inflated and then slowly deflated at a constant rate, an arterial pressure pulse forms. These pressure pulses pass from the arteries, through the arm, and into the pressure cuff itself [8].

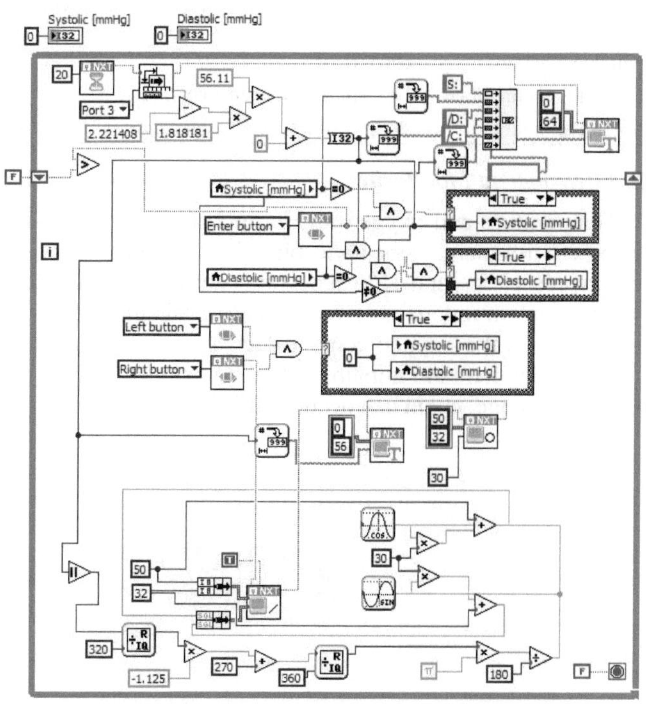

Fig. 7 NXT VI for Blood Pressure Measurement

C. Pulmonary Function Tests (PFTs)

The Spirometer (Figure 3C) can be used to perform a variety of experiments and medical procedures related to air flow and lungs volume, like: FEV (forced expiratory volume), FVC (forced vital capacity) or TV (tidal volume) [9]:

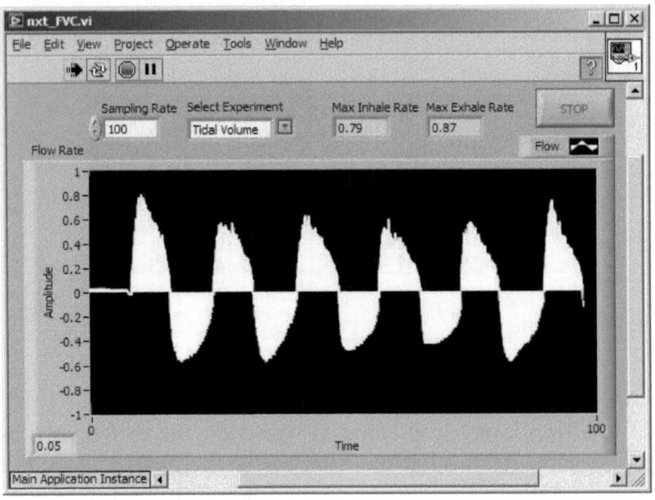

Fig. 8 PC user interface for Spirometer application

Table 3 Vernier Spirometer Specifications [9]

Flow rate range:	±10 L/s
Dead space:	93 mL
Nominal Output:	60μV/[L/s]
Default Sampling Rate:	100 samples/s on computer
Sored Calibration:	slope= 7.1869 (L/s)/V; intercept= -17.9672 L/s

D. Environment Monitoring

Temperature and oxygen level are critical aspects of the living environment. If the atmosphere's oxygen content falls to between 19.5% and 15%, a person's ability to think clearly or work strenuously is reduced. Coordination may be impaired. As the oxygen content decreases further, perception and judgment are impaired. If the O_2 content falls to the 6% to 4% range, coma can occur within seconds [10].

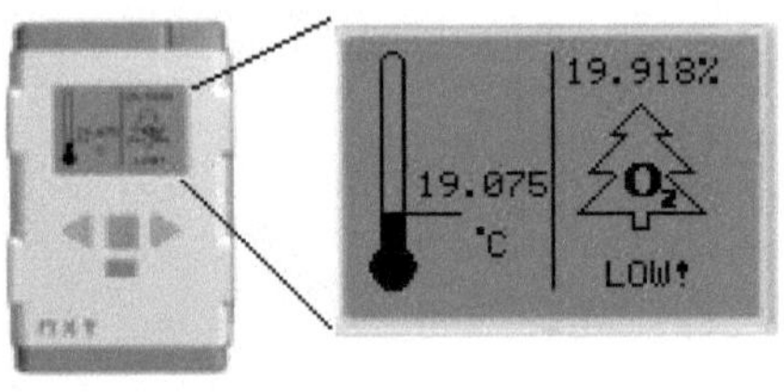

Fig. 9 NXT User Interface for Environmental Analysis

IV. Conclusions and Future Work

The purposed solution offers roughly the same features of a dedicated device, while keeping the freedom and versatility of a dedicated prototyping platform, but for a fraction of the cost.

The recently released third generation Mindstorms platform, LEGO EV3 provides key features like a faster CPU, more memory, WLAN compatibility (via USB device), superior sampling-rate, Linux OS compatibility and most important, it is hardware compatible with the NXT sensors. These advantages will further improve the results, especially for time sensitive measurements like EKG or NIBP.

The described platform is solely intended for educational purposes. It was not intended for medical purposes such as diagnosis, industrial or commercial applications.

Conflict of Interest

The authors declare no conflicts of interest. We do not have any personal relationships with other people or organizations which can have any influence or bias on our work.

References

1. Yu-Fang Chung, Chia-Hui Liu (2013) Design of a Wireless Sensor Network Platform for Tele-Homecare, Sensors (Open Access) 13, 17156-17175; DOI 10.3390/s131217156 at http://www.mdpi.com/journal/sensors
2. S. H. Kim and J. W. Jeon, (2009) Introduction for freshmen to embedded systems using LEGO Mindstorms, IEEE Trans. Educ., vol. 52, no. 1, pp. 99–108
3. S. Moreland, A. Wellman, A. Goldenberg (2007) The Development of an Autonomous GPS Guided Mobile Robot, Department of Mechanical and Industrial Engineering, University of Toronto; http://www.flcinnovation.org
4. M. Gasperi, P. Hurbain, I. Hurbain (2007) Extreme NXT: Extending the LEGO MINDSTORMS NXT to the Next Level, Apress®, ISBN-13 (pbk): 978-1-59059-818-4 at http://www.apress.com
5. *** (2011) Interfacing VIs for Vernier Biosensors, National Instruments, Publish Date: Dec 06, 2011; http://www.ni.com
6. K. Redding, D. Masterman (2007) Biology with Vernier (1st Edition), ISBN-13: 978-1-929075-43-0, ISBN: 1-929075-43-X, Vernier Software & Technology
7. D.E. Becker (2006) Fundamentals of Electrocardiography Interpretation, Anesthesia Progress 2006 summer; 53(2): 53–64; doi: 10.2344/0003-3006(2006)53[53:FOEI]2.0.CO;2 available at http://www.ncbi.nlm.nih.gov/pmc/articles/PMC1614214/
8. *** (2012) Blood Pressure Sensor Manual, Rev. 5.16.2012, Vernier Software & Technology; http://www.vernier.com
9. *** (2010) Spirometer Manual, Rev. 2/17/10, Vernier Software & Technology; http://www.vernier.com
10. P Yanisko, D Croll (2012) Use Nitrogen Safely, Chemical Engineering Progress, Air Products and Chemicals, Inc. pp 44–48, March 2012; http://www.airproducts.com.

Towards Improving Situation Awareness during Emergency Transportation through Ambulance-2-X Communication and Semantic Stream Reasoning

A. Groza , A. Marginean , and B. Iancu

Department of Computer Science, Technical University of Cluj-Napoca
Baritiu 28, 400391, Cluj-Napoca, Romania
{Adrian.Groza,Anca.Marginean,Bogdan.Iancu}@cs.utcluj.ro

Abstract—**With the recent introduction of the eCall system, the cars involved in accidents exchange relevant information directly with the emergency healthcare services. For road safety, Vehicular Ad-hoc Networks can be used to exchange safety information between cars and ambulances, via vehicle-2-x communication. In this paper, we exploit recent advances in vehicle-2-x communication and the advantages of knowledge representation and reasoning in order to deploy cooperative communication for medical emergency services. The developed system continuously matches data retrieved from inter-vehicular communication with structured knowledge from vehicular ontologies and open street maps.**

Keywords— **emergency medical services, Car-2-X communication, stream reasoning, semantic web**

I. Introduction

With the adoption by the European Commission of the directive ensuring that, by October 2015, cars will automatically call emergency services in case of serious accident. The "eCall" system automatically dials 112 and communicates the vehicle's location to emergency services. From the technical viewpoint, the eCall system introduces some challenges, but also many opportunities to employ emerging technologies (like vehicular communication) for emergency healthcare services.

Vehicular Ad-hoc Networks (VANETs) use vehicles as mobile nodes able to self-configure in order to create a communication network. In VANETs, cars are able to employ secure and reliable communication to ensure innovative intelligent transport systems. For emergency services and road safety, VANETS can be used to exchange safety information between cars and ambulances, via vehicle-to-vehicle (V2V) and vehicle-to-infrastructure (V2I) communications, without being restricted by weather conditions or distance [1].

Vehicle-2-X technology has just solved low level aspects with respect to ad-hoc networks or regulatory norms and standards. Thus, much work remains at the application layer, to seamlessly integrate the newly developed services. In this paper we exploit the advances in *knowledge representation and reasoning* to deploy cooperative communication for medical emergency services. Our solution aims to increase situation awareness of the vehicles closed to the ambulance, thus increasing safeness during medical emergency services. The emergency vehicle moving to a crash site will take advantage of the VANET infrastructure to establish the fastest route, to communicate with the vehicles in the path to ensure a clear route, and also to maintain a permanent connection with the hospital and the damaged vehicle.

Table 1 KRSS syntax and semantics of $\mathcal{ALC}$

Constructor	Syntax	Semantics
negation	(not C)	$\Delta^I \setminus C^I$
conjunction	(and C D)	$C^I \cap D^I$
disjunction	(or C D)	$C^I \cup D^I$
existential restriction	(some r C)	$\{x \in \Delta^I \| \exists y : (x,y) \in r^I \wedge y \in C^I\}$
value restriction	(all r C)	$\{x \in \Delta^I \| \forall y : (x,y) \in r^I \rightarrow y \in C^I\}$
individual assertion	(instance a C)	$\{a\} \in C^I$

II. Enacted Technologies

A. Description Logics

In the description logic $\mathcal{ALC}$, concepts are built using the set of constructors formed by negation, conjunction, disjunction, value restriction, and existential restriction [2], as shown in table 1. Here, C and D represent concept descriptions, while r is a role name. The semantics is defined based on an interpretation $I = (\Delta^I, \cdot^I)$, where the domain Δ^I of I contains a non-empty set of individuals, and the interpretation function $\cdot^I$ maps each concept name C to a set of individuals $C^I \in \Delta^I$ and each role r to a binary relation $r^I \in \Delta^I \times \Delta^I$. The last column of table 1 shows the extension of $\cdot^I$ for non-atomic concepts.

Definition 1. *A concept C is satisfied if there exists an interpretation I such that $C^I \neq \emptyset$. The concept D*

S. Vlad and R.V. Ciupa (eds.), *International Conference on Advancements of Medicine and Health Care through Technology*,
IFMBE Proceedings 44,
DOI: 10.1007/978-3-319-07653-9_20,

subsumes the concept C, represented by (implies C D) if $C^I \subseteq D^I$ *for all interpretations I.*

Definition 2. *An assertional box ABox is a finite set of concept assertions (instance a C) or role assertions (related a b r), where C designates a concept, r a role, and a and b are two individuals. Usually, the unique name assumption holds within the same ABox. A terminology TBox is a finite set of terminological axioms of the forms (equiv C D) or (implies C D).*

Constraints on concepts (i.e. *disjoint*) or on roles (*domain*, *range*, *inverse* role, or *transitive* properties) can be specified in more expressive description logics[1].

B. Vehicle-2-X Communication

Communication among vehicles relies on the Wireless Access in Vehicular Environments (WAVE) protocol and the IEEE 802.11p wireless standard. The WAVE architecture provides interoperable wireless V2V and V2Infrastructure (V2I) services. The IEEE 1609.1 details the management activities required for the proper operation of the applications, while IEEE 1609.3 deals with communication security. Two main message types are used to enable V2X communication [3]: periodic and event-driven messages. A vehicle advertises its current status (i.e., position, speed, direction of travel)to other vehicles, by sending periodic messages in the network. Event-driven messages are emergency messages sent to other vehicles if hazardous situations are detected.

Geocast ad hoc routing protocol is introduced as the core networking protocol for vehicular communication based on IEEE 802.11 technology promoted by the Car-to-Car Communication Consortium (C2C-CC) in Europe [4]. Geocast protocol presumes that vehicles have information regarding their geographic location position by use of GPS or other positioning system. The three key components of Geocast protocol are beaconing, location service and forwarding. Beaconing allows nodes to continuously and periodically broadcast information to all neighbors in the reception range, to permit cooperative awareness. The location service can map a node's ID to its geographical position. Forwarding enables relaying data through VANET network to a certain destination, using GeoUnicast - provides data delivery between two nodes via multiple wireless hops, or GeoBroadcast - distributes data packets by flooding, where nodes re-broadcast the packets if they are located in the geographical region determined by the packets.

[1] We provide only some basic terminologies of description logics in this paper to make it self-contained. For a detailed explanation about families of description logics, the reader is referred to [2].

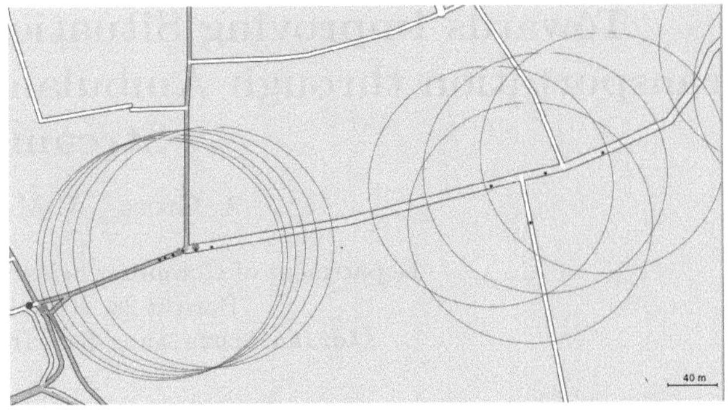

Fig. 1 Simulating an eCall on Ion Creanga street

III. Event Recognition

Our illustrative scenario simulates an eCall triggered by a car accident that took place on the IonCreanga street in Cluj-Napoca, with the ambulance approaching from the Republicii street (see Fig. 1). Our system makes use of: i) the VANET simulator [5], ii) the AllegroGraph system for geospatial reasoning, and iii) RacerPro server [6] for semantic and temporal reasoning. The vehicles communicate within a range of 200 meters. The following subsections describe: i) how the communication between vehicles was designed; ii) how domain knowledge is represented within the emergency vehicle; iii) how the emergency vehicle continuously reason on the data available to recognize traffic events; and iv) queries enacted to increase situation awareness.

A. Communication Protocol

For communication between vehicles, we employ reasoning in description logic on top of the above Geocast protocol to determine the location and status of the vehicles situated in the geographic area where the accident took place. By complementing the location table and the information from the periodically beaconing messages with domain knowledge, a vehicle is able to infer a wide range of information about an approaching ambulance: (i) based on the node ID and the speed entries in the location table, the system can infer if the ambulance is moving or it is stationary; (ii) based on the node ID, the geographical position, speed and heading entries in the location table compared to vehicle data, the system infers if an ambulance is approaching or it is in the rear/front, or if the ambulance is traveling from the

```
1.  (in-tbox emergency-vehicles)
2.  (define-primitive-role on-same-street
      :inverse om-same-street :domain vehicle :range vehicle)
3.  (implies bus vehicle)
4.  (implies emergency-vehicle vehicle)
5.  (implies ambulance emergency-vehicle)
6.  (disjoint bus emergency-vehicle)
7.  (in-abox emergency-vehicles-cluj)
8.  (instance a1 ambulance)
9.  (instance b1 bus)
10. (related b1 a1 on-same-street)
```

Fig. 2 Sample of the ontology in the emergency-vehicle domain

opposite direction; (iii) if the beaconing signal includes lane information, than the system is able to detect lane-changing of the moving ambulance.

When the ambulance is approaching an accident, it sends GeoBroadcast signals enhanced with intended path/route information. The messages sent by the emergency vehicle are selected accordingly to the current situation and running events:

Stop	*Ambulance vehicle crossing!*
Drive right	*Ambulance vehicle in oncoming traffic!*
Drive right	*Ambulance vehicle overtaking!*
Form corridor	*Ambulance vehicle approaching!*

B. Domain Knowledge

To facilitate situation awareness, we empower the vehicular agents with several knowledge sources.

The agent rely on various *vehicular ontologies*, as the one exemplified in Fig. 2. The ontology consists of the tbox *emergency-vehicles* (line 1), which defines the main concepts and relationships among them. The role *on-same-street* is symmetric. Buses and emergency vehicles are subsumed by the more generic concept *vehicle* (lines 3 and 4). If a vehicle is identified as a *bus*, it cannot be interpreted as a emergency-vehicle in future instances of time, constrained by the disjoint property in line 6. In the abox *emergency-vehicles-cluj*, the ontology contains assertions about a particular situation, in which the bus $b1$ is in front of ambulance $a1$ (line 10). Based on axiom 2, both vehicular agents can deduce that $a1$ is on the same street with $b1$. Note that the domain and range restrictions of the *on-same-street* role are satisfied, because the system is aware that $b1$ and $a1$ are vehicles (from axioms 3, 4, and 5).

Street topology data was obtained using *OpenStreetMap*, which gives to vehicular agents the possibility to choose an area by its coordinates and to export it in RDF format.The RDF tuples include knowledge about the selected traffic area: the location of semaphores, number of lines, one way street, etc.

Table 2 Temporal predicates in vehicular streams

Temporal predicate	Informal semantics
((move ?o) t_{start} t_{end}*)*	object *?o* is known to be moving between time t_{start} and time t_{end}
((approach ?o1 ?o2) t_{start} t_{end}*)*	*?o1* is approaching object *?o2* during the time interval $[t_{start}, t_{end}]$
((behind ?o1 ?o2) t_{start} t_{end}*)*	*?o1* is behind object *?o2* during the time interval $[t_{start}, t_{end}]$
((beside ?o1 ?o2) t_{start} t_{end}*)*	*?o1* is beside object *?o2* during the time interval $[t_{start}, t_{end}]$
((in-front-of ?o1 ?o2) t_{start} t_{end}*)*	*?o1* is beside object *?o2* during the time interval $[t_{start}, t_{end}]$

```
11. (define-event-assertion ((move a1) 5 60))
12. (define-event-assertion ((move b1) 1 50))
13. (define-event-assertion ((approach a1 b1) 10 20))
14. (define-event-assertion ((behind a1 b1) 10 20))
15. (define-event-assertion ((beside a1 b1) 20 30))
16. (define-event-assertion ((in-front-of a1 b1) 30 60))
17. (define-event-assertion ((recede a1 b1) 30 40))
```

Fig. 3 Asserting primitive events from vehicular communication about the ambulance $a1$ and the bus $b1$

C. Event Recognition

Stream data received from the vehicular network triggers rules that assert volatile facts about the current situation. Assertions about vehicles are valid only within a certain time interval. The vehicles have to decide: i) if the ambulance approaces or not; or ii) if the ambulance comes from front or behind. The temporal assertions in table 2 have been used in model the above specifications.

The reasoning engine combines contiguous facts in a single temporal assertion. Given two assertions *((behind ?o1 ?o2* t_0 t_k*)* and *((behind ?o1 ?o2)* t_{k+1} t_n*)*, the merged information is stored as *((behind ?o1 ?o2)* t_0 t_n*)*. Assume the assertions in Fig. 3 have been stored. Ambulance $a1$ is moving between instance 5 and 60 (line 11), while bus $b1$ between 1 and 50 (line 12). Between time-steps 10 and 20, ambulance is approaching the bus (line 13). Both vehicular agents are aware that the $a1$ is approaching from behind of the bus (line 14). Between 20 and 30, the vehicles are beside each other, as identified in line 15. After time 30, ambulance is in front of the bus (line 16), while between 30 and 40 ambulance is moving away from b1 (line 40). These assertions are obtained reasoning on the data obtained from vehicular communication.

Rules on top of description logic are enacted to recognize various traffic events such as lane changing, vehicle stopping, or emergency vehicle approaching. The rule for car overtaking event [6] appears in fig. 4. Here, primitive volatile facts from table 2 represent premises of the rule.

```
21. (define-event-rule ((overtake ?o1 ?o2) ?t1 ?t2)
22.       ((?o1 ambulance) ?t0 ?tn)
23.       ((?o1 ?o2 on-same-street) ?t0 ?tn)
24.       ((move ?1) ?t0 ?t2)
25.       ((move ?2) ?t1 ?t2)
26.       ((approach ?o1 ?o2) ?t1 ?t3)
27.       ((behind ?o1 ?o2) ?t1 ?t3)
28.       ((beside ?o1 ?o2) ?t3 ?t4)
29.       ((in-front-of ?o1 ?o2) ?t4 ?t2))
```

Fig. 4 Complex event recognition: identifying when the ambulance overtakes a vehicle

```
select * {GEO SUBTYPE
        <prefix:/spherical/degrees/-180.0/180.0/-90.0/90.0/5.0>
        POLYGON (RESOURCE x:w7934417 ){?a ex:location ?b.}
        Where{}}
ORDER BY <prefix:/fn/haversineKilometers>(?o,POINT(23.58,46.76))
```

Fig. 5 SPARQL query for retrieving the vehicles on the street

D. Querying the Vehicular Network

To retrieve all the vehicles in the same street with the ambulance, the query in Fig. 5 is enacted. Here the street is modeled as a polygon. The role *on-same-street* is used to store the obtained answers (recall line 10 in Fig. 2). To check if the ambulance $a1$ overtakes the bus $b1$, the query q_1 is used: *(timenet-retrieve ((overtake a1 ?v) ?t1 ?t2))*. From axiom 8 in Fig. 2, $a1$ satisfies precondition 22 of the overtaking rule. The precondition 23 is satisfied by the answers obtained from query in figure 5. The preconditions 24 to 29 are satisfied by the assertions in figure 3. The obtained answer *(((?o2 b1) (?t1 (10 19)) (?t2 (31 50))))* confirms that the ovartake event took place between the ambulance $a1$ and the identified vehicle $b1$. For time variables *?t1* and *?t2* an interval for the lower and upper-bound is returned [6]. The overtaking starts between $t1 \in [10,19]$ and it ends at $t2 \in [29,50]$.

IV. Discussion and Related Work

Several studies in mobile telemedicine has concluded that patient survival during a health emergency situation [7] depends on the effective pre-hospital healthcare [8]. In order to achieve a complete system that covers all telemedicine elements, VANETs are seen as the missing link. V2V and V2I communication capabilities of VANET added to existing mobile telemedicine systems can ensure rapid intervention and thus patient survival. Combining V2X technology, communication, and semantic stream reasoning, we proposed an efficient method for telemedicine services. By facilitating different communication channels during ambulance transportation, we aimed at minimizing collision hazards and decreasing intervention time by inter-vehicular collaboration.

V. Conclusion

We proposed a method to increase situation awareness during emergency transportation of patients. Our approach combines semantic reasoning with the emerging Car-2-X technology. We employed reasoning in description logic on top of data collected continuously from vehicular communication. The developed system performs temporal reasoning on real topological maps imported from OpenStreetMap. Our approach is a step towards minimizing hazards during medical emergency services.

Conflict of Interest

The authors have no conflict of interest.

Acknowledgements

This research is supported by Technical University of Romania through the research project "GREEN-VANETS: Improving transportation using Car-2-X communication and multi agent systems".

References

1. Martinez Francisco J, Toh Chai-Keong, Cano J-C, Calafate Carlos T, Manzoni Pietro. Emergency services in future intelligent transportation systems based on vehicular communication networks *Intell. Trans. Systems Mag., IEEE.* 2010;2:6–20.
2. Baader Franz, Calvanese Diego, McGuinness Deborah L., Nardi Daniele, Patel-Schneider Peter F.. , eds. *The Description Logic Handbook: Theory, Implementation, and Applications.* Cambridge University Press 2003.
3. Olariu Stephan, Weigle Michele C. *Vehicular networks: from theory to practice.* CRC Press 2010.
4. Festag Andreas, Baldessari Roberto, Zhang Wenhui, Le Long, Sarma Amardeo, Fukukawa Masatoshi. Car-2-x communication for safety and infotainment in europe *NEC Technical Journal.* 2008;3:21–26.
5. Tomandl Andreas, Scheuer Florian, Federrath Hannes. Simulation-based evaluation of techniques for privacy protection in VANETs in *WiMob*:165-172,IEEE 2012.
6. KG Racer Systems GmbH & Co.. Racer user guide 2.0 2012.
7. Naja Rola. *Wireless vehicular networks for car collision avoidance.* Springer 2013.
8. Batistatos MC, Tsoulos George V, Athanasiadou Georgia E. Mobile telemedicine for moving vehicle scenarios: Wireless technology options and challenges *Journal of Network and Computer Applications.* 2012;35:1140–1150.

Materiovigilance and Medical Devices

S. Mirel[1], L. Colobatiu[1], E. Fasniuc[1], A. Boboia[1], C. Gherman[2], V. Mirel[3], and D. Muresan[2]

[1] University of Medicine and Pharmacy "Iuliu Hatieganu", Faculty of Pharmacy, Cluj-Napoca, Romania
[2] University of Medicine and Pharmacy "Iuliu Hatieganu", Faculty of Medicine, Cluj-Napoca, Romania
[3] National Institute for Research and Development of Isotopic and Molecular Technologies, Cluj-Napoca

Abstract— **The medical devices may have caused serious events for patients and could have contributed to healthcare costs. The post-market surveillance, as part of Medical Device Vigilance Systems, lead to improve the safety of patients and users by reducing the reoccurrence of the incidents. Furthermore, the existing incidents argue that it must continuously monitoring medical devices in use, in order to protect the patients' health. The current regulations and guidance documents regarding medical devices focused on post market vigilance framework. were examined and discussed. The post-market surveillance data was evaluated in order to synthesize and compare the EU state members for their active implication. In this context, Romanian regulations concerning medical devices are described and analyzed. This study aims to identify if Romania is harmonizing its medical device vigilance system with respect to those of the European Directives.**

Keywords— **medical devices, materiovigilance, incidents, device regulation**

I. Introduction

Nowadays, medical devices - defined as all articles (instruments, apparatus, materials, etc) which are intended to be used for a medical purpose - are an integral part of health system, to healthcare providers and patients. These health products have a well-known role in the diagnosis, prevention, monitoring and treatment of diseases [1, 2]. There are over 500,000 different types of devices worldwide available [3], with a large area of application because of the diversity of products and technologies implemented. The progress made over the last twenty years in areas such as electronics, information technology and materials had a direct impact on supply care more sophisticated and in the increasing number of devices. Furthermore, the medical technology industry is considered to be a leader in innovation with over 10,000 patent applications in Europe in 2012, more than any other technical field [4]. In this context, in order to assure and to improve the level of safety for users, the general standards for the quality and safety of medical devices were established.

The available regulations [5-8] stipulate that the medical devices must be manufactured in such a manner so that used under the conditions and intended purposes they will not compromise the patients' health.

The potential risk and benefit of all medical devices must be assessed across all stages of the product life cycle. Thus, the risk-management systems, which include pre-market (pre-approval studies) and post-market surveillance, improved the protection of health. The manufacturer must perform the conformity assessment, but this not always guarantee the patient safety [9]. The large number of recall reports proves that the pre-market review process cannot identify all possible malfunctions of all different medical devices currently on the world- market.

As an example, from 2006 to 2010, 2124 field safety notices registered were reported in UK, with an increase of 1220% number of devices recalled over the 5-year period [3]. In USA, only in 2006, a number of 116 086 potential device-related injuries and 2830 potential device-related deaths were registered [10]. In according with the same report, 4146 recall actions were registered from 2000 to 2006. Other study concerning 2005 -2009 period, mentioned 115 names of recalled devices (involving millions of units) on their high-risk recall list [11]. In Australia, only from 2000 to 2011, 6812 incidents involving medical devices were reported, but in the same time period, there were only 35 medical device recalls and 34 medical device alerts issued [12]. This explains why the post-market surveillance – as part of Medical Device Vigilance Systems – is the key factor [13] and led to improve the safety of patients and users by reducing the reoccurrence of the incident elsewhere. Initiated in 1970 by the Food and Drug Administration (FDA -US), the post-market surveillance of medical devices must be a part of device-regulation process over the world [14].

This article has the desire to focus on the particularities of a vigilance system according to medical devices Directives and the aspects of the implementation of data exchange system in the field of medical device vigilance.

The study was initiated in order to examine the available framework and its implication for the Romanian medical device vigilance system according with European Directives and Global Harmonization.

S. Vlad and R.V. Ciupa (eds.), *International Conference on Advancements of Medicine and Health Care through Technology*, IFMBE Proceedings 44,
DOI: 10.1007/978-3-319-07653-9_21, © Springer International Publishing Switzerland 2014

II. METHODS

The study was divided into two parts.

The first part consisted of reviews of current regulations of medical devices and guidance documents regarding medical devices focused on postmarket surveillance.

For the second part, a dataset of the medical devices incidents which had been reported over the 10-years period (1990-2010) was created in order to facilitate a comparison between different systems. The information and records from publically available data were colected and standardized. We used the official Websites of the regulatory authorities (http://ec.europa.eu/health/medical-devices, http://www.mhra.gov; http://www.bfarm.de; http://ansm.sante.fr, http://www.anm.ro).

The statistical reports posted as part of annual reporting of mentioned authorities and reported studies published in peer-reviewed journals or disseminated in accessible media searches were considered as eligible for inclusion. The study synthesized the post-market data by year. Statistical analyses were performed using Excel.

III. RESULTS AND DISCUSSIONS

A. Current Regulations of Medical Devices: Post- Market Vigilance Systems Framework

Generally, all over the world, there should be available policies and specific regulations regarding medical devices. But, according to the 2010 WHO Baseline Country Survey on Medical Devices, only 65% of 145 responding countries have a national authority responsible for implementing and enforcing medical device regulations [15].

At global level, the Global Harmonization Task Force (GHTF) has been available since 1993. The GHTS represent medical device regulatory authorities and industry from the European Union (EU), US, Australia, Canada and Japan, which established the international standards for harmonized regulatory processes to assure the safety, quality and performance of medical devices available to all countries [16]. Its goal is to provide opportunities to maintain the access to safe and effective healthcare technologies.

The GHTF principal objectives and rules were considered and transposed into the different region/country context, in order to develop the national medical device regulations. Even if the devices regulations are different in different regions and countries, there are several similarities. One of the important points is the classification of medical devices, in graduated categories, using the risk criteria (table 1).

Table 1 Classification of medical devices in EU

Risk class	Criteria	Conformity assessment procedures	Vigilance system
Class I	low risk	+/-	+
Class IIa	moderate risk	+	+
Class IIb	Potential high risk	+	+
Class III	high risk	+	+

Thus, the risk based classification system available - applies to all products and throughout the world - is correlated with to the conformity assessment procedures (for higher classification the greater the level of assessment is required (tab. 1).

But, regardless the class of the device, all devices must be subject to the reporting requirements under their specific vigilance system.

In the European Union (EU), the medical devices are regulated by 3 main Directives [6-8]:

- Council Directive 93/42/EEC – concerning medical devices generally (MDD)
- Council Directive 90/385/EEC –concerning active implantable medical devices (AIMDD)
- Council Directive 98/79/EC –concerning in vitro diagnostic medical devices (IVDMD)

The MDD establish specific procedures which the national authorities need to follow in the case of unsafe medical device according of vigilance criteria described in the EU Guidelines on Medical Devices Vigilance System (MEDDEV 2 12-1 rev. 8) [17]- applicable for all 3 Directives. As a part of the health vigilance system, the Medical Device Vigilance Systems has as key objective to improve the safety of patients and users.

The major control point for medical devices is post market testing [18] knowing as materiovigilance [19]. The vigilance system is designed to generate information for identify the problems related to the use of the health products, in order to facilitate the development of safety devices.

The *materiovigilance* refers to medical devices whereas *pharmacovigilance* refers to medicines. It must be mentioned that the regulation of medical devices are less developed and had appeared later than the one of medicines [18]. But, contrary to medicines, the medical devices do not usually require a national marketing authorization (in Europe, it must have the CE mark in order for free circulated). Moreover, while for all medicines, the benefit must be proved in clinical evaluations, the medical devices can enter the market without trials (asked only for those considered to high risk).

Materiovigilance is the monitory of incidents or potential incidents that may result from the use of medical devices after their placing on the market. According to Article 10 of the MDD, the incidents that must be notified are:

- any malfunction or deterioration in the characteristics or performance of a medical device
- any inaccuracy in the labeling or
- any inaccuracy in the instructions for use

which have led (or could have led) to the death or serious deterioration in the state of health of a patient or users [17].

MEDDEV guidance document describes the system for:

- the notification (reported incidents),
- evaluation of incidents,
- -information (disseminated as National Competent Authority Reports (NCARs) and
- adoption - if necessary- the field safety corrective actions (FSCA).

In the same time, each state member, must inform the European Commission (EC) and the other EU member states regarding the taken measures in order to minimize the risk of incidents. This guidance is implemented both by manufacturers and each national Competent Authorities [16]. Several countries –through their National Competent Authorities – have elaborated their Guidance on the operation of the EU vigilance system.

Therefore, in the second part of the present study, we analysed the available data from european statistics [20] regarding the NCARs sent by countrys and exchanged at European level in the last 10 years (between 2003 and 2012). From all 4588 NCARs registred at European level, the majority were raported by Germany (1741), folowed by UK (981), while 10 countries reported under 10 NCARs in the same periode. According to the same available reports, between 2003-2012, only 5 out of 32 contries included in the list of „"vigilance contact points" had never had any report. Romania is one of those countries, together with Estonia, Lithuania, Latvia and Slovenia.

It might be seen that there are diferencess concerning the NCARs' exchanged number. This leds to questions regarding not the quality of medical devices used (assuming that in Germany, UK, Ireland, France or Swiss performing devices are beeing used) but the political implementation of materiovigilence in each countries.

In figure nr. 1 was graphically represented the number of NCARs exchanged at EU level for Germany, France and UK, 3 of the most active countries in the vigilance European system.

Starting from this note, we searched information about nationale rules in the field and materiovigilence reports registrated in those contries. According to the Devices Bulettin of Adverse Incidents of each Competent Authorities [21-23], collaborated with the data presented in parallel studies [18, 24] the number of the reports related to the events associated with the use of medical devices is enormous (over 10.000 reports in 2010 in UK). In fig. 2 was graphically represented the number of incidents report involving medical devices in Germany, France and UK.

It can be noticed that the reporting numbers are much higher than the number of NCARs exchanged at EU level. This is due to the fact that the relation of the accident with the use of medical devices was not proved for all the signaled incidents. Of course, device incidents (approximately 300 deaths each year "associated" with a medical device), are not necessarily caused by the devices [25].

The majority of the reports had been registered in UK, followed by French and Germany, countries where we can see a continuous increased in the number of incidents which could be associated to the use of medical devices.

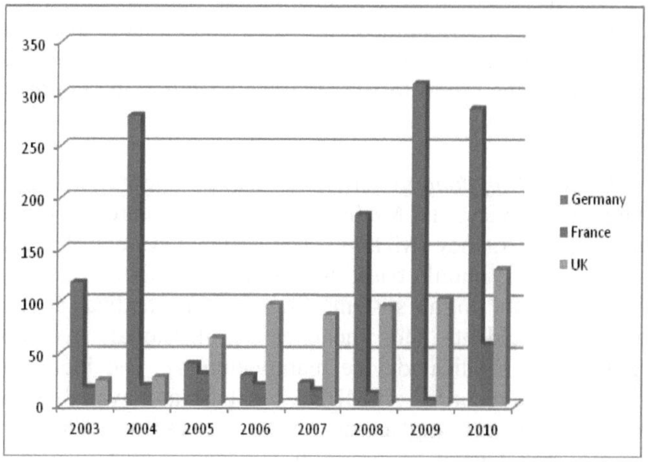

Fig. 1 No of NCARs exchanged at EU level

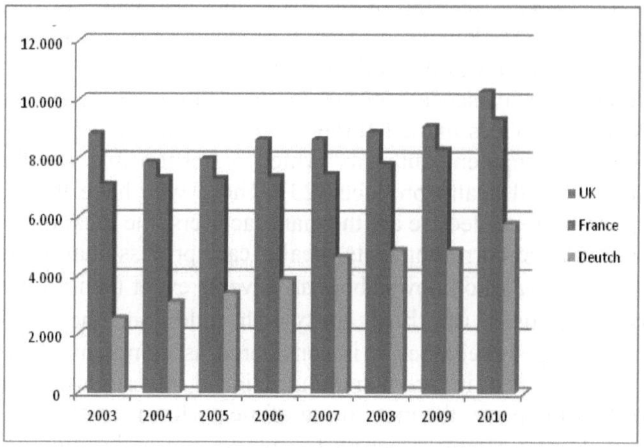

Fig. 2 Number of incidents report involving medical devices

It must be mentioned that for both graphics we have chosen the period between 2003 and 2010 because the UK bulletins for 2011and 2012 are not available yet on MHRA website.

Several countries adopted their own rules on the manner of reporting adverse effects during the use of medical device, as well as the manner of organizing the system of their monitoring. Generally, a minimum dataset required for a reportable accident/incident: an adverse event (with details), a susceptible medical product, an identifiable patient, and an identifiable reporter (patient, healthcare workers, manufacturer, etc). The value of incident information can increase when the data are collected and analyzed at national level, and exchanged at an international level.

In *Germany,* according with the German Safety Plan for Medical Devices, the Federal Institute for Drugs and Medical Devices (BfArM) -through Medical Devices Division - is responsible for medical devices and ensures the central collection, analysis and evaluation of risks arising from their use [26]. Manufacturers, distributors, and also the professional users notify BfArM of incidents. A recent analysis of the report to BfArM concluded that the majority of incidents are caused partially by errors of device handling. [27]

United Kingdom government agency the regalements Medical Devices is Medicines and Healthcare products Regulatory Agency (MHRA). The national system of vigilance in UK is mainly based in online reporting system with three separate online systems for reporting medical device adverse incidents (for healthcare-professional, patients /public and medical device manufacturers). The incidents reported are recorded on MHRA database and available for specialists to investigate and review. An estimated top ten of medical devices involved in incidents reports are also annually published in the Device Bulletin in the official website [28].

In *France,* starting with 2012, the National Security Agency of Medicines and Health-products (ANSM) replaces the former health products safety agency (AFSSAPS - Agence française de sécurité sanitaire products of santé). Medical devices market survey is one of the main tasks of French competent authority which is responsible for the safety of all health products [23]. Those who have the responsibility to declare are the manufacturers, the local materiovigilance correspondents (health care professionals) and also anyone who knows about an adverse event (whether a patient, user or third party). In addition, the post-marketing surveillance it is considered as complement the data collected in pre-marketing clinical investigation. In order to improve the monitoring of the performance of medical devices supplied across the world, the authorities encourage the reporting of adverse events by users of devices.

The Medical Devices Directive (93/42/EEC) stipulates that manufacturers have the legal obligation to report adverse events associated with medical devices. In several countries the healthcare professionals and consumers have the obligation of reporting adverse effects and adverse events associated with the use of medical devices. Furthermore, in several countries not reporting is considered a matter for disciplinary actions for healthcare professionals and manufacturer (in France).

In UK and France the patients were encouraged to report adverse events that could be caused by the use of medical devices. But in other countries their specific legislation stipulates that only manufacturers have the legal obligation to report the adverse events associated with medical devices.

B. Romanian Regulatory System

Romanian agency that regalements all activities linked to medical devices is The National Agency for Medicines and Medical Devices (NAMMD), operating under the Ministry of Health (set up in 2010 as a result of the merger of the National Agency for Medicines and the Technical Office for Medical Devices). The surveillance of the safety of medicinal products for human use –including medical devices - is one of the missions of the NAMMD [29]

The medical devices activities is specifically regulated by the Romanian legislation - Law no. 176/2000 regarding medical devices / republished and its implementation norms (Order 1636/2004, Government Decision no. 54/2009), which implements among others the Council Directive 93/42/EEC [30]. According to the Law 176/2000, the term of „materiovigilence" is not directly used, being defined as monitoring, referring to measures that assure and confirm usage safety and the performances of the medical device as long as it used [31].

According with our national legislation, the Romanian Ministry of Health must ensure the registration and the evaluation of any information received in relation to medical devices incidents. The obligation to report all the incidents is to be performed by the healthcare professionals, sanitary units and also the manufacturers. After report, the Ministry of Health should inform the manufacturer (or its authorized representative) about the "suspect" medical device and the related incident. After analysis and evaluation, the Ministry must inform immediately the EC and the EU member states about the taken measures.

Although the regulations mention this specific reporting, it is not indicated the way in which it should be actually realized. On ANDM site, pharmacovigilance reporting is possible (for drugs), but no options are available in order to report incidents related to medical devices. There are no reports, published statistics or studies related to the number or the severity of such incidents.

On the website of the European Commission, our country appears to be included in the section dedicated to Medical Devices, Vigilance and Surveillance (as vigilance contact points) [32]. But according to European statistics publically available [20], there was no Romanian reporting available in the last 10 years.

Therefore, the question is whether in Romania there are no such accidents/incidents or none of them are being reported. It is difficult to argue that medical devices used in our country are better than the ones used in UK, France or Germany and that these devices have never generated any risks to human health.

In a previous work [33], we established the steps for the procedure of reporting undesirable effects during the use of medical devices, in order to organize a national system of monitoring medical devices' effects. The questions regarding the proper way to manage and asses such problems related to the safety of our patients still remain.

A lack of available transparent data makes full analyses of the safety impact of reported incident devices in Romania to be impossible. We considered that this kind of information could be made available openly for the public (by publishing information). Also, it would be better to have our own databases (data collection and analysis) and voluntary recording systems. In order to increase the easiness of reporting it is important to develop an application that facilitates the reporting system, which must be implemented in each hospital, ambulatory settings, and also in the public pharmacy. In addition, the rules and regulations of the vigilance system should be integrated into the medical education.

IV. Conclusions

All over the world, the medical devices are regulated by specific rules. The goal of post-market surveillance is to reduce the risk associated with the use of medical devices. Reporting adverse incidents provides valuable information that could prevent similar future incidents. Due to the diversity and complexity of medical devices, it is necessary to have in all countries the standard procedure to notify incidents to the authorities (by developing a national incident reporting systems) and these obligations must be applicable immediately. In order to enhance the efficiency of the Medical Device Vigilance System, it is necessary to encourage the reporting of incidents. Taking as a model the European countries which are active and involved in the assurance of patients' safety, Romania must begin to introduce an adverse event reporting system relate to medical devices and to have an available transparent data. It is necessary to have and to implement specified strategies.

The limit of this study is given by the information available, in different formats, and by the fact that some countries have no open access to the data regarding the use of medical devices. Also, the information on the causes of incidents was not available in all annual reports or on the competent authorities' websites.

Conflict of Interest

The authors declare that they have no conflict of interest.

References

1. Audry A, Ghislain JC (2009) Le dispositif médical. Editure PUF, Paris
2. Mirel, S. Pop, E. Onaca, S. Domnita, V. Mirel (2011) The use of Medical Devices in Self Monitoring of Chronic Diseases, IFMBE Proc. MediTech 2011, Cluj-Napoca, Romania, 36: 48–53
3. Heneghan C, Thompson M, Billingsley M et al. (2011) Medical-device recalls in the UK and the device-regulation process: retrospective review of safety notices and alerts, BMJ Open; 342:d2973;
4. Financial impact of the Revision of the EU Medical Devices Directives on European SMEs and industry, at http://www.eucomed.be/uploads
5. French-Mowat E, Burnett J (2012) How are medical devices regulated in the European Union? J R Soc Med 105: S22 DOI: 10.1258/jrsm.2012.120036
6. Medical Device Directive, MDD (93/ 42/EEC) at http://www.ce-marking.com/medical-devices.html
7. Active Implantable Medical Device Directive, AIMDD (90/383/EEC) at http://www.ce-marking.com/medical-devicesactive-implantable.html
8. In Vitro Diagnostic Medical Device Directive, IVDMDD (98/79/EC) at http://www.ce-marking.com/medical-devices-invitro-diagnostic.html
9. German National Associations of Statutory Health Insurance Funds. Medical devices: the myths and the truth, 2013 at http://www.aok-bv.de/imperia/md/aokbv/politik/versicherte/thesenpapier_gross_0913_engl_1.pdf
10. CDRH FY 2006 Annual Report, at http://www.fda.gov/downloads/AboutFDA/CentersOffices/CDRH/CDRHReports/ucm129258
11. Zuckerman DM, Brown P, Nissen S.E (2011) Medical device recalls and the FDA approval process, Arch Intern Med., 13; 171(11):1006-11.
12. McGee RG, Webster AC, Rogerson TE, Craig JC (2012) Medical device regulation in Australia: safe and effective?, Med J Aust; 196 (4): 256-260 DOI 10.5694/mja11.11261
13. Higson GR (2002) Medical Device Safety: The Regulation of Medical Devices for Public Health, IOP Publishing, London
14. Guidance for Industry and FDA Staff: postmarket surveillance under section 522 of the Federal Food, Drug and Cosmetic Act. at http://www.fda.gov/downloads/MedicalDevices/DeviceReg ulatio-nandGuidance/GuidanceDocuments/ucm072564.pdf
15. Medical devices regulations, at http://www.who.int/medical_devices/safety/en/
16. Role of Standards in the Assessment of Medical Devices Endorsed by: The Global Harmonization Task Force www.imdrf.org/.../ghtf-sg1-n012r10-standards

17. Guidelines on a Medical Devices Vigilance System, MEDDEV 2 12-1 rev. 8 Vigilance, http://ec.europa.eu/health/ medical-devices/files/meddev/2_12_1_ol_en.pdf
18. Jefferys DB (2001) The regulation of medical devices and the role of the Medical Devices Agency. Br J Clin Pharmacol 52 (3):229-235.
19. Canivet N, Hollander K, Mousnier JP, Quaranta JF (2000) La matériovigilance, une vigilance exercée sur l'utilisation des dispositifs médicaux. Transfusion Clinique et Biologique 7(1) : 96–100
20. Vigilance reports at http://ec.europa.eu/health/ medical-devices/documents/vigilance-reports/index_en.htm
21. Anzahl-Risikomel at http://www.bfarm.de/DE/Medizinprodukte/risikoerfassung/wissauf/ statist/statist-Auswert_quartalsweise_Anzahl-Risikomel.html?nn=3497578
22. Annual Report on Devices Adverse Incidents, at http://www.mhra.gov.uk/Publications/Safetyguidance/ DeviceBulletins/CON111657
23. Dispositifs-medicaux at http://ansm.sante.fr/Produits-de-sante
24. Angot H (2011) Matériovigilance. Gestion des incidents. Gestion des alertes, at http://www.synprefh.org/rc/org/synprefh/htm/Article/2011/ 20111223-145916-711/src/htm_fullText/fr/
25. Murray A (2013), Design, Development, Training and Use of Medical Devices; with Practical Examples from Cardiovascular Medicine and Surgery, IFMBE Proc. vol.41, 2014, XIII, Mediterranean Conference on Medical and Biological Engineering and Computing, Spain, 2013, pp 3-6
26. BfArM at http://www.bfarm.de/EN/medDev
27. Rölleke, T (2009) Incident reports to BfArM support the importance of usability for patient safety. IFMBE Proc. vol.25, 2014, XIII, World Congress on Medical Physics and Biomedical Engineering, 2009, Germany, pp. 298-300.
28. Amual Report on Devices Adverse Incidents at http://www.mhra.gov.uk/Howweregulate/Devices/index.htm
29. Dispozitive medicale at http://www.anm.ro/anmdm/
30. Puia V (2010) Cercetări privind legislația dispozitivelor medicale în România.Clujul Medical 83 (3): 468-472.
31. Lege Nr. 176 / 2000 (Republicată), Monitorul Oficial 79 (2005)
32. Vigilance contact points within the national competent authorities at http://ec.europa.eu/health/medical-devices/ links/vigilance_contact_points_en.htm 10.
33. Mirel S, Neag F (2008) Medical Devices Risk Management. International Conference on Automation, Quality and Testing, Robotics, Cluj-Napoca, Romania, 2008, Proc. pp 28-31

Author: Mirel Simona
Institute: UMF Cluj-Napoca
Street: N. Pascaly 9
City:Cluj Napoca
Country: Romania
Email: smirel@umfcluj.ro

Content Marketing in Dentist's Websites. An Empirical Comparative Study between Romania and the UK

A. Constantinescu-Dobra

Technical University of Cluj-Napoca, Electrical Engineering Faculty, Department of Electric Power Systems and Management, Cluj-Napoca, Romania

Abstract— **The dental industry is one of the most attractive segments of the healthcare industry because it has experienced constant growth, in recent years. Existing studies concerning healthcare marketing activity reveal that Internet marketing has become a more important strategy than in the last decade. Moreover, content marketing can be an effective strategy for dental providers.**

This paper aims at identifying the core elements concerning content marketing for dental websites. Furthermore, the main goal is to comparatively analyze those website content items that contribute to establishing trust and an educational relationship between patients and dentists. The empirical research is both a quantitative and a qualitative one, based on the assessment of 57 items clustered into nine categories: trust enhancing information, brand awareness, service information, related, educational information, non-related information, mapping, targeting of visitors, feedback tools. The sample consists of 50 Romanian websites and 50 websites from the United Kingdom (UK). We have chosen this sample because, according to [1], UK has the most efficient public oral health care service. The research outcomes exclusively reflect the propensity for education and prevention of UK sites and the propensity rather toward marketing communication of the Romanian ones. The main finding is the following: the degree of content marketing penetration in UK sites is 57%, while in Romanian's ones, only 23%. The significant disparity between the dental sites from the two countries is encountered in brand awareness content (17% UK vs. 3% RO) and feedback (15% UK vs. 1% RO).

Keywords— **content marketing, websites content, dental industry, dental education**

I. INTRODUCTION

The dental industry today is rapidly growing and it is facing many challenges. The most important of them are the shifts in patients' behavior, doubled by the high level of technological progress of apparel and materials used in this field. Some reasons that explain the constantly expanding demand for dental services are the growing acceptance for cosmetic dental surgery [2] strong competition in materials and equipment production, price reduction of cosmetic treatments and finally, media coverage that has created a high level of consumer interest in such procedures and services. The transactions on dental services have annually increased with 4.5% market growth [3] [4].

From a different perspective, researchers also reveal that Internet is becoming a rich source of health care information for the public [5]. More than 70 000 websites disseminate health information and more than 50 million people seek health information online [6]. The Internet offers widespread access to health information and the advantages of interactivity, customized information and anonymity.

Although Romanian dental industry is at its early stage of development, patients also choose cosmetic dental surgeries apart from basic procedures. The latest studies on Romanian Dental Market [7] [8] highlight a great potential for future growth on the base of affordable pricing, short treatment period, usage of advanced state-of-the-art technology and well-trained professionals. In the last ten years, ageing population, along with rising awareness for oral health, aesthetics and improved dental treatments have increased this segment by 17%.

The above-mentioned researches suggest that dental marketing strategy will be the key to success in the future for most stakeholders in this field.

Thus, innovative technologies along with stronger and more esthetic materials are making work easier for clinicians and laboratory technicians and strengthening their relationships with customers and patients. Experts in the fields [9] agree that, in 2013, the following trends have influenced the dental industry:

- the mass digitization of dentistry. Patient's treatment becomes more effective and the subjectivity in dental services decreases as dentists and laboratory technicians use digital processes and procedures in an extensive manner. Furthermore, communication becomes faster and more critical;
- the economic crisis. The economic regression has driven many patients to seek more cost-effective solutions;
- the dental insurance companies` strategy has changed: in the sense of them identifying new ways to lower healthcare costs by offering dental care packages for employers to give to their employees.
- *Content marketing* is a relatively recently implemented strategy in dental field, marketers recommend it especially to service providers as one of the most powerful tools in order to achieve loyal customers.

S. Vlad and R.V. Ciupa (eds.), *International Conference on Advancements of Medicine and Health Care through Technology*, IFMBE Proceedings 44,
DOI: 10.1007/978-3-319-07653-9_22, © Springer International Publishing Switzerland 2014

Given this, it is a fact that, in the last decade, dental marketing became more and more oriented to image building, especially through Internet channels. Nowadays, attracting attention to a dentist's website is as important as the practice itself and contributes to how patients perceive the overall value. Posting informative articles and interacting via social media allows dentists to show a more personal and approachable side, to strength the relation with patients and customers. Social media profiles can also reveal more information about the persons involved in the medical act. The medical provider is thus seen as a trusted consultant and partner in patients' health. In addition, trough Internet marketing, patients can share their positive experiences in dental practices with their reference group. Furthermore, specialists agree that recommendations from a trusted family member or friend continue to be among the most powerful advertising [10]. Patient referrals and recommendations are no longer limited to one-to-one interactions, but can now effectively be broadcast as one-to-many communications via social media. Recent studies found that E-learning, in all of its many guises, becomes increasingly important [11].

In Romania, dental stakeholders slowly begun to adapt to the global dental trends presented above [12]. Romanian dental suppliers are implementing just a few of online tactics, combining direct sales with brand consolidation.

Another reason to analyze content marketing pattern in the dental field was determined by the findings [13] [14] according to which Internet holds the future for dental marketing. Thereby, along with the trends towards globalization, networking, mass customization, and digitization, companies must align their practice. Nowadays, websites represent an efficient tool for distributors, general dentists, specialists, educators, and consultants in the dental field.

All of the above facts are the reasons why our study aims at identifying the strategic differences between content marketing strategies of Romanian and UK companies acting in dental industry. Specifically, we try to assess content marketing items of providers' websites that determine image consolidation. We chose the dental care sector because the online techniques, materials used and procedures are rapidly evolving in this particular branch of the healthcare industry.

In order to achieve our goal, the paper examines the state of the art in websites assessment and content marketing. A customized methodology was elaborated. The pilot study is using both the qualitative and quantitative approach: contents analysis. For websites analysis, the sample consists of 100 Romanian and UK companies from the dental industry.

The originality of the paper mainly consists in the specific methodology built to reach the objective and the results of content marketing practice in Romania and the UK.

This study can be useful especially for dental entrepreneurs interested in undergoing a self-check for the various areas indicated in the study and recommends actions on how the gaps can best be minimized. We believe that content marketing can help dental entrepreneurs improve their customer service and performance.

II. CONTENT MARKETING AND WEBSITES CONTENT

The term content marketing was used as early as 1996 [15] but in the last decade has enriched with other meanings, due to the various channels provided by the Internet. There are a lot of definitions of these terms, meaning researchers and practitioners are still looking at ways to apply it. Content Marketing Institute states that [15] content marketing is "the marketing and business process for creating and distributing relevant and valuable content to attract, acquire, and engage a clearly defined and understood target audience – with the objective of driving profitable customer action".

According to [16] content marketing is not a tactic, but a strategy that is especially created for online tools. It can [17] encompass all forms of content that add value to consumers thereby directly or indirectly promoting a business, brand, products or services. Additionally, it offers to the business-client or to the end-user prospective trustful, meaningful, tailored and needed information. Basically, content marketing supports companies in disseminating information that makes the buyer more intelligent instead of pitching the products or services.

The advantage of content marketing in an advertisements-crowded environment is that the main goal is not to sell, but to provide brand recognition, authority, credibility, loyalty and authenticity.

The most important tactics of content marketing are: social-media posts, e-mail newsletters, blog posts/Guest blog posts, e-books, PowerPoint presentations, podcasts, standard videos/Micro-videos, live presentations; webinars, white papers. Research conducted in 2010 [18] found that nowadays small and medium companies spend 33% from the total marketing budget for content marketing and over 60% of marketers planned to increase this percentage in the future. Moreover, 90% of US companies are implementing content strategy in the marketing mix.

In our opinion, in addition to content marketing, the online marketing is a 'generic term' that includes in the same extent online advertising, viral marketing, e-mail marketing, search engine marketing, direct response marketing. We believe, also that the websites marketing can comprise the content marketing tools, only if:

1) the provided content has not the purpose to sell but is focused on delivering information to make the buyer more intelligent (hence, without e-stores, e-forms, web-marketing advertising) and
2) the websites is an integrative platform for social media, blogs, live seminars, videos etc. (if on the websites there is a link for these tools)

A great number of authors have put forward recommendations about how to create a quality online content [18][19][20][21]. The most used criteria encountered in almost every specialists approach include elements such as purpose, source/authority, and information about products and company.

Liu and Arnett [22] explained the quality factors for content marketing such as accuracy, completeness, relevancy, reliability, customization and interactivity, and organization. Experts argue that 62% of the final score given by a visitor to a site is related to its content [23]. Bradley [23] describes features to look for when assessing and evaluating the authority of a resource. Among others, these include authority, domain name, company logo, contact details, currency, awards, page design, the owners of the site etc. However, it is also noted that assessing the content quality is not a straightforward procedure involving an identification of the presence or absence of different features or facilities. Methodologies focused on the Websites content quality approach emphasize hypermedia Web design and the importance of the interface in order to facilitate information access and to improve the overall human-computer interaction. [23]

III. Methodology

A. Research Objectives

The main goal of this research is to investigate the degree of content marketing usage in Romanian and UK dental websites. The main objectives derived from this goal are:

- Assessing the penetration of content marketing tools in the dental field;
- Evaluating the degree of implementation of content marketing tools in Romania vs. the UK dental websites.

B. Research Methodology

The performed research is a qualitative one, based on content analysis of dental websites information and a quantitative one, analyzing 57 variables of each assessed website.

The data was collected between November and December 2013. The random sample was planned to enclose 50 Romanian dental websites and 50 from the UK. We have assessed the first 50 sites for each countries displayed by local Google search engine by the words "dental services". We choose a sample from UK and Romania because, according to [1], UK has the most efficient public oral health care service. Children and young people in UK now have Europe's best oral health in terms of mean DMFT (decayed, missing or filled teeth), with 10% lower in 2009 to 1973. In addition, [24] found that UK marketers use content marketing tactics more than North American and Australian marketers.

From the listed websites, during the assessment period, 20% were dental portals (that are not owned by a dental practitioners and are listing many possibilities to find dentist practitioners by category of provided services), 35% belonged to clinics (which provide more dental care services and more dental practitioners are involved) and the majority of them were websites of private practitioners and clinician.

In order to assess the content, we have clustered the variable founded in previous section into nine categories. Examples of variable are given:

1.) Trust enhancing information (12 items): list of employees e-mail addresses and phones, information about CEO, Owners, practitioners and technicians (names, personal values, CV, projects, photos), other employees photos, annual report, investments information, social responsibility, company history, vision;
2.) Brand awareness (6 items): leisure activities (specific games for different target groups), possibility to download logo, commercials icons for mobiles, greeting cards with visual-audio identifications systems, press release;
3.) Service information (9 items): descriptions of services, information about treatment procedures, about used materials, comparison of different type of treatments with arguments, testimonials, patients program, support group, prices, payment modality;
4.) Related information (3 items): information about insurances, donations, links to health care organizations;
5.) Educational information (6 items): general health care information, oral care information, prevention, oral procedure, oral hygiene, cosmetic procedure, chirurgical procedures;
6.) Other information (non-related) (3 items): general news, tips and tricks, links to non-health care organizations;
7.) Mapping (5 items): navigation path, search full text, index, help function, sitemap;
8.) Targeting the group of website visitors (5 items): specific information for payers, suppliers, partners, customer, and team;
9.) Feedback tools (8 items): social networking, blog, forum, online consultation, intranet, newsletter, guestbook.

For each website, every variable was evaluated in a binary system and the final score resulted from the total amount of all existing variables in a website. It is worth mentioning that we do not take into consideration those tabs (variables) that exist in the websites but they were not functional or the information was obsolete. For example we do not aggregate the score of an empty (or with no relevant information) link (even if the tab exists) or for a no-updated Facebook page (with no information).

In the evaluation process, every variable was considered equally important.

IV. FINDINGS AND DISCUSSION

The data was processed in the statistic software SPSS 16. In evaluating the content marketing for dental websites we assessed the above listed variables by clusters. The results are depicted in Figure 1 and Table 1.

In the beginning, we have analyzed the percentage of the each nine characteristics in dental content marketing. Figure 1 presents the aggregate score by the three types of websites: dental portals, dental clinic websites and clinicians' sites.

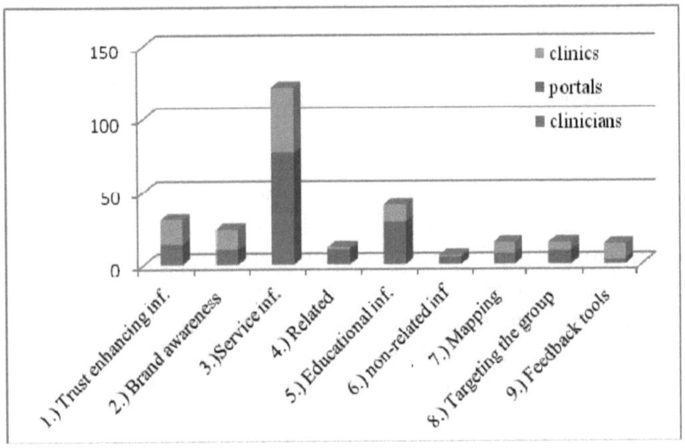

Fig. 1 The content marketing dimensions of the sample

The highest score was obtained by the characteristic service information (39%), followed by trust enhancing information (13%), and brand awareness, respectively, educational information (12%). Feedback, mapping and targeting are not so important for dental marketers (or practitioners), obtaining just 8%, 7%, respectively 5% in total content marketing implementation. The most neglected characteristics are related to information of health care and general information. When evaluating the three types of dental websites (portals, clinics' websites and clinicians/practitioners websites) in depth, one can notice that big actors such as clinics pay more attention to building trust and credibility and to brand reinforcement as opposed to clinicians' websites and portals. The differences reach 7% and, respectively, 3% percentages. In clinics' websites, navigation tools are more performing by targeting the public. Hence, the prospective customers have the possibility to access the needed information rapidly. In the case of dental portals, content marketing is abundant in educational information. The disparity in comparison with clinicians is quite large: with 10% more information in dental portals than in clinics websites or 15% than in private clinicians' websites. On the one hand, dental portals are targeting better the group segments providing tailored information but, on the other hand, pay less attention to mapping and feedback tools. The portals in this particular case can be considered an intermediary, as portal owners are perceived as having more expertise in marketing which allows for the customization of the information provided to different clients. Nevertheless, they do not encourage the feedback process probably because they are not dental professionals.

Private clinicians usually small companies, disseminate service information, contact information and do not consider it significant, in most of cases, to educate customers in terms of prevention, segments targeting or informing online visitors about dental news.

Table 1 reveals the most or least used variables of content marketing of the sample. All the companies in the sample describe the services they are providing in detail. Many of the dental websites comprise content marketing variables such as: corporate information, inside photos, treatment procedure, insisting on the materials used and their characteristics/benefits for patients.

Table 1 The most often used and the less used content marketing (MK) variables of dental websites in the sample

***Top ten* content MK Variables**	(%)	**The *last ten* content MK variables**	(%)
Services descriptions	100	Personal value of practitioners	0
Corporate information	96	Investments information	0
Inside Photos	88	Downloads ringtone/icons	0
Patients' program	87	Annual report	0
Company contacts	87	Donations	0
Equipment/material Inf.	78	Press release	1
Treatment procedure	74	Leisure activity	3
Names of practitioners	72	Information about CEO/owner	3
Prices	70	Support group	4
Payment modality	69	Social responsibility	5

Source: computed data form empirical study, N=100

Conversely, the content of accessed sites is very weak in what concerns the following variables: *personal* believes/values of practitioners (0%), investment information etc.

The degree of content marketing penetration in UK sites is 57%, while in Romanian's ones, only 23%.

Figure 2 presents disparities between the nine characteristics of dental Romanian sites and those from the UK.

The biggest gap in content marketing of the two analyzed countries is revealed in *brand awareness content* (17% UK vs. 3% RO) and *feedback* (15% UK vs. 1% RO).

Dental websites from the UK insist on displaying video-audio identification systems in many forms and websites' places.

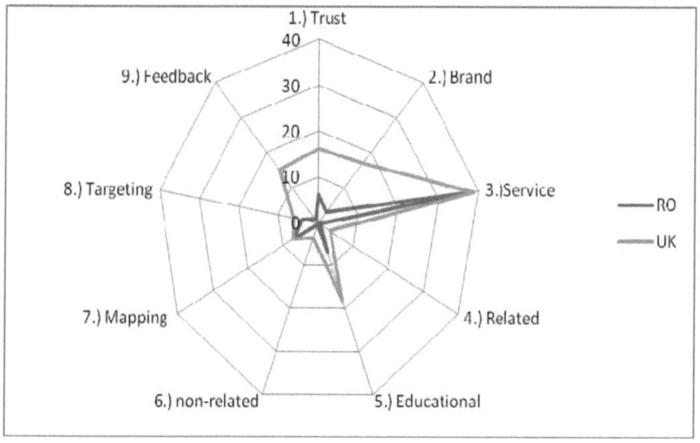

Fig. 2 The comparatively content marketing study by countries

A percentage of 37% of UK sites offer the possibility to download some useful (or funny) applications which emphasize the company's colors, name and logo, like: dental theme school schedules/diplomas for kids, post- its, brushing timers, interesting or original commercials as ring tone, applications for smart phones (personalized with logo) helping to plan the dental treatment, to archive chronologically dental problems/facts, processing images (adding to a photo library and create, send, and print them). More than that, the prospects can access dedicated soft in order to simulate their teeth whitening or their aspects with braces.

Neither Romanian nor UK sites use many online tools for feedback in their websites. Only 4 dental sites from the UK have links to social networks and none have a forum, blog or chat. 4 Romanian sites display a feedback form and 2 the possibility to ask online solution for a dental problem.

Education information from UK sites point out a disparity of 11%. Romanian sites list mainly information regarding upper-mass dental services: implants (49%), orthodontics (36%) or cosmetic dentistry (whitening, teeth veneers) (32 %) but hygiene information is almost neglected. Only 12% of Romanian sites display general information about prevention and teeth care. The study found little information about brushing, especially for kids. It is known that Romanians are not very educated in terms of health prevention in comparison with patients from more developed countries [25]. Hence, the un-educative websites could be an answer to market behavior. Thereby, Romanian practitioners write about top edge dental services which are accessed by a documented customer who affords to pay a skimming price.

In the UK dental websites, education information is provided in a very dynamic manner. The existing animation allows dentists to illustrate the effects of dental conditions such as periodontal disease, decay, cracks, and other conditions over time. Moreover, 24% of UK websites offer access to educative applications for smart devices regarding dental care. Most of them refer to:

- containing challenging questions that cover a wide variety of subjects from radiography, odontology, diet and prevention, children's dentistry and many other dental aspects especially for kids, teenagers and students;
- teaching patients the correct way to brush;
- containing a dental glossary, diagram and symptom checker;
- containing dictionary of all things Dentistry;
- allowing patients to see all teeth in X-ray format.

Finally, the last significant gap is encountered in *trust building information* (16 % UK vs. 6% RO). UK sites offer more details of clinicians and their expertise than Romanian ones. The detailed information about companies is insignificant in all sites from the sample.

V. CONCLUSIONS

The degree of content marketing penetrations in dental field is quite small – 40%. In conclusion, dental practitioners are implementing content marketing strategies with some particularities: emphasis on service information, trust enhancing, brand awareness and dental care education, neglecting feedback tools, mapping, target tools and general information. Romanian websites are focusing particularly on the most specialized (also expensive) services, while UK sites are moving toward providing interactive applications in order to make site navigation more accessible and enjoyable. We consider that content marketing could help dental marketers increase patients' loyalty especially in the case of the young generation which is "digitally native". We sugest for UK and Romanian marketers and dental practitioners to display more educative and customized information for prospects by target segments, not only from the field of dental care, but in a holistic manner, with links on the general healthcare. In order to strenght the relations with their public, and make them loyal, the owners/clinicians must interact more through online means: to reveal their personals values, beliefs on blogs and comments the dental news on forums or using social media. They can offer some gust book for patients and the feedback must be provided promptly. For partners, sending relevant newsletters can be a solution in order to maintain a good business relation.

Webminars, study cases, quizes can be very usefull for dental students, segment that will become in the future oppinion leader for specialized procedure.

VI. Limitation and future research

The limitation of the present study consists in the small sample of dental websites. The author`s future actions will be: 1) to validate the methodology on a larger sample, taking into account the size and the market share of investigated dental companies.

2) to check through specific marketing research if the dimensions are equally efficient and defining weights for each dimension

Acknowledgment

This study has been performed in the framework of PN II-RU research grant “Development of an electronic marketing plan for Romanian SMEs in order to increase their competitiveness”, PD 58/2010, supported by CNCSIS-UEFISCSU.

Conflict or Interest

The author declares that she has no conflict of interest.

References

1. Oral Health in Europe Report Commissioned by the Platform for Better Oral Health in Europe, http://www.oralhealthplatform.eu/sites/default/files/field/document/Report%20-%20the%20State%20of%20Oral%20Health%20in%20Europe.pdf
2. De Jongh A., Oosterink F., van Rood Y. and Aartman I. (2008) Preoccupation with ones appearance: A motivating factor for cosmetic dental treatment? *British Dental Journal* 204 (12): 691
3. Press J, Simms C (2010) Segmenting cosmetic procedures markets using benefit segmentation: A study of the market for tooth whitening services in the UK, *Journal of Medical Marketing* (2010) 10, 183–198
4. Global Dental Industry: An Analysis (2009) http://www.reportlinker.com/p0167104/Global-Dental-Industry-An-Analysis.html
5. Tickotsky N., Moskovitz M. and Caspi A. (2011) Dentists' attitudes toward discussing Internet health information with their patients – does professional self-efficacy matter?, *Journal of Public Health Dentistry,* 71,(2) pp. 102–105
6. Cline R and Haynes KM (2001). Consumer health information seeking on the Internet: the state of art. Health Educ Res 2001 Dec;16(6), pp. 671–692
7. Euromonitor International (2010) Romania : economy statistics and industry reports, http://www.reportlinker.com/r0792/Romania-industry-reports.html
8. Institutul National de Statistica, www.insse.ro
9. Roger P. Levin, DDS, (2012) Trends in Dentistry, *Inside Dental Technology,* December 2012, Volume 3, Issue 11, Published by AEGIS Communications, https://www.dentalaegis.com/idt/2012/12/trends-in-dentistry
10. Catana G A (2009) Marketingul serviciilor de ocrotire a sanatatii, Alma Mater, Cluj-Napoca
11. Downes P. K. (2007) Putting it all together; dentistry and the Internet, *British Dental Journal* 203, pp.75 - 86 ,published online: 28 July 2007 | doi:10.1038/bdj.2007.633
12. Constantinescu-Dobra A. (2012) The internet marketing and the SMEs. A comparative analisys of dentistry strategy for online and printing advertising. Proceedings of International Conference on Marketing, *"Marketing from information to decision" 5-th edition*, Universitatea Babes-Bolyai, Cluj-Napoca, Facultatea de Stiinte Economice si gestiunea Afacerilor, Ed. Risoprint, p. 75-88
13. Baldwin, A. and Sohal A. (2003) Service quality factors and outcomes in dental care, *Managing Service Quality*, Vol. 13 Issue: 3, pp. 207 – 216
14. Chandler, E.W. and Weller, R.B. (2004)The practice of marketing by dentists, *Health Marketing Quarterly* 1994; 12(1), pp.73-96.
15. Pulizzi, J. (2012) Six Useful Content Marketing Definitions, *Chief Content Officer Rewiev*, June 6, 2012, http://contentmarketinginstitute.com/2012/06/content-marketing-definition/
16. Lieb, R. (2011) Content Marketing: Think like a publisher-How to use content marketing online and in Social Media, Que Publishing
17. Gunelius S. (2011) *Content Marketing*, John Wiley & Sons Inc, pp.4-6
18. Head, A. J. (2000). Design Wise: A guide for evaluating the interface design of information resources. New Jersey: CyberAge books.
19. Mich, L., Franch, M. & L. e Gaio (2003). ‚Evaluating and Designing Web Site Quality’. *IEEE Multimedia*, Janeiro-Março 2003, pp.34-43.
20. Nielsen, J. (2002) Homepage usability: 50 websites deconstructed. Indianapolis: New Riders.
21. www.profnet.de
22. Liu, C. and K.P. Arnett (2000). ‘Exploring the factors associated with web site success in the context of electronic commerce. *Information and Management*, **38**(1), 23-33
23. Bradley, P. (2002) *The Advanced Internet Searcher’s Handbook.* 2-nd edition. London: Library Association Publishing.
24. http://contentmarketinginstitute.com/2013/12/uk-2014-content-marketing-research
25. IRES (2012) Institutul Roman de Evaluare si Strategie, Medicii dentisti– Percepţii publice. Atitudinile şi comportamentele de igienă dentare ale românilor, http://www.comunicatemedicale.ro/upload/docs/443.pdf

Author: Constantinescu-Dobra Anca
Institute: Technical University of Cluj-Napoca
Street: Memorandumului, no. 28
City: Cluj-Napoca
Country: Romania
Email: anca.constantinescu@eps.utcluj.ro

Reliability Indicators and a Failure Mode and Effect Analysis Calculation for a Holter Recorder

D. Iudean[1], R.A. Munteanu[1], P. Bechet[2], C. Mureşan[1], and A. Creţu[1]

[1] Faculty of Electrical Engineering, Technical University of Cluj-Napoca, Cluj-Napoca, Romania
[2] "Nicolae Balcescu" Land Forces Academy, Sibiu, Romania

Abstract— **Product reliability is very important nowadays, and everyone seeks products that will last very long without failing. It is hard to make a product good and reliable without investing in reliability research from the early stages of the design. This paper presents a reliability analysis for a Holter Recorder for home use, and also a Failure Mode and Effect Analysis using Relex software. This approach can be used for any similar device and helps the manufacturer design a better product.**

Keywords— **Reliability, FMEA, Holter Recorder**

I. Introduction

The probability that a system or an element to function in certain conditions is denoted by R(t) and it represents the probability that the operating time in good conditions of the system or element to be at least equal to the operating time given by the manufacturer.

The probability of good operating is given by the equation [1][2]:

$$R(t) = \frac{N(t)}{N} \quad (1)$$

where:

- N represents the total number of elements;
- N(t) represents the number of elements which have not failed during time t.

The probability of failure of a system or element is given by:

$$Q(t) = 1 - R(t) \quad (2)$$

The failure rate has an important role in reliability analysis. It is denoted by λ(t) and represents the probability of failure for a system or element after a certain period of time.

The failure rate is given by the equation [1][2]:

$$\lambda(t) = \frac{Q(t)/dt}{R(t)} \quad (3)$$

In case the failure rate is considered constant the probability of operating without failure is given by the equation [1][2]:

$$\lambda(t) = \frac{Q(t)/dt}{R(t)} \quad (4)$$

The mean time to failure is denoted by MTTF and is given by the equation [1][2]:

$$MTTF = \int_0^\infty R(t)dt \quad (5)$$

The mean time between failures is denoted by MTBF and is given by the following equation when the failure rate is constant [1][2]:

$$MTBF = \frac{1}{\lambda} \quad (6)$$

A FMEA (failure mode and effect analysis) is part of the inductive methods of evaluating the reliability and security of systems. FMEA provides a method to analyze the system and to evaluate the potential failures. It consists in breaking the system into components to determine what can fail, how it fails (failure modes), why it fails and, in the end, to determine the effects of each failure. An important part of a FMEA includes the analysis of the criticality of the end effects of failure modes. FMEA represents one of the most frequently used instruments in reliability evaluation. [3][4]

Usually FMEAs are made accordingly to standards published and accepted all over the world. The most frequent standards used are MIL-STD-1629 and SAE ARP5580 [3][4][5].

The existing reliability standards require a qualitative approach to criticality. Table 1 [3][4][5] defines the criticality groups when a qualitative approach is used.

The criticality values from Table 1 are calculated using the following equation [3][4][5]:

$$Cm = \beta * \alpha * \lambda p * t \quad (7)$$

where:

- Cm - criticality number for the failure mode;
- β - conditional probability of loss, or failure effect probability;

S. Vlad and R.V. Ciupa (eds.), *International Conference on Advancements of Medicine and Health Care through Technology*, IFMBE Proceedings 44,
DOI: 10.1007/978-3-319-07653-9_23, © Springer International Publishing Switzerland 2014

- α - failure mode ratio;
- λp - part failure or hazard rate;
- t - number of operating cycles expressed in hours.

Table 1 Qualitative Approach to Criticality Analysis

Criticality Group	Probability Criteria
Level A – Frequent	Failure mode probability is greater than 0.20 of the overall probability of failure
Level B – Reasonably Probable	Failure mode probability is greater than 0.10 but less than 0.20 of the overall probability of failure
Level C – Occasional	Failure mode probability is greater than 0.01 but less than 0.10 of the overall probability of failure
Level D – Remote	Failure mode probability is greater than 0.001 but less than 0.01 of the overall probability of failure
Level E – Extremely Unlikely	Failure mode probability is less than 0.001 of the overall probability of failure

A technique used for analyzing the risk associated with potential problems identified during a FMEA is the Risk Priority Number (RPN).

Risk Priority Number uses three rating scales: the first one is Severity which rates the severity of the potential effect of the failure; the second one is Occurrence which rates the likelihood that the failure will occur and the third one is Detection which rates the likelihood that the problem will be detected before it reaches the end-user/customer [6]:

$$RPN = severity * occurence * detection \tag{8}$$

II. RELIABILITY INDICATORS CALCULATION

To analyze a system with the Relex Reliability Studio 2007 software (now Windchill Prediction) it is important that the system, its components and the operating environment to be known. The data gathering was made analyzing data supplied by the manufacturer: the operating conditions and the technical parameters of the recorder.

To calculate the reliability indicators a system tree was defined (Holter Recorder). For each component composing element of the recorder, a data set was assigned: the category and subcategory of the element, number of units and the standards (the most common standards used were: MIL-STD-1629 and SAE ARP5580) according to which the indicators were calculated. Thus, in Figure 1 is shown the failure rate percentage, the reliability, the failure rate calculated in fpmh (failure per million hours) and the mean time between failures (MTBF).

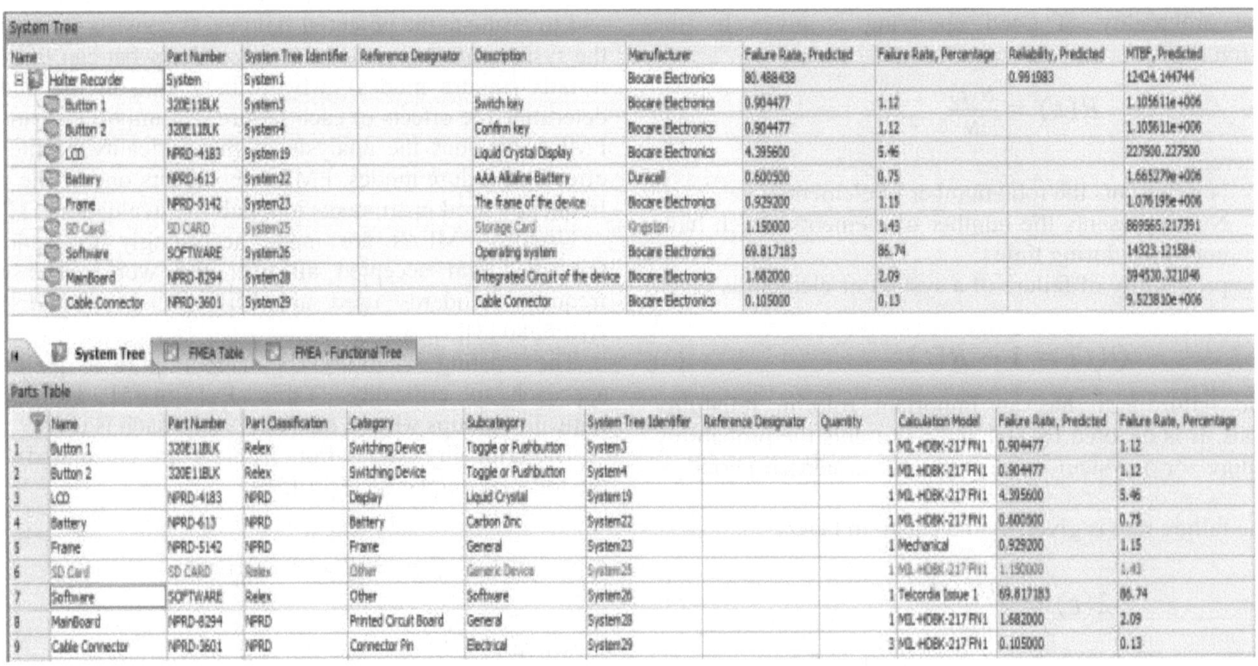
System Tree

Name	Part Number	System Tree Identifier	Reference Designator	Description	Manufacturer	Failure Rate, Predicted	Failure Rate, Percentage	Reliability, Predicted	MTBF, Predicted
Holter Recorder	System	System1			Biocare Electronics	80.488438		0.991983	12424.144744
Button 1	320E11BLK	System3		Switch key	Biocare Electronics	0.904477	1.12		1.105611e+006
Button 2	320E11BLK	System4		Confirm key	Biocare Electronics	0.904477	1.12		1.105611e+006
LCD	NPRD-4183	System19		Liquid Crystal Display	Biocare Electronics	4.395600	5.46		227500.227500
Battery	NPRD-613	System22		AAA Alkaline Battery	Duracell	0.600900	0.75		1.665279e+006
Frame	NPRD-5142	System23		The frame of the device	Biocare Electronics	0.929200	1.15		1.076195e+006
SD Card	SD CARD	System25		Storage Card	Kingston	1.150000	1.43		869565.217391
Software	SOFTWARE	System26		Operating system	Biocare Electronics	69.817183	86.74		14323.121584
MainBoard	NPRD-8294	System28		Integrated Circuit of the device	Biocare Electronics	1.682000	2.09		594530.321046
Cable Connector	NPRD-3601	System29		Cable Connector	Biocare Electronics	0.105000	0.13		9.523810e+006

System Tree | FMEA Table | FMEA - Functional Tree

Parts Table

	Name	Part Number	Part Classification	Category	Subcategory	System Tree Identifier	Reference Designator	Quantity	Calculation Model	Failure Rate, Predicted	Failure Rate, Percentage
1	Button 1	320E11BLK	Relex	Switching Device	Toggle or Pushbutton	System3		1	MIL-HDBK-217 FN1	0.904477	1.12
2	Button 2	320E11BLK	Relex	Switching Device	Toggle or Pushbutton	System4		1	MIL-HDBK-217 FN1	0.904477	1.12
3	LCD	NPRD-4183	NPRD	Display	Liquid Crystal	System19		1	MIL-HDBK-217 FN1	4.395600	5.46
4	Battery	NPRD-613	NPRD	Battery	Carbon Zinc	System22		1	MIL-HDBK-217 FN1	0.600900	0.75
5	Frame	NPRD-5142	NPRD	Frame	General	System23		1	Mechanical	0.929200	1.15
6	SD Card	SD CARD	Relex	Other	Generic Device	System25		1	MIL-HDBK-217 FN1	1.150000	1.43
7	Software	SOFTWARE	Relex	Other	Software	System26		1	Telcordia Issue 1	69.817183	86.74
8	MainBoard	NPRD-8294	NPRD	Printed Circuit Board	General	System28		1	MIL-HDBK-217 FN1	1.682000	2.09
9	Cable Connector	NPRD-3601	NPRD	Connector Pin	Electrical	System29		3	MIL-HDBK-217 FN1	0.105000	0.13

Fig. 1 Holter Recorder System and Parts Table

Following, the results of the analysis of the Holter Recorder are presented. The reliability indicators that must be tracked are: reliability over time, failure rate and MTBF.

From the results of the calculation, it can be seen that the reliability of the module, analyzed for 15000 hours of operating is good, sticking to the ideal path. After the considered period of time, the product reaches its end of life. The chart for the reliability over time is presented in Figure 2.

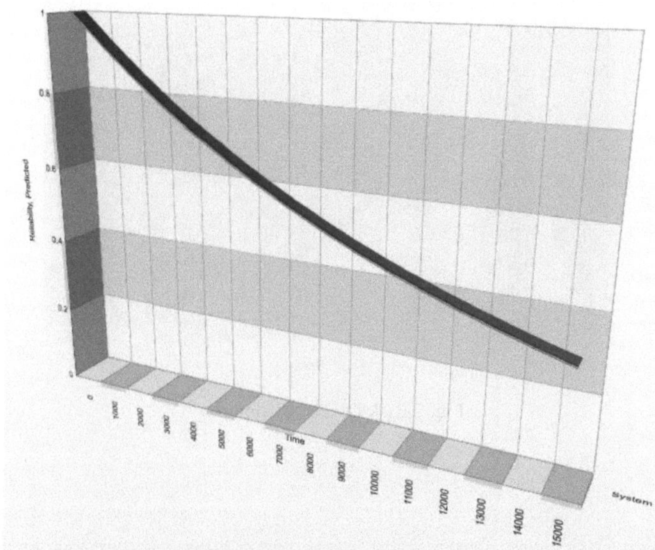

Fig. 2 Reliability over time

The Holter Recorder can operate in different environments like fixed, mobile or benign. For all these environments the reliability remains relatively high and constant like shown in Figure 3.

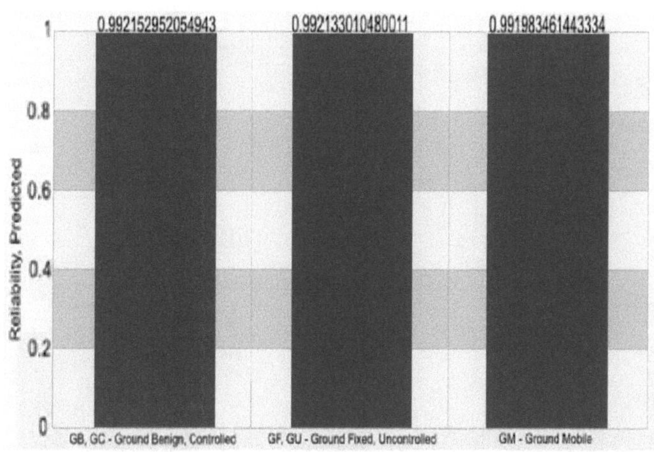

Fig. 3 Reliability over environments

Where the system is subjected to stress, it can be seen that the failure rate has a slightly increasing characteristic (Figure 4), but still at intensive use the level of the failure rate is low. The stresses are expressed in percent.

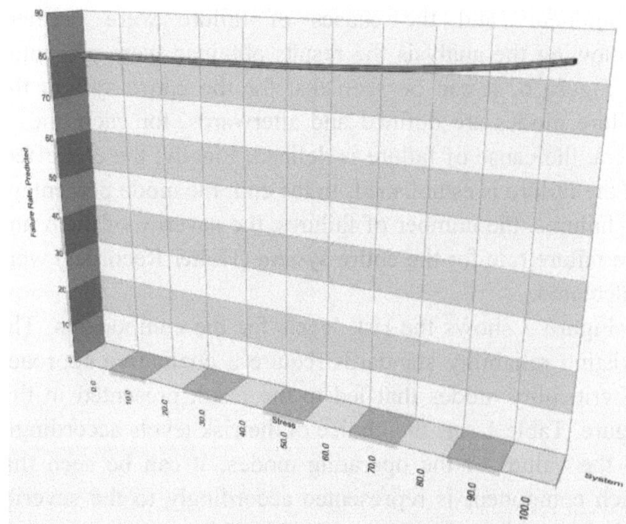

Fig. 4 Failure rate over Stress

The MTBF characteristic (Figure 5) is relatively constant in terms of stresses. It can be seen that at around 12000 hours of operating, a failure may appear. For increasing stresses MTBF decreases but it remains around 12000 hours. The stresses are expressed in percent.

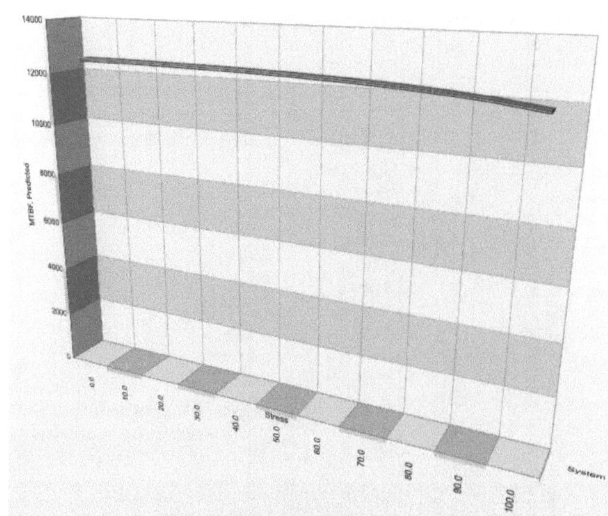

Fig. 5 MTBF over Stress

III. FAILURE MODE AND EFFECT ANALYSIS

This paper provides an original study in order to conduct the Failure Mode and Effect Analysis for the Holter Recorder. For the recorder, the failure modes of the components and the causes of failure were defined. Following the analysis the results obtained were presented in Figure 6. It can be seen that for the entire system the failure modes are defined and afterwards, for each one of them, the cause of failure is defined. Finally, the end effect of the failure is established. In the end, the mode percentage of failures, the number of failures, the severity of them and the failure rate for the entire system (Holter Recorder) were calculated.

Figure 7 shows the risk levels for the components. The existing reliability standards require a qualitative approach of criticality modes that led to the result presented in this figure. Table 1 sets the choice of the risk levels accordingly to the values of the operating modes. It can be seen that each component is represented accordingly to the severity and the number of occurrences of the failures.

For the Holter Recorder the criticality values of the components are presented in Figure 8. These values are calculated using equation (7). It can be seen that the software has the highest probability of failure, followed by the SD Card and the rest of the components.

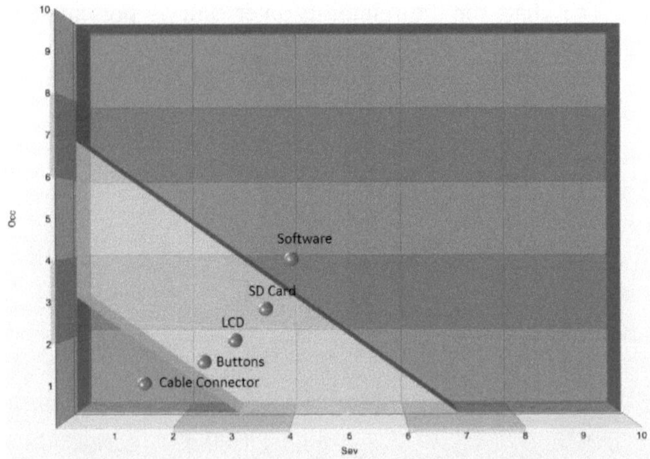

Fig. 7 Risk Levels distribution

FMEA Worksheet

	Item Identifier	Item Name	Item Description	Mode Identifier	Failure Mode	Cause of Failure	End Effect	Mode Percentage	Occurence	Detection	Severity	RPN	Item Failure Rate
1	System	Holter Recorder	Holter Recorder is a device which performs ECG recording and blood pressure for adults and kids above 12 years of age	Buttons	Not responding to action	Bad contact	Not able to select the needed settings	3.44	Remote	9	Critical	1575	80.488438
2						Faulty buttons							
3				SD Card	The recorder shows the message "ACTV Card Failed" or "Erase Card Error, Check SD Card!"; The PC doesn't find the card or the documents	The card was not properly inserted	Not able to store documents on SD card; Not able to read the documents stored on the SD card	32.57	Reasonably Probable	9	Catastrophic	6750	
4						Problems with the device							
5						Faulty memory card							
6						The format of the card is not corresponding							
7						Faulty SD card reader							
8						USB connection is unstable							
9						PC operating systems take a while until finding the recorder, if it is removed before finding it, the documents can't be shown							
10				LCD	Incorect display	LCD faulty	Incorrect viewing of values; Hard to read and view the values	7.46	Remote	9	Critical	1575	
11				Software	Not showing the parameters on the PC; Incorect display of values; Not responding to commands	Software improperly installed or setup error	Not able to use the recorder	55.40	Reasonably Probable	10	Catastrophic	7500	
12						Software error							
13						Recorder error							
14						Improper connexion with the PC							
15				Cable Connector	Interferences; Poor signal quality	Problem with the wires	The recorder won't display the values	1.13	Remote	8	Critical	1400	
16						Poor contact between electrodes and skin							

Fig. 6 FMEA Worksheet for the Holter Recorder

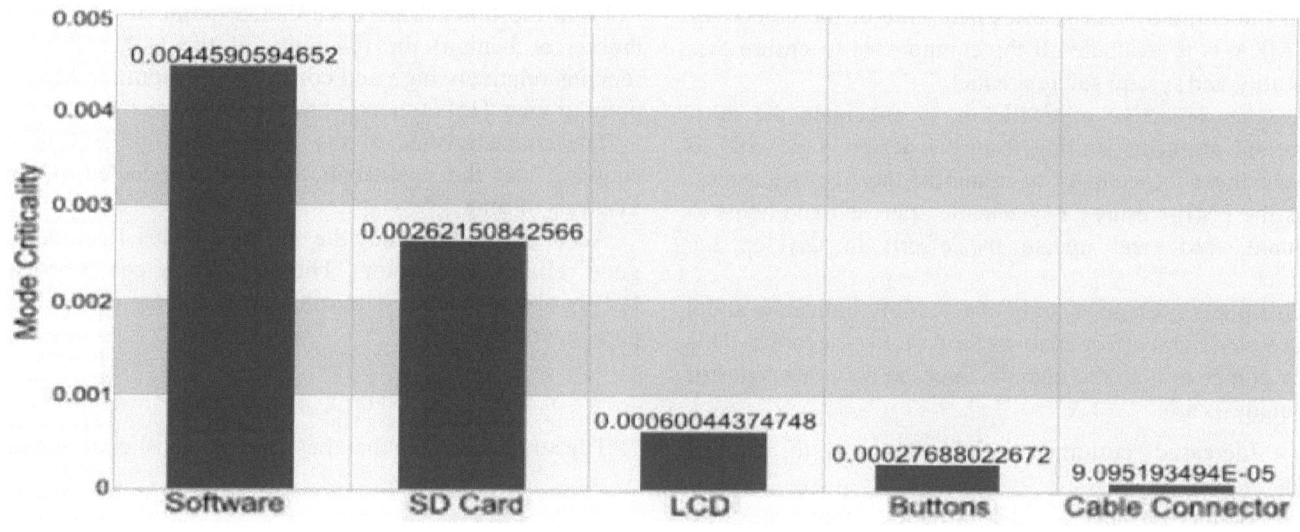

Fig. 8 FMEA Mode Criticalities

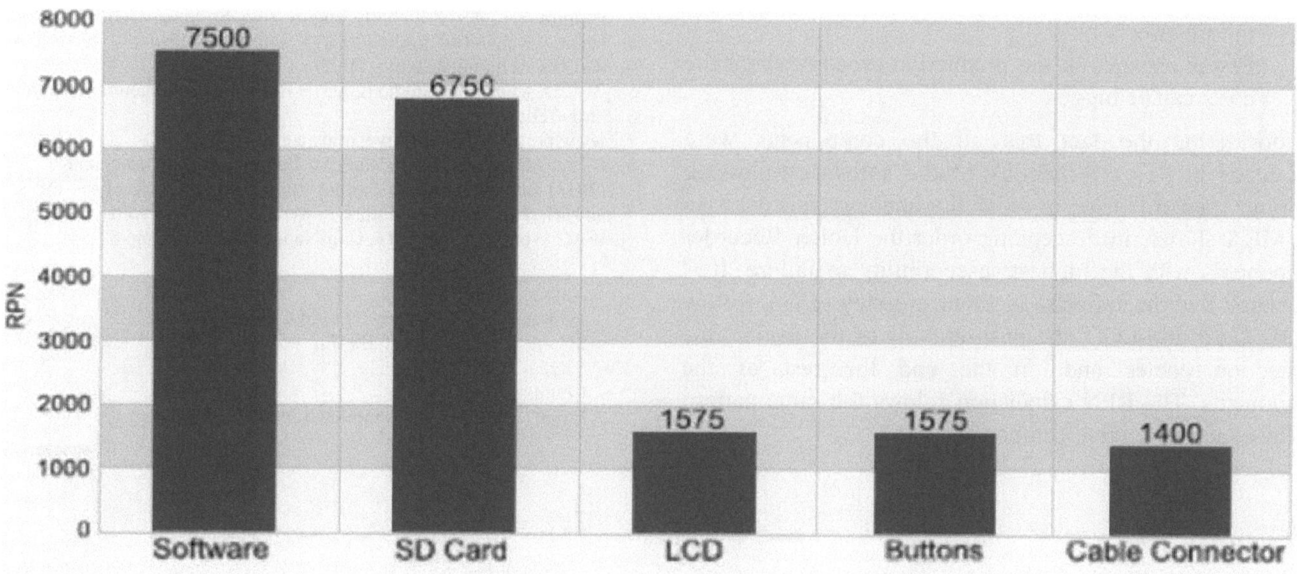

Fig. 9 Risk Priority Number Analysis

A Risk Priority Number (RPN) analysis has also been conducted, thus for the considered system the values presented in Figure 9 were obtained. It can be seen that the hierarchy remains unchanged like in the previous case (Mode Criticality) which validates the obtained results.

IV. Conclusions

All the reliability analysis and FMEAs concentrate on design and impact evaluation that failure has over performance and system safety. However FMEAs can be clasified in two categories: it either analyzes the product, or the process involving the manufacturing and the assembling of the product. [3][4][5]

The FMEA process represents a bottom up analysis of the system. The analysis starts from the lowest desired level, such as a component or a process step and than determines all the failure modes. The following step is to determine the effect of the failure. Than it determines the severity and the probability of occurence. The process ends when the entire system is evaluated. One of the objectives of FMEA is to evaluate all the components to ensure that reliability and system safety are met.

Another objective of FMEA is to anticipate the most important problems starting from the design stages and to prevent them to occur, or to minimize their consequences. Thus the FMEA esures a systematic approach and helps to evaluate, track and update the efforts to develop the product.

This paper presents a study of reliability indicators and a failure mode and effect analysis for a Holter Recorder. This study comes to help the manufacturer, so the advantages of this analysis are:

- Increased customer satisfaction due to product improvement;
- Better design of the products that considers operating enviroments that are not ideal;
- Efficient tests on products;
- Better maintenance based on the importance of failure effects;
- Fewer changes in the production process where the costs can be bigger.

Considering the fact that all the components were introduced in Relex Reliability Studio software following common standards used in reliability analisys, this analisys of FMEA shows, in descending order the Holter Recorder components with the highest susceptibility to failure. It is calculated that the software is the most likley to fail, follow by SD Card, the LCD, the push buttons of the device, the connection cables and, in the end the rest of the components. The RPN calculation folows the same pattern for the exactly the same components.

From the functioning environment point of view (fixed, mobile or benign) the reliability of the Holter Recorder remains relatively high and constant, and from the life time point of view (15000 hours) has a good value.

The characteristics of the failure rate and MTBF are showing that the maintenance can be conducted at large intervals of time.

According to this study the analyzed Holter Recorder has good reliability indicators. The most likely components to fail are also presented. The values obtained are in standard's parameters.

Conflict of Interest

The authors declare that they have no conflict of interest.

References

1. Leitch R. D. (1995) Reliability Analysis for Engineers, Oxford University Press
2. Birolini A. (1999) Reliability Engineering, Springer, Germany
3. RELEX Reliability Studio (2007) – Reference Manual
4. RELEX Reliability Studio (2007) – Getting Started Guide
5. RELEX Reliability Studio (2003) – Reliability, A Practitioner's Guide
6. http://reliabilityweb.com
7. www.ptc.com (former www.relex.com)
8. R. A. Munteanu, D. Iudean, V. Zaharia, C. Muresan and T. Cretu (2013) Implementing an Failure Mode and Effect Analysis for Small and Medium Electric Motors Powered from Photovoltaic Panels, 2nd IFAC Workshop, ICPS'13, Cluj-Napoca, Romania, pg. 81-84

Author: Dan IUDEAN
Institute: Technical University of Cluj-Napoca
Street: 26-28, George Baritiu
City: Cluj-Napoca
Country: Romania
Email: dan.iudean@ethm.utcluj.ro

Patient Satisfaction with Healthcare – A Focus Group Exploratory Study

M.A. Coţiu[1], I.M. Crişan[2], and Gh.A. Catană[3]

[1] Faculty of Economics and Business Administration/Marketing Department, Babeş-Bolyai University, Cluj-Napoca, Romania
[2] Regional Institute of Gastroenterology and Hepatology Prof. Dr. Octavian Fodor/Iuliu Haţieganu University of Medicine and Pharmacy, Cluj-Napoca, Romania
[3] Faculty of Electrical Engineering/Electroenergetics and Management Department, Technical University of Cluj-Napoca, Cluj-Napoca, Romania

Abstract— **Patient satisfaction has been increasingly recognized as an important aspect in healthcare especially in the last decades when system reforms, increased competition for patients or an increased attention given to the quality of care have attracted more attention to patients' needs and expectations. At the same time patient satisfaction is closely associated with various benefits such as greater patient involvement and compliance, increased staff morale, positive word of mouth or a decrease in patients' litigation intent. The subject is also a very challenging one due to the particular nature of healthcare as a highly complex professional service. This often makes it difficult for scholars and professionals in the field to agree on a common definition or a common set of measures and determinants for patient satisfaction. The article takes on this challenge and aims to explore patients' perspectives on aspects affecting their satisfaction with healthcare through four focus groups conducted on patients admitted to two teaching medical facilities in Cluj-Napoca, Romania. Patient views are explored using focus groups as they provide the opportunity of eliciting rich quality data through spontaneous interactions. This also permits the uncovering of unanticipated issues that surveys may fail to identify. Results are obtained through qualitative analysis. Participants highly value positive interactions with the medical staff, expect a correct diagnosis and treatment and appear to be less influenced by administrative procedures or accommodation facilities. Most patients seem highly aware of the funding limitations pressuring the Romanian healthcare system. This awareness tends to make them limit their expectations to the point where they are satisfied with simply receiving treatment.**

Keywords— **patient satisfaction, hospital healthcare, expectations**

I. Introduction

Patient satisfaction has gained considerable attention over the last decades in the context of increasing competition and quality of care monitoring determined by system reforms and increased scrutiny of public services [1]. A multidimensional concept [2], patient satisfaction has a series of benefits from both a marketing and a medical point of view. As such, previous research shows that patient satisfaction is important in promoting healthcare and well-being as it is associated with improved patient compliance, a decrease in patients' intentions to seek a second opinion, file a complaint or seek treatment elsewhere as well as increased staff morale [3] [4]. From a marketing point of view, patient judgments on their satisfaction represent the basis for their future choices or recommendations with regard to a certain facility [5], as well as contributing to creating a positive image of the organization and thus supporting its "financial viability" [4]. This is especially important in the context of current increasing pressures on the medical systems due to increased competition, sustained pressure on health expenditure because of the ageing population, rising public expectations or the growing emphasis being placed on provider accountability [6] [7]. Furthermore, current pressures to reform the healthcare system often affect it fundamentally as they frequently imply "reforming and changing it on any scale – from details of remuneration to the very principles it is based on like the public or private provision of services" [8].

In spite of all these and although patient satisfaction has been extensively researched in the past decades [9] [10], there is still no consensus in the literature as to its definition, determinants or measurement methods [10]. Moreover, findings of different studies are often contradictory, especially with regard to patient satisfaction determinants and measurement [11] [12] [3]. Healthcare aspects affecting satisfaction identified in the literature include perceptions of stay, understanding of discharge instructions [13], physical comfort, emotional support and patient preferences [10], waiting times [14] or overall health status and the presence of pain [15]. At the same time, some conflicting results have been obtained, especially with regard to age, perceptions of care and health status correlation with patient satisfaction [15] [16] [13]. This not only impedes advancements in its conceptualization [9], but also hinders practical developments in improving patients' healthcare experiences.

The purpose of this article is therefore to explore patients' perspectives on different aspects of healthcare delivery and their relation to patient satisfaction. We try to discover what matters to patients with regard to five aspects

S. Vlad and R.V. Ciupa (eds.), *International Conference on Advancements of Medicine and Health Care through Technology*, IFMBE Proceedings 44,
DOI: 10.1007/978-3-319-07653-9_24, © Springer International Publishing Switzerland 2014

of care (caring and reassurance, interactions with the medical staff, facility procedures, medical outcome and attention given to family and friends) as well as exploring their views on the ideal admittance and current level of satisfaction. In order to reach this goal, four focus groups were conducted in two university hospitals in Cluj-Napoca, Romania.

The study is conducted at a time when patient satisfaction with the healthcare system in Romania ranks lower than in other European countries. Only 25% of Romanians evaluate the national healthcare system positively which places Romania last among the countries analyzed [17]. With regard to hospital services, satisfaction is higher, but still below most European countries (only around 50% of inhabitants evaluate services positively) [17]. Some of the main challenges of the Romanian public healthcare system include: patients' dissatisfaction with regard to service quality, lack of funding and the inefficient usage of resources, poor management, low staff morale, an increased level of bureaucracy or a depersonalized service [18]. The research is also conducted at a time of considerable debate regarding the Romanian national healthcare system in the view of the system reform started in 2008 which aims to tackle, among other things, aspects of costs, quality of services and patient satisfaction [19].

The added value of this article lies in its exploratory nature which allows us to obtain original, spontaneous information and insights about healthcare services. While questionnaires may too narrowly frame the range of possible answers or not give patients the possibility for real input into how they would like to be treated [1], focus groups allow researchers to gain valuable information on what patients expect and value in a healthcare experience and what changes they would like to see made through spontaneous interactions and debates [1] [20]. The results will be further used for the development of both qualitative and quantitative research with the aim of reaching a thorough, in depth understanding of what drives patients' satisfaction, expectations, experiences and perceptions of healthcare and suggest concrete improvement measures.

II. Materials and Methods

A. Rationale for the Use of Focus Groups

We chose to use focus groups as they represent a qualitative research method, emphasizing interactions between group members which elicit spontaneous, valuable data regarding their perceptions, knowledge, perspectives or beliefs on the topic [21] [20]. Moreover, this also allows researchers to "tap into different day-to-day forms of communication including jokes, anecdotes, teasing and arguments" [21] thus obtaining rich, authentic, even novel data communicated in a natural, instinctive manner [21] [22].

Furthermore, as opposed to questionnaires where the use of closed-ended questions may not cover all aspects important to patients or may not give respondents the chance to offer real input, discussions on open ended questions are recommended for engaging patients in satisfaction and quality improvement studies [1]. At the same time, as healthcare in itself is closely related to a social context and a social environment, focus groups can be used to gain deeper insights into people's various experiences [21].

As the research we conducted is part of a larger project aimed at analyzing patient satisfaction determinants and suggesting concrete improvements, focus groups enable us to explore patients' perspectives for new approaches, insights, knowledge and attitudes while also allowing for the uncovering of different feelings associated with healthcare services [20]. This type of exploration is even more important if we consider the contradictory findings and lack of consensus in the patient satisfaction literature discussed above.

The article is mainly addressed to public policy analysts, healthcare managers, practitioners and users. We believe research in this area to be helpful in assisting healthcare providers and planners to improve the services they provide for the well-being of both patients and the healthcare providers.

B. Focus Group Participants and Protocol

The research was conducted through four focus groups (N=21) on patients admitted to the gastroenterology and internal medicine departments of two university teaching hospitals in Cluj-Napoca, Romania with 31 and 45 beds, respectively. Two focus groups were conducted in each medical unit between 6 and 9 January 2014. The number of focus groups is considered sufficient for research relevance as per [22]. At the same time, information saturation has been reached during the four focus groups with regard to the major themes approached.

Focus group participants were recruited using convenience sampling from admitted patients considering their illness and health status. Patients were not included in the focus groups if their health status did not permit them to take part.

Focus groups were conducted in a comfortable setting, which allowed all participants to be part of the research without interference from medical staff or visitors, while at the same time not affecting their treatment in any way. All participants were presented with the details of the focus group, its duration and purpose. In the introductory part, participants were assured that all answers would be recorded anonymously, would not affect their medical treatment and that they were confidential. This was important in order to avoid bias being introduced by such fears. Participants consented to the focus group being audio recorded. They were also informed that participation was voluntary and that they had the right to withdraw if they wished to do so. Participants filled in a Patient Consent Form and demographics questionnaire to allow for a comprehensive and comparative analysis of the data. The study was conducted in accordance with the Helsinki Declaration.

The focus group guide was designed to explore aspects of health care delivery with regard to five aspects of care (caring and reassurance, interactions with the medical staff, facility procedures, medical outcome and attention given to family and friends) that had been identified in previous research [23], as well as exploring participants' views on the ideal admittance and current level of satisfaction.

Two pretests of the focus group guide were conducted for questions clarity. These resulted in no major alterations being made to the initial focus group guide.

Focus group participants were homogenous under aspects of gender and disease severity, while differences existed in terms of period of admittance, age, income and level of education. In total, 21 patients participated in the four focus groups, 6 men and 15 women aged between 30-82 years, from both urban and rural areas. Regarding the level of education, patients from rural areas graduated from secondary school, while those from urban areas had a high school diploma. Only three participants in the focus groups earned a university degree. Most of the participants were either employed or retired, with a monthly income ranging from under 350 lei (approx. 80 euro) to 3000 lei (approx. 680 euro). Patients were either admitted by appointment or underwent emergency hospitalization. Most of them had not been admitted before for their current complaints. Hospitalization time ranged between one and 14 days in the respective unit.

Conversation and input from all focus group participants was encouraged by the moderator at all times. Qualitative analysis was then performed on the data obtained.

III. Results

The first major theme approached by the moderator was that of caring and reassurance in the healthcare network. When asked what influenced their level of satisfaction in the hospital setting regarding the aforementioned aspect, most patients responded amiability and being talked nicely without having known or having offered material gifts to the medical and paramedical staff in advance.

Another important aspect was the promptness of the consult and procedures irrespective of the way of admittance (appointment/emergency). One patient said that "if you wait while in pain, you become desperate, hopeless", thus emphasizing a psychological negative effect of waiting time.

Patients also agreed on moral support, patience and encouragement from the medical team as a satisfaction determinant under this theme. "I found my peace and touch of health" one patient said, while another one commented: "The way they treat you and look at you, it helps me, it gives me hope" which suggests a positive effect caring and reassurance has on patients. Many of the patients also indicated a professional approach and not having to give informal payments in order to be cared for as being important to their level of satisfaction.

While most patients were pleased with the individual time and attention given to them by the hospital personnel in general and suggested this as a satisfaction determinant, some participants were dissatisfied with the long waiting times they were subjected to when requiring the service of a nurse or paramedical staff. One of the patients said "I called her three or four times and then I had to ask one of my ward colleagues to go call the nurse because I couldn't move" while another one commented that the nurses had not been willing to offer her extra tea although she was not allowed to drink anything else because of her illness. "They told me to bring it from home!", she added. Both patients then explained that such a situation made them feel even more helpless than they were already feeling because of their illness. However, despite recognizing that they sometimes needed to wait a bit longer, some of the patients also seemed to empathize with the medical personnel as they acknowledged a shortage of staff and suggested more medical staff be hired.

Questions in section two referred to the interaction with the medical staff. For the majority of patients the kindness of the doctor/nurse was crucial in communicating medical information. One patient said "Talking kindly is half of the treatment" and another one added "It gives you a ray of hope". Some of the patients also commented that they often felt stressed or scared so that doctors and nurses speaking kindly was important.

All patients found understandability of diagnostic steps and discharge instructions to be very important; one patient emphasizing that "This is why one comes here, to have a check-up, to know about him". Male patients seemed to appreciate moral support from the doctors' part more. As one patient pointed out there is a need for a "doctor-patient relationship".

Being informed about their condition and the diagnostic procedures was essential to every participant. "The fact that the doctor informs you about your state of heath's lower and upper limit gives you psychological comfort" one patient added. However, a few patients considered they needn't be explained why they had to undergo certain medical tests, as long as their doctors said they were necessary.

The third theme of the focus group questionnaire regarded medical outcome. Being asked what they expected from their current admission, all patients agreed on receiving a sure diagnostic and having their health status improved. Some expected receiving medication, one participant adding that "medication should be the same for the same illness, not some patients receiving preferential treatment" in the sense of better medication. A few patients also added it was important for their satisfaction levels not to be discharged before their health status had improved with one participant saying about her experience in a different medical facility "They let me go and I was still ill".

Questions in section four referred to facility procedures. Asked about what influenced their satisfaction with hospital accommodation, almost all patients responded that clean conditions, bathroom hygiene and hospital renovation were very important. One patient said "They should repaint; there must be so many germs in these walls that we now inhale". However, a few disagreed about this matter, one participant noting that "when you are ill, sometimes you overlook it". The ideal number of beds in the ward would be three or four for most patients. None of them desired to stay in a single-bed ward because of boredom and because it would preclude forming patient solidarity. One patient also suggested better linings as the current ones were old. He explained this aspect was not of outmost importance, but better ones would make him feel better. Some of the female patients also noted the material mattresses were made of which allowed the lining to move and they had to rearrange it quite often. Although this was not of outmost importance to them, they still found it annoying.

While for all patients hospital meal quantity sufficed, for most of them the food lacked diversity and could have been better in terms of taste. This was especially obvious with patients who had been admitted longer. Some patients disagreed, stating that food was good compared to the large number of patients. For example one patient said defensively "Being so many, I'm surprised they still have food for all of us". However, most patients considered noise in the ward disturbing. "Patients with psychological issues should be separated from the others or calmed with medication" carefully added one patient not to offend the others. Two male patients also noted the lack of parking facility and of a TV set in the ward as influencing their satisfaction level with the hospital stay. "You come from a different city by car and you have to leave it in a private parking. For five days that costs about two or three hundred lei (approx. 50-60 euro). If you chose to invest in a good car you can't just park it anywhere."

With regard to the person performing medical procedures (an expert or a trainee) almost all patients said it did not matter to them, as young doctors or nurses had to learn too. Participants also commented on how the privacy of the consult or medical maneuvers influenced their level of satisfaction with the admission. While none of them was disturbed by the presence of other patients in the ward, the presence of other persons or the door being open during the maneuvers were major complaints.

Asked whether hospital bureaucracy represented a problem to their admission, almost all patients were satisfied with the admittance paperwork, finding waiting time acceptable. One patient stated empathically that "you are not alone, you have to wait" in the sense that everyone should be aware that other patients also need to be taken care of.

Attention given to family and friends was another major theme of the discussion. The manner in which the hospital staff addressed and paid respect to family members or friends was an admittance satisfaction prerequisite. Moreover, even though relatives did not respect visiting hours, "nobody stopped them and this matters a lot" one patient noted with gratitude, later adding "they [family and friends] come when they can, they are busy, and they have jobs". For almost all patients it was not important whether they or their families were informed first about their condition as long as information was transmitted.

The last section of the focus group asked participants to rank the items that had been discussed as satisfaction determinants until then and choose the three most important to them. Ranking appeared to be difficult to the majority of patients, most of them naming the first and second and having difficulties choosing a third element. This was despite the fact that all of them had commented many factors during the previous sections. Patients with lower income particularly found this question difficult to answer as they seemed to feel they could anyhow not afford more. As one patient put it "You can`t be poor and also expect too much". Cleanliness/hygiene appeared to be the most important factor. It ranked first (six patients) and second (eight patients). One patient even said "I`ll buy what they don`t have, but they should at least do the toilets". This was followed by treatment and access to medication ranked first by five patients and second by three and medical staff interactions and professionalism ranked first by two patients, second by six and third by seven patients.

Participants were then asked to imagine an ideal admittance. This also proved to be a difficult question to answer, most of them saying the current admittance was good enough. One participant added "It is ok, for what's happening in Romania now, it is ok" while others were grateful they received treatment. "It's good enough they have doctors to treat us" one patient said, while another one added "I know what hard work is, I have cooked for one hundred people so I am satisfied with what I have, that I have a bed to sleep in". A few of the patients however, had higher expectations and imagined the ideal admittance "like in the West" or "like in the movies" or said it should have "better accommodation" or "better equipment". One of the patients reacted to vague responses and said "Come on, if we don't say how we would like it to be, they won't change anything", but this did not affect the generally weak expectations of the other participants. One patient also said she would like to be able to have the procedures for free, not pay for a CT for example, while a few added that an ideal admittance would imply hot water and cleaner facilities, new windows and the walls painted. One of the male participants also added the existence of parking for patients, while another one suggested doctors should be paid higher wages. One of the female participants suggested chapels should be kept inside hospitals because they helped maintaining hope.

In terms of participants' level of satisfaction with the current admission, patients were asked to give a mark from 1 (least satisfied) to 10 (very satisfied). 81% of participants were very satisfied with the current admission awarding grade 10 (48%) and 9 (34%), about 30% higher than the rates recorded in other studies [17]. Grades awarded were between 7 (4%) and 10 (48%). One patient awarded grade 7 (4%) also commenting that "conditions are awful".

IV. Discussions

Patients seem to be very aware of the current limits of the Romanian healthcare system which keeps their expectations low. This has been visible during all of the four focus groups we conducted and was especially noted when patients found themselves unable to imagine an ideal admittance, most of them invoking the system's lack of money. Few patients imagined the ideal admittance implying the positive side of the aspects they had complained about. Patients also had difficulties in dotting the i when suggesting improvements or thinking about rankings of factors that affected their satisfaction. They generally tended to respond with a vague "better" without naming concrete improvements unless specifically asked to give details by the moderator. Even then, patients seemed to have difficulties suggesting improvements. This may be because most of them do not believe things will change in the near future as the lack of funding is perceived very strongly, while others were already grateful that they were receiving any kind of treatment. Another explanation might be that some of the patients seemed to have had negative experiences either with previous admittances or in other aspects of life so that they appreciated any help they were getting, especially as they regarded the current treatment as a professional one.

We noted no major variations in factors affecting satisfaction between the groups. Male participants tended to emphasize the importance of only being discharged with a correct diagnosis and treatment while also emphasizing the need for emotional and psychological support from the medical staff more than female participants. Expectations and the level of satisfaction did not vary significantly with income, gender, and rural/urban status, level of education or marital status. This may be because patients generally expected an improvement of their health status, irrespective of demographics. Although health status improvement was the main and sometimes sole expectation of most patients, they did agree other factors that influenced their satisfaction with the current admittance. Younger patients, both male and female, seemed to find it easier to suggest concrete improvements and valued the accommodation services more.

With regard to the ideal admittance wealthier male participants presented more improvement ideas, some of which included parking places for patients or a TV set in the ward, whereas female participants and patients with lower or medium income generally referred to hospital facilities in terms of cleanliness and equipment availability. An interesting note is the fact that patients did not want single or double wards, but three or four beds in order to prevent boredom. All participants showed empathy for their colleagues and acknowledged the fact that other patients may be in a more serious condition and thus, selfness if required.

The study also reveals a high degree of passivity among patients who accept the time and funding limitations of the system and greatly appreciate what they get. It is interesting to note, that only two participants complaint of the fact that they had to pay for medications or procedures and that this point was not raised by those with lower incomes, but by those with medium income. It may be that participants regard this as the state of the system that cannot be changed at this point. We do however find it odd that access to medication was not mentioned as a dissatisfier, having been mentioned only once prior to the moment when patients were asked to imagine an ideal admittance.

The high level of satisfaction reported by patients may be due to the fact that the study was conducted in teaching centers where hospital diagnostic and accommodation facilities might be superior to those of smaller units, thus increasing the level of patients' satisfaction with healthcare. Also, their satisfaction could have been higher because of a contrast between the care received and the general healthcare system image in the Romanian media.

V. Limitations

A limitation of the study was the relatively small number of participants. Only two focus groups could be organized at each hospital due to the poor health status of the other inpatients admitted to the respective departments. A larger number of focus groups could have allowed for a deeper understanding of the issues discussed. However, we do not believe this to have affected the study negatively with regard to the information obtained as information saturation has been reached during the four focus groups. The focus group number is also sufficient for research relevance as per [22].

VI. Conclusions

The focus groups we conducted allowed for the exploration of various factors affecting patient satisfaction. Results showed that although patient expectations mostly related to improved health or a correct diagnosis, other aspects also improve their satisfaction levels. Cleanliness/hygiene together with treatment and access to medication and staff interactions and professionalism were ranked as the most important factors influencing satisfaction. Discussions also revealed the high degree of patient awareness with regard to the Romanian healthcare limits and their difficulties in suggesting concrete improvements. Patient satisfaction appeared to be high, yet its causes are worth further investigation. We believe further qualitative and quantitative research is needed in order to further explore the relation between various aspects of healthcare and patient satisfaction. We also believe careful consideration should be given to the particularities of the Romanian healthcare system with regard to its image in the media, patients' awareness of system limitations and other negative life experiences and the way these factors affect patients' expectations and evaluations of the treatment and the conditions that they receive.

Conflict or Interest

The authors declare that they have no conflict of interest.

References

1. Schwarz M, Landis S E, Rowe, J E, Janes C L and Pullman N (2000) Using Focus Groups to Assess Primary Care Patients' Satisfaction. Eval Health Prof 23: 58 DOI 10.1177/01632780022034480
2. Crow R, Gage H, Hampson S. et al (2002) The measurement of satisfaction with healthcare: implications for practice from a systematic review of the literature. Health Technol Assess 6(32) (Executive Summary)
3. Taylor C, Benger J R (2004) Patient satisfaction in emergency medicine. Emerg. Med. J. 21: 528-532 DOI 10.1136/emj.2002.003723
4. Boudreaux E D, O'Hea E L (2004) Patient Satisfaction in the Emergency Department: A Review of the Literature and Implications for Practice. J Emerg Med. 26(1): 13-26 DOI 10.1016/j.jemermed.2003.04.003
5. Magaret N D, Clark T A, Warden C R et al (2002) Patient Satisfaction in the Emergency Department – A Survey of Pediatric Patients and Their Parents. Acad Emerg Med. 9(12): 1379-1387
6. Aiken L H, Sermeus W, Heede K et al (2012) Patient safety, satisfaction, and quality of hospital care: cross sectional surveys of nurses and patients in 12 countries in Europe and the United States. BMJ 344: e1717 DOI 10.1136/bmj.e1717
7. Larson C O, Nelson E C, Gustafson D et al (1996) The Relationship Between Meeting Patients` Information Needs and their Satisfaction with Hospital Care and General Health Outcomes. International J Qual Health Care 8(5): 447-456 DOI 10.1093/intqhc/8.5.447
8. Kotzian P (2009) Determinants of Satisfaction with Health Care System. The Open Political Science Journal 2: 47-58
9. Gill L,White L (2009) A critical review of patient satisfaction literature. Leadership in Health Services 22(1): 8-18
10. Jenkinson C, Coulter A, Bruster S et al (2002) Patients' experiences and satisfaction with health care: results of a questionnaire study of specific aspects of care. *Qual Saf Health Care* 11: 335-339 DOI 10.1136/qhc.11.4.335
11. Wolf M H, Putnam S, James S A et al (1978) The Medical Interview Satisfaction Scale: development of a Scale to Measure Patient Perceptions of Physician Behavior. J Behav Med. 1(4): 391-401
12. Sitzia J, Wood N (1998) Response rate in patient satisfaction research: an analysis of 210 published studies. *Int J Qual Health Care,* 10(4): 311-317 DOI 10.1093/intqhc/10.4.311
13. Boudreaux E, Ary R D, Mandry C V et al (2000) Determinants of Patient Satisfaction in a Large, Municipal ED: The Role of Demographic Variables, Visit Characteristics, and Patient Perceptions. *AJEM* 18(4): 394-400 DOI 10.1053/ajem.2000.7316
14. Booth A J, Harrison A J, Gardener G J et al (1992) Waiting times and patient satisfaction in the accident and emergency department. *Archives of Emergency Medicines,* 9: 162-168
15. Rahmqvist M (2001) Patient satisfaction in relation to age, health status and other background factors: a model for comparisons of care units. Int J Qual Health Care 13(5): 385-390 DOI 10.1093/intqhc/13.5.385
16. Jackson J L, Chamberlain J, Kroenke K (2001) Predictors of Patient Satisfaction. Soc. Sci. Med. 52: 609-620
17. Jankauskiene D, Jankauskaite I (2011) Access and quality of healthcare system by opinion of patients in ten European countries. Management in health, XV/3:31-39
18. Catană Gh A (2009) Marketingul serviciilor de ocrotire a sănătății (S.O.S.). Alma Mater, Cluj-Napoca
19. Voinea L, Pamfilie R (2009) Considerations Regarding the Performance Improvement of the Hospital Healthcare Services from Romania by the Implementation of an Integrated Management System. Amfiteatrul Economic XI(26): 339-345
20. Jamieson L, Williams L M (2003) Focus group methodology: Explanatory notes for the novice nurse researcher. Contemporary Nurse 14: 271-280
21. Wong L P (2008) Focus group discussion: a tool for health and medical research. Singapore Med J 49(3):256
22. Rabiee F (2004) Focus group interview and data analysis. Proceedings of the Nutrition Society (0029-6651) 063(004):655 DOI: 10.1079/PNS2004399
23. Coţiu, M A (2013) Consumer Satisfaction in the Healthcare Sector. A Critical Review of Some Empirical Studies. IJEPT "in press"

Author: Mădălina-Alexandra Coţiu
Institute: Faculty of Economics and Business Administration, Babeş-Bolyai University
Street: Teodor Mihali, no. 58-60
City: Cluj-Napoca
Country: Romania
Email: madalina.cotiu@gmail.com

Simulation Based Training for Medical Staff from Department of Pediatrics and Neonatology

R. Ciorap[1], C. Luca[1], C. Corciovă[1], and E. Moraru[2]

[1] "Gr.T.Popa" University of Medicine and Pharmacy, Bioengineering Faculty, Iaşi, Romania
[2] "Gr.T.Popa" University of Medicine and Pharmacy, Department of Mother and Child Medicine, Iaşi, Romania

Abstract— **In this paper we presents our experience in training medical staff using high fidelity simulator. We train 500 physicians and nurses from 10 County Hospitals that cover a large area of Romania.**

Appropriate assessment and resuscitation is an important part of neonatal care provided during the first minutes of life. "Senior" and "junior" medical staff are often in the frontline of neonatal resuscitation. Appropriate education and training of medical staff is therefore essential if the standard of care delivered to babies in the delivery suite is to be improved and maintained. Evaluation of any such educational interventions is necessary to assess their effectiveness.

Practical courses in neonatal resuscitation can contribute to improvements in the quality of care provided to babies immediately after birth. These courses are more effective than theoretical teaching alone. Our goal is to evaluate the results of a course in neonatal resuscitation that we sustained on a neonatal simulator and to see the effects of the course on the medical staff.

Keywords— **Simulation based training, neonatal resuscitation, medical simulation**

I. Introduction

According to the World Health Organization, nearly one million babies die each year due to birth difficulties. As many as 10 percent of all newborns have breathing difficulties at birth and require some assistance. With proper training and minimal equipment, many of the deaths of newborns due to breathing problems can be avoided.

Perinatal asphyxia, a potentially modifiable cause of neonatal mortality and morbidity affects over four million newborns in developing countries annually. About 1.2 million of affected infants die and at least the same number develop severe consequences such as cerebral palsy.

Skills needed for resuscitating newborns are taught in training courses, which contain a combination of textbooks, lectures and scenarios using resuscitation equipment and manikins. Simulation based medical education offer a safe environment for physicians and nurses to gain practical skills [1], [2], [3].

A neonatal staff nurse or doctor, works in either a Level I, II, or III nursery [Note: These levels of care are set forth by the Perinatal Regionalization Model and are also described in the Guidelines for Perinatal Care, 4th ed., published by the American Academy of Pediatrics and American College of Obstetrics and Gynecology, 1997, Elk Grove Village.].

Level I is usually a healthy newborn nursery largely nonexistent now because mothers and babies have a very short hospital stay these days and often share the same room.

Level II is an intermediate care or special care nursery where the baby may be born prematurely or may be suffering from an illness; these babies may need supplemental oxygen, intravenous therapy, specialized feedings, or more time to mature before discharge.

Level III neonatal intensive care unit (NICU) admits all neonates (during the first 28 days of life) who cannot be treated in either of the other two nursery levels. These babies may be small for their age, premature or sick term infants who require high technology care, such as ventilators, special equipment, incubators, or surgery. The Level III units may be in a large general hospital or part of a children's hospital. Neonatal nurses provide the direct patient care to these infants.

II. Methodology

The new, extensively updated Neonatal Resuscitation Program (NRP) offers a rich array of teaching and learning aids based on the 2010 American Academy of Pediatrics (AAP)/American Heart Association (AHA) "Guidelines for Cardiopulmonary Resuscitation and Emergency Cardiovascular Care: Neonatal Resuscitation Guidelines."

All program components reflect the AAP/AHA guidelines' increased emphasis on evidence-based treatment recommendations, as well as the new International Liaison Committee on Resuscitation (ILCOR) evidence-based consensus on science.

We developed a program for training physicians and nurses who work in Department of Pediatrics and Neonatology from 10 County Hospitals. This project was based on experience of Clinical Simulation Laboratory from Medical Bioengineering Faculty of Iasi [4].

Beginning March 2011 physicians and nurses enrolled in this training program had to self-study the e-learning

S. Vlad and R.V. Ciupa (eds.), *International Conference on Advancements of Medicine and Health Care through Technology*, IFMBE Proceedings 44,
DOI: 10.1007/978-3-319-07653-9_25, © Springer International Publishing Switzerland 2014

platform and to attend on the resuscitation course and simulation. After these courses the trainees had to complete the online examination. Up to 9 hours of Continuing Education Credit will be offered for the examination for physicians and nurses.

On this paper we evaluate only the medical maneuver that the medical staff made on the neonatal simulator on these courses.

Developed by the METI and named BabySim, our neonatal simulator is a self-directed educational tool for health care professionals that teaches hands-on resuscitation skills. The neonatal simulator BabySim, shown in figure 1, is equipped with squeeze bulbs to simulate spontaneous breathing, palpable brachial and femoral response, crying, a simulated equipment panel, feeding tube, 50-mL syringe, clamp, stethoscope, oxygen tubing, monitoring system of vital signs, and equipment for endotracheal intubation.

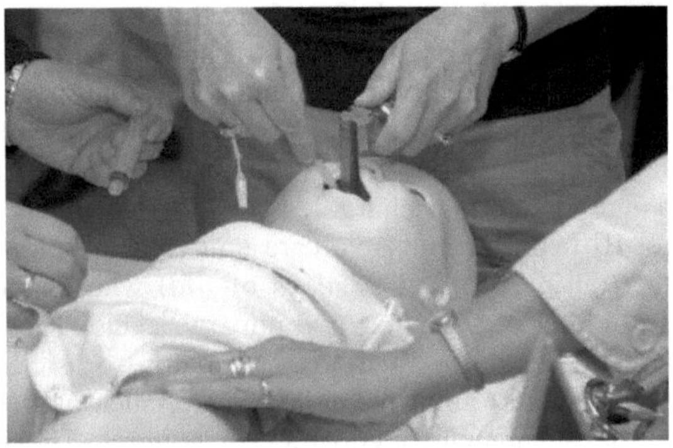

Fig.1 BabySim neonatal simulator

Various methods have been used to evaluate the performance of neonatal resuscitation. These include written tests, practical performance tests and video recording of an actual resuscitation. The participants in the course demonstrated their skills gained in simulated conditions.

Our study evaluated the efficacy of a neonatal resuscitation program aimed at the staff in our hospital and other hospitals by comparing the pre and post training period to assess the highest level of the pyramid-action or how staff actually provided care. The outcome of babies in the developed world is so good that to show an improvement in mortality outcome due to these courses would require a multinational study with very large numbers of babies enrolled, ideally in a randomized controlled trial.

The ethics of this would be difficult to justify. As an effect on mortality itself has not been shown, we chose certain proxy markers to assess the quality of resuscitation. The results of our study show that the quality of care given to neonates can be improved as shown by a decrease in the use of inappropriate drugs and a decline in the incidence of hypothermia on admission to special care baby unit. Our study suggests that these courses are superior to previously delivered theoretical training.

It can be difficult to establish a link between an intervention and its impact on patient care. The presence of resuscitation teachers and a focus on resuscitation are confounding factors but this was a pragmatic assessment, which has demonstrated a change in practice. There is, however, little data available on the efficacy of these courses and our study has clearly shown an improvement in practices.

III. Results

Train-the-trainer model was used to train health professionals at 2–3 day workshops from 2011 to 2012. Obstetric Anticipatory Care and Basic Neonatal Care modules were taught as part of Neonatal Resuscitation Training package. Neonatal Resuscitation Program was adapted to the clinical role of participants and local resources. Cognitive knowledge was evaluated by written pre- and post-training tests.

This study evaluated the knowledge gained and retained by neonatal practice physicians and nurses who participated in the Neonatal Resuscitation Program (NRP) course. We train 177 physicians and 323 nurses from 10 neonatal departments from all over the country as shown in table 1. Knowledge attainment and its retention was assessed by the administration of pre-, post-, tests using the standard NRP written examination.

Table 1 Distribution of course participants

Medical centres (county)	No. of physicians form III level clinics	No. of physicians form II level clinics	No. of nurses form III level clinics	No. of nurses form II level clinics
Timis	25	15	30	50
Cluj	8	4	8	0
Mures	10	20	10	30
Bucuresti	5	15	10	50
Oradea	10	5	15	10
Sibiu	10	0	20	10
Iasi	18	2	20	5
Vaslui	0	5	0	25
Neamt	0	10	0	15
Botosani	0	5	0	15

In the simulation part of the training program we have built neonatal resuscitation scenarios covering a wide range of neonatal pathologies like: resuscitation, administration of adrenaline, bleeding with blood transfusion, intraventricular hemorrhage grade IV, cardiorespiratory stop, pneumothorax.

Participants were physicians and nurses from neonatal units, residents in obstetrics and pediatrics and medical officers in secondary level health facilities.

Each workshop had 20 participants. The first workshop was conducted by a neonatal resuscitation training instructors from Iasi- Regional Center for Neonatal Intensive Care.

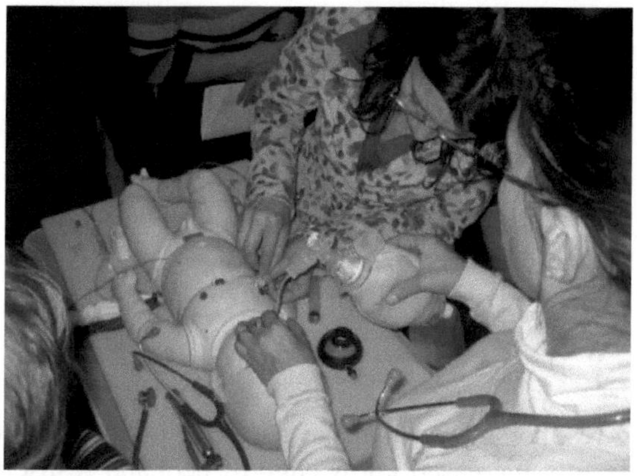

Fig.2 Physician and nurse using bag and mask ventilation

We taught the lessons of NRP: (i) principles of resuscitation; (ii) initial steps in resuscitation; (iii) bag and mask ventilation; (iv) chest compressions; (v) endotracheal intubation; (vi) medications; (vii) special considerations. Figure 2 illustrated the practical training for bag and mask ventilation. The Special Considerations lesson was adapted to local context.

We ensured comprehension of the subject by: (a) teaching a maximum of three lessons per day and spending more time on practical sessions; (b) discussion of test questions for each lesson after presentation and evaluation of that lesson.

IV. Discussion

We have shown that NRP can be used to improve the cognitive knowledge of health professionals on neonatal resuscitation in Romania. The highest improvement occurred in nurses and physicians but the performance of midwives at primary health facilities was significantly lower than those at secondary and tertiary facilities.

The "train-the-trainer" model sustained the program. Our holistic approach to incorporate the 3 modules was to enable participants to understand the complex relationship between obstetrics and newborn care and modern concepts of neonatal resuscitation. This adaptation is consistent with NRP recommendations of targeting training to conform to the professional roles of learners.

An important finding in our cohort is that nurses and physicians who are the vanguard of acute obstetric and ne natal care in Romania had the highest percentage increase in cognitive knowledge. We speculate that concerted effort to train them in emergency perinatal care will improve clinical skills that save newborn lives. The performance of midwives at primary health facilities may have resulted from the extensive information we presented in a relatively short period of time. Many of these participants were not familiar with current newborn resuscitation principles and some had never used a resuscitation bag; however, 66% achieved pass post-test scores after one workshop. We ensured that all participants had satisfactory practical skills irrespective of their test score. In table 2 we analyzing the time needed for executing different clinical maneuver

Table 2 Analysis of time for executing different clinical maneuver

Clinical maneuver	Normal time	Subject execution time				Correct maneuver executed			
		Physian L. II	Physian L. III	Nurse L. II	Nurse L. III	Physian L. II	Physian L. III	Nurse L. II	Nurse L. III
During the execution of a script	23.5 min.	47.3 min.	30.03 min.	54.6 min.	42.3 min.	-	-	-	-
External cardiac massage maneuver	30 sec.	60 sec.	58 sec.	85 sec.	76 sec.	20.08%	58.9%	29.10%	57.6%
Endotracheal intubation maneuver	30 sec.	75 sec.	35 sec.	-	-	10.09%	49.56%	-	-
Balloon and mask ventilation	30 sec.	62.5 sec.	57 sec.	83.5 sec.	75.4 sec.	15.09%	60.89%	15.02%	59.56%
Fluid administration support	2 min.	-	-	2.4 min.	2.05 min.	-	-	60.9%	89.05%
Blood administration	3 min.	-	-	4.02 min.	3.9 min.	-	-	62.9%	85.45%
Observation bulging fontanelle (newborn evaluation)	10 sec.	120 sec.	87 sec.	210 sec.	174 sec.	-	-	-	-
Observation curved chest (newborn evaluation)	10 sec.	102 sec.	58 sec.	174 sec.	140 sec.	-	-	-	-
Airway permeability	15 sec.	10 sec.	13.6 sec.	9.4 sec.	11.5 sec.	60.73%	84.64%	67.84%	85.4%
Tactile stimulation	15 sec.	10.9 sec.	12.6 sec.	10.4 sec	14.5 sec.	63.64%	85.,5%	63.64%	82.6%
Drain pneumothorax	15 min.	48.6 min.	37.7 min.	-	-	1.4%	27.4%	-	-

"Train-the-trainer" model increases knowledge, promotes ownership, builds capacity and enables sustainability of programs. These qualities are important for sustaining clinical skills in Romania health professionals.

However, the real test is whether the knowledge and skills are retained over time to improve practices that save newborn lives in labor rooms.

The data were analyzed using repeated measures analysis of variance and Student's test and are showed in figures 3 to 7.

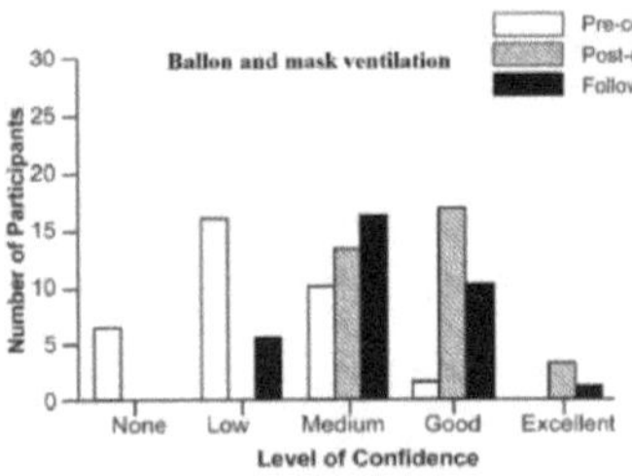

Fig. 3 Data analysis for balloon and mask ventilation

Analyzing the data for balloon and mask ventilation we observed that the majority of participants had medium or good results post-course and at follow-up.

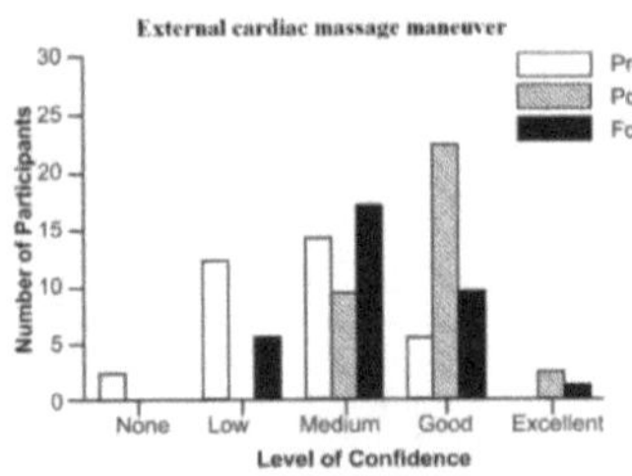

Fig. 4 Data analysis for external cardiac massage maneuver

Data analysis for external cardiac massage maneuver showing us that the majority of participants had good results post-course but at follow-up their skills are partially lost

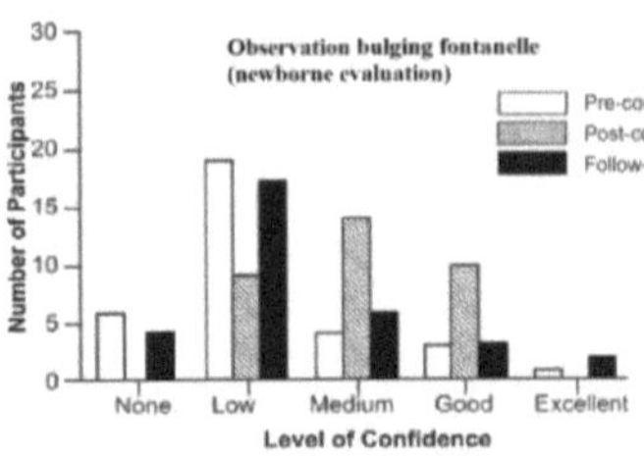

Fig. 5 Data analysis for observation bulging fontanelle

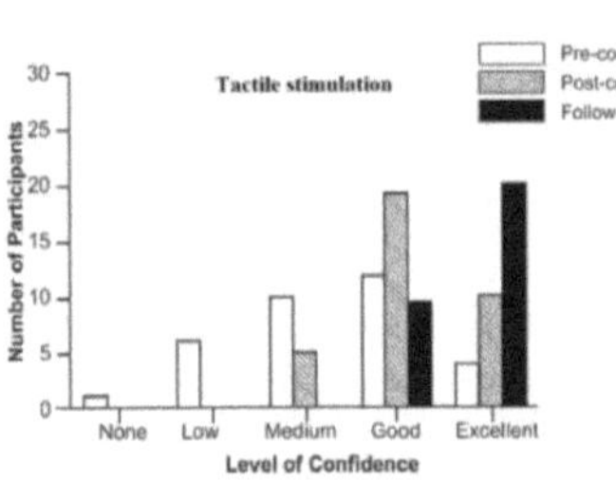

Fig. 6 Data analysis for tactile stimulation

For drain pneumothorax maneuver the majority of participants had bad results given the complexity of the maneuver.

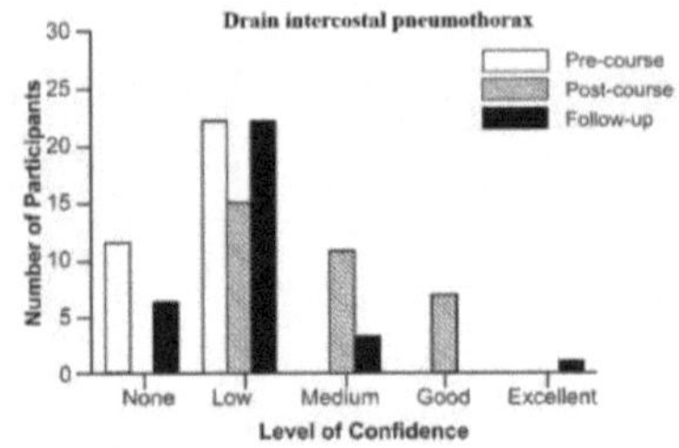

Fig. 7 Data analysis for drain pneumothorax

V. CONCLUSIONS

The results suggest that participation in an NRP course significantly increased knowledge of neonatal resuscitation by family practice residents, but that knowledge may decrease over time.

All groups of the 500 professionals (323 nurses and 177 physicians) who completed the course showed significant improvement ($p < 0.001$) in median post-training test scores. Evidence-based neonatal resuscitation training adapted to local resources significantly improved cognitive knowledge of all groups of health professionals.

CONFLICT OF INTEREST

The authors declare that they have no conflict of interest.

REFERENCES

1. Lippert A., Dieckmann P.G., Oestergaard D. (2009) Simulation in Medicine, Notfall Rettungsmed + Suppl 2 12:49-52, DOI 10.1007/s10049-009-1208-z
2. Murphy J.G., Cremonini F., Kane G.C., Dunn W. (2007), Is simulation based medicine training the future of clinical medicine, European Review for Medical and Pharmacological Sciences 11:1-8
3. Small S.D., Wuerz R.C., Simon R., Shapiro N, Conn A., Setnik G. (1999) Demonstration of High-fidelity Simulation Team Training for Emergency Medicine, Academic Emergency Medicine 6:312-323, DOI: 10.1111/j.1553-2712.1999.tb0395.x
4. Zaharia D., Ciorap R.(2009), Bioengineering Education in Romania, World Congress on Medical Physics and Biomedical Engineering, 7-12 September 2009, Munich, Germany, pp.275-276

Author: Ciorap Radu
Institute: "Gr.T.Popa" University of Medicine and Pharmacy, Bioengineering Faculty
Street: M. Kogalniceanu 9-13
City: Iasi
Country: Romania
Email: radu.ciorap@bioinginerie.ro

Polymer Based Nanostructures for Innovative Bio and Immunosensors Development

L. Fritea[1], A. Florea[1], M. Tertiş[1], A. Cristea[2], R. Săndulescu[1], and C. Cristea[1]

[1] Analytical Chemistry Department, Faculty of Pharmacy,
Iuliu Haţieganu University of Medicine and Pharmacy, Cluj-Napoca, Romania
ccristea@umfcluj.ro
[2] Dept. of Building Services, Faculty of Building Services, Technical University of Cluj-Napoca
Cluj-Napoca, Romania

Abstract— **Different types of electrochemical bio and immunosensors are reported based on conductive polymers and nanoelements like carbon nanotubes, graphenes, cyclodextrines. Two model molecules are detected with those sensors and an innovative way to obtain an immunosensor for MUC4 cancer biomarker detection is presented.**

Keywords— **polyethyleneimine, polypyrrole, polyanthranilic acid, carbon based and gold electrodes, nanomaterials**

I. Introduction

The development of electrochemical sensors has attracted a great interest due to their high sensitivity. By including an enzyme in the sensors they gain also high specificity. They have been widely investigated for the detection of molecules of biomedical, food and environmental interest [1] due to their inherent advantages respect to the conventional techniques, such as high sensitivity, high selectivity, low cost, fast analysis and miniaturization.

The immobilization of the biorecognition element on the sensing electrode surface is of paramount importance in the sensor design. Various nanomaterials have been succesfully applied for the immobilization of bioelements, such as gold nanoparticles [2], TiO_2 nanotubes [3], nanosilver coated magnetic beads [4] etc. Among all these, due to their unique physiochemical features, carbon nanotubes (CNTs) have gained special attention in the last years [5]. A number of immunosensors for the detection of tumor markers have been developed in recent years based on CNTs. For example, Gao et al fabricated a simple and sensitive immunosensor for the detection of carcinoembryonic antigen based on a chitosan-carbon nanotubes-gold nanoparticles nanocomposite as antibody immobilization matrix achieving a limit of detection of 0.04 ng mL^{-1} [6].

Conducting polymers have attracted wide attention for the fabrication of immunosensors due to their excellent compatibility with biomolecules in a neutral aqueous solution [7]. CNTs/Ppy films have been investigated for the construction of immunosensors proving high stability, enhaced conductivity and better electron transfer reactions of biomolecules [8]. An electrochemical immunosensor was reported for the detection of Hepatitis B surface antigen based on CNTs-conducting polymer three dimensional network. A poly (pyrrole propionic acid) film was used to integrate the CNTs into a stable network reaching a detection limit of 0.01 ng mL^{-1} [9].

Polypyrrole (PPy) has been the focus of several recent studies during the last two decades, due to its high conductivity and good environmental stability, being easily overoxidized to create an electrically insulating layer [10, 11].

Besides polypyrrole, polyethyleneimine (PEI), a cationic polymer is used for the entrapment of several molecules in various biosensors configurations [12, 13]. During the development of the novel biosensors for acetaminophen detection, the use of PEI offered the advantage that the retention of the biomolecule at the electrode surface was made without stressing it with a supplementary electropolymerization process.

Poly *o*-aminobenzoic acid (PAA), an aniline based conductive polymer capable of self-doping is of interest as a soluble derivative of polyaniline [14]. Its carboxylic acid group serves as a functional group that can be used as a matrix material for immobilization onto substrates or for covalent bonds with biomolecules such as proteins and antibodies. Therefore, functionalized polymers are widely used as a platform to immobilize enzymes and primary antibodies on the electrode surface.

Two model molecules, acetaminophen and dopamine were used as target analytes, taking into account that the detection of drugs from pharmaceutical products or biological fluid by using fast and accurate methods is of great interest. N-acetyl-*p*-aminophenol (4-acetamidophenol, known as acetaminophen-APAP) is an acetylated aromatic amide that has been used as an analgesic for over 30 years, being a very effective treatment for the relief of pain and fever. Dopamine is a neurotransmitter involved in Parkinson disease, schizophrenia, attention deficit hyperactivity disorder (ADHD), and restless legs syndrome (RLS).

Mucin4 (MUC4) is a tumor marker with elevated levels in various types of cancer such as such as pancreatic [15],

S. Vlad and R.V. Ciupa (eds.), *International Conference on Advancements of Medicine and Health Care through Technology*, IFMBE Proceedings 44,
DOI: 10.1007/978-3-319-07653-9_26, © Springer International Publishing Switzerland 2014

lung [16], gastro-intestinal [17], breast [18] or ovarian cancer [19]. The sensitive detection of MUC4 can play an important role in the early diagnosis of cancer and during follow-up therapy.

Hence, in the work reported herein, we try to demonstrate the potential of different types of nanocomposites based on the combination of CNT/graphene/cyclodextrine and polymers as immobilization platform for innovative devices. The obtained electrochemical sensors were applied for the drug analysis and cancer biomarkers detection.

II. Experimental

A. Reagents and Materials

The multiwall carbon nanotubes (MWCNT) were provided by NanoLab Inc. (USA). Graphene and graphene oxide solutions were purchased from Dropsens and graphene oxide (solid powder) was purchased from Aldrich. The horseradish peroxidase enzyme (HRP 1.11.1.7 type II, 180 U/mg solid) and tyrosinase from mushroom (3150 U/mg solid) were provided by Sigma. The Rabbit polyclonal MUC4 antibody was purchased from Novus Biologicals (CO, USA). 1-Ethyl-3-(3'-dimethylaminopropyl) carbodiimide hydrochloride (EDC) and N-hydroxysuccinimide (NHS) were obtained from Alfa Aesar (Germany).

β-cyclodextrin (β-CD) and acetaminophen were purchased from Merck and dopamine was from Sigma. 0.1 M phosphate buffer solution at pH 7.2 was used (sodium dihydrogen phosphate and sodium monohydrogen phosphate from Sigma). All aqueous solutions were prepared with ultrapure water (MilliQ Barnstead EASY pure). All the measurements were performed at room temperature.

Polyethyleneimine (MW 60000) (PEI) (used without further purification) and pyrrole (Py) (reagent grade, 98%) were purchased from Aldrich. The hydrogen peroxide 30%, anthranilic acid and H_2SO_4 were purchased from Sigma Aldrich and KCl was provided by Merck.

The stock solutions of the acetaminophen were dissolved in phosphate buffer and kept in the refrigerator while the dopamine solutions were freshly prepared each day.

The 1 mg/mL PEI solution was prepared by dissolving the necessary amount of PEI in water: alcohol (1:1) mixture. The 1% β-CD solution was obtained by dissolving the necessary amount of β-CD in the above described 1mg/mL PEI solution. Glassy carbon electrodes (GCEs, d=4 mm) were modified as follows: 6 µl of solution 1mg/mL PEI with and without 1% β-CD were dropped onto the electrodes surface and then dried for 30 minutes at room temperature.

50 mg graphene oxide solid powder was suspended in 100 mL H_2O followed by 2 h sonication, then mixed for 30 minutes together with 0.4 % β-CD aqueous solution. The obtained suspension is then mixed with 1000 mg ascorbic acid and stirred for 48 h. The solid obtained after filtration, washing and drying is then used to obtain a more homogenous suspension. The preparation of unmodified reduced graphene oxide was similar to the procedure mentioned above without the addition of β-CD [20, 21].

All reagents were of analytical grade, and used as received.

The screen printed electrodes (SPE) were provided by DropSens and they had a graphite or gold working electrode, a graphite auxiliary electrode and a silver pseudo-reference electrode.

The glassy carbon electrode (GCE) used as working electrode in the conventional three electrode cell was provided by BAS Inc. (USA) and was carefully washed with demineralized water and polished with diamond paste (BAS Inc., West Lafayette, USA).

B. The Preparation of HRP Based Biosensors

1 mg MWCNT was suspended in 1 mL PEI solution, 1mg/mL (prepared in 50:50 v/v ethanol/water) followed by 15 min sonication. Equal amounts of the MWCNT-PEI suspension and a 0.3 mg/mL HRP solution in phosphate buffer solution (PBS) (pH 7.4; 0.1 M) were mixed with vortex for 5 min. 10 µL mixture was deposited on the working electrode and dried at room temperature for 2h.

1 mg MWCNT was suspended in 1 mL 5mM pyrrole solution in 0.1 M $LiClO_4$, followed by 15 min sonication. Equal amounts of the MWCNT-Py suspension and a 0.3 mg/mL HRP solution in PBS (pH 7.4; 0.1 M) were mixed with vortex for 5 min. 20 µL from this mixture was deposited on the working electrode and dried at room temperature. The electropolymerization of pyrrole was carried out by cycling the potential between 0 and +0.8V, at 100 mVs^{-1} for 20 cycles, in 0.1 M $LiClO_4$, followed by an overoxidation by cycling between 0 and +1.2V, for another 5 cycles.

C. The Preparation of Tyrosinase Based Biosensor

Prior to the biosensor preparation, the GCE was polished with alumina slurry and rinsed thoroughly with ultrapure water between each polishing step. Then it was washed successively with acetone and water in ultrasonic bath and dried in air. Aliquots of 5 µL of 1 mg/mL reduced graphene oxide suspension in water were carefully dropped on the electrode surface and dried at 40°C. 5µL of 1 mg/mL β-CD solution was then dropped on the electrode and allowed to dry in air followed by fourteen additions of 5 µL of 1 mg/mL tyrosinase solution, and finally 5 µL of 1 mg/mL tyrosinase solution in 1mg/mL of PEI solution. The obtained biosensor was then well dried for one hour and kept in PBS (pH 7.4; 0.1 M) before using to maintain the enzyme hydration.

D. Preparation of PAA Nanostructured Platform

Various nanocomposites based on MWCNTs and gold nanoparticles (AuNPs) in PAA matrix were employed for the development of a MUC4 immunosensor.

In a first approach, a one-step deposition of a MWCNT/PAA film was performed on the surface of graphite SPEs by electropolymerization in a solution containing 1mg/mL MWCNT and 50 mM anthranilic acid in 1M H_2SO_4 and 0.1M KCl, cycling the potential between 0 and +0.8 V, at a scan rate of 50 mVs^{-1} for 15 cycles. Prior to electrodeposition, MWCNT were sonicated in PBS (pH 7.4; 0.1 M) for 2h.

In another approach, PAA was electrodeposited on the surface of MWCNTs and AuNP modified graphite electrodes purchased from DropSens, Spain. The electropolymerization of PAA on AuNP/MWCNT-modified SPEs was achieved through CV, by applying 15 polymerization cycles at 0 to +0.8 V with 50 mVs^{-1} scan rate, in 50 mM anthranilic acid solution prepared in 1M H_2SO_4 and 0.1M KCl.

To investigate if the prepared polymer nanocomposite is able to bind the antibody, after activation of the carboxylic groups of PAA with a solution of 0.4 M EDC/0.2 M NHS, the modified electrodes were incubated with a solution of 50 µg/mL MUC4 capture antibody overnight at 4°C.

E. Analytical Methods

The electrochemical experiments were carried out with an Autolab PGSTAT 12 potentiostat equipped with GPES 4.9 software and FRA for EIS experiments, using a standard three electrode cell.

The β-CD+PEI/Graphene modified GCEs were used for EIS studies and the results were compared with those obtained on bare GCE. Electrochemical impedance experiments were carried out in the presence of 10 mM $K_3[Fe(CN)_6]$ and $K_4[Fe(CN)_6]$ redox probes prepared in PBS (0.1 M; pH 7.2) with Ag/AgCl as reference electrode and a platinum wire as the counter electrode. A voltage of 10 mV in amplitude (peak-to-peak) was applied in a frequency range of 100 kHz-10 mHz. The dc potential was the open circuit potential.

During chronoamperometry the potential applied was kept at -0.2 V for the acetaminophen and at -0.3V vs. Ag/AgCl for the dopamine, under continuous stirring conditions. The working potential was imposed and the background current was allowed to arrive at a steady state value. Different amounts of acetaminophen or dopamine standard solution were added, every 100 seconds, into the stirred electrochemical cell and the current was recorded as a function of time. The data obtained using chronoamperometry were used to determine the linear range and detection limits. In the case of HRP based biosensor used for acetaminophen, the chronoamperometry experiments were performed in the presence of hydrogen peroxide 0.2 mM.

III. Results and discussions

A. Polymers Based Nanostructures Developed for Acetaminophen Analysis

The first example consists in a biosensor based on glassy carbon electrodes modified with carbon nanotubes and HRP entrapped in polymeric films used for acetaminophen detection.

MWCNT (lenght 30±10µm; diameter 1-5µm) was used as modifier for glassy carbon electrodes (d=3mm) in order to obtain nanostructures for the acetaminophen biosensor's development. Two types of polymers: PEI and Ppy were used to entrap the MWCNTs and HRP onto the electrode surface and the experimental protocol was optimized (see II. EXPERIMENTAL).

The amperometric response obtained after the addition of constant volumes (20 µL) of 0.01 M acetaminophen solution in 0.2 mM H_2O_2 in PBS (pH 7.4; 0.1 M) under constant stirring in the case of MWCNT-HRP-Ppy/GCE and MWCNT-HRP-PEI/GCE nanocomposite biosensors is presented in Figure 1.

The applied potential was -0.2 V vs. Ag/AgCl and the enzyme concentration in the MWCNTs suspension was 0.3 mg/mL. It can be observed that in the case of the biosensor obtained using electrogenerated polypyrrole film (Figure 1, curve b) the amperometric signal is better defined that in the case of the PEI based biosensor (Figure 1, curve a). The results obtained with MWCNT-HRP-Ppy/GCE tested in the presence of 0.2 mM H_2O_2 allowed us to have a calibration plot with the parameters: I(A) = 0.0164 [acetaminophen](M) -1.025 10^{-6}; $R^2 = 0.984$ while for MWCNT-HRP-PEI/GCE the parameters obtained are: I(A) = 0.008 [acetaminophen](M) -0.186·10^{-6}; $R^2 = 0.913$.

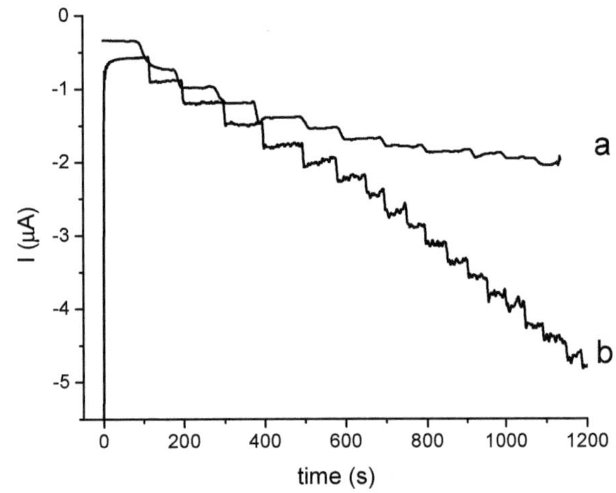

Fig. 1 Chromoamperograms for acetaminophen at (a) MWCNT-HRP-PEI/GCE and (b) MWCNT-HRP-Ppy/GCE

B. Polymers Based Nanostructures Developed for Dopamine Analysis

A second example uses dopamine as target molecule and the determination was made by using a tyrosinase biosensor based on glassy carbon electrodes modified with graphenes and β-CD entrapped in polyethyleneimine.

Figure 2 shows the Nyquist plots of bare GCE and modified with reduced graphene oxide in contact with the redox probe consisting in 10 mM $K_3[Fe(CN)_6]$ and $K_4[Fe(CN)_6]$ prepared in PBS (0.1 M; pH 7.2) in the range 100 kHz to 10 mHz.

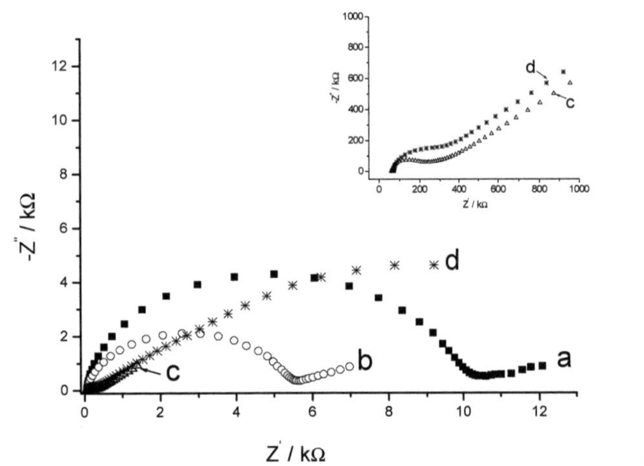

Fig. 2 EIS spectra registered for 10 mM $[Fe(CN)_6]^{3-}/[Fe(CN)_6]^{4-}$ in 0.1 M PBS (pH 7.2) at: bare GCE (a); GCE modified with reduced graphene oxide deposited by spin coating (b); layer by layer method (c) and layer by layer deposition together with β-CD (d)

The EIS spectra showed that the reduced graphene oxide presence at the electrode surface decreases the charge transfer resistance (R_{ct}) (Figure 2, curves b, c and d) compared with bare GCE (Figure 2, curve a). The lowest resistance is obtained if the reduced graphene oxide is deposited using layer by layer technique (curve c). The β-CD presence in the graphene based nanostructure lead to a small increasing of the R_{ct} value, meaning that the modification of the electrode conductivity is mainly due to graphene presence to the electrode surface.

SWV experiments were performed in order to demonstrate the utility of the GCE surface modification with graphene.

The reduced graphene oxide induces a significant increasing of the oxidation peak intensity for the dopamine electrochemical oxidation, (Figure 3). The SWV determinations were performed with β-CD/PEI modified GCE and β-CD/Graphene/PEI modified GCE in the presence of 1 mM dopamine solution in PBS (0.1M; pH 7.2).

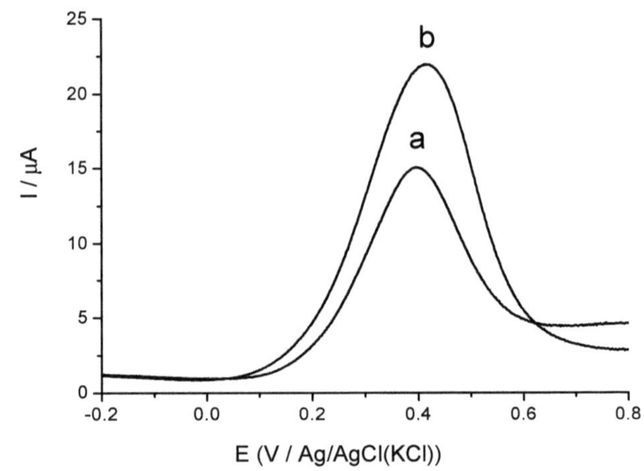

Fig. 3 SWVs registered for 1 mM dopamine solution PBS (0.1M; pH 7.2) at: β-CD/PEI modified GCE (a) and β-CD/Graphene/PEI modified GCE (b)

The tyrosinase does not cause any significant improvement of the signal intensity at the β-CD/Graphene/PEI modified GCE, but the dopamine oxidation potential is shifted to more negative values with about 200 mV.

The layer by layer technique was chosen for the reduced graphene oxide deposition on the electrode surface before the enzyme immobilization. The number of the graphene layer deposited on the electrode was optimized using SWV and EIS determination and the best results were obtained using three layers (data not shown).

The amperometry allowed the estimation of the current response which is linear with dopamine concentration in the range of 30 to 2500 μM. The sensitivity of enzyme sensor is 0.073 $\mu A\ \mu M^{-1}$ and the detection limit 10.42 μM.

C. Polymers Based Immunosensor for MUC4 Detection

EIS measurements were performed in order to characterize the modified electrodes, in 10 mM $[Fe(CN)_6]^{3-/4-}$ in PBS pH 7.4. It was observed that after the electropolymerization of PAA on the surface of graphite electrodes the charge transfer resistance increased (data not shown). Polyanthranilic acid is a carboxylated derivative of polyaniline. Although it possesses some advantages over polyaniline, such as increased solubility over a wide range of pH, it exhibits low conductivity compared to polyaniline, which explains the increased charge resistance. The incorporation of MWCNTs in the PAA film resulted in an excellent electron-transfer advantage given the well-known unique physicochemical proprieties of MWCNTs.

Although promising results in terms of conductivity were obtained for the prepared polymer nanocomposite, the reproducibility after incubation with antibody proved to be poor, probably due to inhomogeneous incorporation of MWCNTs in the film during the polymerization step and the loss of MWCNTs, therefore the second approach was tested for further incubation.

The Nyquist plots of the electrodes prepared according to the second approach are illustrated in Figure 4.

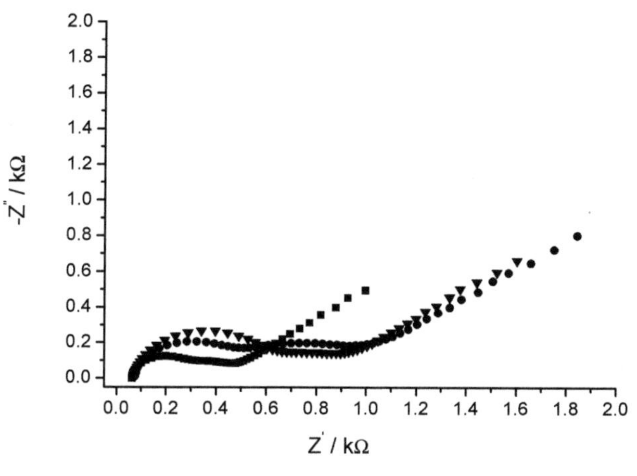

Fig. 4 The Nyquist diagrams obtained with 10 mM $[Fe(CN)_6]^{3/4-}$ in PBS (pH 7.4) at MWCNT/AuNP-modified (■), PAA-MWCNT/AuNP (●) and PAA-MWCNT/AuNP-Ab graphite based SPEs (▲)

After the deposition of PAA films the charge transfer value increases due to the coverage of highly conductive MWCNTs/AuNPs with a relatively low conductivity film (curve ●). The resistance value further increased after the immobilization of the capture antibody (curve ▲) owing to the blocking effect of the antibodies, which have nonconductive proprieties, reducing the electron transfer from the redox mediator to the electroactive area, confirming the binding of the antibodies at the carboxyl groups of PAA.

IV. Conclusions

The major goal of the study is the development of new, innovatives devices for early diagnosis of cancer and for the detection of some pharmaceuticals. In this respect different types of polymers were used in order to retain at the surface of the electrodes several nanostructures (like carbon nanotubes, graphene or cyclodextrines) and bioelements (enzymes and antibodies). The easiness of electrode surface modification combined with the sensitivity and specificity enhancements represents a good alternative to the currently used methods in pharmaceutical and biomedical analysis.

Acknowledgment

The authors are grateful for the financial support to the Romanian National Authority for Scientific Research, CNCS-UEFISCDI for the Project PN-II-ID-PCE-2011-3-0355.

Conflict of Interest

The authors declare that they have no conflict of interest.

References

1. Wilson GS, Hu Y (2000) Enzyme-Based Biosensors for In Vivo Measurements. Chem. Rev 100:2693-2704
2. Florea A, Taleat Z, Cristea C, Mazloum-Ardakani M, Săndulescu R (2013) Label free MUC1 aptasensors based on electrodeposition of gold nanoparticles on screen printed electrodes. Electrochemistry Commun 33:127–130
3. Gao Z D, Guan FF, Li C Y, Liu H F, Song Y Y (2013) Signal-amplified platform for electrochemical immunosensor based on TiO_2 nanotube arrays using a HRP tagged antibody-Au nanoparticles as probe. Biosens Bioelectron 41: 771-775
4. Chen H, Tang D, Zhang B, Liu B, Cui Y, Chen G (2012) Electrochemical immunosensor for carcinoembryonic antigen based on nanosilver-coated magnetic beads and gold-graphene nanolabels. Talanta 91:95-102
5. Vashist S K, Zheng D, Al-Rubeaan K, Luong J H T, Sheu F S (2011) Advances in carbon nanotube based electrochemical sensors for bioanalytical applications. Biotechnology Advances 29(2):169-188
6. Gao X, Zhang Y, Wu Q, Chen H, Chen Z, Lin X (2011) One step electrochemically deposited nanocomposite film of chitosan-carbon nanotubes-gold nanoparticles for carcinoembryonic antigen immunosensor application. Talanta 85 (4):1980-5
7. Zhu Y, Son J I, Shim Y B (2010) Amplification strategy based on gold nanoparticle-decorated carbon nanotubes for neomycin immunosensors. Bionsens Bioelectron 26(3):1002-1008

8. Tam P D, Hieu N V (2011) Conducting polymer film-based immunosensors using carbon nanotube/antibodies doped polypyrrole. Applied Surface Science 257(23): 9817-9824
9. Hu Y, Zhao Z, Wan Q (2011) Facile preparation of carbon nanotube-conducting polymer network for sensitive electrochemical immunoassay of Hepatitis B surface antigen in serum. Bioelectrochem 81(2): 59-64
10. Tertiş M, Florea A, Săndulescu R, Cristea C (2013) Carbon Based Electrodes Modified with Horseradish Peroxidase Immobilized in Conducting Polymers for Acetaminophen Analysis. Sensors 13:4841-4854
11. Fritea L, Tertiş M, Cristea C, Săndulescu R (2013) New β-Cyclodextrin Entrapped in Polyethyleneimine film Modified Electrodes for Pharmaceutical Compounds Determination. Sensors 13:16312-16329
12. Sima V, Cristea C, Bodoki E, Duțu G, Săndulescu R (2010) Screen-printed electrodes modified with HRP-zirconium alcoxide film for the development of a biosensor for acetaminophen detection. Centr Eur J Chem 8(5): 1034-1040
13. Sima V, Cristea C, Lăpăduş F, Marian I O, Marian A, Săndulescu R (2008) Electroanalytical properties of a novel biosensor modified with zirconium alcoxide porous gels for the detection of acetaminophen. J Pharm Biomed Anal 48(4):1195-1200
14. Rao P S, Sathyanarayana D N (2002) Synthesis of electrically conducting copolymers of aniline with o/m-amino benzoic acid by an inverse emulsion pathway. Polymer 43: 5051–5058
15. Swartz M J, Batra S K, Varshney G C, Hollingsworth M A, Yeo C J, et al. (2002) MUC4 expression increases progressively in pancreatic intraepithelial neoplasia. Am J Clin Pathol 117: 791–796
16. Karg A, Dinç Z A, Başok O, Üçvet A (2006) MUC4 expression and its relation to ErbB2 expression, apoptosis, proliferation, differentiation, and tumor stage in non-small cell lung cancer (NSCLC). Pathol Res Pract 202(8): 577–583
17. Bruyère E, Jonckheere N, Frénois F, Mariette C, Van Seuningen I (2011) The MUC4 membrane-bound mucin regulates esophageal cancer cell proliferation and migration properties: Implication for S100A4 protein. Biochem Bioph Res Co 413(2): 325-329
18. Workman H C, Miller J K, Ingalla E Q, Kaur R P, Yamamoto D I (2009) The membrane mucin MUC4 is elevated in breast tumor lymph node metastases relative to matched primary tumors and confers aggressive properties to breast cancer cells. Breast Cancer Res 11(5):R70
19. Ponnusamy M P, Lakshmanan I, Jain M, Das S, Chakraborty S, Dey P, Batra S K (2011) MUC4 stabilizes HER2 expression and maintains the cancer stem cell population in ovarian cancer cells. J Ovarian Res 26 (4):7-11
20. Guo Y, Guo S, Li J, Wang E, Dong S (2011) Cyclodextrin–graphene hybrid nanosheets as enhanced sensing platform for ultrasensitive determination of carbendazim. Talanta 84: 60–64
21. Lu D, Lin S, Wang L, Shi X, Wang C, Zhang Y (2012) Synthesis of cyclodextrin-reduced graphene oxide hybrid nanosheets for sensitivity enhanced electrochemical determination of diethylstilbestrol. Electrochim Acta 85 :131– 138

Author: Cecilia Cristea
Institute: University of Medicine and Pharmacy "Iuliu Hatieganu"
Street: 4 Pasteur
City: Cluj-Napoca
Country: Romania
Email: ccristea@umfcluj.ro

Study Regarding a System for Evaluation of the Sportsmen's Balance

L.D. Milici, M.R. Milici, and N. Dumitrasca

"Stefan cel Mare" University of Suceava, Romania

Abstract— **This paper aims to analyze the possibility of using wireless peripherals for studying the motor skills, study which is necessary both for the athletes and people who have suffered an accident of locomotor system and are within the recovery period. For some athletes a very important aspect is the equal distribution of force on both legs and thus the maintaining a balance as close to perfection. Patients who have suffered musculoskeletal accidents can measure and monitor the progress during recovery, and if they have sequels after trauma suffered they can, using the peripherals presented in this paper, to learn more easily and quickly how to compensate these sequels in the aim to maintain a balance as good. In order to achieve the intended purpose was need to develop an application which retrieves the data from the Wii balance board, processes them and then to displays them on the screen, so that the user can interpret them and make then the necessary corrections. To develop this application it was used the LabVIEW software.**

Keywords— **balance, motivity, equilibrium, virtual instrument**

I. INTRODUCTION

About balance it is spoken often but, most of the time, it is referred to the inner balance and mental balance. Without giving less attention to these issues compared to body balance, a definition of balance is our report about inner and outer world. When we have the ability to process and maintain the balance, we can free the consciousness and subconsciousness in order to use the energy for other purposes. A harmonious development of an individual refers to the dynamic equilibrium of living in the context of a limited energetic environment in which works, as a factor of regulating, its relationship with everything around him.

Endogenous performance factors are essential in training a sportsman and they are those that affect the performance inside the body and represent the base of the structure of performance in sport. In this group are: the predispositions on basic psychomotor skills (strength, resistance, speed, coordination), predispositions on coordinative psychomotor skills (balance, coordination, motive intelligence, response speed and predictive speed, spatial-temporal perceptions, ambidextrous ability), intellectual predispositions (memory, attention, judgment, thinking, imagination, etc.), psycho-affective predispositions (emotional stability, resistance to stress), volitional psycho-adjusting predispositions (voluntary effort, perseverance, combativity, resistance to pain), functional predispositions (oxygen consumption, energy substances and enzyme reserves, blood and oxygen flow, striated muscle structure, muscle innervation, supplying with nutrients, assimilation and de-assimilation), sportsman's character and temperament, his physical condition (physical, technical, tactical, psychological and theoretical training). [2]

When referring to the model of connections and interactions between the need to maintain balance during competitions and the chance to get the desired victory, we can evaluate the chance S_t of getting higher yields for a period of time t using the relation

$$S_t = \alpha(a_{t,x} + a_{t,y}) + \beta(b_{t,x} + b_{t,y}) + \mu\left[1 - (m_{t,x} - m_{t,y})^2\right] \quad (1)$$

where $a_{t,x}$ is the evolution of the coefficient of concentration in the first period of the competition, $b_{t,x}$ is the capacity to maintain the motive parameters during the first period of the competition, $m_{t,x}$ is the probability to obtain a major result within that competition since its start, and the terms in y refers to the last period of the competition. The coefficients $\alpha \in (0\ ,\ 1)$ are the values of the coefficient of equilibrium due to concentration, $\beta \in (0\ ,\ 1)$ represents the value of the balance coefficient due to the motility, μ express the sportsman's wish to win. [1]

The probability that the sportsman to obtain a favorable result in a competition is given by the relation:

$$m_{t,x} = \begin{cases} \varepsilon \frac{a_{t,x}}{a_{t,x}+a_{t,y}} + \omega \frac{b_{t,x}}{b_{t,x}+b_{t,y}} & if\ a_{t,x} + a_{t,y} > 0 \\ \frac{b_{t,x}}{b_{t,x}+b_{t,y}} & if\ a_{t,x} + a_{t,y} = 0 \end{cases} \quad (2)$$

where ε, ω are normalization coefficients and $\varepsilon+\omega = 1$. [1]

II. ELEMENTS OF MOTIVITY EVALUATION

Specific and nonspecific means used in sports influences the development bio-motive qualities: strength, power, speed, ability, mobility and psycho-behavioral abilities in the cognitive sphere (attention, specialized perceptions, imagination and creativity), volitional (energy, fortitude, perseverance, combativeness, resistance to physical pain), affective (emotional balance, self-control, restoring after success/failure/accident, resistance to stress), social (cooperation, teamwork, communication ability and self-evaluation), attitudinal and behavioral (motivation for victory, interest for

S. Vlad and R.V. Ciupa (eds.), *International Conference on Advancements of Medicine and Health Care through Technology*, IFMBE Proceedings 44,
DOI: 10.1007/978-3-319-07653-9_27, © Springer International Publishing Switzerland 2014

performance, sense of responsibility, critical and self-critical spirit, discipline, positive traits of character, professionalism). [2]

Equilibrium is defined as the function of keeping the unipodal position or the functional stretching from upright standing.

A very important factor in sport is the coordination. Coordination involves the optimum resolving of the complex situations offered by the changing conditions of the competition situations. The manifestation forms of coordination are: general, specific and within the regime of other motive qualities [6]. The coordination components are [1][3][4][5]:

- ability to motive learn;
- rapid response ability;
- ability to manage and control;
- rhythm and tempo ability;
- ability to combine and to differentiate the movements;
- ability for spatial and temporal orientation;
- ability to adapt the movements and to transform them;
- bi-laterality;
- balance, static or dynamic;
- accuracy, another component of coordination, which, within the sportive styles of combat, plays an extremely important role, because the target missing leads to the loss of the opportunity to obtain points and therefore of the match.

Psychological preparation in sport training is the action systematic and continue (in the aim to cultivate the personality traits) that includes all psychomotor abilities (which educates the kinesthetic sense, laterality, coordination, balance) and the system of the adaptive adjusting abilities (which refers to the cognitive, volitional, affective and behavioral sphere). [7]

The concept of motricity is defined as expressing a quality of the human being, innate and acquired, to react, with the locomotor system, to the internal and external stimuli, as a movement. Motricity brings together all the motive acts performed to maintain the relations with the natural and social environment, inclusive through performing skills specific to the sport areas. It's about the motive acts performed by skeletal muscle contraction. [9]

In summary, we define the motive activity as a process of satisfying a need (functional requirement) or, from a structural perspective, a sum of actions, operations, acts or gestures directed to achieve a particular goal. Therefore, the theory of motive activities corresponds to a system of knowledge on the origin, essence and laws of doing movements, highlighted in the theories biological, psychological, physical and social, which have studied and study the man moving, from particular perspectives, specific to them. [8]

Neuromuscular coordination plays an important role in the successful implementation of extremely rapid and precise techniques. In this way, muscle chains and groups used within a specific technique will therefore be controlled to work synergistically or, contrary, asynchronously, to achieve the motion, the tensioning of some joints involved in the technique, to achieve the balance needed in the body stability, a decisive factor in its effectiveness. On the background of its development, the neuromuscular coordination improves the mechanisms of some complicated movements, condition to learn correctly and rapidly the technical and tactical skills and to use them in different situations. [6]

III. Equipment description and experimntal data

The recent years have been marked by significant developments in the field of semiconductor sensors and transducers, among them being also the acceleration, gyro and force sensors. These sensors have found from the most diverse uses, in addition to the traditional uses, appearing uses less conventional, such as their integration in the controllers of the various video game consoles. A good example is the Wii video game console, produced by the Japanese company Nintendo, console proposing several types of controllers, such as the Wii Remote, which has included acceleration and gyro sensors, or the Wii balance board, which is based on four force sensors, disposed in each corner of the plate. The two peripherals use the Bluetooth protocol to communicate with the console, a protocol used currently for all mobile phones, tablets and other devices that need wireless transfer, on short distances. Some users of the console began to search for alternative uses of the accessories, in science rather than in video games (figure 1).

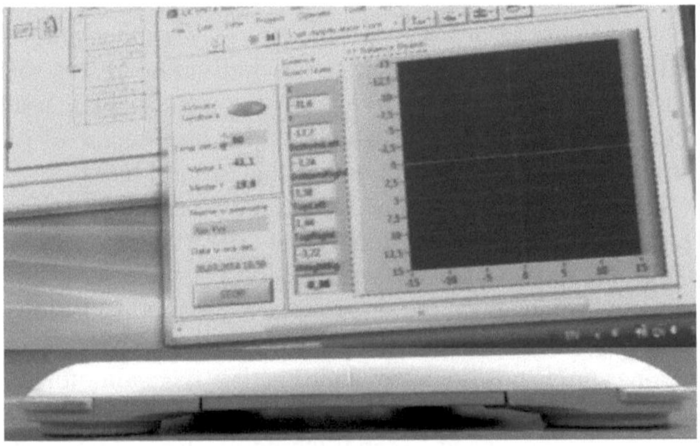

Fig. 1 Experimental platform

Virtual instrument developed, uses a sequential structure that initializes the Bluethoot communication port, open sequence acquisition, takes data in a repetitive While structure, process the data acquired, save them in a document and finally closes the communication port. The front panel allows customization of the experiment (and the time interval for testing), shows a chart for the position of the center of gravity for the subject, allows the registration of its name and data derived from measurements, provide information about the file with data saves.

The purpose of the above mentioned study was to examine the effects of the real-time viewing of the asymmetry influenced by loading in very well trained sportsmen and healthy individuals. It was hypothesized that the visual reaction will reduce the asymmetry during the genuflections and that the trained sportsmen will have a lower asymmetry than the healthy individuals of the same age but untrained. The results showed that the both categories have reduced the asymmetries influenced by loading from an initial factor of 2,8 - 9 to a final factor of 1,9 - 6,5 at the end of the study, using the real-time feedback provided by the two balance plates. Asymmetries were measured and, generally, were reduced using the balance plates from the Nintendo Wii consoles, equipments inexpensive, portable and widely available and which are relatively easy incorporated into the training program of sportsmen. [10]

The tests set has been established with the coaches of the athletes lots from Suceava University and it tries to highlight the effectiveness of exercises for the balance maintaining in the case of novice athletes. It was measured, in centimeters, the average deviation of the center of gravity from the central position, for a period of 60 seconds, in seven distinct situations:

- support on both feet, eyes opened, with feedback (viewing by the subject the position of the center of gravity on the computer screen);
- support on both feet, eyes open, without feedback;
- support on both feet, eyes closed;
- support on the left/right leg with the eyes opened, without feedback, and respectively with the eyes closed.

Measurements were made on a total of 100 subjects classified by level of education and different situations of stress and physical fatigue. In figure 2 are some diagrams obtained.

It can be observed the dispersion of results in case (*b*) (evaluation with eyes closed) in comparison with the case *a* in which the determination was made with feedback. The subject (*A*) has a high dispersion recorded in the first case; in the second case it has a higher dispersion than the average of the subjects. It can be seen and the role that each member has on maintaining balance. Thus, from diagram (*a*) it is seen that the right foot is generally more involved in balance control with feedback, and from diagram (*b*) we identify the role of the right foot to always control the position when there is no visual feedback.

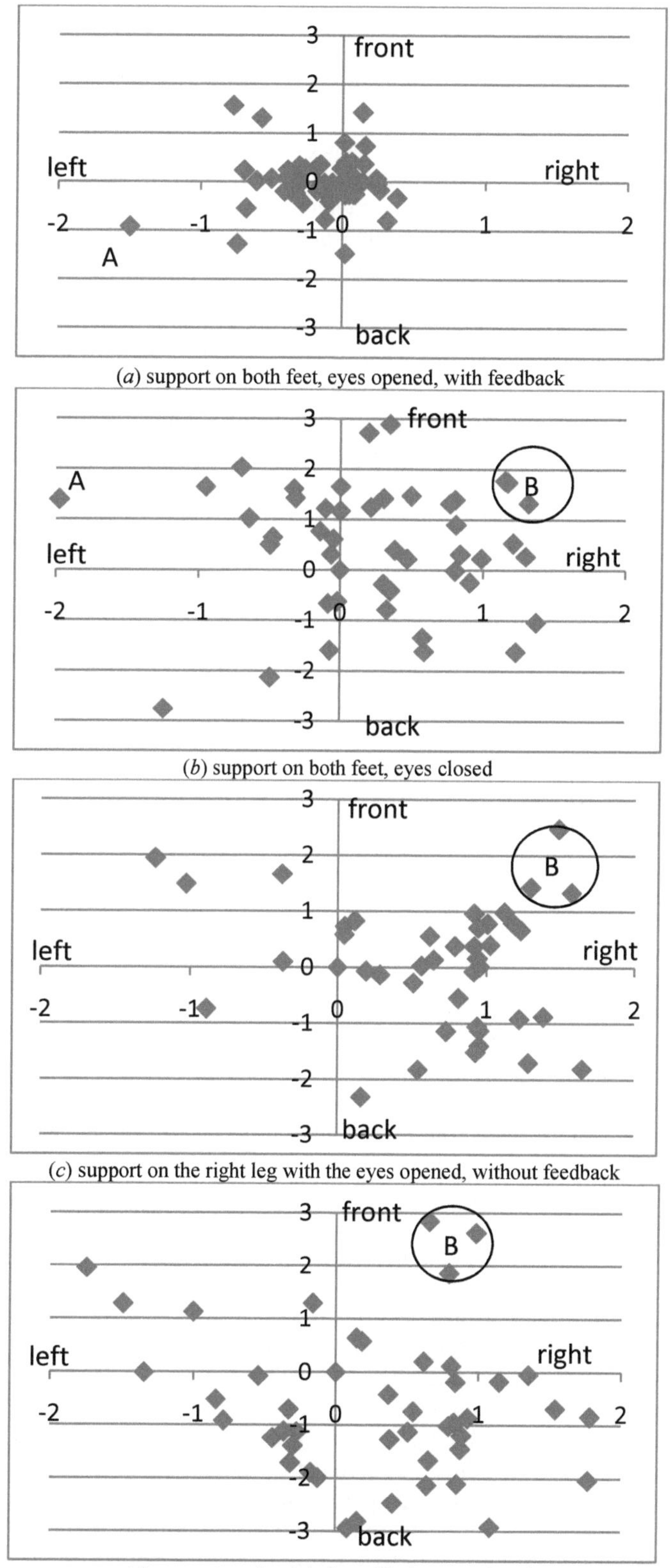

(*a*) support on both feet, eyes opened, with feedback

(*b*) support on both feet, eyes closed

(*c*) support on the right leg with the eyes opened, without feedback

(*d*) support on the right leg with the eyes closed.

Fig. 2. Experimental data

For the case in which subjects support only on the right foot it can find the same high dispersion when the measurements were made with the eyes closed (d) in comparison with the measurements made with the eyes opened (c), and the difference from the case (a) can be explained by the complexity of measurements and the lack of feedback. There are cases where the subjects have a constant dispersion, regardless of the valuation (group B), which is explained by a lack of training on balance.

To highlight the influence of physical fatigue and external disturbing factors for the same subject, the same set of measurements was done for an athlete before and after its evolution into a sports competition (figure 3). It can be seen the dispersion of experimental data as an effect of the muscle fatigue and noises coming from the sporting arena.

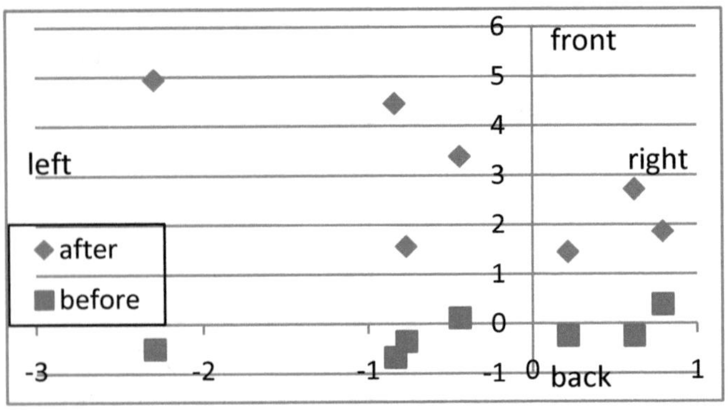

Fig. 3 Influence of fatigue in maintaining the balance for a sportsman (both legs, without feedback)

IV. Conclusions

During the effort, sometimes appear imbalances in the muscular work and in the ability of autonomic systems, especially the respiratory and circulatory, of supplying with oxygen and energetic substances. The imbalance called "dead point" can be installed within the range of 30 seconds and 6 minutes of an effort, depending on the effort intensity and degree of sportsman's training. The occurrence of the "dead point" can be felt as an accentuate tiredness in muscles and brain, a tiredness due to lack of oxygen, the respiratory and circulatory system not being able to ensure the necessary oxygen in a short time. This unpleasant sensation disappears through the sportsman desire to continue the activity, desire which can overcome the "dead point" if it is intense and sustained. To avoid the "dead point", it is recommended a thorough preparing of the body before starting the effort, especially in training and competitions. [2] The proposed system allows to determine the moment before the installing the "dead point".

From the studies done we can draw the following conclusions:

- the equipment used has the advantage of wireless connection which allows the use and placing it away from the computer system that makes the monitoring;
- the shape and the characteristics of the device are optimally chosen so as to allow an easy measurement with high accuracy;
- the virtual instrument developed can be modified so as to easily adapt to a particular type of determination/measurement;.

The continuation of studies can be done by:

- identification of new tests and new types of tests (evaluation the motive parameters during the genuflections or during the jumping with beat);
- the concomitant using of the balance board and of the manual Wii console to do complex tests related to human motive performance;
- the computing of some parameters which to allow the accurate quantitative estimation of the monitoring done.

References

1. P. DeCezara (2012) Human psycho-motric modelling, MIT Publishing House;
2. B. Zabet, B.A. Zabet, (2006) Curs de caiac-canoe (Kayak-canoe course), Universitatea Bacău;
3. B. Voiculescu (2007) Anatomia şi fiziologia omului (Human anatomy and physiology), Ed. Corint, Bucureşti;
4. Л.П. Матвеев (2008) Теория и методика физической культуры (Theory and Methodology of Physical Education). 3-е изд., перераб.и доп. – Мо: Физкультура и спорт, СпортАкадемПресс;
5. A. Dragnea, M. Teodorescu (2002) Teoria educaţiei fizice şi sportului (Theory of physical education and sport), Ed. FEST Bucureşti;
6. C. Ivan (2006) Alcoolul în activităţile sportive (Alcohol in sport), Analele Universitatii Spiru Haret, an. III, nr. 3, pp. 23-26;
7. E.L. Sidenco (2006) Evaluarea generală şi funcţională în kinetoterapie şi recuperarea medicală (General and functional evaluation in kinetotherapy and medical rehabilitation), Analele Universitatii Spiru Haret, an. III, nr. 3, pp. 67-72;
8. Teoria activităţilor motrice (Theory of the motive activities) (iunie 2012) at http://mariananu.wordpress.com/psihologie;
9. Tonusul muscular (The muscle tone) (iunie 2012) at http://www.elipetromed.ro/tonusul-muscular.html;
10. Testarea încărcării asimetrice a membrelor (Testing of asymmetric loading of the limbs) (mai 2012) at http://w4.ub.uni-konstanz.de/cpa/article/viewFile/5011/4653;

Author: L. Dan MILICI
Institute: "Stefan cel Mare" University of Suceava
Street: Universitatii Street, 13
City: Suceava
Country: Romania
Email: dam@eed.usv.ro

SQUID Gradiometer for Biomagnetic Fields

O. Baltag and C.M. Rau

"Grigore T. Popa" University of Medicine and Pharmacy,
Biomedical Engineering Department, Iasi

Abstract— **This work presents theoretical and experimental results of the research concerning the design and characteristics of a 1st and 2nd order SQUID gradiometer with electronic subtraction. The SQUID biogradiometer was used for recording the magnetic field of the heart in laboratory conditions. The MCG signal was recording using a complex installation composed from a non ferromagnetic shielded room, a large triaxial Helmholtz coil system and the SQUID gradiometer reconfigured from a triaxial sensor in a three 1st order and one 2nd order gradiometer. The MCG signal and its characteristics is presented.**

Keywords— **SQUID, biogradiometer, biomagnetic fields**

I. Introduction

Measurement of the biomagnetic fields is confronted with certain difficult aspects, given the very small value of the measured parameters, which is about 10^{-15} T (the smallest) for the field generated by foetal heart, and hardly 10^{-12} T (the highest) corresponding to the field generated by the biocurrents of an adult heart. No wonder that solutions have been searched to measure them, solutions that need to be accessible from both technical and material standpoints. The existence of natural or artificial environmental electromagnetic fields, much higher than the biomagnetic fields, determines the necessity to carry out the biomagnetic field measurements in spaces where these are diminished to smaller values or comparable with the measured field.

The environmental electromagnetic field spectrum is very complex; therefore the methods to diminish it are very complex from a conceptual and constructive standpoint. There are several measuring methods used to measure magnetic fields in terms of field intensity, measurement precision and resolution, equipment complexity, measurement duration, cost price etc. Yet, none of these methods was completely satisfactory when the biomagnetic field measurement was desired. Given their very small values, ranging from nT to fT, systems with very high sensitivity threshold have been developed going to 10^{-17} T, very versatile, named Superconducting Quantum Interference Device (SQUID). These are flux-voltage converters and are the sensors with the highest sensitivity and the lowest sensitivity threshold known up to now, for weak magnetic field measurement. The width of the operational band is big, from quasi-static measurements to values exceeding 1 GHz.

They are able to measure any physical parameter that can be converted in magnetic flux: magnetic field and gradient, magnetic susceptibility, voltage, current, mechanical displacement.

Being the sensor with the lowest sensitivity threshold for magnetic flux measurement, it is the mostly used in the design and construction of biomagnetic field measurement devices.

A standard SQUID sensor consists of a ring of semiconductor material, interrupted by one or more Josephson junctions which convert the magnetic flux into voltage. The noise level for axial magnetometers or gradiometers can reach values ranging between 5 $fT/Hz^{1/2}$ and 10 $fT/Hz^{1/2}$ at low frequencies in a magnetically screened room, and sensitivity smaller than 2 $fT/Hz^{1/2}$.

One of the mostly known methods to improve the signal/noise ratio is using a *1st, 2nd* or *3rd* gradientmeter structure instead of magnetometer classical structures [1], [2]. In biomagnetism are using SQUID gradiometers mainly because of their ability to detect magnetic field gradients and reject common vector of magnetic field.

In 1971, Zimmerman was the first which introduce the concept of gradiometer with which it can be remove the ambient electromagnetic interference. He made the first SQUID gradiometer for magnetocardiographic measurements in unshielded rooms [3]. Experiments with SQUID gradiometers were performed by other research groups from China, Japan and Germany [4] - [12].

II. Theoretical Issues

The magnetic field originates in the movement of the electric charges within the volume of the heart tissue. The heart morphology and physiology are very complex, such that an integral analytical description is practically impossible from this point of view. If one considers several simplifying hypotheses related to the considered volumes, can imagine the heart as a magnetic dipole whose field is determined by the movement of electrical charges. The magnetic field generated in one point by the movement of a number *i*

S. Vlad and R.V. Ciupa (eds.), *International Conference on Advancements of Medicine and Health Care through Technology*, IFMBE Proceedings 44,
DOI: 10.1007/978-3-319-07653-9_28, © Springer International Publishing Switzerland 2014

of electric charges q_i with the velocities $\vec{v}_i$ situated at the distance $\vec{r}_i$ is given by the equation:

$$\vec{B} = \frac{\mu}{4\pi}\sum_i \frac{q_i \vec{v}_i}{r_i^3} \times \vec{r}_i \quad (1)$$

For small enough time intervals and distances, one can consider that the movement of the charges q_i is linear. In fact, this movement occurs within a conducting volume with variable geometry and structure that presents a time and space dynamics of the electric properties. The presence of electric dipoles with a special dynamics determines a complex system of magnetic dipoles with variable magnetic moments, position, distribution and spatial orientation. At a distance bigger than the magnetic dipoles basis, the entire heart system can be considered as a dipole with variable magnetic moment and spatial orientation, correlated during a cardiac cycle.

Due to this complex character, one can not speak about the heart isoelectric or isomagnetic axis, as these axes are in fact virtual complex volumes described by electric and magnetic vectors, in permanent motion, that describe imaginary volumes during the cardiac cycle. The relation between these can be approximated with a quite high degree of error, such that they can be considered as two conical regions relatively perpendicular to each other, each of them corresponding to the electric and magnetic fields respectively, Figure 1.

If the resultant of the isoelectric and isomagnetic axes is projected on the vertical and horizontal planes, one can determine for a certain moment a non-linear „axis" that can be interpreted as „isoelectric".

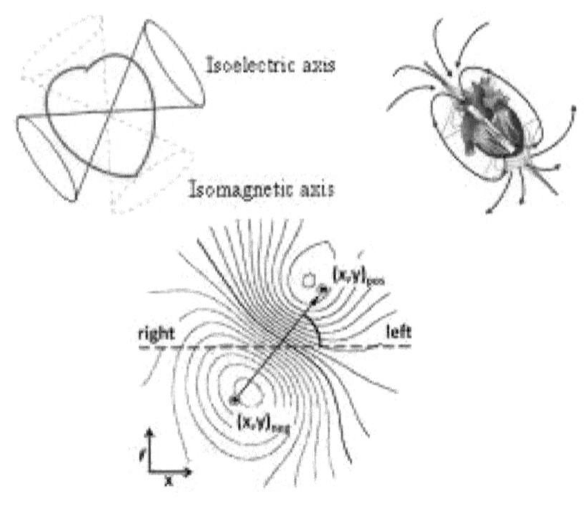

Fig.1 Isoelectric and isomagnetic axis

The magnetic field energy is determined by the energy density produced by the cardiac activity, according to the equation:

$$W_B = \frac{1}{2\mu_0} B^2 \quad (2)$$

Considering a magnetic induction with the value of 100 pT, we obtain for the energy density:

$$W_B = 4 \bullet 10^{-15} J/m^3 = 4 \bullet 10^{-21} J/cm^3 = 4 \bullet 10^{-9} pJ/cm^3$$

By comparing the magnetic energy density of biological origin with the density of ambiental magnetic fields, one can find that their level is in an especially disadvantageous ratio for the biologic magnetic fields. Therefore, it is preferably to use gradient type techniques for the reduction of the common mode vector of the disturbing field. We consider that the biomagnetic field source and the disturbing source produce fields subjected to the same laws specific for the magnetic dipole.

The easiest gradiometry structure is composed of two coils, coaxial, located in parallel planes with same number of turns and identical sections, located at a fixed distance, named baseline, connected in opposition in flux transformer circuit. This is the 1st order gradiometer. Starting from this structure, one can obtain 2nd, 3rd.... n^{th} order structures. They deliver a signal proportional with the 2nd, 3rd,... n^{th} order gradient of the measured field.

One can realize a gradiometer of any order making use of gradiometers of a lower order: two magnetometers (0th order gradiometers) which deliver signals of opposite polarity can make a first order gradiometer; two gradiometers of first order that deliver signals with opposite polarities can make together a 2nd order gradiometer; two 2nd order gradiometers can form a 3rd order gradiometer.

Gradiometry problem is concerned with both increasing the sensitivity of the physical system and the precision of measurement. Certainly, the physical gradiometric structure introduces an error with respect to the derivative computed in the points at the ends of the corresponding interval *z*. The increase of sensitivity can be accomplished by increasing the basis (with the possibility to introduce an additional error), increasing the basis also implying a diminution of gradient measurement precision.

We have analyzed the distribution with distance of the magnetic field and the 1st and the 2nd order gradients produced by two sources, one of disturbances and the other of biosignal, as well as the effect of the gradiometer basis in measuring the gradient of the biomagnetic field in the presence of a magnetic disturbance. There are differences between the mathematical definition of the gradient and the physical structure through which the magnetic field gradient is measured, resulting in the appearance of measurement and interpretation errors. Different configurations of the field and biofield sources, as well as their layout in the measurement space have been chosen. A structure was considered for gradient measurement, consisting of three identical coaxial coils, positioned in parallel planes, which form a 1st order gradiometer with the basis *d*, a 1st order gradiometer with the basis *2d* and a *2nd* order gradiometer with the basis d. These gradiometers are located in the fields generated by a source of biomagnetic field *Bs* and by a disturbance source *Bp* respectively, Figure 2.

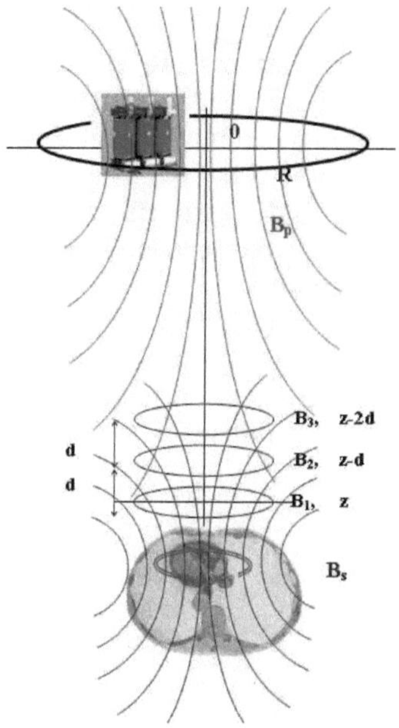

Fig.2 Simulation of perturbation and biomagnetic fields

For the analysis of the contribution to the signal detected by gradiometers, it has been considered that the imaginary sources (the disturbance and biofield sources were assimilated with circular spire with magnetic moments *Mp* and respectively, *Ms*) are coaxial with the gradiometers, which is a disadvantageous disposal in terms of disturbance signal, but favorable in terms of the biofield signal [13]. The centre "*O*" of the disturbance spire was considered as reference; the signal coil *B1* is located at a distance *z*, the other coils *B2* and *B3* being located at the distances z-d and *z-2d* respectively. The signal coil is located in the endmost point from the disturbance source and in proximal position as related to the biomagnetic field source. A theoretical study was performed concerning the spatial distribution (the gradient) of the biomagnetic field source, on the one side, and of the disturbing sources on the other side. As the result of this study, differences were found with respect to the field and the *1st* and *2nd* order gradients distribution with the distance, which permit to diminish the disturbance effects by an adequate choice of the gradiometer type measuring structure.

As the result of the law of field and gradients variations with distance, the gradient of the biomagnetic source has bigger values in the area of the measuring coil, while the gradient of the disturbing sources has much smaller values. The gradient spatial variation shows that the measurement of the 1st order gradient is more advantageous (as compared to the field measurement) in terms of the signal induced by the distant disturbing source; this variation shows that if one takes the measuring basis into account, inconveniences can appear at small distances from the biomagnetic field source, mainly as the size of the biomagnetic field source is comparable with the distance between the measuring coil and the source.

We have analyzed the distribution with the distance of the magnetic field and of the *1st* (Figure 3) and *2nd* order gradients (Figure 4) produced by two sources (for different *Ms/Mp* ratios), one of disturbances – *Mp* magnetic moment and one of biosignal - *Ms* magnetic moment. We found out that it is more advantageous to measure the *2nd* order gradient than the *1st* order gradient, as the signal/noise ratio is improved.

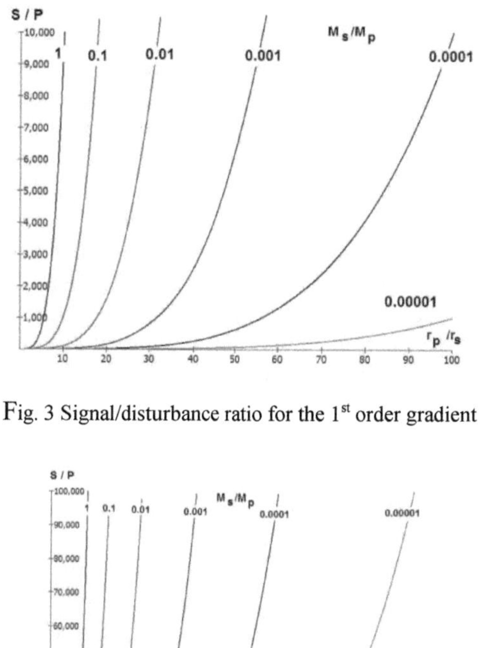

Fig. 3 Signal/disturbance ratio for the 1st order gradient

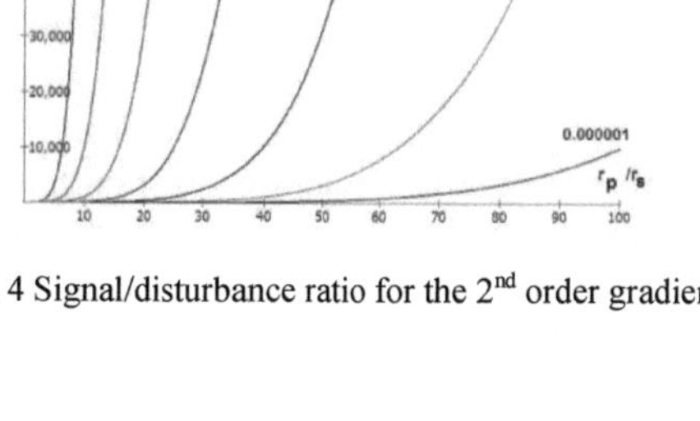

Fig. 4 Signal/disturbance ratio for the 2nd order gradient

The assimilation of the disturbance source with a dipole having a magnetic moment leads to the same conclusions concerning the advantage of measuring the *2nd* order gradient as compared to *1st* order gradient, an obvious advantage in the case when there are several disturbance sources, since the resulting magnetic disturbance vector changes its amplitude, phase and spatial orientation. The gradient measured by using two coils is smaller than the gradient resulting from calculation by the measuring coil. This difference increases as the gradiometer basis increases.

Taking into account a symmetrical structure of the proximal and distal coils as related to the biomagnetic field source presents some calculus facilities, besides providing a diminished gradient dispersion. The complexity of the methodology used to approach the biomagnetic measurements is determined by the complexity of the biofield source, imprecision in the knowledge of field and gradient spatial distribution, assimilation of bio-sources with multipolar sources, as well as by the small distances between the imaginary centres of the bio-sources and the position and configuration of the gradiometer structure. The theoretical results demonstrate the advantage of biomagnetic measurements by means of the *2nd* order gradiometer systems, as compared to the utilization of the *1st* order gradiometers, even if these are more complex and need a more tidy construction. It has been demonstrated that, irrespective of its order, the gradiometer coils must satisfy certain conditions: they have to be perfectly aligned and their sections and turn numbers must satisfy the relation: $S_1N_1= S_2N_2$. Due to the small dimensions of the coils used in SQUID, the alignment condition is quite difficult to satisfy, such that usually the external magnetic fields give a signal component that represents about 1% of the value of the gradient signal. From the construction standpoint, the conditions concerning misalignment and non-identity of the magnetic flux can be accomplished using adequate technologies and adjustments, which permit to obtain a high rejection factor.

III. Experimental resuls

Following the results of the performed theoretical studies, it was realize a SQUID gradiometer by converting a triaxial SQUID magnetometer type „Tristan HTS SQUID Magnetometer model 703". The magnetometer provides the noise-related performances, but it can not operate in the environmental electromagnetic medium of the laboratory. The triaxial SQUID magnetometer was transformed from a complex triaxial gradiometer system by changing the positions of the three SQUID sensors corresponding to the *Ox*, *Oy* and *Oz* axes. The coils were re-positioned at equal distances from one another, in a vertical direction, axially and in three parallel planes.

The coils were fastened with small brass screws; the material used for screws is not superconductive at the liquid nitrogen temperature and therefore there is no danger of introducing parasite fields produced by the superconducting currents induced by screws. With this aim in view, the SQUID sensors were moved from their initial coaxial position in three coaxial holders positioned vertically, this being thus converted in a system of 1st and 2nd degree gradiometers for the measurement of vertical components of magnetic field gradient.

The magnetometer sensors are connected through flux transformers to three independent electronic modules, such that to obtain three magnetometric channels. With the magnetometric signals processed by means of the electronic subtraction three *1st* order gradient channels and one *2nd* order gradient channel were accomplished. We present the three SQUID sensors directed vertically along the *Oz* axis, for the measurement of the *B(z)* magnetic field component. The distance between two neighboring sensors is of 4 cm and it represents the gradient measuring basis. The distance between the proximal and distal sensors, located at extremities, is of 8 cm, Figure 5.

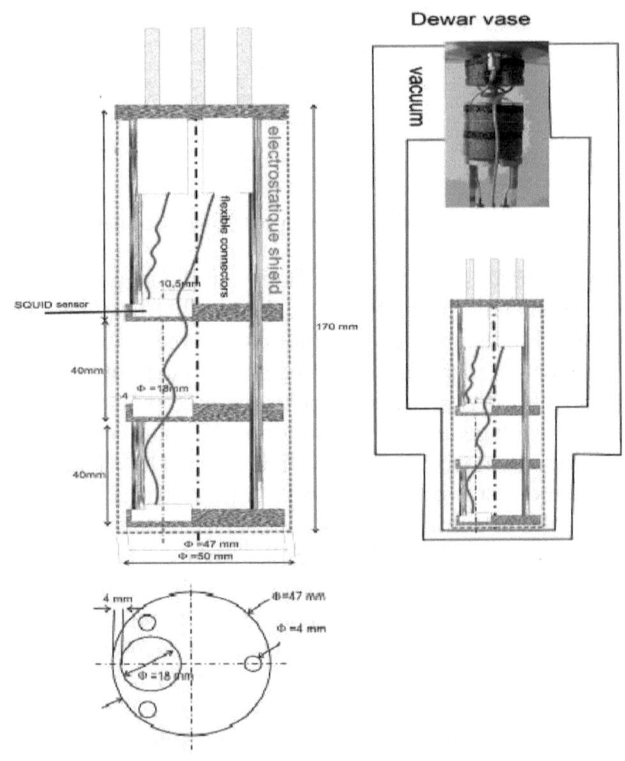

Fig. 5 SQUID Gradiometer

These gradiometers differ from the classical ones accomplished with sensors (superconducting coils) connected in opposition. The three magnetometric channels are galvanically separated from each other. These transmit the analogical signal to a conversion circuit that communicates at distance with the electronic blocks through optical fiber cable. The optical interface communicates with digital / analogical conversion circuits and delivers an analogical signal proportional with the measured field. The adopted solution is advantageous due to the fact that, from the three SQUID magnetometer channels, one can realize several SQUID gradiometers by using the electronic subtraction of the signal arrived from the three individual magnetometric channels. By electronic subtraction produced at the output of the three channels, a four channels gradiometer was obtained, Figure 6.

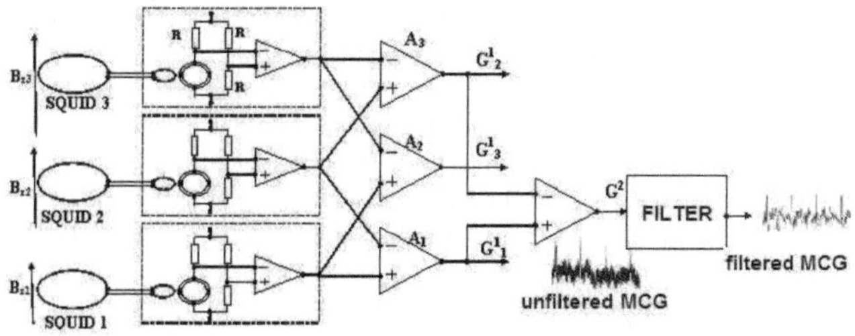

Fig. 6 First and second order SQUID gradiometers with electronic subtraction

After electronic subtraction, the gradient signals are filtered through of low-pass filter with the cut-off frequencies of 38 Hz, 60 Hz and 120 Hz. The adopted solution is advantageous due to the fact that one can produce several SQUID gradiometers from the three SQUID magnetic channels, by using the electronic subtraction of the signal delivered by the three individual magnetometric channels.

Using the operation of electronic subtraction occurring at the output of the three channels, a four-channels gradiometer was realized, namely:

- two 1st order gradiometers with baseline *dz = 4 cm*,
- one 1st order gradiometer with baseline *dz = 8 cm*,
- one 2nd order gradiometer with baseline *dz = 4 cm*.

The modification of the structure of the three SQUID sensors, as well as of the afferent electronics, implies both the problem of proper noises of the three realized SQUID sensors, as well as of the gradient measurement errors. The noise of the SQUID sensor is $50\,fT / Hz^{1/2}$ at the frequency of *1 Hz*. The global gradiometric sensitivity is $14.4 \bullet 10^{-9}$ *T/V*. Since the three magnetometric channels have different sensitivities, in order to perform the electronic subtraction three electronic circuits were introduced, which perform the leveling of the transfer coefficients or factors (channels sensitivity). With this SQUID gradiometer was recorded the first magnetocardiogram (MCG) performed in Romania, at the Bioelectromagnetism Laboratory of the Medical Bioengineering Faculty, Iasi, Figure 7.

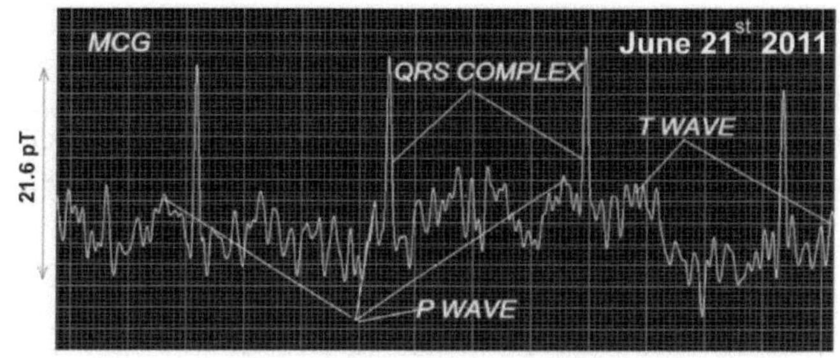

Fig. 7 Magnetocardiogram signal

The gradiometric channels were adjusted as follows: using a Helmholtz magnetic field generator, a known field is applied to each channel and the amplification factors are individually adjusted until the sensitivity of the three channels becomes equal to each other. The signals arrived from the three magnetometric channels are applied to the three channels of analogical subtraction accomplished with operational amplifiers. At the output of the analogical circuits three signals are obtained, proportional with the gradient of the magnetic field determined by the intensity of the field by the three SQUID sensors of the magnetometric channels. The SQUID gradiometers thus configured are installed in the centre of the shielded room and of the Helmholtz coils system, above the bed mobile in the horizontal plan. In order to calibrate the gradiometers system we have used a field and field gradient generator of small dimensions, relatively easy to manipulate, with a useful volume adequate to the size of the gradiometer basis. Simultaneously with magnetocardiogram recording, an electrocardiogram was executed, with standard derivations. The utilized electrodes are not magnetic (non-magnetic). The magnetograms were measured within the following regions: the Vth left intercostals space, on the medio-clavicular line and in the xiphoid appendix zone, Figure 8.

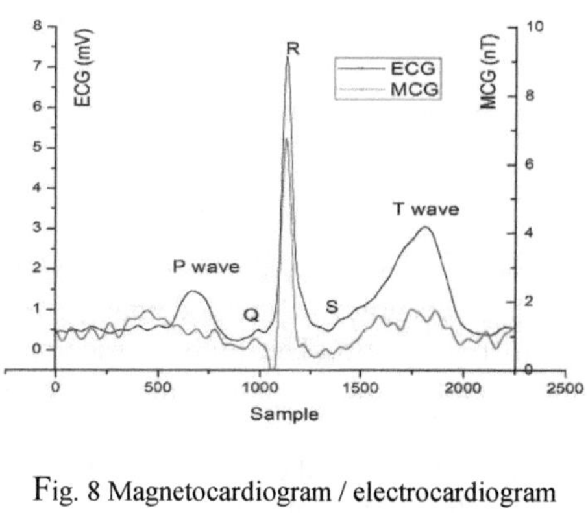

Fig. 8 Magnetocardiogram / electrocardiogram

The recorded MCG signal was processed using the coherent averaging with a number of 34 samples. One can notice the presence of disturbances with the frequency of 50 Hz and its harmonics on the MCG signal. The QRS complex has the amplitude higher than the P and T waves; accordingly, is less affected by the external magnetic disturbances (5.5 pTpp). The Pearson correlation between the EKG reference signal and MCG signal has the value of 0.82, Figure 9.

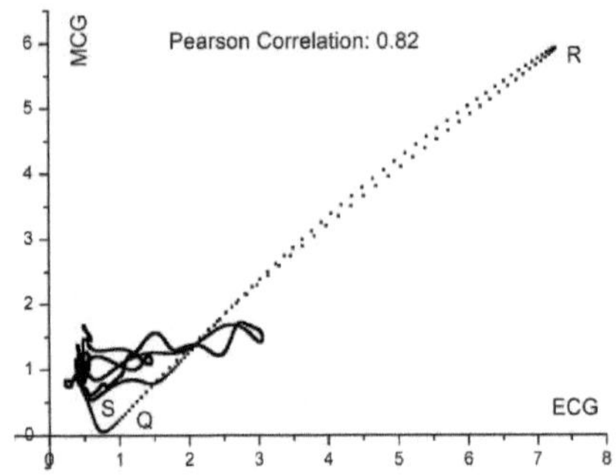

Fig. 9 Pearson correlation MCG / EKG signals

The distribution cloud is intensely populated in the zone of low intensity signals, disturbing the recorded P and T waves. A correlation coefficient of 0.99 is obtained if one analyses the MCG/EKG correlation of the QRS complex, Figure 10.

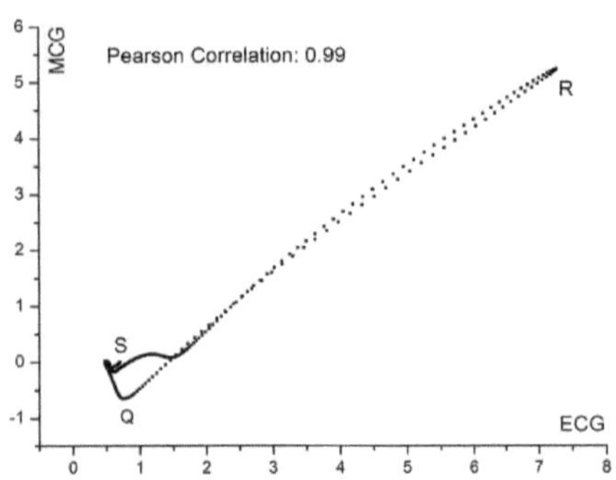

Fig. 10 Pearson correlation of the QRS interval

IV. Conclusions

It is preferable to perform the biomagnetic field measurements using the gradient method that permits a very good signal to noise ratio. The higher order gradiometers improve the signal to noise ratio, but they diminish the measurement sensitivity.

The correlation between the reference EKG signals and the MCG signals has very high values, quite close to identity by the QRS complex.

The correlation coefficients diminish for the P and T waves due to the low level MCG signal and to some residual magnetic disturbances; the magnetic disturbances diminish the signal to noise ratio within the intervals of the P and T waves.

Conflict of Interest

The authors declare that they have no conflict of interest.

References

1. Hwang Y., Jong Rok Ahn (2001) et al. Balancing of the single-layer second-order high-Tc SQUID gradiometer, IEEE Trans. on Applied Superconductivity, pp. 1343-1344
2. Uzunbajakau S. A., Rijpma A. P. (2005) et al. Optimization of a Third-Order Gradiometer for Operation in Unshielded Environments, IEEE Trans. on Applied Superconductivity, pp. 3879-3883
3. Zimmerman J.E., Frederick N.V. (1971) Miniature ultrasensitive superconducting magnetic gradiometer and its use in cardiography and other applications", Appl. Phys. Lett. 19 (1):16-19G
4. Lee Y. H., Yu K.K. (2008) 64-channel second-order axial gradiometer system based on DROS for magnetocardiogram in a thin shielded room", Physica C: Superconductivity 1942–1945
5. Liao S. H., Hsu S. C. (2003) High Tc SQUID gradiometer system for magnetocardiography in an unshielded environment", Supercond. Sci. Technol. 1426-1429
6. Bick M., Sternickel K., et al. (2001) SQUID gradiometry for magneto-cardiography using different noise cancellation techniques", IEEE Trans.on Applied Superconductivity 673-676
7. Becker W., Dickmann V. et al. (1993) First experiences with a multi-channel software gradiometer recording normal and tangential components of MEG, Physiol. Meas A45-A50
8. Seki Y.,, Kandori A.,, et al. Two-dimensional gradiometer, Japanese Journal of Applied Physics 3397-3401
9. Stolz R,, Bondarenko N. et al. (2003) Integrated gradiometer-SQUID system for fetal magneto-cardiography without magnetic shielding, Sci. Technol. 1523-1527
10. Drung, D., Absmann C. et al (1995) The PTB 83-SQUID System for Biomagnetic Applications in a Clinic, IEEE Trans. Appl. Supercond. 2112-2117
11. Zhang Y., Panaitov G. et al (2000) A HTS SQUID gradiometer using superconducting coplanar resonators for operation in unshielded environment", Chinese Journal of Physics 330-338
12. Nenonen J., Ilmoniemi R.J. et al. (2001) The 8-layered magnetically shielded room of the PTB: Design and construction in Biomag 2000, Proc. 12th Int. Conf. on Biomagnetism, eds. (Helsinki Univ. of Technology, Espoo, Finland,2001, pp. 970-973
13. Rau M.C. (2012) Researches in Biomagnetic Fields Measurements, Ph.D. Thesis, „Gh. Asachi" Technical Univ of Iasi, Romania

Author: Miuta Carmina Rau
Institute: "Grigore T. Popa" University of Medicine and Pharmacy, Biomedical Engineering Department, Iasi, Romania
Street: Universitatii, 16
City: Iasi
Country: Romania
Email: miuta.carmina@gmail.ro

A Method to Determine the Nominal Diameter for Hip Joint with No "Pre-wear" Data

C. Neamţu, F. Popişter, R. Ghinea, and V. Tompa

Technical University of Cluj-Napoca, Department of Design Engineering and Robotics, Romania

Abstract— **This paper presents a methodology for determining the initial diameter of the explanted hip prosthesis based on scanning/measuring using coordinate measuring machines (CMM) and CAD processing of the obtained data. ISO 14242-2:2000 shows two methods for determining wear of hip joint: gravimetric and measuring using CMMs. Only the second method (measuring using a CMM) can provide information regarding the position and the geometry of the wear print. Using CMMs to determine the hip joint's wear with no "pre-wear" data involves finding the initial diameter of the prosthesis and then comparing the ideal surface with the real one which was determined using the explained scanning procedure. Most times there is no accurate measurement of the prosthesis before implantation to determine the real surface of the prosthesis. The presented methodology involves scanning the sphere so that it can calculate the deviation of the scanned points compared to a theoretical circle determined using CAD or numerical methods (roundness deviation). The scanning of the prosthesis or of a sphere can be done using at least three strategies: one of them offers the possibility of scanning complete circles and the other two only allow the scanning of arcs (½ or ¼ of a complete circle's circumference). The strategy enables the use of scan points for determine the deviation from circularity. Items that have a significant deviation from the nominal circle are the removed in a CAD program using for this purpose the roundness error map. The remaining points are used to calculate the sphere's diameter and the center will then be taken as a reference to determine the area of the prosthesis that has wear.**

Keywords— **hip joint measurement, coordinate measuring machine, initial diameter estimation**

I. INTRODUCTION

An artificial hip joint is a spherical joint that can replace the arthritic human hip. The spherical head of the femur (thigh bone) moves inside the hemispherical socket of the pelvis – acetabulum component of the hip joint. Between femoral head and acetabulum component of the hip joint can be a plastic liner for minimize the wear of this two components. This movement at a rate of typically 1–2 million cycles per year leads to wear within the articulation [1].

These types of prostheses are used in treating the disease suffered by the hip joint (human arthritic hip) (rheumatoid arthritis or osteoarthritis) which involves partial or total replacement of it with artificial elements created from biocompatible material.

The problems associated with prosthetic failure and the consequent need for revision surgery still represent a major clinical issue. The most common reasons for revision surgery include prosthesis loosening, periprosthetic osteolysis, infection, malalignment, stiffness, prosthesis failure or fracture, and wear [2].

The term 'wear' could be defined as an undesirable progressive loss of material from one or both surfaces in relative motion between them. The mechanism of wear is very complex and there are two broad approaches to the classification of wear: the first is descriptive of the results of wear, while the second is based on the physical nature of the underlying processes [3].

Measure the hip joint prostheses in order to determine wear and highlight the area where the wear is generally done in accordance with ISO 14242-2:2000 which regulates two measuring methods: one gravimetric and the second using Coordinate Measuring Machines (CMMs).

Using the gravimetric method, which is the most common and standardized method to evaluate wear volume in hip joints specimen weight is measured before and after wear test and the difference of the two measurement values are calculated and represent the wear volume [4].

The second method of measuring regulated in the standard is the one which measures the prosthesis' volume using a coordinate measuring machine which must ensure that the maximum distance between two points in the horizontal plane or along any arc is no greater than 1 mm [5], based on the scanned points a surface is generated which is then used to determine the radius and the volume of the prosthesis.

Both methods are successfully used by researchers, measurements of the prostheses in parallel using these two methods have demonstrated no significant differences [6-8] between the results obtained with these two methods. Furthermore a number of researchers have begun to develop alternative methods of measuring wear such as PowerPoint method and laser scanning [9] or using computer tomography (CT) [10].

To estimate the wear of hip prostheses there are a number of theoretical developments [11-14] but also new equipment is designed for this kind of measurement such as Artificial Hip Profiler [15].

S. Vlad and R.V. Ciupa (eds.), *International Conference on Advancements of Medicine and Health Care through Technology*, IFMBE Proceedings 44,
DOI: 10.1007/978-3-319-07653-9_29, © Springer International Publishing Switzerland 2014

As shown in [2], the need for eliminating or reducing wear plays a crucial role in refining prosthesis composition and design. Thus the development of measurement procedures that provide not only information about the volume of material lost by the prosthesis but also the geometrical position of the wear print is important. Accuracy and reproducibility of measurement must be extremely high because the wear for these prostheses is about 2 –10 μm per year in case of metal-on-metal hip prosthesis [15, 16].

Besides studies that are done on simulators which determine the volume and geometry of the prosthesis before and after the wear tests there is a separate category of studies that try to determine the amount of wear of a prosthesis with no "pre-wear" data [8, 17-19]. These studies try to determine the wear on prostheses that were actually used on patients and to emphasize the wear mark on the prostheses that were removed from patients. In this way we can determine for each patient the way in which both the femoral head and the acetabulum cups wear as shown in [8, 10, 20].

II. State of the art in measuring hip joint with CMM

Modern manufacturing of resurfacing hip prostheses allows acetabulum and femoral components to be produced with an out of roundness of less than 5 μm [19]. Starting from this premise the researcher have developed and validated a number of methodologies for determining the diameter and initial surface of the femoral head.

In [17] authors propose to determine the initial surface of the prosthesis by acquiring points only in the unworn zones of the bearing surface. After scanning these areas Non-uniform Rational B-splines (NURBS) are used to fit a surface through the unworn zone surface data points. The resulting surface is assumed to be a pre-worn surface and will be used as a reference in determining the wear after scanning the entire prosthesis. In the same paper, the authors propose a second method which involves scanning an identical prosthesis (same batch) but not used for determining the initial shape of the prosthesis.

Other authors in [18] propose to determine the diameter and the center of the femoral head in two stages, the first stage based on seven points : four points tacked at 90° intervals around the full 360° of the equator in the X–Y plane and three points were taken in the Z–Y plane at 25° intervals, and then a sphere is generated (figure 1 left).

For the generated sphere the sphericity is calculated, if the value is less than the tolerance given by the manufacturer the value is considered correct and a provisional reference system is established in the center of the sphere. If the value of sphericity is higher the measurement is repeated in the same conditions only the sphere is rotated by 10° around the Z axis and the procedure is repeated until the value of sphericity reaches the tolerance range given by the standard ISO 7206-2:2011 – 10 μm.

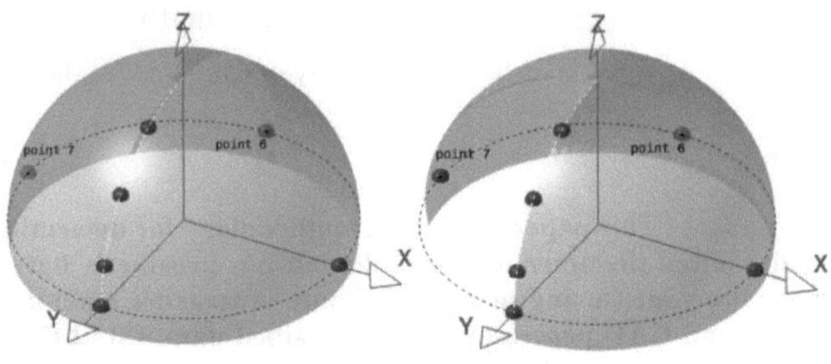

Fig. 1 Procedure for sphericity evaluation in case of 360 (left) and 300 ° (right) according to [18]

If the procedure is repeated 36 times and cannot determine a sphere that has its sphericity deviation in the tolerance range given by the manufacturer the authors propose repeating the procedure with the mention that the first four points will be taken equally distributed on a 300 ° portion of the sphere.

The second step of the methodology involves scanning of 100 points in the YZ plane moving from equator to equator for the femoral heads. Then the reference system is rotated by 22.5° along the Z axis and the procedure is repeated eight times so that finally it acquires a number of 800 points. It generates a second sphere that will represent the reference surface (the surface that is initially unworn) of the prosthesis in relation to which the wear of the prosthesis will then be determined.

To determine the definitive center of the sphere, 100 points were taken but limited to a 120◦ scan about the pole in the case of the acetabular cups (for reasons described above). The coordinate system was then rotated 22.5◦ about the z axis and the process repeated seven times, so that a total of 800 points were taken. Any points which were calculated to be greater than or less than 4 μm deviation from the initial spherical form, as determined from the initial seven points, were discarded as they were unlikely to represent the original surface and so could not be used. All other points were retained and used in the calculation of the second sphere. The center of the second sphere was then taken as the definitive origin.

In [8] the authors propose a visual inspection for identifying the worn area made by two independent observers, they use surface quality and white light for highlighting areas of the prosthesis that are worn. After marking the worn areas, the areas considered not worn are being scanned and the initial surface of the prosthesis is generated.

III. Methodology for estabilsh the un-worn surfcae of hip-joint using CMM in case of no pre-wear data

Scanning a hip join on the CMM can be done using a number of strategies, as shown in figure 2, all of which are used in the different studies: using meridian strategies (a) in [18, 21], using parallel strategies (b) in [8], equator strategies or combinations of these (c) in [17].

To determine the initial surface of a hip prosthesis the authors propose using the scanning method type equator, it scans the hip-joint in planes parallel to the equator (figure 2 c). Using this scanning strategy, the datasets that are obtained are in the form of concentric circles which later can be used to compute the roundness diagram and obtaining the extracted circumferential line as is settled in ISO 12181:1-2011and how is presented in figure 3.

This diagram can be automatically generated using the CMM's software and illustrates based on the Voronoi algorithm [21] the local roundness deviation (positive or negative). Using this diagram will remove in a software solution (CAD or calculus, ex. MSExcel, Mathlab, etc.) all the points that are not in the tolerance range given by the prosthesis' manufacturer or settled by ISO 7206-1:2008.

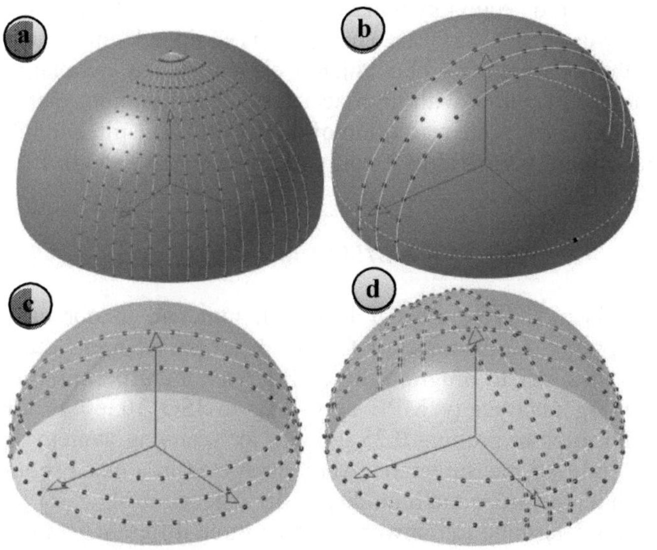

Fig. 2 Scanning strategies of a sphere applicable in case of the hip –joint: a - meridian strategy, b - parallel strategy, c - equator strategy, d - hybrid strategy

The nominal value of the circle associated with each scan of the prosthesis in the equatorial plane is determined by the intersection between a theoretical sphere with a radius equal to the prosthesis and a plane parallel to the XY plane of the reference system associated to the prosthesis.

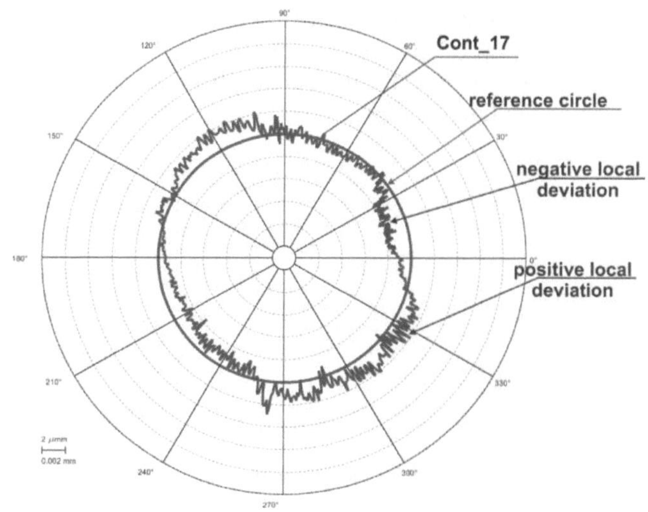

Fig. 3 Roundness diagram for a scan set of data points

The prosthesis is scanned from the plane of the equator toward the pole (figure 4) with a Z-step which should ensure that the space between any two points is no greater than 1 mm in the horizontal plane or along any arc as provided in [5].

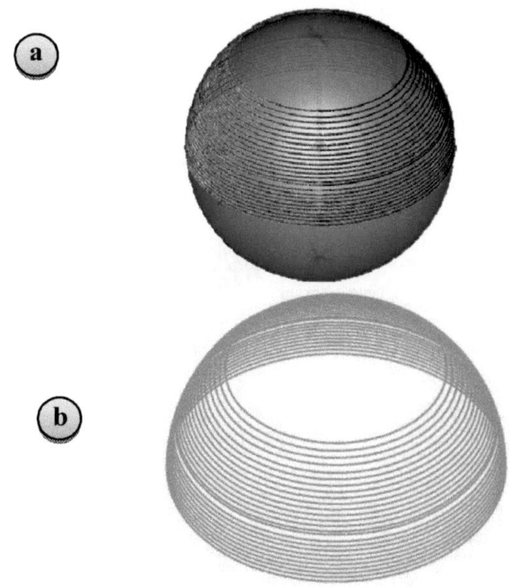

Fig. 4 Hip Joint scanning strategy (a) and the cloud point (b)

For each scanned circle the roundness diagram (figure 3) is built and the points that are not in the tolerance range that is imposed by the manufacturer or the standard are removed (figure 7).

Using this strategy the sphere cannot be scanned entirely, in the pole (top of the sphere) due to “slip” errors of the probe’s ruby sphere on the measured sphere’s surface as can be seen in the figure below.

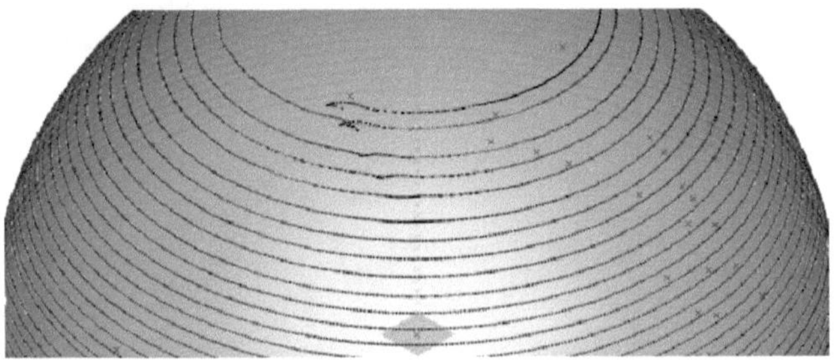

Fig. 5 Error when scanning the femoral head using equator strategy

This is not a drawback because as shown in [8, 18, 22, 23] the wear mark appears in the top of the hip joint (see figure 6). After obtaining the point cloud, it is converted directly into a 3D surface. For the obtained sphere its center is determined which will be used as a reference origin of the coordinate system associated with the 3D model which represents the unworn model of the prosthesis and will be used to scan and determine the wear of the prosthesis.

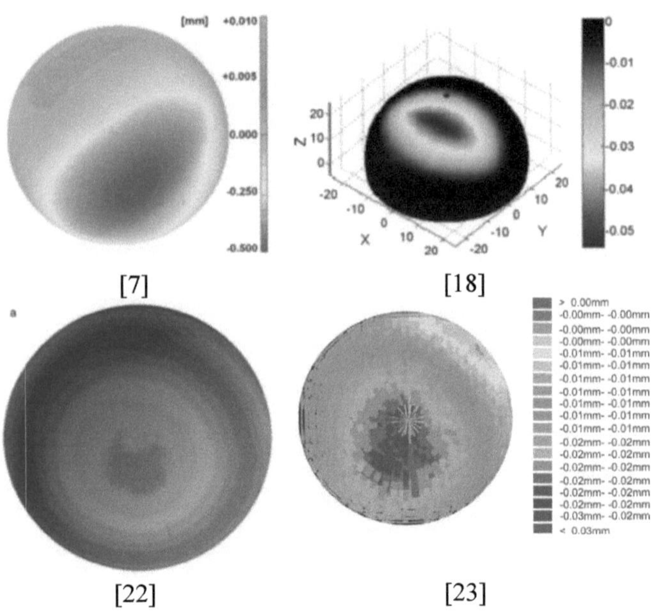

Fig. 6 Wear area on hip-joint according with different researcher

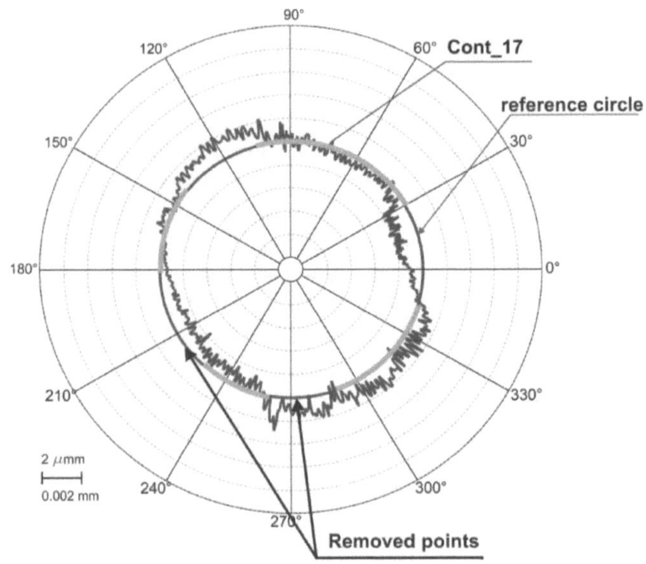

Fig. 7 Removed points which are not in the tolerance

IV. METHOD VALIDATION

In order to validate the method to determine the unworn surface in case of the femoral head, a multisensory CMM was used to accurately measure the geometry in the unworn and worn heads surfaces. The CMM is equipped with a state of the art scanning probe which is capable to acquire a large number of points with high accuracy. The minimum incremental linear scale resolution of the CMM is 0.1 μm and the maximum permissible error (MPE) according with ISO 10360:

$$E1: (1.8 + L/500)\mu m \qquad [1]$$

Where L is measuring length in mm and in our case represents the diameter of femoral head plus 2 mm necessary in order to program the CMM. Maximum permissible probing uncertainty MPE according to ISO 10360 is for point to point probing 0.75 μm and for scanning strategy is 1.9 μm. All measurements were conducted in a clean room with temperature and humidity under strict control.

To determine the unworn surface three different femoral heads have been measured (32, 47 and 50 mm – see figure 8). Before each measurement the CMM’s performances were checked using a calibrated sphere of a 50 mm diameter which was placed in the same device that was used to clamp the prostheses. The caliber was scanned with both the equator strategy to determine the surface that hasn’t been worn and the meridian strategy to determine the worn surface.

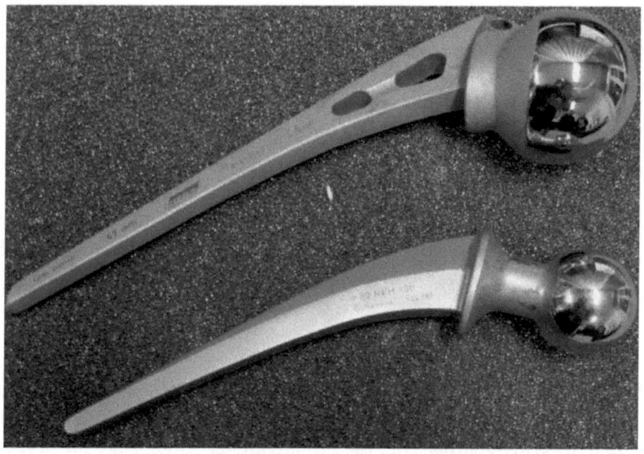

Fig. 8 Two of femoral head used in the study

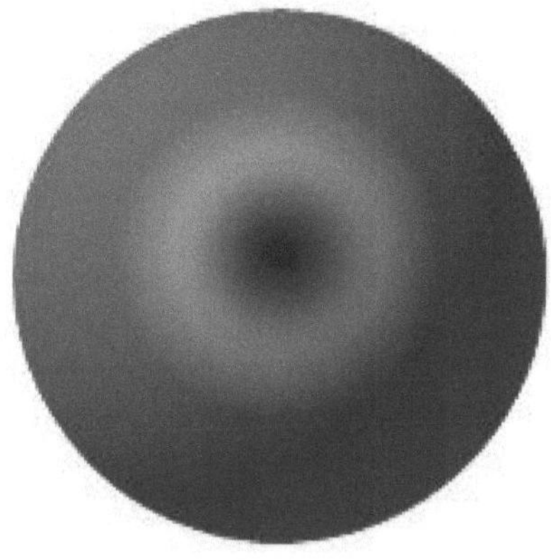

Fig. 9 Wear mark in case of the femoral head with 32mm diameter

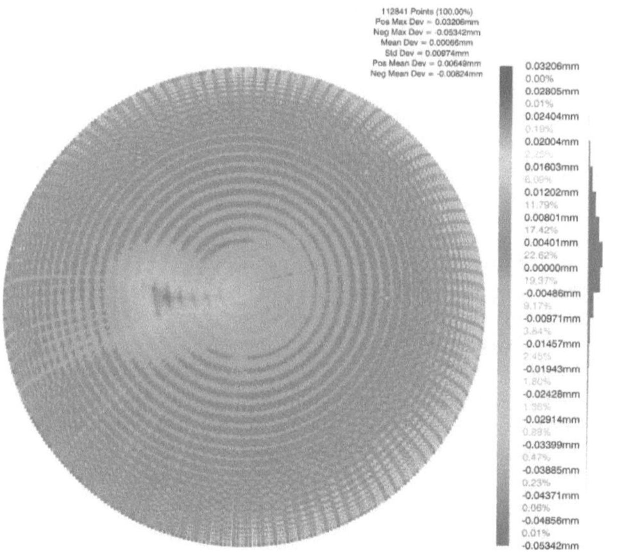

Fig. 10 Wear mark and deviation distribution for the 47 mm diameter femoral head

Both for the calibrated sphere and the femoral head the feed on the Z axis in case of the equator strategy was 0.5mm with a 0.1mm pitch between the scanned points on the circumference of the circle. In case of the scan using the meridian strategy the angular step was 1° and the distance between the points measured on the circle's cord was 0.1mm.

Each femoral head was scanned three times with both strategies, their position being rotated by 120° for each scan, the scan results are listed and can be seen in table 1 (number of points).

After scanning, the points' coordinates were exported for each circle separately and were processed in MS Excel in order to remove the points that were situated on a radius greater than the nominal value ± 5μm. After the elimination of the points from the wear area the rest of the points were imported in Catia V5 where the sphere which represents the surface without wear of the femoral head was generated.

The surface was generated directly base on the points, which helped remove the step of generating a 3D mesh that normally introduces a number of geometric approximations that influence the outcome.

Table 1 Scanning results

Diameter	32 mm	47 mm	50 mm
Strategy		Points	
Ecuator 1	32456	46825	49986
Ecuator 2	32382	46828	49978
Ecuator 3	32422	46796	49964
Meridian 1	723045	106065	112847
Meridian 2	72389	106084	112789
Meridian 3	72364	106112	112823

The second scan of the prostheses was performed to determine the real surface of the worn prostheses, the scanning method used was meridian which offers a high density of points in the area where a worn object appears at such prostheses. The difference between the two surfaces (not worn and worn) was emphasized by a color map as shown in figures 9 and 10.

V. Conclusions

The method used to determine the unworn surface for the femoral head presented in the paper is original and has not been addressed so far in literature. It determines the initial surface without wear of a prosthetic hip joint for which there is no information before it has been removed from the patient.

The method allows for an objective determination of the points which can be used to recreate the initial surface based on the roundness diagram. This is a documented mathematic instrument and it is implemented by the most important CMM manufacturers. Workload associated with this method is higher than in the methodologies presented in Chapter II, as the methodology for determining the diameter and shape of the initial surface is more laborious. The results obtained in case of the three femoral heads scanned are in accordance with the literature which confirms that the methodology is correct.

The use of this method requires mastery of the methodology for measuring and scanning with a CMM, spreadsheets and CAD processing specific to surface reconstruction and reverse engineering.

Conflict of Interest

The authors declare that they have no conflict of interest.

References

1. Silva, M., et al., (2002) Average patient walking activity approaches 2 million cycles per year: Pedometers under-record walking activity, The Journal of Arthroplasty, 17(6): p. 693-697.
2. Grillini, L. and S. Affatato, (2013) How to measure wear following total hip arthroplasty, Hip International, 23(3): p. 233-242.
3. Affatato, S. and D. Brando, (2012), Introduction to wear phenomena of orthopaedic implants, Woodhead Publ Ltd: Cambridge
4. Sagbas, B. and M.N. Durakbasa, (2012) Measurement of Wear in Orthopedic Prosthesis, Acta Physica Polonica A, 121(1): p. 131-134.
5. 14242-2, I., (2000) Implants for surgery - Wear of total hip joint prostheses - Part 2: Methods of measurement
6. Bills, P., et al., (2004) The use of CMM techniques to assess the functionality of total knee replacements, Measure and Quality Control in Production, 1860: p. 73-80.
7. Carmignato, S., et al., (2011) Uncertainty evaluation of volumetric wear assessment from coordinate measurements of ceramic hip joint prostheses, Wear, 270(9-10): p. 584-590.
8. Morris, B., et al., (2011) Quantifying the wear of acetabular cups using coordinate metrology, Wear, 271(7-8): p. 1086-1092.
9. Yun, H.H., et al., (2012) Reliability of a PowerPoint Method for Wear Measurement After Total Hip Arthroplasty A Retrieval Study Using 3-Dimensional Laser Scanning, Journal of Arthroplasty, 27(8): p. 1530-1537.
10. Jedenmalm, A., et al., (2011) Validation of a 3D CT method for measurement of linear wear of acetabular cups, Acta Orthopaedica, 82(1): p. 35-41.
11. Ilchmann, T., M. Reimold, and W. Muller-Schauenburg, (2008) Estimation of the wear volume after total hip replacement - A simple access to geometrical concepts, Medical Engineering & Physics, 30(3): p. 373-379.
12. Wu, J.S.-S., S.-L. Hsu, and J.-H. Chen, (2010) Wear patterns of, and wear volume formulae for, hemispherical acetabular cup liners, Wear, 268(3–4): p. 481-487.
13. Chuter, G.S.J., et al., (2007) Wear analysis of failed acetabular polyethylene - A Comparison of analytical methods, Journal of Bone and Joint Surgery-British Volume, 89B(2): p. 273-279.
14. Mattei, L., et al., (2012), Wear simulation of metal on metal hip replacements: an analytical approach, Amer Soc Mechanical Engineers: New York
15. Tuke, M., et al., (2010) 3D linear and volumetric wear measurement on artificial hip joints-Validation of a new methodology, Precision Engineering-Journal of the International Societies for Precision Engineering and Nanotechnology, 34(4): p. 777-783.
16. Okazaki, Y., Effect of head size on wear properties of metal-on-metal bearings of hip prostheses, and comparison with wear properties of metal-on-polyethylene bearings using hip simulator, Journal of the Mechanical Behavior of Biomedical Materials, .
17. Bills, P., L. Blunt, and X. Jiang, (2007) Development of a technique for accurately determining clinical wear in explanted total hip replacements, Wear, 263: p. 1133-1137.
18. Lord, J.K., et al., (2011) Volumetric wear assessment of failed metal-on-metal hip resurfacing prostheses, Wear, 272(1): p. 79-87.
19. Joyce, T.J., D.J. Langton, and A.V.F. Nargol, (2011) A study of the wear of explanted metal-on-metal resurfacing hip prostheses, Tribology International, 44(5): p. 517-522.
20. Geerdink, C.H., et al., (2008) The determination of linear and angular penetration of the femoral head into the acetabular component as an assessment of wear in total hip replacement - A comparison of four computer-assisted methods, Journal of Bone and Joint Surgery-British Volume, 90B(7): p. 839-846.
21. Kim, K., S. Lee, and H.B. Jung, (2000) Assessing Roundness Errors Using Discrete Voronoi Diagrams, The International Journal of Advanced Manufacturing Technology, 16(8): p. 559-563.
22. Bills, P.J., et al., (2012) Volumetric wear assessment of retrieved metal-on-metal hip prostheses and the impact of measurement uncertainty, Wear, 274: p. 212-219.
23. Blunt, L., et al., (2009) The role of tribology and metrology in the latest development of bio-materials, Wear, 266(3–4): p. 424-431.

Corresponding author:

Author: Neamtu Calin
Institute: Technical University of Cluj-Napoca
Street: Bd. Muncii 103-105
City: Cluj-Napoca
Country: Romania
Email: calin.neamtu@muri.utcluj.ro

Pars Plana Vitrectomy with the 25 + Vitrectomy System

S.D. Nicoară, A. Moroti, L. Sârbu, A. Popeangă, and C. Cristian

"Iuliu Haţieganu" University of Medicine and Pharmacy/Ophthalmology,
Faculty of Medicine, Cluj-Napoca, Romania

Abstract— **The 25+ vitrectomy system was developed with the aim to make vitrectomy a safer, simpler and faster procedure. In our Department, this innovative technique became available in 2011 and since then, we use it exclusively in our cases. The purpose of this paper is to present the outcomes of 25+vitrectomy in various ocular diseases. We conducted a retrospective study including all the 418 vitrectomies that we carried out for the past two years. We discuss the technical characteristics and results according to the clinical condition in which 25+ vitrectomy was performed, as follows: rhegmatogenous retinal detachments - 150 cases (35.88%), vitreous hemorrhages - 105 cases (25.11%), silicone oil extractions - 57 cases (13.63%), tractional retinal detachments- 40 cases (9.56%), epimacular membranes - 20 cases (4.78%), dislocated nucleus/lens/implant into the vitreous cavity - 12 cases (2.87%), intraocular foreign bodies - 15 cases (3.58%), macular holes - 10 cases (2.39%), endophthalmities - 6 cases (1.43%), intraocular inflammations - 3 cases (0.71%). We illustrate the advantages of the 25+ vitrectomy system with the most suggestive clinical conditions. The 25+ vitrectomy has been shown to be a safe and efficient procedure on our series.**

Keywords— **25+ vitrectomy, retinal detachment, vitreous hemorrhage, endophthalmitis, intraocular foreign body**

I. Introduction

Since Robert Machemer invented the modern pars plana vitrectomy in 1972, significant improvements were registered in this field [1]. For more than 30 years, 20G vitrectomy was the only one used for vitreo-retinal surgery.

At the beginning of 2004, the minimally invasive vitrectomy system (MIVS), including 23G and 25G vitrectomy, became available [1, 2]. The rationale for developing small gauge vitrectomy was to make this procedure safer, shorter and easier.

The transition from 20G to small gauge vitrectomy requires several modifications of the technical approach regarding incision making, intraoperative fluidics, use of the vitrector, illumination probes and the accessory instruments. The 25+ vitrector has an opening which is very close to the tip of the instrument. This technical feature, combined with the use of high cutting rates (5000 cpm), allow the surgeon to work very close to the retina, with a very low risk to injure it [1].

For the past two years, we have been using exclusively the 25+ system in our vitrectomy cases.

The aim of this study is to present the outcomes of 25+ vitrectomy in various ocular conditions. The description of our cases will be preceded by the concise exposure of the technical abilities associated with the 25+ vitrectomy system.

II. Technical features of the 25+ vitrectomy

A. Incision Making

The 25+ vitrectomy requires the use of small, sutureless incisions. In order to prevent the postoperative leakage, which is dangerous, as it leads to ocular hypotony and increased risk of infection, the incisions must be water-tight, once the surgery is concluded.

In order to achieve this goal, a trocar insertion system was designed, with a beveled and compact blade and a funnel-shaped, beveled tip trocar.

In the latest available models, the trocars are valved, preventing the exit of fluids when the instruments are removed from the eye. Thus, the risk of inadvertent retinal incarceration at the incision site is considerably diminished [1, 2, 3].

B. Fluid Movement during 25+ Vitrectomy

The most important parameter that determines the vitreous removal is the *transorifice pressure* (TOP) at the tip of the vitrector. A low TOP is associated with slow vitreous removal and long operative times and a high TOP leads to vitreo-retinal traction and risk of iatrogenic retinal breaks.

The efficiency of a vitrectomy system is given by the rate of vitreous removal, meaning the *flow*. This parameter depends on: the viscosity of the material to be removed, the infusion and aspiration pressures, probe geometry and the duty cycle of the vitrector. The latter factor represents the ratio between the length of time during which the vitrector is open and closed.

In order to make the system more efficient, there are several options: to increase the infusion and aspiration pressures and to modify the duty cycle of the vitrector such as the port is open for a longer time [1, 3].

S. Vlad and R.V. Ciupa (eds.), *International Conference on Advancements of Medicine and Health Care through Technology*,
IFMBE Proceedings 44,
DOI: 10.1007/978-3-319-07653-9_30, © Springer International Publishing Switzerland 2014

C. Endoillumination and Accesory Instruments

The decrease of illumination associated with small gauge probes was overcome by the development of xenon and halide metal sources that deliver brighter illumination [1, 2].

The high flexibility of the small gauge accessory instruments (forceps, scissors, picks) limits their torsion capability, which imposed the design of stiffer instruments.

The 25+ vitrectomy system limits the use of multifunction instruments, as they have higher diameters.

One major advantage is that the 25+ system eliminates the need for accessory instruments in many instances, given the technical abilities of the vitrector itself [1, 2].

D. The 25+ Vitrector

The vitrector (cutter) is the most important instrument during vitrectomy. In the 25+ system, the Ultravit High Speed Vitrectomy Probe is used, which has dual pneumatic drives. This means that with the help of pulsed air, the surgeon can regulate the bias of the duty cycle, independently from the cut rate.

One of the three modes can be selected, according to the moment of surgery: core, shave and 50/50.

For core vitrectomy, open bias cutter at 5000 cpm is used. In the proximity of the detached retina, the shave mode is selected, with a closed duty cycle.

The port-biased closed duty cycle with lower cut rate will induce lower flow rate. As the cut rate increases, the flow increases [1, 2, 3].

III. OUTCOMES OF THE 25+ VITRECTOMY SYSTEM

This study was carried out in accordance with the standards of the Ethical Committee of "Iuliu Haţieganu" University of Medicine and Pharmacy and with the Helsinki Declaration of 1975, as revised in 2000 and 2008.

A. General Description of Our Cases

We used 25+ vitrectomy system in 418 cases representing the following clinical conditions: rhegmatogenous retinal detachments, vitreous hemorrhages, tractional retinal detachments, epimacular membranes, macular holes, dislocated lenses, endophthalmities, intraocular foreign bodies, ocular inflammations and silicone oil removals from the eye.

The data of the 418 cases are summarized in table 1.

Table 1 Clinical conditions in which we used the 25+ vitrectomy system

Clinical condition	Number of cases	%
Rhegmatogenous Retinal Detachment	150	35.88
Vitreous hemorrhage	105	25.11
Tractional Retinal Detachment	40	9.56
Epimacular membrane	20	4.78
Macular hole	10	2.39
Dislocated lens	12	2.87
Endophthalmitis	6	1.43
Intraocular foreign body	15	3.58
Ocular inflammation	3	0.71
Silicone oil removal	57	13.63

B. The 25+ Vitrectomy in Rhegmatogenous Retinal Detachment

Rhegmatogenous Retinal Detachment (RRD) was the most common indication of 25+ vitrectomy on our series: 35.88%.

The major goal of a vitrectomy in a RRD is to be as complete as possible, in order to relieve all the vitreo-retinal tractions. This is difficult to achieve in an eye with a detached, mobile retina. The design of the 25+ cutter, with the opening located very close to its tip, allows the surgeon to work in the proximity of the retina, with a very low risk to injure it. The use of high cutting rates (5000 cpm) maintains the port open for a very short time/duty cycle, making the risk of inadvertent cut of the retina very low [4]. Figure 1 displays the 25+ vitrector with the tip very close to the retina, in an eye with retinal detachment.

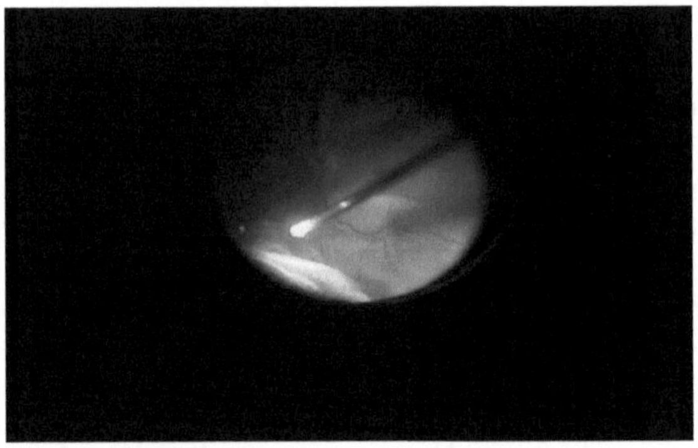

Fig. 1 25+ Vitrectomy in an eye with RRD

The complete vitrectomy in RRD is followed by the drainage of the subretinal fluid by exchange with air and by the treatment of the retinal break with endolaser (Fig. 2)

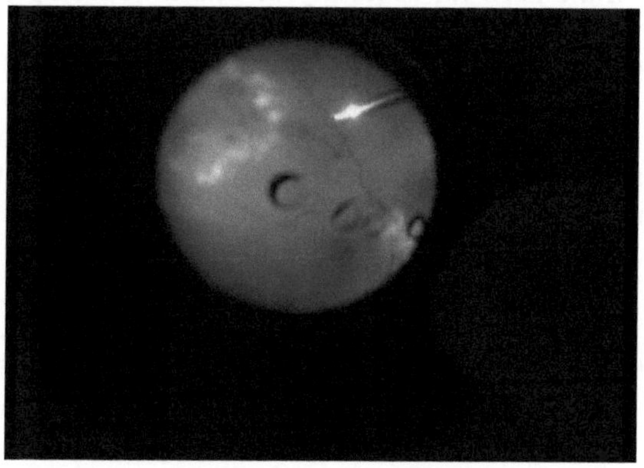

Fig. 2 Laser spots around the retinal break

After the fluid/air exchange is completed and the retina attached, the break is treated by the application of endolaser spots around it, as shown in Fig. 2.

C. The 25+ Vitrectomy in Removing the Epimacular Membranes

In order to remove a membrane from the surface of the macula, a special forceps must be used. The initial inconvenience came from the fact that the small gauge instruments were very flexible and therefore, engineers had to design stiffer forceps, able to perform torsion movements during surgery [5, 6]. Fig. 3 reveals the removal of a thick membrane, visible as a white, opaque tissue, from the surface of the macula.

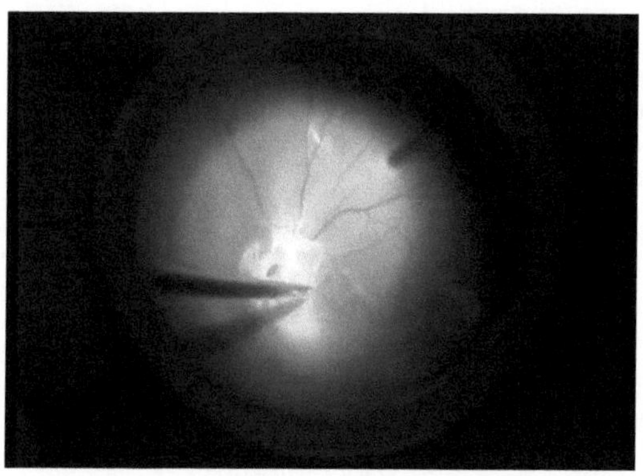

Fig. 3 Removal of an epimacular membrane

D. The 25+ Vitrectomy in Removing the Dislocated Lens

If the dislocated lens is not hard, it can be removed with the 25+ vitrector, using high aspiration and low cutting rates, such as the port of the vitrector remains open longer.

If the nucleus is too hard, a hybrid approach is used: after completing the vitrectomy, one incision is enlarged to 20G, in order to give access to the fragmatome which uses ultrasounds to break the nucleus [7]. For the moment, the fragmatome is available only in the 20G setting.

Of the 12 dislocated lenses, we managed to remove the lens with the vitreotome in 7 cases, as the lens was soft (Fig. 4). In the remaining 5 cases, we had to use the fragmatome, because the hardness of the lens did not allow its removal with the vitreotome.

E. The 25+ Vitrectomy in Removing the Intraocular Foreign Bodies

All the intraocular foreign bodies (IOFBs) on our series (15 cases) were removed by a hybrid approach, either with the intraocular magnet (12 cases - 80%), or with the forceps (3 cases - 20%).

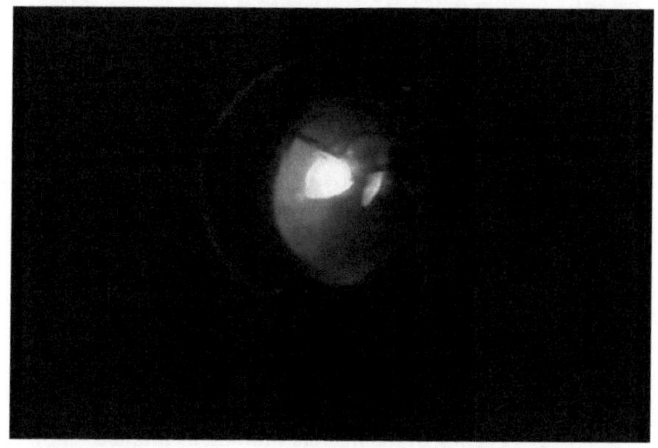

Fig. 4 Removal of the lens from the vitreous cavity with the vitreotome

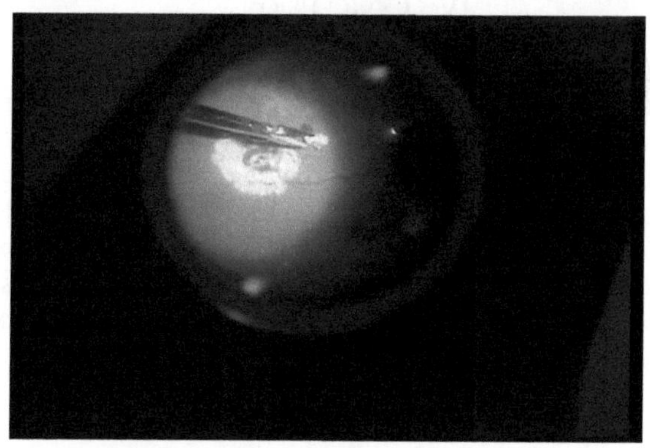

Fig. 5 Removal of an IOFB with the forceps

Fig. 5 shows the removal of an IOFB with the intraocular forceps, after having treated the retinal lesion at the impact site of the foreign body, by laser photocoagulation.

In every case, the IOFB removal was preceded by the dissection of all the adherences between the vitreous /retina and the IOFB. If this maneuver is not performed, during IOFB removal, significant traction is exerted on the retina, with a very high risk of iatrogenic retinal break and subsequent retinal detachment [1].

F. The 25+ Vitrectomy in the Treatment of Macular Hole

The goal of surgery for macular hole is to remove the posterior hyaloid and peel the internal limiting membrane, in order to induce its closure. With this technique, anatomic success rates of 85 - 95% were reported [6].

We treated with 25+ vitrectomy, 10 macular holes, with the anatomic closure of 9 of them.

The peeling of the internal limiting membrane of the retina is illustrated in Fig. 6. This technique is performed with a special 25G forceps, after having colored the membrane with indocyanine green, in order to enhance its visibility.

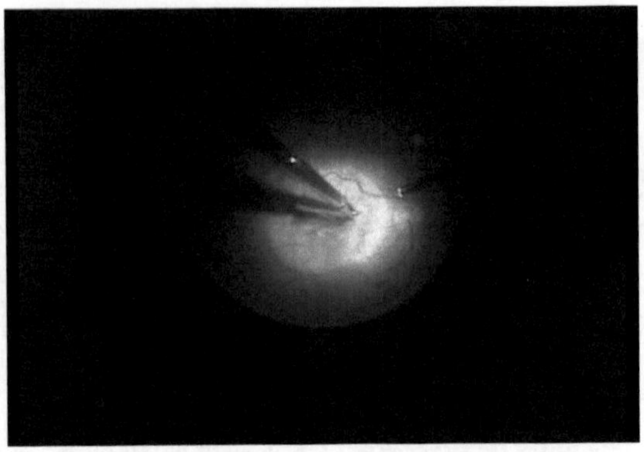

Fig. 6 Peeling of the internal limiting membrane

IV. Conclusion

The 25+ Vitrectomy System proved to be efficient and safe on our case series. Currently, this is the only system that we use for vitreo-retinal surgery.

The most significant impact the 25+ system is revealed in the cases of rhegmatogenous retinal detachment. The location of the port at the tip of the vitrector, combined with the possibility to use high cutting rates (5000 cpm) allows the surgeon to work in the proximity of the detached, mobile retina, with little risk of creating iatrogenic retinal breaks.

When the fibrous tissue needs to be removed from the surface of the retina (tractional retinal detachments, epimacular membranes), the technical abilities of the 25+ cutter diminish the need for accessory instruments: forceps, scissors, picks.

Overall, the use of the 25+ system on our case series, was associated with less invasiveness, fast recovery, high efficiency, short operating times. The future is open for research in developing smaller gauge vitrectomy systems, with higher cutting rates.

Conflict of Interest

The authors declare that they have no conflict of interest.

References

1. Nicoara SD (2013) Innovative Technologies in Pars Plana Vitrectomy - Minimally Invasive Vitrectomy System. IJLSMR 3:129–138
2. Thompson JT (2011) Advantages and limitations of small gauge vitrectomy. Survey of Ophthalmology 56: 162-172
3. Magalhaes O Jr, Chong L, De Boer C, et al (2008) Vitreous dynamics: vitreous flow analysis in 20-, 23-, and 25-gauge cutters. Retina 28: 236-241
4. Ţălu SD, Rus S, Tămăşoi I, and Dragoş C (2011) Innovative Technologies in Vitreo-Retinal Surgery for Rhegmatogenous Retinal Detachment. IFMBE Proceedings, 36: 13-18
5. Yang SJ, YoonSY, Kim JG et al (2009) Transconjunctival suturelsss vitrectomy for the treatment of vitreoretinal complications in patients with diabetes mellitus. Ophthalmic Surg Lasers Imaging 40: 461-4666
6. Patelli F, Radice P, Zumbo G, et al. (2007) 25-gauge macular surgery: results and complications. Retina 27: 750-754
7. Parkes C, Nagpal M, Little B, Prasad S (2011) Drop and stop: the dropping and the dropped nucleus. Retina Today 1:76-80

Author: Simona Delia Nicoară
Institute: "Iuliu Haţieganu" University of Medicine and Pharmacy
Street: V. Babeş
City: Cluj-Napoca
Country: Romania
Email: simonanicoara1@gmail.com

Using Laser Scanning to Measure the Difference between Classical Individual Custom Trays and 3D Ideal Individual Custom Trays in the Totally Edentulous

D. Buhățel[1], Z. Buna[2], R.S. Campian[1], A. Ilea[1], M. Moga[1], V. Țărmure[3], and C. Neamțu[2]

[1] University of Medicine and Pharmacy "Iuliu Hatieganu",
Department of Oral Rehabilitation, Cluj-Napoca, Romania
[2] Technical University of Cluj-Napoca, Department of Design Engineering and Robotics, Romania
[3] University of Medicine and Pharmacy "Iuliu Hatieganu", Department of Maxillofacial Surgery and Radiology,
Cluj-Napoca, Romania

Abstract— **This paper presents a methodology for measuring using laser scanning the differences between ideal individual custom trays and classical individual custom trays obtained in the dental laboratory in the case of treatment steps to achieve total prostheses. The resulted 3D models from the scans can be used to: verify the accuracy of operations performed by the dental technician to create the ideal individual custom trays obtained directly from dental records, in dental prosthesis and for digital dental records storage. In this case study scanning equipment for high precision industrial metrology and engineering CAD software solutions were used to process the scans results.**

Keywords— **custom tray, totally edentulous, 3D scanning, engineering CAD software**

I. Introduction

Full edentation is perhaps the most mutilating pathological state of the stomatognat system, as it perturbs all the latter's functions, bearing consequences on the entire body. In order to speak about success in the prosthetic restoring of the totally edentulous patient, we must start from the thorough knowledge of the prosthetic field, of its respective components, as well as its morphology. The success in achieving individual spoons, covering completely the totally edentulous prosthetic field and which not cause discomfort to formations on the outskirts of the prosthetic field, undoubtedly means that the start of the treatment was favorable [1]. Just making a single proper spoon, we proceed to the final impression stage, solving adhesion problems of future prostheses. Most authors pay attention to imprinting stage [2], [3], [4]. Any imprinting techniques used and any progress we would have made in imprinting materials, whether individual spoon is not made properly, this imprinting stage becomes, at best, one laborious. Using laser scanning in the field of dentistry was addressed to compare digital dental impressions with the classical ones [5], used to evaluate, by indirect methods, the accuracy of computer-designed surgical guides in the oral implant supported rehabilitation of partially or completely edentulous patients [6], for study 3-dimensional changes in the palatine rugae [7]. 3D modeling and engineering CAD software solutions have been successfully used to solve problems such as reliability analysis and the stability of the implant–abutment and implant bone interface with the help of Finite Element Analysis (FEA) [8], study the stresses distribution in dental prosthesis under different loading cases [9], do develop a CAD/CAM framework for the accurate planning of dental implant surgeries based on the integration of Computed Tomography (CT) and surface optical scanning [10] and also the engineering CAD solution is used for digital reconstructions [11], or, in a larger sense, for aiding in the development of advanced medical devices [12], [13].

Various optical scanning systems and software tools have been devised in the field of dentistry and orthodontics for building digital models of single teeth, dental arches, crowns, bridge preparations, full dental casts [14]. In most cases, industrial scanners are used as references in the study of performances (accuracy and reliability) of dental scanners [15].

II. Objectives

The objective of this study is to develop an interdisciplinary methodology of digitization and evaluation of dental trays in order to determine the precision of the execution of the classical version of the individual custom trays.

Development of a work methodology that allows obtaining 3D ideal individual custom trays obtained directly based on digital dental records.

III. Material and Methods

A. The Study Material

A number of 52 patients were diagnosed with full bimaxillary edentation have been included in the study. Each patient had an observation chart drawn out, and they subsequently filled out/signed an informed consent towards the performing of a medical act and a consent for entering in study. The patients have been examined clinically and were then printed

DOI: 10.1007/978-3-319-07653-9_31,

after the classical technique, using standard custom trays of various sizes depending on the size of the prosthetic fields; alginate was used as printing material. On the preliminary prints, we have traced the limits of the prosthetic field by means of a marker, after the known technique (see Figure 1).

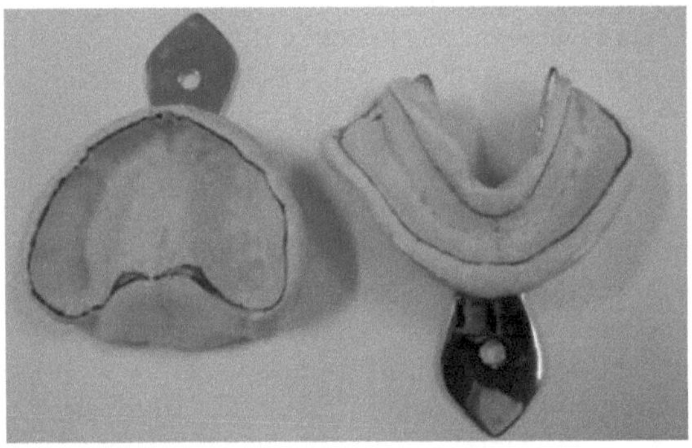

Fig. 1 Dental impressions of a pacient

The authors used the methodology shown in Figure 2 to evaluate the precision of the classical individual custom trays.

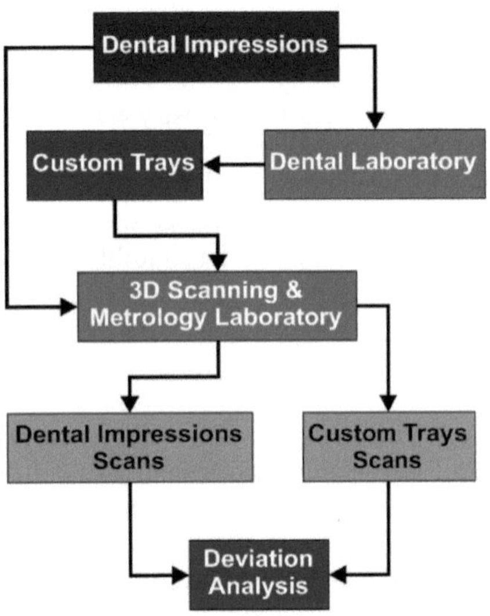

Fig. 2 The methodology

The prints were numbered accordingly to each person who has entered the study and were scanned with a laser scanner which belongs to the Department of Design Engineering and Robotics of the Faculty of Machine Constructions within the Technical University of Cluj-Napoca in order to obtain virtual 3D models, and later 3D ideal individual custom trays.

After scanning, the same prints were cast on the spot in order to obtain preliminary models. Subsequently, classical individual custom trays were thus made. These individual custom trays obtained classically were scanned. Then, the two 3D models, representing the ideal custom tray, and, respectively, the classical custom tray, were compared, in order to visualize the "minuses" shown up in the classical realization in the dental technique laboratory of the custom trays.

B. Digitization and Evaluation of Dental Trays

The most important operation of the methodology proposed by the authors is the digitization of dental trays, the steps that have been completed are:

- Establishment of the position and the holding position of dental trays during the digitization operation;
- Establishment of the reference system;
- Digitization of the dental impressions and the custom trays;
- Point clouds and mesh processing;
- Deviation analysis of the obtained meshes.

After harvesting the dental impressions, these were scanned with a mobile 3D scanner, VIUScan, which has an accuracy of 50 μm.

Before scanning is very important the positioning of the parts that will be digitized, because these cannot be moved after the scanning process is started and it is very important that they be fully scanned in the important areas. Using the scanner and the related software, VX Elements, the dental trays are digitized. In Figure 3 a digitized dental tray can be seen in VX Elements.

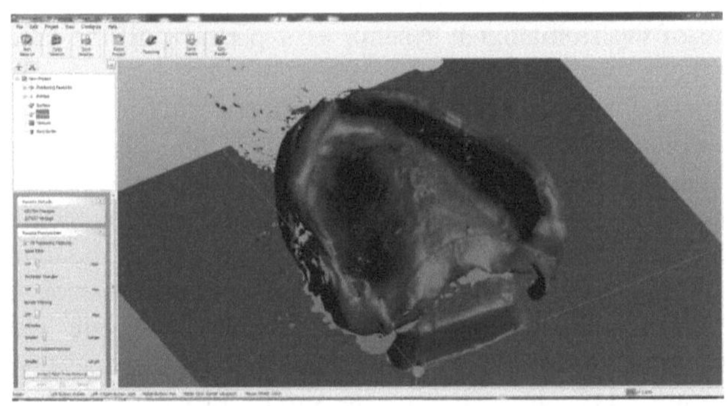

Fig. 3 Scanned dental tray in VX Elements software

After this step a technician creates the classical individual custom tray, which will be scanned with the same method. Using CATIA V5 software both scans are processed and compared with each other within the deviation analysis tool. With the help of the deviation analysis (Figure 4) which is a method used to highlight and measure the differences between two seemingly identical surfaces (the reference surface and the surface which is analyzed) will determine the difference between the 3D ideal individual custom tray and the classical individual custom tray. The differences between the two surfaces are shown as a color map as can be seen in Figure 4. Every gradation of the color map represents a deviation value measured in millimeters.

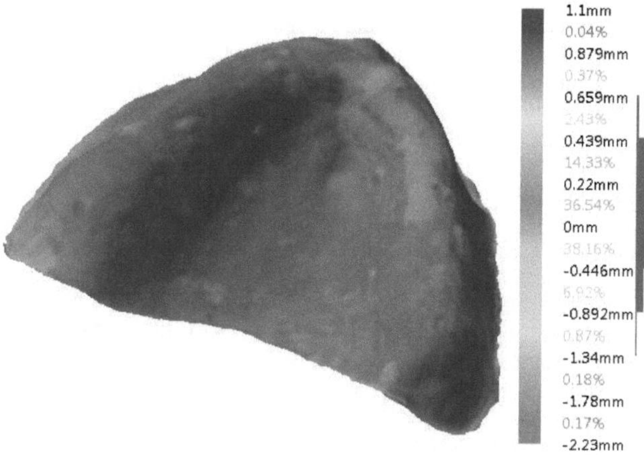

Fig. 4 Deviation analysis

C. Future Work

For a more accurate classical individual custom tray the authors recommend the creation of these trays using rapid prototyping. In the process can be used the scans from the dental impressions to generate the 3D model of an individual custom tray. In order to create the 3D model some steps have to be completed sown in Figure 5.

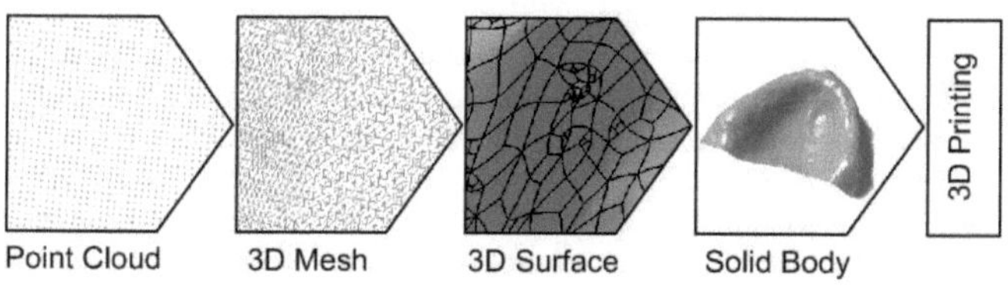

Fig. 5 Methodology to create 3D models from scanning for 3D printing

The 3D printed pieces can be verified for precision using the methodology described above.

IV. Results

In the study group was observed a number of 37 cases that showed a total toothless old crowding between 0 and 2 years. The number of cases in the study surprised toothless old 3-5 years or over 5 years is substantially equal, 7 and 8 subjects. Of the 26 male patients examined, 19 of them showed edentulous with a length between 0 and 2 years. To women, of 26 cases examined, 18 were edentulous with a length in the same range.

Table 1 Edentulous duration distribution in the target group.

Edentulous	Distribution	Years
Total distribution	72%	0-2 years
Total distribution	13%	3-5 years
Total distribution	15%	>5 years
Distribution at men	73%	0-2 years
Distribution at men	15%	3-5 years
Distribution at men	12%	>5 years
Distribution at women	69%	0-2 years
Distribution at women	12%	3-5 years
Distribution at women	19%	>5 years

A few results of the deviation analysis are shown in Table 2, where are shown values as: positive maximum deviation (Pos Max Dev), negative maximum deviation (Neg Max Dev), mean deviation (Mean Dev), standard deviation (Std Dev), positive mean deviation (Pos Mean Dev) and negative mean deviation (Neg Mean Dev).

Table 2 Results of the deviation analysis

Patients	Pos Max Dev [mm]	Neg Max Dev [mm]	Mean Dev [mm]	Std Dev [mm]	Pos Mean Dev [mm]	Neg Mean Dev [mm]
1	0.957	-1.36	0.00448	0.251	0.173	-0.207
2	2.95	-4.06	-0.0619	0.52	0.226	-0.343
3	1.35	-2.32	-0.0523	0.278	0.094	-0.238
4	2.13	-243	-0.00673	0.342	0.186	-0.234
5	1.1	-2.23	-0.021	0.297	0.178	-0.252
6	3.79	-7.27	0.204	0.901	0.0996	-0.468
7	2.11	-3.51	-0.109	0.452	0.167	-0.338
8	2.75	-4.25	-0.305	0.693	0.169	-0.533
9	1.35	-3.72	-0.0976	0.605	0.362	-0.511
10	6.12	-6.09	-0.107	0.79	0.166	-0.354
11	9.99	-8.14	-0.45	1.45	0.383	-0.977
12	2.43	-2.55	-0.048	0.286	0.115	-0.189

The data analysis reveals a removal trend of material from the classical individual custom trays compared to the 3D ideal individual custom trays. After analyzing the results obtained comparing the pairs of custom trays, the authors were not able to identify areas prone to changing geometry during the operation of making these individual classical custom trays.

In the set of custom trays analyzed the average positive mean deviation is about 0.2 mm and the negative is about 0.3 mm, overall the standard deviation for each custom tray indicates an average of 0.5 mm. It can be concluded that the precision of the execution of classical individual custom trays is around ±0.3 mm.

V. CONCLUSIONS

The analysis of the mucous-bone support offers a good perspective of the prognosis for each particular case. Through the results obtained, the analysis of the mucous-bone support constitutes a useful didactic material in order to emphasize the great variability of the prosthetic fields examined. Comparing the scans of the two custom trays, classical and 3D, respectively, shows the imperative necessity of creating ideal custom trays. The creation of the ideal 3D custom trays offers the premises of a final printing of great accuracy.

Based on the data analysis was determined the precision of the execution of the classical individual custom trays, which in the case of the dental technician who made these models is ±0.3 mm. Errors on the individual classical custom trays are completely random and systematic errors have not been identified. The only conclusion that can help the dental technician's activity is that there is a tendency to remove material from the classical individual custom trays in comparison with the initial model obtained after printing the patient.

The methodology presented allows the obtaining of 3D models for 3D ideal individual custom trays which can then be used to obtain some 3D printed individual custom trays on high performance rapid prototyping equipment to ensure an accuracy of around ±0.1 mm.

The obtained 3D models can be used in virtual prosthetic or for digital storing of the dental impressions.

ACKNOWLEDGMENT

In the study were included patients who took part in the "Sanodentaprim Program", a program which promotes Oral Health by increasing the disadvantaged population's access to stomatological services as part of the partnership between University of Medicine and Pharmacy "Iuliu Haţieganu" and the Cluj-Napoca Town Hall. The target group refers to institutionalized persons (old person's homes, children's homes, etc), retired people, unemployed people, and young people under the age of 26 who do not have any income. From this target group of over 1400 patients, registered with the Faculty of Oral Rehabilitation, Oral Health, and the Management of the Dental Office, during April 2010 - February 2012, we have selected patients with bimaxillary full edentation.

CONFLICT OF INTEREST

The authors declare that they have no conflict of interest.

REFERENCES

1. Păuna M., Preoteasa E. Aspecte practice în protezarea edentaţiei totale. Editura Cermaprint Bucuresti, 2002; pp 75-80, pp 113-167
2. Păuna M, Ionescu A. Corectitudinea închiderii palatinale posterioare în protezarea totală superioară. Arta Stomatologică. 1996; 2:10-11.
3. Câmpian RS. Proteze şi aparate chirurgicale oromaxilofaciale. Editura Medicală Universitară "Iuliu Haţieganu", Cluj-Napoca, 2007; pp 62-68.
4. Bratu D, Forna NC, Păuna M. Date de anatomie clinică şi fiziologie orală la edentatul total. In:Bratu D, Forna NC, Lascu L, Păuna M, Popşor S. Protetica dentară. Proteza parţială mobilizabilă. Proteza totală. Bucureşti: Editura Enciclopedică; 2011. pp 379-462.
5. Ender, A. and A. Mehl (2013). "Accuracy of complete-Arch dental impressions: A new method of measuring trueness and precision." Journal of Prosthetic Dentistry Volume: 109 Issue:(2) Pages: 121-128 ISSN: 00223913 (ISSN).
6. Giordano, M., P. Ausiello and M. Martorelli (2012). "Accuracy evaluation of surgical guides in implant dentistry by non-contact reverse engineering techniques." Dental Materials Volume: 28 Issue: (9) Pages: e178-e185 ISSN: 01095641 (ISSN).
7. Kim, H. K., S. C. Moon, S. J. Lee and Y. S. Park (2012). "Three-dimensional biometric study of palatine rugae in children with a mixed-model analysis: A 9-year longitudinal study." American Journal of Orthodontics and Dentofacial Orthopedics Volume: 141 Issue: (5) Pages: 590-597 ISSN: 0889-5406.
8. Kayabaşı, O., E. Yüzbasıoğlu and F. Erzincanlı (2006). "Static, dynamic and fatigue behaviors of dental implant using finite element method." Advances in Engineering Software Volume: 37 Issue: (10) Pages: 649-658 ISSN: 0965-9978.
9. Merdji, A., B. Bachir Bouiadjra, T. Achour, B. Serier, B. Ould Chikh and Z. O. Feng (2010). "Stress analysis in dental prosthesis." Computational Materials Science Volume: 49 Issue: (1) Pages: 126-133 ISSN: 0927-0256.
10. Paoli, A. and A. V. Razionale (2012). A CAD-based methodology for dental implant surgery, Milan.9781467325653 (ISBN).
11. Soltaninejad, M. R., R. A. Zoroofi and G. Shirani (2012). Automatic crown surface reconstruction using tooth statistical model for dental prosthesis planning, Tehran.9781467331302 (ISBN).
12. Pisla, D., Plitea, N., Vaida, C., Hesselbach, J., Raatz, A., Vlad, L., Graur, F., Gyurka, B., Gherman, B., Suciu, M. "PARAMIS parallel robot for laparoscopic surgery." Chirurgia Volume: 105 Issue: (5) Pages: 677-683 ISSN: 1221-9118.
13. Pisla, D., Gherman, B., Vaida, C., Suciu, M., Plitea, N. "An Active Hybrid Parallel Robot for Minimally Invasive Surgery." Robotics and Computer-Integrated Manufacturing Volume: 29 Issue: (4) Pages: 203-221 ISSN: 0736-5845.
14. Brusco, N., M. Andreetto, L. Lucchese, S. Carmignato and G. M. Cortelazzo (2007). "Metrological validation for 3D modeling of dental plaster casts." Medical Engineering and Physics Volume: 29 Issue: (9) Pages: 954-966 ISSN: 13504533 (ISSN).
15. Hayashi, K., A. U. C. Sachdeva, S. Saitoh, S. P. Lee, T. Kubota and I. Mizoguchi (2013). "Assessment of the accuracy and reliability of new 3-dimensional scanning devices." American Journal of Orthodontics and Dentofacial Orthopedics Volume: 144 Issue: (4) Pages: 619-625 ISSN: 08895406 (ISSN).

Corresponding Author: Calin Neamtu
Institute: Technical University of Cluj-Napoca
Address: Muncii Avenue, No. 103-105, Cluj-Napoca, Romania
Email: calin.neamtu@muri.utcluj.ro

Micro-tweezers Based on V-Beam Thermal Actuator

R.S. Chiorean[1], M.C. Dudescu[1], M. Pustan[2], and M. Hardau[1]

[1] Technical University of Cluj-Napoca, Department of Mechanical Engineering, Bdul.Muncii, nr.103-105, 400641, Cluj-Napoca, Romania
[2] Technical University of Cluj-Napoca, Department of Mechanical System Engineering, Bdul.Muncii, nr.103-105, 400641, Cluj-Napoca, Romania

Abstract— **This paper presents some modeling aspects regarding an application of the V-beam thermal actuator in micro-manipulation. The influence of the Micro-tweezers' geometrical parameters on the output gripping force is analyzed in order to provide the basis on the future design of some task oriented structures. Numerical simulations are performed on the complete V-beam thermal actuator – Micro-tweezers assembly in order to evaluate the proposed model. The results provided by the two approaches on this problem proved to be in good agreement. As referred to in the paper, the V-beam thermal actuator's behavior as a separate entity has been previously investigated by both numerical and experimental methods.**

Keywords— **Micro-tweezers, V-beam thermal actuator, gripping force**

I. Introduction

The development of micro-fabrication technologies has led to both the means and the need to manipulate small scale objects. Some of the fields that benefit from and are further enhanced by the advances in micro-manipulation techniques are micro-assembly, micro-robotics, biological (including medical), microelectronics, etc. Some of the solutions viable for general purpose manipulation tasks have some drawbacks in regard to medical applications. Electrostatic and piezoelectric based grippers [1,2] have voltage requirements that exceed 100V, making them unsafe for handling biological samples. Shape-memory-alloy based grippers [3] have limited opening compared to their size, as well as efficiency problems (21.1% efficiency for the gripper presented in the referred paper).

Electro-thermal actuation has the benefit of producing relatively large forces and/or displacements, but it has low operating frequencies because of the time needed to reach thermal equilibrium [4]. The two basic structures capable of performing angular (the bimorph thermal actuator) and linear (V-beam thermal actuator) motion as a consequence of the thermal expansion phenomenon presented in [4] can be implemented as actuators in the structure of micro-tweezers as shown in [5].

II. Analitical Model of the V-Beam Thermally Actuated Micro-Tweezers

Figure 1 shows a schematic geometrical representation of a Micro-tweezers – V-beam thermal actuator assembly. This is used to derive the analytical model and thus revealing the influence of its geometrical parameters on the output gripping force. The initial position of the assembly is represented in solid line, while the dashed line shows the assembly in the deformed state.

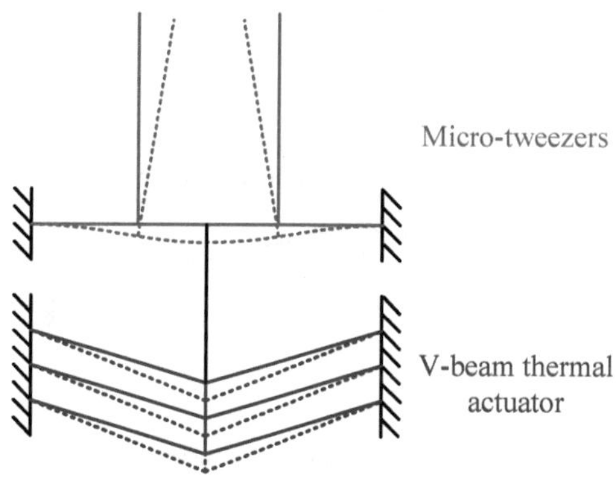

Fig. 1 Schematic representation of a V-beam thermally actuated Micro-tweezers

This problem can be divided into two separate easier problems: A. the determination of the V-beam thermal actuator's force and B. the determination of the Micro-tweezers' gripping force when a known force is applied to the middle of the beam span.

A. Output Force of the V-Beam Thermal Actuator

The geometrical parameters of the V-beam presented in Figure 2 are defined as follows: l – length of the beam; w- width of the beam; t – thickness of the beam; θ – beam inclination angle; d – distance between two consecutive beams.

S. Vlad and R.V. Ciupa (eds.), *International Conference on Advancements of Medicine and Health Care through Technology*, IFMBE Proceedings 44,
DOI: 10.1007/978-3-319-07653-9_32,

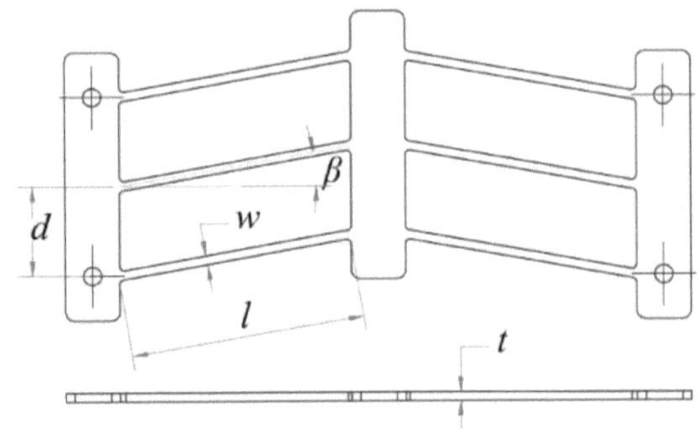

Fig. 2 Geometrical parameters of the V-beam thermal actuator

The problem of actuation force determination can be solved using the superposition principle, namely by considering two distinct situations: the free expansion of the structure under thermal load (see Figure 4) and the deformation of the structure without thermal load but under the presence of an external force that has the same position and direction as the actuation force (see Figure 6). The actuation force can then be determined by imposing the restriction that both the situations described above should generate equal deformations.

The simplified model used to obtain the analytical solution is presented in Figure 3.

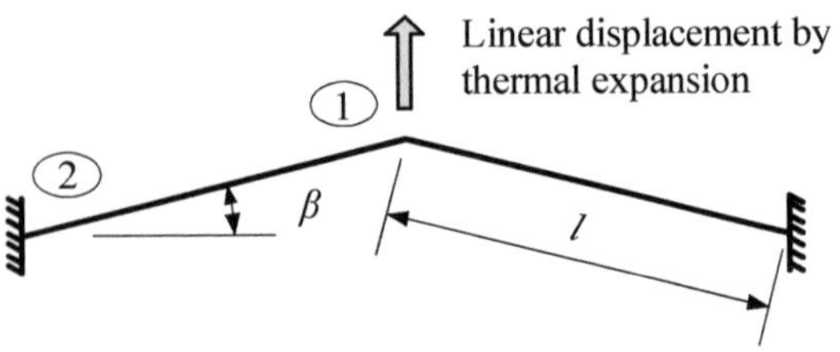

Fig. 3 Theoretical model with boundary conditions

Taking into account the geometrical and loading symmetry, the problem can be solved for a single beam, as shown in Figure 4.

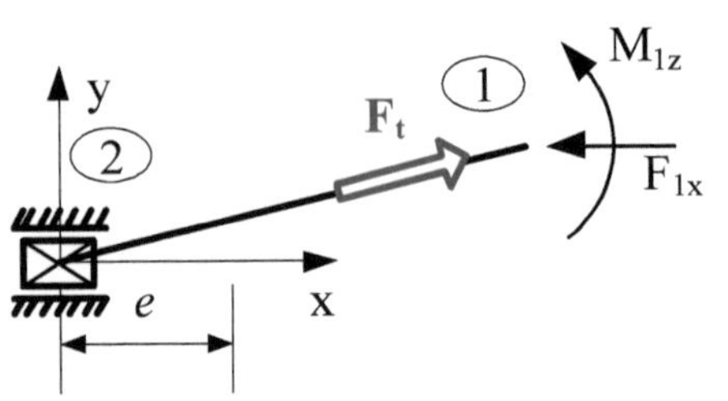

Fig. 4 Half model with thermal load

Equation 1 defines the output deflection of the actuator (the displacement of point 1 along the y-axis) under thermal load and without external forces:

$$u_{1y}^{Fig.4} = \alpha \Delta T l \sin(\beta) + \frac{\sin(\beta)\cos(\beta)(Al^2 - 12I_z)(e + \alpha \Delta T l \cos(\beta))}{12I_z \cos^2 \beta + Al^2 \sin^2 \beta} \quad (1)$$

in which the terms that weren't previously defined are: α – coefficient of thermal expansion of the sensor's material; ΔT – temperature difference between the initial and final deformed states of the sensor; A – cross-section area of the beam; I_z – moment of inertia of the cross-section of the beam; e – imposed displacement along the x-axis. The imposed displacement can include substrate deformation due to the reaction forces in the anchors, thermal expansion of the substrate or even thermal expansion of the central shaft of the actuator along the x-axis.

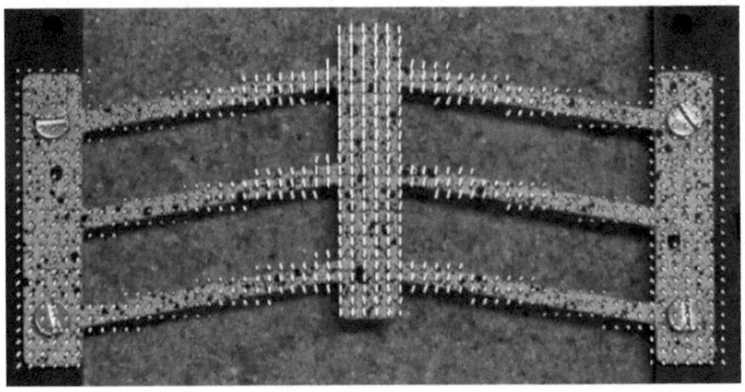

Fig. 5 Full field displacement of the V-beam thermal sensor extracted using VEDDAC 6.0 Digital Image Correlation software

Figure 5 shows the experimental deflection determination by the means of Digital Image Correlation software performed on several macro-scale samples of the V-beam thermal actuator. Further details on the experimental set-up, the geometrical types tested and the numerical simulations that led to the validation of Equation 1 are presented in [6].

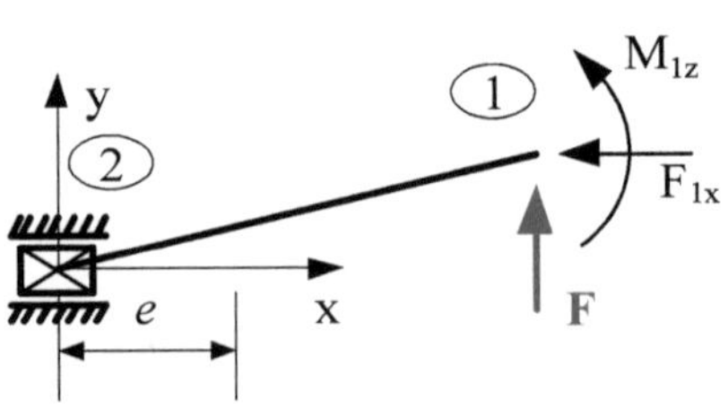

Fig. 6 Half model with external force but without thermal load

The relationship between the external force and the deflection of the structure (shown in Figure 6) is given by the equation below:

$$u_{1y}^{Fig.6} = \frac{Fl^3}{E(12I_z \cos^2 \beta + Al^2 \sin^2 \beta)} \tag{2}$$

in which E represents the elastic (Young's) modulus of the actuator's material.

The output force can be extracted from Equation 2:

$$F = \frac{u_{1y} E(12I_z \cos^2 \beta + Al^2 \sin^2 \beta)}{l^3} \tag{3}$$

The u_{1y} deflection required by Equation 3 in order to determine the output force of one beam is no other than the deflection expressed by Equation 1. The actuation force of the entire V-beam thermal actuator is determined by multiplying the force from Equation 3 by the number of beams. Further details on the geometrical types and the numerical simulations that led to the validation of Equation 3 are presented in [7].

B. The Micro-Tweezers' Gripping Force

The Micro-tweezers' gripping force determination is a symmetrical problem as well, thus allowing for a solution based on the half model of the structure.

The geometry and the boundary conditions for the half model are depicted in Figure 7.

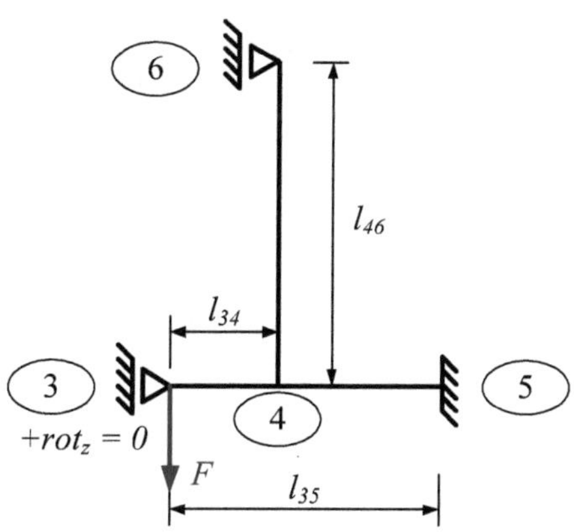

Fig. 7 Geometrical parameters and boundary conditions of the half model schematic representation of the Micro-tweezers

In order to determine the gripping force of the actuator, the supports are replaced with their corresponding reaction forces, as shown in Figure 8.

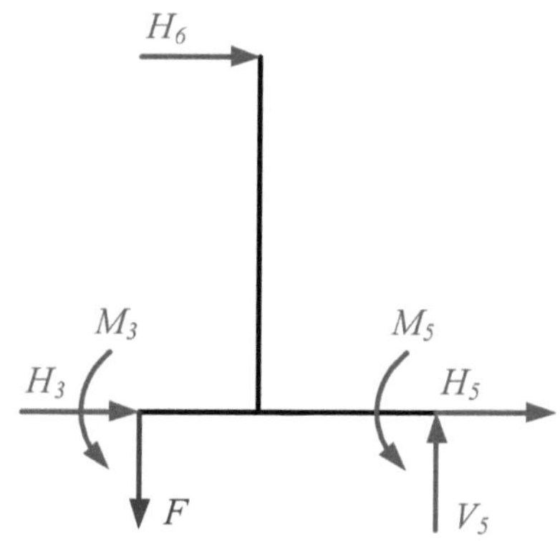

Fig. 8 Half model force equilibrium

The problem has 6 unknowns (the 6 reaction forces and couples shown in Figure 8), making the structure 3 times statically indeterminate. One of these unknowns (H_6) is the gripping force of the Micro-tweezers. Based on Newton's laws of motion, 3 static equilibrium equations can be written for a planar structure. Castigliano's 2nd theorem states that the partial derivative of the strain energy (U_d) with respect to the generalized force Q_i gives the generalized displacement q_i in the direction of Q_i. Taking into account the degrees of freedom that are canceled out by the supports 3 and 6, the relationships presented in Equation 5 can be written in order to make the problem solvable.

$$u_3 = \frac{\partial U_d}{\partial H_3} = 0; \quad \varphi_3 = \frac{\partial U_d}{\partial M_3} = 0; \quad u_6 = \frac{\partial U_d}{\partial H_6} = 0 \tag{5}$$

The resulting gripping force is defined by the relationship given in Equation 6:

$$H_6 = -F \frac{3l_{34}^2 l_{35} l_{46} - 9l_{34} l_{35}^3 + 18l_{34}^2 l_{35}^2}{-36l_{34}^2 l_{35} l_{46} + 18l_{34}^3 l_{46} + 18l_{34} l_{35}^2 l_{46}} \cdots$$
$$\cdots \frac{-3l_{34} l_{35}^2 l_{46} - 9l_{34}^3 l_{35}}{+6l_{35}^2 l_{46}^2 - 6l_{34}^2 l_{46}^2 + 2l_{35} l_{46}^3} \tag{6}$$

in which l_{ij} are the geometrical parameters of the Micro-tweezers defined in Figure 7.

The complete V-beam thermal actuator – Micro-tweezers assembly has been modeled, constrained and loaded. The deflection along the vertical axis, resulted by performing Finite Element Analysis (FEA) using the Static Structural module of ANSYS v12, is presented in Figure 9. The wireframe depicts the undeformed structure.

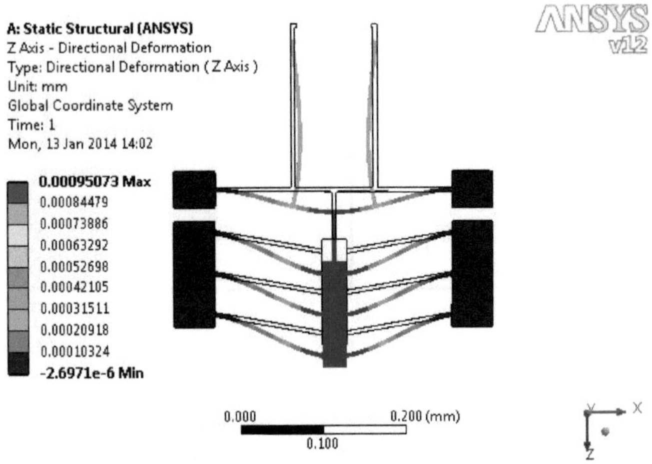

Fig. 9 The displacement along the vertical axis obtained from the ANSYS v12 FEA software

The gripping force is determined by inserting a Reaction Force probe connected to the support that replaces the manipulated object, as shown in Figure 10, and multiplying it by 2, due to the symmetrically opposite support.

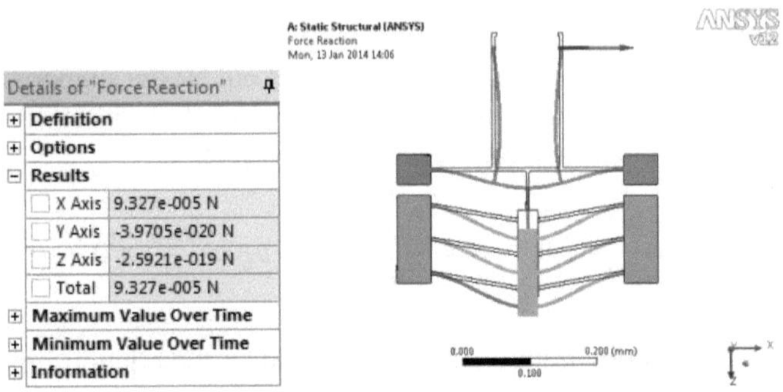

Fig. 10 The output gripping force of the V-beam thermal actuator – Micro-tweezers assembly

III. Results and conclusions

In order to compare the two models, an aluminum sample defined by the following parameters was tested using both the analytical model and the FEA simulation: w=5μm; t=3μm; l=130μm; θ=10°; α=2.3·10^{-5}μm; E=71GPa; l_{34}=50μm; l_{35}=143μm; l_{46}=200μm and ΔT=58°C. The analytical deflection is 953nm while the simulated value is 951nm. As far as the gripping force in concerned, the analytical value is 17.34·10^{-5} N, while the simulated value is 2·(9.33·10^{-5}) = 18.66·10^{-5}N (a 7.6% relative error). The analytical and the simulation results are in good agreement, thus leading to the validation of the proposed model.

The gripping force can be lower or higher than the actuation force by varying the geometrical parameters of the Micro-tweezers. A decrease in force is beneficial for higher precision while an increase in force makes the Micro-tweezers viable for a wider range of manipulation tasks.

Conflict of Interest

The authors declare that they have no conflict of interest.

Acknowledgements

This work was supported by the Reliability design of RF-MEMS switches for space applications (REDEMS) research project founded by the Romanian Space Agency's STAR Program.

References

1. Sujatha L, Vigneswaran N, Mohamed Yacin S (2013) Design and Analysis of Electrostatic Micro Tweezers with Optimized Hinges for Biological Applications Using CoventorWare, Procedia Engineering Volume 64, International Conference on Design and Manufacturing (IConDM2013), ISSN 1877-7058, pp 283-291
2. Bong-Seok Kim, Joon-Shik Park, Byoung Hun Kang, Chanwoo Moon (2012) Fabrication and property analysis of a MEMS micro-gripper for robotic micro-manipulation, Robotics and Computer-Integrated Manufacturing, Volume 28, Issue 1, ISSN 0736-5845, pp 50-56
3. Zhong ZW, Yeong CK (2006) Development of a gripper using SMA wire, Sensors and Actuators A: Physical, Volume 126, Issue 2, ISSN 0924-4247, pp 375-381
4. Lobontiu N, Garcia E (2005) Mechanics of Microelectromechanical Systems, Chapter 4.2.Thermal Transduction, Springer US, ISBN 978-1-4020-8013-5, doi:10.1007/b100026
5. Luo JK, Flewitt AJ, Spearing SM, Fleck NA, Milne WI (2005) Comparison of microtweezers based on three lateral thermal actuator configurations, Journal of Micromechanics and Microengineering, Volume 15, pp. 1294-1302, doi:10.1088/0960-1317/15/6/022
6. Chiorean RS, Dudescu MC, Pustan M, Hardau M (*in press*) Deflection determination of V-beam thermal sensors using Digital Image Correlation, Key Engineering Materials, Trans Tech Publications
7. Chiorean RS, Dudescu MC, Pustan M, Hardau M (*in press*) Analytical and numerical study on the maximum force developed by a V-beam thermal actuator, Procedia Technology, Elsevier

Author: PhD.-stud. Radu Stefan CHIOREAN
Institute: Technical University of Cluj-Napoca
Street: Bdul.Muncii, nr.103-105, 400641
City: Cluj-Napoca
Country: Romania
Email: *Radu.Chiorean@rezi.utcluj.ro*

Recording of Biomedical Parameters during Magnetotherapy

R. Ciorap[1], D. Andrițoi[1,2], C. Corciovă[1], and V. David[2]

[1] "Gr.T.Popa" University of Medicine and Pharmacy, Iaşi, Romania
[2] "Gh. Asachi" Technical University, Iasi, Romania

Abstract— **In this paper we presents some results of our studies regarding the modifications of biomedical parameters during magnetotherapy. We recorded and analyzed the ECG and EEG signals for patients who follow a regular session of magnetotherapy. The aim of this study was to observe the electrical activity of the heart and brain during pulse magnetotherapy taking into account that this procedure is frequently used for a lot of diseases. We analyzed the EEG and ECG signals recorded in frequency domain and various measures of HR dynamics, such as time-domain, spectral, and non-linear measures of HR variability.**

Keywords— **biomedical measurements, ECG, EEG, magnetotherapy, signal processing, Heart Rate Variability (HRV)**

I. INTRODUCTION

Magnetotherapy is one of the most commonly used physiotherapy procedures. This therapy is based on application of a static magnetic field, an alternating magnetic field of a frequency of 50 Hz usually derived from sinusoidal mains voltage or using a pulse magnetic field characterized by fast changes of field and the intensity [1]. In nowadays, when the chronic disease affects individuals in their peak mid life years disrupting the future of the families dependant on them, magnetotherapy is used for treatment of spread area of diseases like cardiovascular, neuropschiatric or rheumatic. Monitoring of phisiological parameter during therapy for optimisation of treatment is one of the major problems of the health care system [2].

Many studies have been made regarding the effects of extremely low frequency (ELF) electromagnetic field on human biological systems [3]. The extremely low frequency (ELF) refers to the range of electromagnetic field frequencies less than 100 Hz [3] or, according other opinion below 300 Hz [4]. Baldi et al. [5] study on the influence of pulsed electromagnetic field exposure on heart rate variability revealed a variation in all cases. Sastre et al. [6] analyze the influence of earth magnetic field on EEG signal.

The aim of this study is to observe the brain electrical activity and the heart electrical activity during pulse magnetotherapy.

Our department has established a research effort in the biomedical engineering area, with a focus on Medical Devices, Measurement and Instrumentation.[1,2,7,8,9,10]

II. SIGNAL RECORDING PROCEDURE

In study were involved 13 subjects (9 female and 4 male) with age between 22 and 40 years. For selected procedure it was used only the cylindrical coil with a diameter of 60 cm placed in lumbar region. The design of this applicator was adapted for creating a linear magnetic field as large as possible part of the applicator. For each subject we use two kind of pulse magnetic field using sinusoidal pulses.

The EEG and ECG signals were recorded using Data Acquisition device BIOPAC Inc., which consisted of MP150 system with EEG100 (Electroencephalogram amplifier) and ECG100 (Electrocardiogram amplifier). The electrodes were placed on the scalp in the occipital region (O1-Cz and O2-Cz leads) and D2 chest lead as shown in figure 1.

As magneto therapy device we used BTL-4000 a well-known medical device with proven effects on pain, anti-inflammatory control and acceleration of healing. BTL-4000 have recommended applications for different medical fields. For selected procedure it was used only the cylindrical coil with a diameter of 60 cm placed in lumbar region.

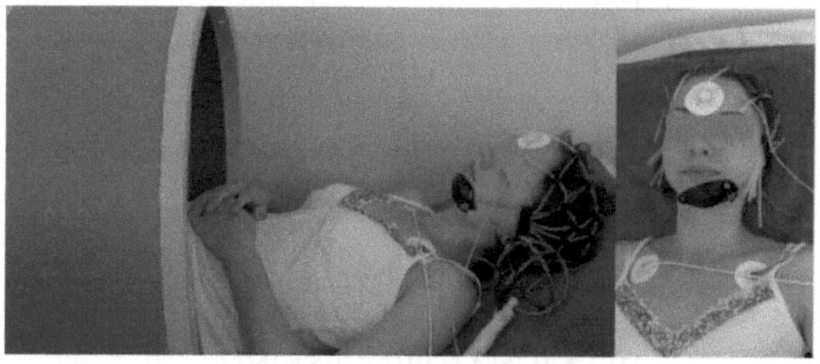

Fig.1 Subject during magneto therapy session

All signals were recorded for 300 seconds. First 60 second was recorded without magnetic field, the next 180 seconds of recording was made in the presence of magnetic field and the last 60 seconds after the magnetic field exposure.

The basic task of ECG processing is R-peaks detection. There are some difficulties one can encounter in processing ECG: irregular distance between peaks, irregular peak form, presence of low-frequency component in ECG due to patient breathing etc. To solve the task the processing pipeline should contain particular stages to reduce influence of those factors. In order to filter the ECG signals, they were

S. Vlad and R.V. Ciupa (eds.), *International Conference on Advancements of Medicine and Health Care through Technology*, IFMBE Proceedings 44,
DOI: 10.1007/978-3-319-07653-9_33, © Springer International Publishing Switzerland 2014

used some IIR filters and also wavelet denoise method. Figure 2 illustrated a samples of ECG signal recorded. After these signal processing, we determined QRS complex and RR intervals from recorded ECG signals.

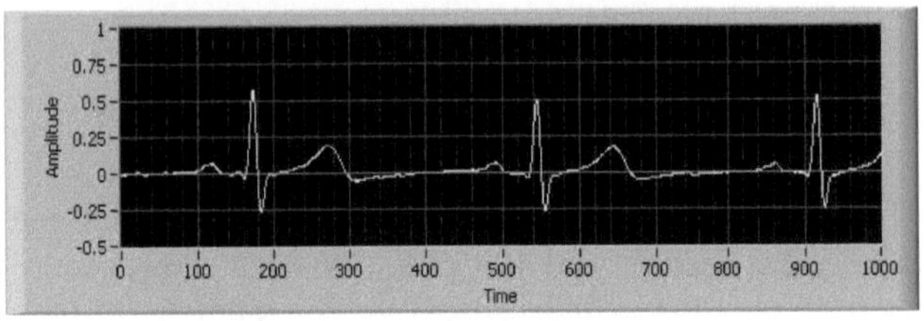

Fig.2 Samples of ECG signals recorded

The EEG recorded from O1-Cz and O2-Cz leads is presented in figure 3.

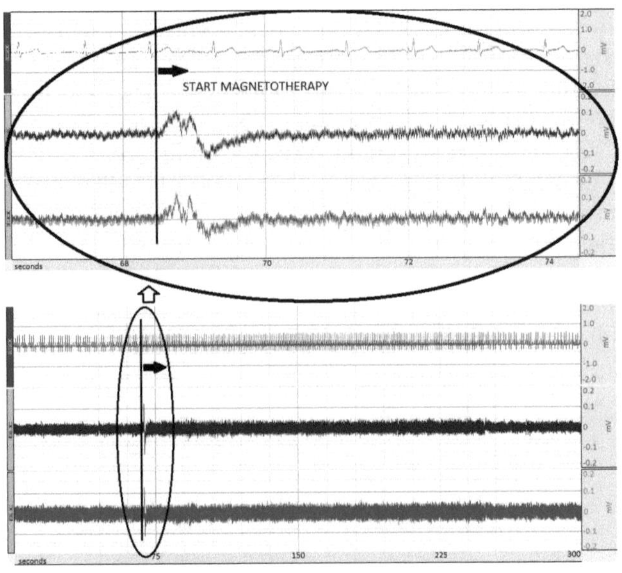

Fig.3 Samples of ECG signals recorded

III. SIGNAL PROCESSING

The detection of the R-peaks and consequently of the QRS complexes in an ECG signal provides information about the heart rate, the conduction velocity, the condition of tissues within the heart as well as various abnormalities. For this reason, it has drawn considerable attention in the ECG signal processing. However, the presence of noise and time-varying morphology makes the detection difficult. Thus, ECG signal is processed and analyzed in order to calculate the heart rate. In order to describe oscillation in consecutive cardiac cycles, other terms have been used in the literature, for example cycle length variability, heart period variability, RR variability and RR interval tachogram, as shown in figure 4, and they more appropriately emphasize the fact that it is the interval between consecutive beats that is being analyzed rather than the heart rate per sec.

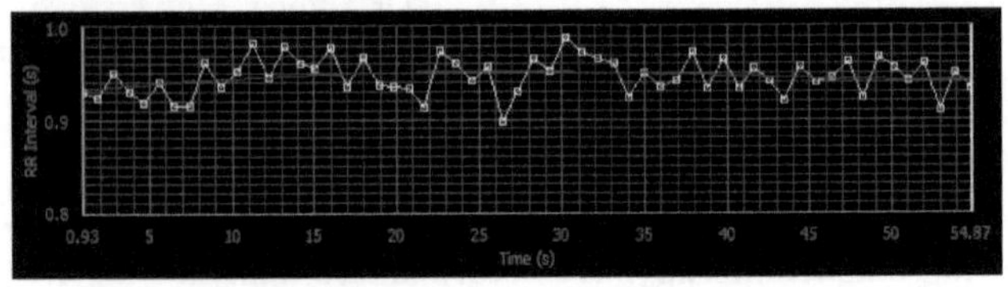

Fig.4 R-R interval variation over 1 minute

The predictive value of heart rate variability alone is modest, but combination with other techniques substantially improves its positive predictive accuracy over a clinically important range of sensitivity (25% to 75%) for cardiac mortality and arrhythmic events.

The most commonly used measures derived from interval differences include *RMSSD,* the square root of the mean squared differences of successive NN intervals, *NN50,* the number of interval differences of successive NN intervals greater than 50 ms, and *pNNSO* the proportion derived by dividing NN50 by the total number of NN intervals. All these measurements of short-term variation estimate high frequency variations in heart rate and thus are highly correlated. Figure 5 illustrated a sample of analysis of R-R interval variation from the statistical point of view.

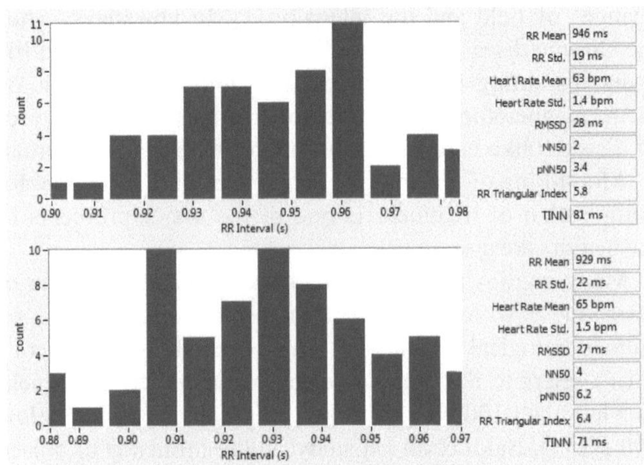

Fig.5 Statistic analysis of R-R interval variation over 1 minute

Three main spectral components are distinguished in a spectrum calculated from short term recordings of 2 to 5 min: very low frequency (VLF), low frequency (LF), and high frequency (HF) components. The distribution of the power and the central frequency of LF and HF are not fixed but may vary in relation to changes in autonomic modulations of the heart period.

Measurement of VLF, LF and HF power components is usually made in absolute values of power (ms2), but LF and HF may also be measured in normalized units (n.u.) which represent the relative value of each power component in proportion to the total power minus the VLF component. The representation of LF and HF emphasizes the controlled and balanced behavior of the two branches of the autonomic nervous system. Moreover, normalization tends to minimize the effect on the values of LF and HF components of the changes in total power as shown in figure 6.

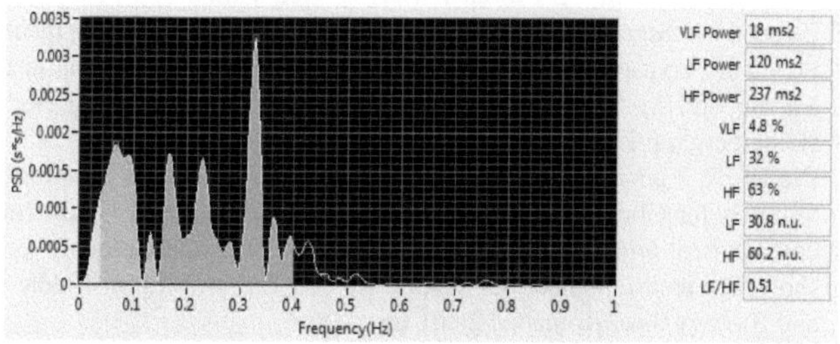

Fig.6 VLF, LF, MF, LF and HF representation of one minute recording

LF and HF can increase under different conditions.

We manage to observe an increased LF and VLF (expressed in normalized units) during magneto therapy session and several minute after. (Table.1)

Table 1 Main spectral components representation

	1 min.	2 min.	3 min.	4 min.	5 min.
VLF Peak (Hz)	0.00	0.00	0.00	0.00	0.00
LF Peak (Hz)	0.13	0.04	0.09	0.09	0.05
HF Peak (Hz)	0.22	0.39	0.38	0.36	0.36
VLF Power (ms^2)	7.53	21.04	864681.28	876442.74	855913.06
LF Power (ms^2)	184.68	68.08	481.64	584.09	737.75
HF Power (ms^2)	91.88	115.44	121.81	179.12	191.91

These changes may indicate a shift of sympatho-vagal balance towards sympathetic predominance and reduced vagal tone. Similar conclusions were obtained by considering the changes in the LF/HF ratio.

For the experiment we set the frequency band of EEG amplifier between 0 to 100 Hz. The EEG recorded signals were first processed using high pass filter (0.1 Hz) for rejecting the DC component and after that using notch filter for 50 Hz. After that the signals were analyzed for calculate FFT and PSD.

After the denoising the signals we perform a EEG frequency analysis using band pass filter for delta (0.5-4 Hz), theta (4-8 Hz), alpha (8-13 Hz) and beta (13-30 Hz) rhythms. We also calculate for all recordings the PSD in three situations: before, during and after magnetotherapy. A sample of the results during magnetotherapy with type 1 pulses (sinusoidal shape 10ms pulse, 10 ms pause) is showed in figure 7

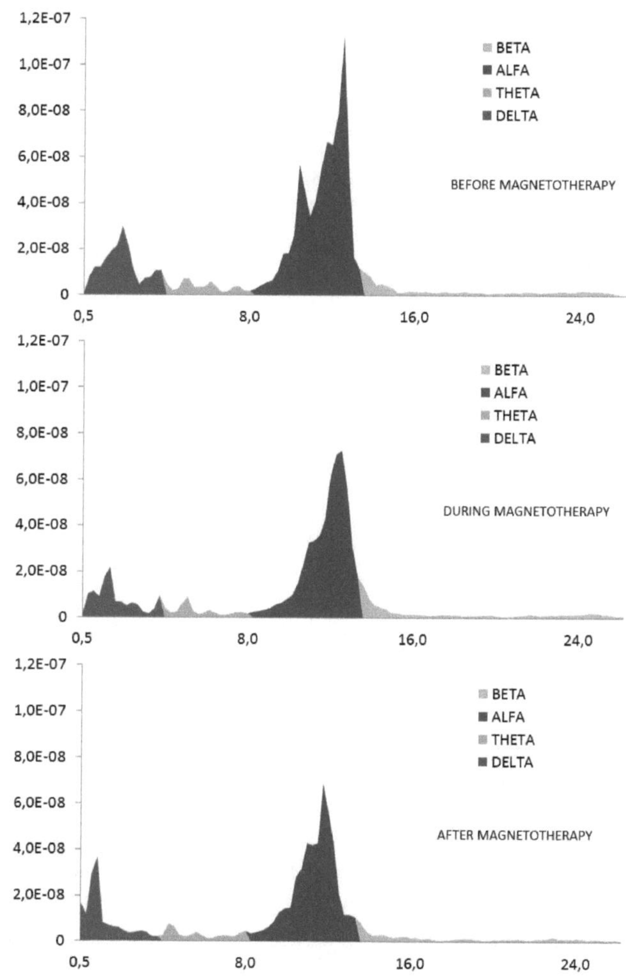

Fig.7 Sample of PSD for O1-Cz with type 1 pulses

We estimated the total power for each EEG wave calculating the area of PSD waveform in establishes frequency domains (delta 0.5-4 Hz, theta 4-8 Hz, alpha 8-13 Hz and beta 13-30 Hz). The results for delta and alpha wave are presented in table II and IV. The statistical analyses for these data are synthetized in table 2 and 3.

Table 2 Total power of delta wave

Record	A_δ before magnetotherapy	A_δ with magneto-therapy	A_δ after magneto-therapy
1	1.76E-08	1.47E-08	3.18E-08
2	2.78E-08	1.74E-08	1.97E-08
3	1.30E-08	1.68E-08	1.88E-08
4	1.31E-08	4.35E-08	1.89E-08
5	1.27E-08	1.70E-08	2.14E-08
6	1.28E-08	4.37E-08	1.93E-08
7	7.19E-10	6.05E-10	6.51E-10
8	1.75E-10	2.34E-09	6.76E-10
9	1.61E-10	1.19E-10	1.39E-10
10	4.48E-10	5.02E-10	7.81E-10
11	1.33E-09	6.56E-10	1.42E-09
12	6.64E-09	6.67E-09	7.39E-09
13	1.30E-08	9.46E-09	1.22E-08

Table 3 Total power of alpha wave

Record	A_α before magnetotherapy	A_α with magneto-therapy	A_α after magneto-therapy
1	1.45E-07	1.1600E-07	1.0200E-07
2	1.46E-07	1.12E-07	9.51E-08
3	6.12E-08	6.34E-08	8.31E-08
4	5.69E-08	6.41E-08	8.50E-08
5	6.11E-08	6.34E-08	7.61E-08
6	5.96E-08	6.37E-08	6.81E-08
7	9.08E-09	7.74E-10	5.46E-10
8	1.94E-09	1.76E-09	1.54E-09
9	2.77E-09	2.84E-09	1.94E-09
10	5.83E-09	4.95E-09	3.07E-09
11	9.64E-09	7.42E-09	4.34E-09
12	9.38E-09	1.50E-08	1.44E-08
13	1.28E-08	1.77E-08	1.49E-08

IV. Conclusions

In this study was recorded and analyzed EEG signals for 13 subjects before, during amd after a session of magnetotherapy. EEG signals was decomposed in four rhythms that cover 0 to 30 Hz domain. It was analyzed the total power of delta and alpha waves for each recording. For alpha waves has been observed that the mean of alpha power during magnetotherapy is lower that before and after.

It is known that casual editing of the RR interval data is sufficient for the approximate assessment of total HRV by the geometric methods. Thus when using the statistical time-domain and/or frequency-domain methods, the manual editing of the RR data should be performed to a very high standard ensuring correct identification and classification of every QRS complex. Automatic 'filters' which exclude some intervals from the original RR sequence (e.g. those differing by more than 20% from the previous interval) should not replace manual editing as they are known to behave unsatisfactorily and to have undesirable effects leading potentially to errors.

Conflict of Interest

The authors declare that they have no conflict of interest.

References

1. David V, Sălceanu A, Ciorap R (2013), Acquisition and Analysis of Biomedical Signals in Case of Peoples Exposed to Electromagnetic Fields in Pervasive and Mobile Sensing and Computing for Healthcare Mukhopadhyay S.C., Postolache A.O. (Eds.), Springer-Verlag Berlin Heidelberg, pp 269-296
2. Ciorap, R, Andritoi, D, Corciovă C et al (2010) Integrated Monitoring Solution for Chronic Diseases Management, International Conference on Electrical and Power Engineering - EPE 2010, International workshop on Electromagnetic Compatibility and Engineering in Medicine and Biology, Iasi, Romania, 2010, pp
3. Marino A.A, Becker R.O (1977) Biological effects of extremely low frequency electric and magnetic fields: A review, Physiol. Chem. Phys. 9:131-147
4. Cvetkovic D, Übeyli E.D, Cosic I (2008), Wavelet transform feature extraction from human PPG, ECG, and EEG signal responses to ELF PEMF exposures: A pilot study, Digital Signal Processing 18:861-874
5. Baldi E, Baldi C, Lithgow B. J (2007), A Pilot Investigation of the Effect ok Extremely Low Frequency Pulsed Electromagnetic Fields on Humans Heart Rate Variability, Biomagnetics 28:64 – 68
6. Sastre A., Graham C., Cook M.R et al (2002) Human EEG responses to controlled alterations of the earth`s magnetic field , Clin. Neurophys, 113: 1382-1390
7. Ciorap R, David V, Ciorap M et al (2013) Analisys of Brain Activity in case of Magnetic Stimulation, Environmental Engineering and Management Journal, 12: 1967-1974
8. Andriţoi D, David V; Ciorap R et al (2013) Recording and Processing ECG Signal During Magnetotherapy Procedures, Environmental Engineering and Management Journal, 12:1231-1238
9. Ciorap R.; Corciova C.; Ciorap M et al.(2011) Optimisation of the Treatment for Chronic Disease Using an e-Health Sistem, 7th International Symposium on ADVANCED TOPICS IN ELECTRICAL ENGINEERING 2011, Bucureşti, Romania, pp
10. Corciova, C.; Ciorap R. ; Zaharia, D.; Salceanu, A., Influence of Ambient Temperature on Central and Peripheral Impedance Measurements of the Human Body, ENVIRONMENTAL ENGINEERING AND MANAGEMENT JOURNAL, 10: 511-517

Author: Ciorap Radu
Institute: "Gr.T.Popa" University of Medicine and Pharmacy, Bioengineering Faculty
Street: M. Kogalniceanu 9-13
City: Iasi
Country: Romania
Email: radu.ciorap@bioinginerie.ro

An Argumentative Approach to Assessing Safety in Medical Device Software Using Defeasible Logic Programming

S.A. Gómez[1], A. Groza[2], and C.I. Chesñevar[1]

[1] Artificial Intelligence Research and Development Laboratory (LIDIA)
Department of Computer Science and Engineering, Universidad Nacional del Sur
Av. Alem 1253, (8000) Bahía Blanca, Argentina
{sag,cic}@cs.uns.edu.ar
[2] Intelligent Systems Group (ISG)
Department of Computer Science, Technical University of Cluj-Napoca
Baritiu 28, 400391, Cluj-Napoca, Romania
Adrian.Groza@cs.utcluj.ro

Abstract— **Modern health-care technology depends to a large extent on software deployed in medical devices, which brings several well-known benefits but also poses new hazards to patient safety. As a consequence, assessing safety and reliability in software in medical devices turns out to be a critical issue. In this paper we outline a method for safety assessment of medical devices based on Defeasible Logic Programming (DeLP), which provides an argumentative framework for reasoning with uncertain and incomplete knowledge. We contend that argumentation theory as defined in DeLP can be used to integrate and contrast different evidences for assessing the approval and commercialization of medical devices, aiming at increasing transparency to all the stakeholders involved in their certification. The outlined framework is validated by modeling the infamous Therac-25 accident.**

Keywords— **medical software, safety assurance, argumentation theory**

I. INTRODUCTION

Modern health-care technology depends nowadays to a large extent on software deployed in medical devices, which brings several well-known benefits but also poses new hazards to patient safety. Computer-related errors have played a significant role in serious injury or even death involving medical devices [1]. With more complex software employed in such devices [2], there is no possibility to perform exhaustive testing or formal methods. As a consequence, assessing safety and reliability in software in medical devices turns out to be a critical issue. The manufacturers of medical devices are expected not only to achieve an acceptable assurance level, but also to convince regulatory bodies that safeness has been achieved. In order to do this, identifying relevant evidence is not enough, as there might be conflicting or incomplete information involved. Consequently, structured, domain-based, safety *arguments* are needed to demonstrate that safety can be ensured.

In this paper we outline a method for safety assessment of medical devices based on Defeasible Logic Programming (DeLP), which provides an argumentative framework for reasoning with uncertain and incomplete knowledge. We contend that argumentation theory as defined in DeLP can be used to integrate and contrast different evidences for assessing the approval and commercialization of medical devices, aiming at increasing transparency to all the stakeholders involved in their certification. Our approach in this paper will aim at two particular issues: (i) how defeasible logic programming can be used to describe safety requirements of medical devices, and (ii) how argumentation theory can detect and solve inconsistencies or safety related doubts.

Our hypothesis is that argumentation theory (in this paper implemented via DeLP) can contribute to improve safety assurance in medical devices, providing a promising research topic (see e.g. [3, 4]). Safety arguments[1] should address at least two issues: (i) to show that all health-related hazards have been analyzed and how the assigned control measures contribute to risk mitigation, and (ii) to prove compliance with safety medical standards or guidelines.

It must be remarked that over the past few years there have been several formal complaints and court trials concerning the approval of medical devices [6], and several studies have shown that the regulatory system is opaque, fragmented and largely privatized [7]. We contend that argumentation theory as defined in DeLP can be used to integrate and contrast

[1] A safety case is defined in UK Defense Standard 00-56 as [5]: *"A structured argument, supported by a body of evidence that provides a compelling, comprehensible and valid case that a system is safe for a given application in a given operating environment." In our case, a safety case should present strong arguments that a medical device is safe to operate within a particular context [3].*

S. Vlad and R.V. Ciupa (eds.), *International Conference on Advancements of Medicine and Health Care through Technology*, IFMBE Proceedings 44,
DOI: 10.1007/978-3-319-07653-9_34, © Springer International Publishing Switzerland 2014

different evidences for assessing the approval and commercialization of medical devices, aiming at increasing transparency to all the stakeholders involved in their certification.

The rest of the paper is structured as follows: Section II presents the fundamentals of argumentation and DeLP, along with a simple motivational example. Section III explains and models the Therac-25 overdose radiation accident using DeLP. We illustrate how the arguments associated with this particular accident can be automatically obtained from the DeLP inference engine. Section IV reviews related work. Finally, in Section V we summarize the main contributions of our proposal.

II. Fundamentals of Defeasible Logic Programming

Defeasible Logic Programming (DeLP) [8] provides a language for knowledge representation and reasoning that uses *defeasible argumentation* [9, 10] to decide between contradictory conclusions through a *dialectical analysis*. Codifying knowledge by means of a DeLP program provides a good trade-off between expressiveness and implementability for dealing with incomplete and potentially contradictory information. In a DeLP program $\mathscr{P} = (\Pi, \Delta)$, a set Π of strict rules $P \leftarrow Q_1, \ldots, Q_n$, and a set Δ of defeasible rules $P \prec Q_1, \ldots, Q_n$ can be distinguished. Defeasible rules account for tentative knowledge, and provide the basis for defining *arguments*.[2]

Definition 1 (Argument) *An* argument $\langle \mathscr{A}, H \rangle$ *is a minimal non-contradictory set of ground defeasible clauses* $\mathscr{A}$ *of* Δ *that allows to derive a ground literal* H *using rules from* $\Pi \cup \mathscr{A}$.

Since arguments may be in conflict (concept captured in terms of a logical contradiction), an attack relationship between arguments can be defined. A criterion is usually defined to decide between two conflicting arguments. If the attacking argument is strictly preferred over the attacked one, then it is called a *proper defeater*. If no comparison is possible, or both arguments are equi-preferred, the attacking argument is called a *blocking defeater*. Generalized specificity [11] is typically used as a syntax-based criterion among conflicting arguments. However, other alternative partial orders can also be valid such (see [8, Sect. 3.2.2]). In this paper we will abstract the comparison criterion and will suppose fthe existence of a relation $\succ$ for comparing two conflicting arguments.

In order to determine whether a given argument $\mathscr{A}$ is ultimately undefeated (or *warranted*), a dialectical process is recursively carried out, where defeaters for $\mathscr{A}$, defeaters for these defeaters, and so on, are taken into account forming a *dialectical tree*. The argument $\mathscr{A}$ is the root of its dialectical tree $\mathscr{T}$, its defeaters the first level of $\mathscr{T}$, the defeaters of these defeaters the second level, and so on. In a dialectical tree nodes are labeled as either defeated (D) or undefeated (U). Leaves are always labeled as undefeated; a node is labeled as undefeated iff all of its children are labeled as defeated, otherwise a node is labeled as defeated. Given a DeLP program $\mathscr{P}$ and a query H, the final answer to H w.r.t. $\mathscr{P}$ takes such dialectical analysis into account. The answer to a query can be: *yes* (when there exists a warranted argument $\langle \mathscr{A}, H \rangle$), *no* (when there exists a warranted argument $\langle \mathscr{A}, \sim H \rangle$), *undecided* (neither $\langle \mathscr{A}, H \rangle$ nor $\langle \mathscr{A}, \sim H \rangle$ are warranted), or *unknown* (H does not belong to $\mathscr{P}$).

In [12], Williams & Hunter define an Ontology Argumentation Framework which combines ontologies and Defeasible Logic Programming in order to reason on a medical scenario regarding the treatment of cancer patients. Next we present a simplified version of that scenario in order to illustrate how DeLP can be used to generate arguments useful for clinical practice.

Example 1 *Consider the DeLP program* $\mathscr{P}_1 = (\Pi_1, \Delta_1)$ *presented in Fig. 1. The set of strict rules* Π_1 *says that there are two treatments for cancer: based on Anastrazole and a program of five years administration of Tamoxifen, Ms. Jones has a disease named* d_1 *which is both a ER positive disease and can be identified as breast cancer. A person who is a man or a woman is among people, early breast cancer is a type of cancer and a treatment with Tamoxifen can be performed either by a three year or a five year program. The set* Δ_1 *of defeasible rules is a very simplified version of what was presented by [12]. The rules are ordered according to the priorities* $r_2 \succ r_1 \succ r_2$ *(meaning that an argument based on* r_2 *will be considered stronger that one based on* r_1 *and so forth). From* $\mathscr{P}_1$ *we can build the following arguments:* $\langle \{r_1\}, has\_treatment(ms\_jones, t) \rangle$, $\langle \{r_2\}, \sim has\_treatment(ms\_jones, t) \rangle$ *and* $\langle \{r_3\}, \sim has\_treatment(ms\_jones, a) \rangle$. *Comparing arguments by using a criterion based on rule priorities, we can see that* $\langle \{r_1\}, has\_treatment(ms\_jones, t) \rangle$ *is defeated by* $\langle \{r_2\}, \sim has\_treatment(ms\_jones, t) \rangle$, *which in turn is defeated by* $\langle \{r_3\}, \sim has\_treatment(ms\_jones, a) \rangle$. *The dialectical trees from program* $\mathscr{P}_1$ *can be seen in Fig. 2*

[2] For space reasons, we provide only some basic DeLP definitions in this paper to make it self-contained. For a detailed explanation of DeLP, the reader is referred to [8].

DeLP program $\mathscr{P}_1 = (\Pi_1, \Delta_1)$**:**

Facts and strict rules Π_1**:**

$anastrazole(a).$
$tamoxifen5Yr(t).$
$woman(ms\_jones).$
$has\_disease(ms\_jones, d).$
$er\_positive\_disease(d).$
$early\_breast\_cancer(d).$
$people(X) \leftarrow man(X).$
$people(X) \leftarrow woman(X).$
$breast\_cancer(X) \leftarrow early\_breast\_cancer(X).$
$tamoxifen(X) \leftarrow tamoxifen3Yr(X).$
$tamoxifen(X) \leftarrow tamoxifen5Yr(X).$

Defeasible rules Δ_1 **with priorities** $r_2 \succ r_1 \succ r_3$**:**

$r_1 : has\_treatment(X,Z) \prec woman(X), has\_disease(X,Y), early\_breast\_cancer(Y), er\_positive\_disease(Y), tamoxifen5Yr(Z).$
$r_2 : \sim has\_treatment(X,Z) \prec woman(X), has\_disease(X,Y), breast\_cancer(Y), tamoxifen(Z).$
$r_3 : \sim has\_treatment(X,Z) \prec woman(X), has\_disease(X,Y), breast\_cancer(Y), anastrazole(Z).$

Fig. 1 DeLP program $\mathscr{P}_1$ on cancer treatment medical trials

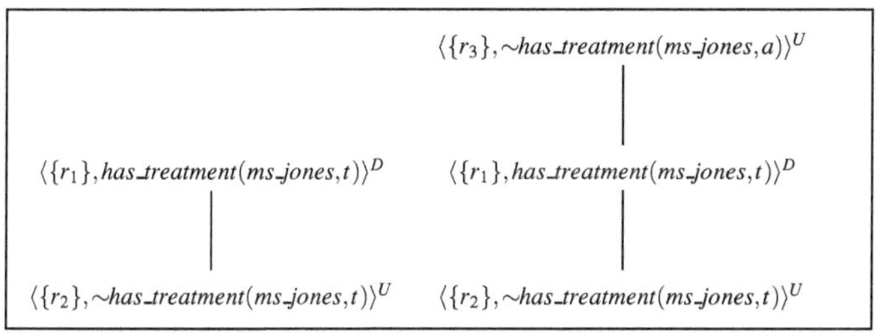

Fig. 2 Dialectical trees from $\mathscr{P}_1$

III. ARGUING IN THE THERAC-25 ACCIDENT

We now present a case study modeling the infamous Threrac-25 accelerator incident in which five people died of radiation overdose due to a malfunction during their cancer treatment sessions [13].

We discuss a DeLP program $\mathscr{P}$ for defining a safety verification system for such a system, we base our modeling in the extensive documentation regarding the Therac-25. Despite knowing that it is a somehow old case (it dates from 1987), we chose to show how DeLP can be used to perform a safety verification on a such a system as the Therac-25 accelerator problem can be considered a benchmark problem due to the extensive analyses it went through.

The main system safety verification is determining if using the accelerator is safe.

Definition 2 (Safety verification system) *A* safety verification system $\mathscr{V}$ *is a pair* $(\mathscr{P}, \mathscr{S})$ *where* $\mathscr{P}$ *is a DeLP program establishing logical criteria for assuring safety and* $\mathscr{S}$ *is a set of literals containing sensor information of the environment. The language* $\mathscr{L}_{\mathscr{V}}$ *of the safety verification system is the set of all literals in* $\mathscr{P} \cup \mathscr{S}$.

Definition 3 (Prospective safety decision) *Let* $\mathscr{V} = (\mathscr{P}, \mathscr{S})$ *be a safety verification system. A* prospective safety decision *is a literal in* $\mathscr{L}_{\mathscr{V}}$.

Definition 4 (Safety recommendation) *Let* $\mathscr{V} = (\mathscr{P}, \mathscr{S})$ *be a safety verification system and* $\mathscr{D}$ *be a prospective safety decision. A safety recommendation for* $\mathscr{D}$ *is either one of:*

- *Conform: If there is a warranting argument for* $\mathscr{D}$ *w.r.t. the DeLP program* $\mathscr{P} \cup \mathscr{S}$.
- *Do not Conform: If there is a warranting argument for* $\sim\mathscr{D}$ *w.r.t. the DeLP program* $\mathscr{P} \cup \mathscr{S}$.
- *Unable to Decide: There is neither a warranted argument for* $\mathscr{D}$ *nor* $\sim\mathscr{D}$ *w.r.t. the DeLP program* $\mathscr{P} \cup \mathscr{S}$.
- *Not Applicable:* $\mathscr{D}$ *does not belong to* $\mathscr{L}_{\mathscr{V}}$.

We will consider the modeling of a safety recommendation system $\mathscr{V} = (\mathscr{P}, safe(therac\_25))$, where the literal $safe(A)$ refers to whenever it is safe to use the accelerator A.

The rest of the section discusses the program $\mathscr{P}$ along with the dialectical analysis that can be derived from it w.r.t. the query $safe(therac\_25)$ in order to reach a safety recommendation for $\mathscr{V}$. We consider three accelerator models built by the AECL company named Therac-6, Therac-20 and Therac-25, represented by three facts: $accelerator(therac\_6)$, $accelerator(therac\_20)$, and $accelerator(therac\_25)$.

There were no reported cases of radiation overdose malfunction neither in Therac-6 nor in Therac-20 accelerator and an accelerator A is normally considered safe if it has a radiation overdose history with no reported cases. This is modeled as DeLP defeasible rules and facts as shown in Fig. 3.

$radiation\_overdose\_misfunction\_reported\_cases(therac\_6, 0).$
$radiation\_overdose\_misfunction\_reported\_cases(therac\_20, 0).$
$safe(A) \prec accelerator(A), \sim problems\_history(A).$
$\sim problems\_history(A) \prec radiation\_overdose\_misfunction\_reported\_cases(A, 0).$

Fig. 3 Overdose history in Therac-25

At this point we can deduce an argument for the Therac-6 accelerator supporting the tentative conclusion that it is safe as no cases of radiation overdose have been reported $\langle \mathscr{A}_1, safe(therac\_6) \rangle$ where

$$\mathscr{A}_1 = \left\{ \begin{array}{l} (safe(therac\_6) \prec accelerator(therac\_6), \\ \quad \sim problems\_history(therac\_6)), \\ (\sim problems\_history(therac\_6) \prec \\ \quad radiation\_overdose\_misfunction\_reported\_cases(\\ \qquad therac\_6, 0)). \end{array} \right\}.$$

It is straightforward to see that the same is valid for the Therac-20 accelerator.

The initial assumption with the case of the Therac-25 accelerator was that an accelerator is usually considered safe whenever its software is based on a library written for a previous accelerator that is known to be problem-free, the software in each accelerator was tested in each respective device, and the Therac-6, Therac-20, Therac-25 were produced in chronological order, and it is also known that the software running on Therac-25 accelerator was based on Therac-6 and Therac-20 software packages (see Fig. 4). So, from all this information we are now able to build an argument $\langle \mathscr{A}_2, \mathit{safe}(\mathit{therac\_25}) \rangle$ where

$$\mathscr{A}_2 = \left\{ \begin{array}{l} (\mathit{safe}(\mathit{therac\_25}) \;\text{—}\!\!\prec\; \mathit{accelerator}(\mathit{therac\_25}), \\ \quad \mathit{software\_inside}(\mathit{therac\_25}, \mathit{therac\_25\_software}), \\ \quad \mathit{software\_based\_on}(\mathit{therac\_25\_software}, \\ \qquad \mathit{therac\_6\_package}), \\ \quad \mathit{software\_module}(\mathit{therac\_6\_package}), \\ \quad\; \mathit{tested}(\mathit{therac\_6\_package}, \mathit{therac\_6}), \\ \quad\; \mathit{accelerator}(\mathit{therac\_6}), \mathit{older\_model}(\mathit{therac\_6}, \mathit{therac\_25}), \\ \quad\; {\sim}\mathit{problems\_history}(\mathit{therac\_6})), \\ (\mathit{older\_model}(\mathit{therac\_6}, \mathit{therac\_25}) \;\text{—}\!\!\prec \\ \quad\; \mathit{next\_model}(\mathit{therac\_20}, \mathit{therac\_25}), \\ \quad\; \mathit{older\_model}(\mathit{therac\_6}, \mathit{therac\_20})), \\ (\mathit{older\_model}(\mathit{therac\_6}, \mathit{therac\_20}) \;\text{—}\!\!\prec \\ \quad\; \mathit{next\_model}(\mathit{therac\_6}, \mathit{therac\_20})), \\ ({\sim}\mathit{problems\_history}(\mathit{therac\_6}) \;\text{—}\!\!\prec \\ \quad\; \mathit{radiation\_overdose\_misfunction\_reported\_cases}(\\ \qquad \mathit{therac\_6}, 0)) \end{array} \right\}$$

supporting the tentative conclusion that the Therac-25 accelerator is a safe device because its software was based on a Therac-6 module, which in turn was a problem free accelerator.

```
safe(A) —< accelerator(A), software_inside(A,P),
           software_based_on(P,M),
           software_module(M), tested(M,OA),
           accelerator(OA),
           older_model(OA,A), ~problems_history(OA).
software_module(therac_6_package).
software_module(therac_20_package).
tested(therac_6_package, therac_6).
tested(therac_20_package, therac_20).
next_model(therac_6, therac_20).
next_model(therac_20, therac_25).
older_model(X,Y) —< next_model(X,Y).
older_model(X,Y) —< next_model(N,Y), older_model(X,N).
software_inside(therac_25, therac_25_software).
software_based_on(therac_25_software, therac_6_package).
software_based_on(therac_25_software, therac_20_package).
```

Fig. 4 Software modules in Therac-25

Another fact that came up during the Therac-25 incident was that the system had been programmed and tested by the same programmer and that it was not possible to determine if that programmer had had formal training in computer science. According to [13] the programmer could not be identified because at the time of the hearings in court he had left the AECL company who built the accelerators. So we will refer to him as John Doe (see Fig 5). In this regard, an argument $\langle \mathscr{A}_3, {\sim}\mathit{safe}(\mathit{therac\_25}) \rangle$ where

$$\mathscr{A}_3 = \left\{ \begin{array}{l} {\sim}\mathit{safe}(\mathit{therac\_25}) \;\text{—}\!\!\prec\; \mathit{accelerator}(\mathit{therac\_25}), \\ \quad \mathit{software\_inside}(\mathit{therac\_25}, \mathit{therac\_25\_software}), \\ \quad \mathit{developed\_by}(\mathit{therac\_25\_software}, \mathit{john\_doe}), \\ \quad \mathit{tested\_by}(\mathit{therac\_25\_software}, \mathit{john\_doe}), \\ \quad \mathit{programmer}(\mathit{john\_doe}), \\ \quad \mathit{no\_background\_information\_on\_programmer}(\mathit{john\_doe}). \end{array} \right\}$$

(defeating argument $\mathscr{A}_2$) against the safety of the Therac-25 accelerator can be built.

```
~safe(A) —< accelerator(A), software_inside(A,S),
            developed_by(S,P), tested_by(S,P),
            programmer(P),
            no_background_information_on_programmer(P).
developed_by(therac_25_software, john_doe).
tested_by(therac_25_software, john_doe).
programmer(john_doe).
no_background_information_on_programmer(john_doe).
```

Fig. 5 Rules describing that there was no background on the programmer

Other criteria suggested that an accelerator is safely tested if its software module has gone through extensive unit, integration and simulator testing; otherwise, it cannot be considered safe. In the case of the Therac-25 software, it was used about 2700 hours without incidents and audits determined that the software in the Therac-25 went through an extensive integration testing but the unit testing was not that appropiate. No extensive simulator testing was performed either (see Fig. 6). In this case, it is easy to see that another argument in favor of the safety of the system based on the amount of hours of usage without incidents can be found but another one against the safety can be built on the grounds that it was proved that no extensive unit testing was performed on the Therac-25 software.

Another criteria for accelerator safety pointed out by [13] is that the Therac-20 accelerator included hardware safety interlocks as an additional safety mechanism to stop the machine in case of a malfunction, thus making Therac-20 a safe device. Those hardware safety interlocks were taken out in Therac-25 for cost reasons, thus making it unsafe (see Fig. 7).

A software module is unsafe if it runs on an unsafe operating system and an unsafe operating system is an operating system which is not safe. From [13], we know that the Therac-25 main bug was based on having a program running in a PDP-11 real time system that allowed concurrent access

```
safe(A) -<
    accelerator(A),
    software_inside(A,S), safe_software_testing(S).
safe_software_testing(S) -<
    used_hours_without_problems(S,H),
    H > 2000.
safe_software_testing(S) -<
    software_module(S),
    extensive_unit_testing(S),
    extensive_integration_testing(S),
    extensive_simulator_testing(S).
~safe_software_testing(S) -<
    ~extensive_unit_testing(S).
~safe_software_testing(S) -<
    ~extensive_integration_testing(S).
~safe_software_testing(S) -<
    ~extensive_simulator_testing(S).

software_module(therac_25_software).
~extensive_unit_testing(therac_25_software).
extensive_integration_testing(therac_25_software).
use_hours_without_problems(therac_25_software, 2700).
```

Fig. 6 Rules describing failed testing

```
safe(A) -< accelerator(A),
    includes_hardware_safety_interlocks(A),
    radiation_overdose_misfunction_reported_cases(A,0).
includes_hardware_safety_interlocks(therac_20).
~safe(A) -< accelerator(A),
    ~includes_hardware_safety_interlocks(A),
    based_on_previous_accelerator(A,PA),
        accelerator(PA),
        includes_hardware_safety_interlocks(PA).
based_on_previous_accelerator(A,PA) -< older_model(PA,A).
~includes_hardware_safety_interlocks(therac_25).
```

Fig. 7 Rules for expressing lack of safety interlocks

to shared variables but it did not allow to test and set for variables as indivisible operations (see Fig. 8). From this point of view, an argument for the non-safety of Therac-25 can be derived.

Finally, if we add the information establishing that at least one patient died, then we get only one tree formed by a single argument based on the strict rule that establishes that an accelerator is not safe if a patient died. So, an accelerator is not definitely safe if a single overdose problem is reported. In the case of Therac-25, five people died of radiation overdose (see Fig. 9). On the light of this final evidence, the safety decision would be that the accelerator is not safe as the safety recommendation of $\mathscr{P}$ w.r.t. to *safe*(*A*) is *Do not Conform.*

IV. Related Work

A software controller for radiological devices has been simulated in [14], aiming at fine-tunning the radiological

```
~safe(A) -< software_inside(A,M), unsafe_module(M).
unsafe_module(M) -< software_module(M),
    runs_on(M,S),
    unsafe_operating_system(S).
unsafe_operating_system(S) -<
    ~safe_operating_system(S),
    operating_system(S).
~safe_operating_system(S) -<
    real_time_operating_system(S),
    allows_concurrent_access_to_shared_variables(S),
    ~test_and_set_for_variables_as_indivisible_operations(S).
real_time_system_operating_system(pdp_11_os).
allows_concurrent_access_to_shared_variables(pdp_11_os).
~test_and_set_for_variables_as_indivisible_operations(pdp_11_os).
```

Fig. 8 Rules for expressing unsafe operating system

```
~safe(A) <- accelerator(A),
        problem_detected(A, overdose, Place, Date).
problem_detected(therac_25, overdose, marietta_georgia, jun_1985).
problem_detected(therac_25, overdose, yakima_washington, dec_1985).
problem_detected(therac_25, overdose, hamilton_ontario, jan_1986).
problem_detected(therac_25, overdose, tyler_texas, mar_1986).
problem_detected(therac_25, overdose, tyler_texas, apr_1986).
```

Fig. 9 Rules and facts expressing overdose reported cases

equipment. Complementary, the results as those obtained in [14] represent inputs of our argumentation machine. Thus, the pieces of evidence collected from [14] feed the DeLP system to reason about safeness of radiological devices.

A model driven approach improves the safety of Patient-Controlled Analgesic infusion pumpsin [15]. The UPPAAL formally verifies the safety properties of the controlling software. By enacting argumentation theory, we aimed to fill the gap between such low level safety specifications and high level safety cases required by conformance decisioneers.

Similar to our work, the goal in [16] has been to increase confidence in the medical-related software by enacting argumentation theory. A safety pattern is proposed for generic infusion pumps, modeled in the Goal Structuring Notation [17] graphical argumentation language. By employing defeasible logic, we additionally perform reasoning on the given model.

The rewrite logic has been used in [18] to verify safety of life-critical medical devices such as pacemakers, ventilator machines, or infusion pumps for pain medication. With the goal to establish safe medical design patterns, the work in [18] focuses on the programmers perspective. We argue that, the defeasible logic better supports decisions of different actors involved in the approval of medical device software.

One line to prove that medical-related software is safe emphases the need of traceability. The Med-trace method [19] identifies the requirements for traceability through each phase in the medical software life-cycle. Similar to our work, the need to increase transparency of health-care software was addressed in [19]. Different from our work, the focus in [19] is on the development life-cycle of software from the project management perspective. We focus on organizing evidence from different perspectives, by enacting a formal method based on argumentation semantics of defeasible logic.

V. CONCLUSIONS

By using argumentation theory, we aimed at structuring the available evidence to demonstrate compliance with medical safety requirements and avoidance of hazards. Our method is able to automatically identify inconsistencies in the argumentation chain. Identifying inconsistencies or flaws in the justification chain signals a possible breach in the functionality of the medical device.

The benefits of using argumentation theory regard the improvement of comprehension of the safety argument among all the key stakeholders (software developers, safety engineers, medical certification bodies, physicians, operators of the device).

CONFLICT OF INTEREST

The authors declare that they have no conflict of interest.

ACKNOWLEDGEMENTS

Part of this work was supported by the Romania-Argentina Bilateral Agreement entitled "ARGSAFE: Using argumentation for justifying safeness in complex technical systems" (MINCYT-MECTS Project RO/12/05) and Universidad Nacional del Sur, Argentina. Adrian Groza is supported by the intern research project at Technical University of Cluj-Napoca, Romania: "GREEN-VANETS: Improving transportation using Car-2-X communication and multi agent systems". Carlos Chesñevar is funded by Consejo Nacional de Investigaciones Científicas y Técnicas (CONICET).

REFERENCES

1. Fu Kevin, Blum James. Controlling for cybersecurity risks of medical device software *Communications of the ACM*. 2013;56:35–37.
2. Olah P., Dobru D., Ciupa R.V., Marusteri M., Bacarea V., Muji M.. Database External Level Architecture for Use in Healthcare Information Systems in *Int. Conf. on Advancements of Medicine and Health Care through Technology* (Vlad Simona, Ciupa RaduV.. , eds.);36 of *IFMBE Proceedings*:36-39Springer Berlin Heidelberg 2011.
3. Graydon Patrick J., Habli Ibrahim, Hawkins Richard, Kelly Tim, Knight John C.. Arguing Conformance *IEEE Software*. 2012;29:50-57.
4. Chung Paul, Cheung Larry, Machin Colin. Compliance Flow - Managing the compliance of dynamic and complex processes *Know.-Based Syst.*. 2008;21:332–354.
5. Defence UK Ministry. 00-56 Safety Management Requirments for Defence Systems *UK Ministry of defence*. 2007;4.
6. Campillo-Artero Carlos. A full-fledged overhaul is needed for a risk and value-based regulation of medical devices in Europe *Health Policy*. 2013;113:38 - 44.
7. McCulloch Peter. The EUs system for regulating medical devices *BMJ: British Medical Journal*. 2012;345.
8. García A., Simari G.. Defeasible Logic Programming An Argumentative Approach *Theory and Prac. of Logic Program.*. 2004;4:95-138.
9. Chesñevar Carlos Iván, Maguitman Ana, Loui Ronald. Logical Models of Argument *ACM Computing Surveys*. 2000;32:337-383.
10. Bench-Capon Trevor J. M., Dunne Paul E.. Argumentation in Artificial Intelligence *Artificial Intelligence*. 2007;171:619–641.
11. Simari G., Loui R.. A Mathematical Treatment of Defeasible Reasoning and its Implementation *Artificial Intelligence*. 1992;53:125-157.
12. Williams M., Hunter A.. Harnessing ontologies for argument-based decision-making in breast cancer *Proc. of the Intl. Conf. on Tools with AI (ICTAI'07)*. 2007:254–261.
13. Leveson Nancy, Turner Clark. An Investigation of the Therac-25 Accidents *IEEE Computer*. 1993;26:18–41.
14. Roman N.M., Colosi H., Pusca M.. Digital Simulation for Computer Control of Radiological Devices: A Preliminary Model Using Partial Differential Equations in *Int. Conf. on Advancements of Medicine and Health Care through Technology* (Vlad Simona, Ciupa RaduV., Nicu Ancal.. , eds.);26 of *IFMBE Proceedings*:37-42Springer Berlin Heidelberg 2009.
15. Kim BaekGyu, Ayoub Anaheed, Sokolsky Oleg, et al. Safety-assured development of the gpca infusion pump software in *Proceedings of the ninth ACM international conference on Embedded software*:155–164ACM 2011.
16. Ayoub Anaheed, Kim BaekGyu, Lee Insup, Sokolsky Oleg. A safety case pattern for model-based development approach in *NASA Formal Methods*:141–146Springer 2012.
17. Spriggs John. *GSN - The Goal Structuring Notation: A Structured Approach to Presenting Arguments*. Springer 2012.
18. Sun Mu, Meseguer José, Sha Lui. A formal pattern architecture for safe medical systems in *Rewriting Logic and Its Applications*:157–173Springer 2010.
19. Regan Gilbert, Caffery Fergal Mc, Daid Kevin Mc, Flood Derek. Medical device standards' requirements for traceability during the software development lifecycle and implementation of a traceability assessment model *Computer Standards and Interfaces*. 2013;36:3 - 9.

Sensorial System for Visually Impaired Individuals

V.D. Zaharia, S. Crişan, B. Ţebrean, V.T. Popa, and R.A. Munteanu

Department of Electrotechnics and Measurements, Faculty of Electric Engineering,
Technical University of Cluj-Napoca, Cluj-Napoca, Romania

Abstract— **Designing precise and efficient interfacing methods for visually impaired individuals has been a concern of various research groups for decades. Over time, multiple concepts have been designed and presented, each of them introducing different detection and warning methods. This paper presents an upgrade for the classic long cane used by the visually impaired.**

The design will provide the user with additional information about the surrounding environment, thus increasing the user's awareness and safety level. The module will be able to detect obstacles 4 meters in front of the user at lover body level and 2 meters at upper body level with the help of ultrasonic sensors. Another feature of the device is to signal the user's presence and intentions by powering up an array of LEDs in low light environments or when the cane is positioned parralel to the ground.

Keywords— **Obstacle, detection system, visually impaired, walking plane, head level obstacles**

I. INTRODUCTION

Blindness is the phenomena of partial or total loss of sight due to neurological or physiological causes. In order to assess an individual's degree of blindness, several measurement scales have been developed [1].

Social integration and awareness concerning visually impaired individuals is of relative recent concern. To be more specific, the issue became of interest at the same time Braille alphabet was introduced to the public in the first half of the 19th Century. Since the introduction of the Braille alphabet, objects and techniques intended to integrate the visually impaired in day to day activities have been developed [1],[7], addressing two main approaches: daily use objects adapted for visually impaired individuals and obstacle detection and orientation devices. Some of the devices found in the second category also have the purpose of signaling the people around the person using them about the user's condition.

The purpose of this paper is to present a concept device for obstacle detection meant to be used by visually impaired individuals. The concept is based on the classic long cane used by the visually impaired and it features additional obstacle detection, user interaction and signaling functions.

II. ANALYSIS OF EXISTING DEVICES AND IDENTIFYING NEEDS

Daily use objects for the visually impaired are adaptations of general use objects with Braille markings, which make them usable by blind people. Objects in this category stretch from currency and packaging to watches, entertainment and electronic and communication devices.

Most of the devices in obstacle detection and orientation category are based on the well known long cane used by the visually impaired, with additions in terms of obstacle sensing and user positioning [3],[5],[7]. From the multitude of obstacle detection devices described in literature, the ones based on the classic cane are equipped with ultrasonic or infrared sensors for the purpose of obstacle detection, and tactile or acoustic user interfacing. Most of these devices are designed to detect obstacles up to waist level, placed mainly in the user's horizontal walking plane [2],[4]. Such devices can enhance the user's perception on the obstacles placed on the desired walking path by providing information on the obstacles' existence with a wider range compared to the classical long cane. However, obstacles placed at waist height and above are imperceptible to such devices, therefore posing a possible threat to the user.

In order to detect obstacles above waist level, several head-worn devices have been designed. Such devices detect obstacles by means of ultrasound sensors and interact in a tactile fashion with the user. However, these devices are only complementary to a handheld device for primary obstacle detection.

With the advance and higher availability of GPS tracking devices, some existing obstacle detection devices have also been equipped with such technology, giving them an additional orientation function.[5]

A series of discussions have been conducted with a group of 18 visually impaired individuals who use the classic long cane. The interviewed persons consider the long cane as being very useful for obstacle detection at a lower level and for warning purposes. However, they have pointed out the lack of obstacle detection above ground level (parked cars, barriers etc.). This lack of detection accuracy can result in a possible damage of the cane and the user's injury.

When asked about the features considered to be useful in a modern detection device, the interviewed individuals manifested their interest in long distance detection of obstacles placed on the walking surface, the possibility of detection range selection according to the user's height and movement speed and the implementation of both acoustical and tactile interaction with the device. The suggested design also featured light weight, water tightness and shock

S. Vlad and R.V. Ciupa (eds.), *International Conference on Advancements of Medicine and Health Care through Technology*, IFMBE Proceedings 44,
DOI: 10.1007/978-3-319-07653-9_35, © Springer International Publishing Switzerland 2014

resistance for high reliability at prolonged use in various environments.

III. The Proposed System

Following the analysis of available devices and the discussions conducted with the visually impaired individuals, a design for the proposed system has been conceived.

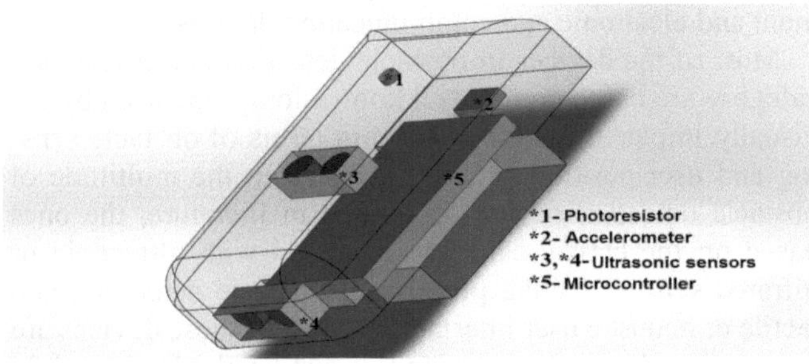

Fig. 1 The device's proposed design

The proposed design consists of a module hosting two ultrasonic sensors, a photoresistor, an accelerometer, a piezoelectric speaker, an Arduino microcontroller and a Lithium-Polymer battery as the system's main power source. The module is attachable to a classic long cane used by the visually impaired, providing an upgrade to an existing device. In addition, a led strip is attached along the cane in order to visually signal the user's presence and intentions to other people (by-passers or drivers). The usage of the detection system in enclosed spaces can result in false detections by the ultrasonic sensors, therefore the cane will be used as secondary detection device, also providing redundancy in case the battery is depleted.

The two ultrasonic sensors are used for obstacle detection. The lower sensor (Fig. 1 – 4) is meant to detect obstacles which may come in contact with the user's lower body, having a maximum detection range of four meters. When an obstacle is detected, the user is warned by means of an electromagnetic vibrator placed on the cane's handle. The vibratory output has three levels of intensity, starting from the lowest level for obstacles detected at a longer distance and increasing as the distance between the obstacle and the detection system decreases.

The other ultrasonic sensor (Fig. 1 – 3) is used for detecting obstacles targeted at the user's upper body, with a maximum detection range of two meters. In order to provide the user with accurate and usable information regarding the surrounding environment, when obstacles are detected by the upper sensor warnings are issued by means of a piezoelectric speaker, therefore eliminating possible confusions between obstacles placed in lower or upper body sections.

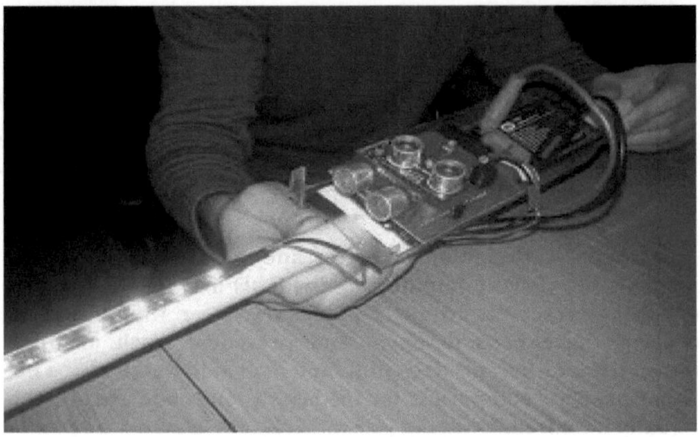

Fig. 2 The implemented prototype

The obstacle detection system based on the two ultrasonic sensors both increases the detection range of the classic long cane (lower sensor) and provides detection of up to head level obstacles (upper sensor), which is not granted by the classic device.

Another function of the proposed device is to signal the user's intention of crossing the street. Usually, visually impaired individuals raise their canes up to a parallel position with the ground when they want to cross the street, therefore making drivers aware of their intention. In order to increase the awareness of the traffic participants, the cane has been equipped with a white LED strip which gets powered up when the accelerometer placed in the attachable module senses that the user has modified the inclination of the device up to a position parallel to the ground, therefore showing the intention of crossing the street. The LED strip is powered off when the cane is repositioned in normal usage position. In addition to this function, the accelerometer constantly monitors the device's movement. Weather no motion is detected for more than ten seconds, the obstacle detection system is powered off in order to preserve battery life, when the accelerometer senses motion, the obstacle detection system is automatically resumed.

In order to signal the user's presence to other individuals in dark environment, the system has been equipped with a photoresistor. When the illumination level detected with the photoresistor drops under the 200 lux value, the microcontroller powers on the LED strip placed along the cane, making the device and its user more visible to other individuals, pedestrians and drivers alike. When the illumination level grows above the mentioned value, the LED strip is automatically powered off by the microcontroller in order to increase battery life. At each system start-up a battery check is conducted, giving the user information about the battery's charge level by means of the piezoelectric speaker.

IV. The Experimental Device

The system's sensors' output signals are acquired by the Arduino microcontroller which analyses and interprets the measurement data accordingly to the programming algorithm written in its memory. After the input data has been processed according to the algorithm, the microcontroller generates output signals which command the system's active components. The device's block diagram is shown in the following figure.

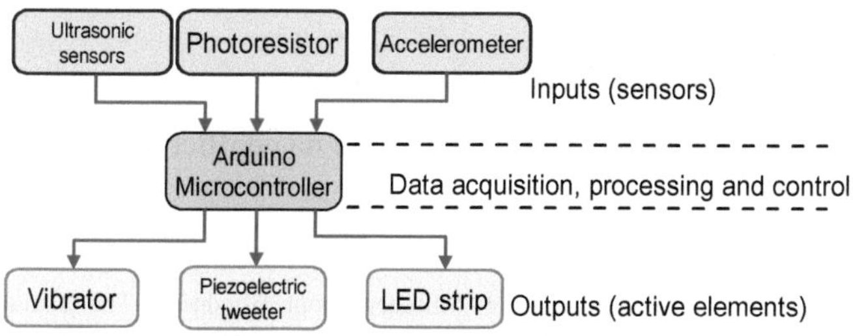

Fig. 3 The proposed system's block diagram

In order to keep the dimensions of the final device to a minimum, a custom circuit board has been designed and implemented, having the same size and connection pin display as the microcontroller development board, allowing the superposition of the two and connecting all the sensors and the active elements to the device's processing unit.

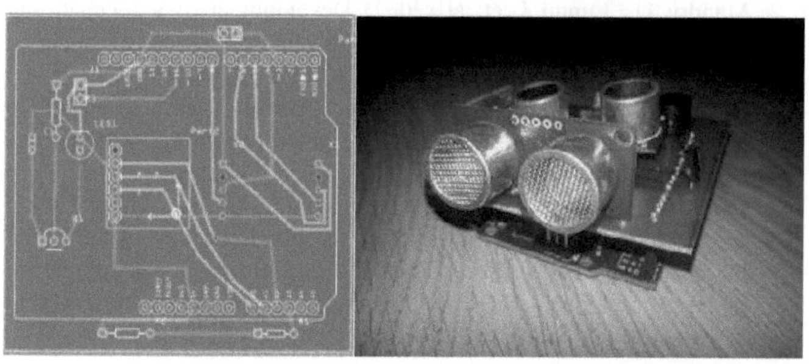

Fig. 4 The PCB design and its implementation

After attaching the proposed device to a 150 centimeters cane, a series of measurements have been conducted in order to determine the system's obstacle detection capabilities and accuracy. Tests have been conducted in an environment in which various types of obstacles have been simulated. The choice for the simulated obstacles has been made considering daily real-life situations an individual might get confronted with while using the detection device both in indoor and outdoor environments. These objects have been placed in the horizontal walking plane as well as above the ground, simulating possible situations where the user could encounter obstacles which might harm the upper section of the body. The objects considered as obstacles placed in the walking plane are a rectangular box facing the user with a flat surface and an edge, a PVC pipe with a 15 centimeters diameter placed at 10 centimeters above the ground and an office chair, while the ones considered for the upper section are a branch, an irregular object (wooden plank covered with wire mesh), a horizontal pipe with a 10 centimeters diameter, a vertical porous flat surface and a flat wooden board positioned both vertically and inclined at a 45° angle towards the detection device. The measurements have been conducted in the mentioned intervals, with the obstacles being placed at distances starting from the range's lower limit and covering the whole interval in 20 centimeters steps. Due to the high volume of measurement data, only the information considered as the most relevant will be presented in the following tables.

The absolute and relative errors presented in the tables are computed between the detection distance given by the ultrasonic sensors and the actual distance the object has been placed from the detection device.

Table 1 Measurement results for obstacles placed in the horizontal walking plane

Object	Maximum detection distance [cm]	Maximum absolute error [cm]	Maximum relative error [%]
Rectangular box – flat surface	400	23	11.33
Rectangular box – edge	200	44	18.03
PVC pipe	220	18	10.11
Office chair	280	18	6.98

Out of the simulated obstacles, detection of the rectangular box with an edge facing the user has the poorest accuracy. This obstacle is detected at 200 centimeters from the user, which can be considered as a safe detection distance for an object placed in the horizontal walking plane, since the sensorial system is also backed-up by the long cane.

Table 2 Measurement results for obstacles placed at head level

Object	Maximum detection distance [cm]	Maximum absolute error [cm]	Maximum relative error [%]
Branches	200	22	12.09
Irregular object	180	19	11.95
Horizontal pipe	200	14	9.09
Vertical porous surface	200	21	13.04
Vertical wooden board	160	29	17.95
Inclined wooden board	200	12	7.89

The lowest detection distance for obstacles placed at the user's head level is observed in the case of the vertical wooden board, which is detected only at a distance of 160 centimeters, which however can be considered as safe for the user at a normal walking speed.

The same measurements have been conducted with the obstacles and the sensors placed at the same level with considerably lower detection errors, due to the fact that the sensors used in the experimental system are designed to have maximum detection accuracy when positioned in the same plane as the obstacle. In spite of this slight inconvenient, the detection distances for obstacles placed both in the user's walking plane as well as the ones placed at head level are considered to be satisfactory.

V. Conclusions

The paper introduces an experimental device consisting of an attachable module with a classic long cane used by visually impaired individuals for obstacle detection. The main purpose meant for the device was to enhance the obstacle detection function of the classic long cane in the user's walking plane, as well as introducing additional functions such as detection for possible obstacles which may occur in the user's upper body section. The obstacle detection is signaled by means of both acoustical and tactile stimuli generated by the system's active elements. Furthermore, an optical warning system has been included in the experimental device. Its purpose is to signal the user's presence, raising the awareness of other traffic participants (both pedestrians and drivers) about the user's intentions. Other features of the presented device are the battery monitoring function and the automatic stand-by switching which has been devised for energy saving reasons.

The main advantage of the presented concept consists in the fact that the experimental module is attachable to a classic long cane used by visually impaired individuals which requires minimum adjustments to an existing device. Furthermore, all the detection functions and the auxiliary ones are integrated and performed by a single device, making the system easy to implement and to use.

Given the fact that the presented device is a conceptual prototype resulted from preliminary discussions conducted with visually impaired individuals, it may lack the robustness intended for usage on a daily basis. However, it is the authors' intention to present the prototype in its present form to a group of visually impaired individuals for further assessment of the functionality and to implement features based on the group's feedback in a device which would be suitable for daily use. Further studies are intended to determine improvements for the proposed device's functions and to reduce the classic long cane users' learning curve.

Acknowledgment

The authors wish to thank Dr. Roxana Cziker, Headmaster of the High School for the Visually Impaired Cluj-Napoca, for the help and valuable information provided during the design and implementation of the prototype presented in the present paper.

Conflict of Interest

The authors declare that they have no conflict of interest.

References

1. Bell E (2009) Measuring Attitudes about Blindness: The Social Responsibility about Blindness Scale, Professional Development and Research Institute on Blindness Louisiana Tech University
2. Dunai L, Peris-Fajarnés G, Lluna E, Defez B (2013) Sensory Navigation Device for Blind People. The Journal of Navigation, 66, 349–362; DOI 10.1017/S0373463312000574
3. Gahrieb W., Nagib G., (2007) Robotic Cane for Blinds
4. Guerrero L, Vasquez F, Ochoa S (2012) An Indoor Navigation System for the Visually Impaired. Sensors 2012, 12, 8236-8258;
5. Madad Ali Shah et. al (2010) Blind Navigation via a DGPS-based Hand-held Unit, Australian Journal of Basic and Applied Sciences, 4(6), pp 1449-1458
6. Mândru D., Lungu I. et. al (2007) Development of a Mechatronic blind Stick, Annals of The Oradea University, Fascicle of Management and Technological Engineering, Volume VI (XVI)
7. Reid F, Simkiss P (2009) The Hidden Majority. A study of economic inactivity among blind and partially sighted people in Sweden, Germany and Romania, RNIB
8. Serrão M, Rodrigues J.M.F., Rodrigues J.I., du Buf J.M.H (2012) Indoor localization and navigation for blind persons using visual landmarks and a GIS. Proceedings of the 4th International Conference on Software Development for Enhancing Accessibility and Fighting Info-exclusion (DSAI 2012) Procedia Computer Science 14, 65 – 73

Author: Valentin Dan ZAHARIA
Institute: Faculty of Electric Engineering, Technical University of Cluj-Napoca
Street: George Barițiu 26
City: Cluj-Napoca
Country: Romania
Email: Valentin.Zaharia@ethm.utcluj.ro

Assessment of Peripheral Diabetic Neuropathy: New versus Conventional Methods

G.V. Inceu[1] and I.A. Veresiu[1,2]

[1] "Iuliu Hatieganu" University of Medicine and Pharmacy, Cluj-Napoca, Romania
[2] Clinical Center of Diabetes, Nutrition, Metabolic Diseases, Cluj-Napoca, Romania

Abstract— **Diabetic peripheral sensory neuropathy is a common complication of diabetes that can cause considerable morbidity and mortality in diabetic patients. It increases the risk for complications of diabetes such as amputations and foot ulcers, thus it is important to detect peripheral neuropathy early so that diabetic foot care education can be provided and protective measures can be used to avoid devastating complications with the diabetic foot. Our aim of this paper was to study the incidence and extent of peripheral sensory neuropathy in diabetic patients with <5, 5–10 and >10 years duration of diabetes using two different modalities of testing: 5.07 Semmes-Weinstein Monofilament Testing (SWMT) and Rapid-Current Perception Threshold (R-CPT) measurements using the Neurometer. Our study population consisted of 60 patients treated for diabetes mellitus in the Unirea Medical Center. Thirty-five, 15 and 5 patients had duration of diabetes of 5, 5–10 and 10 years, respectively. All patients were tested for sensory neuropathy using SWMT and the Neurometer.**

Our results showed that a higher incidence of sensory neuropathy was found in patients with a longer duration of diabetes, especially in those who have been diagnosed for >10 years. Even for patients with <5 years duration of diabetes, the incidence of sensory neuropathy detected was considerable. The incidence of neuropathy detected continued to increase with length of duration of diabetes. Hence, we recommend screening of patients for neuropathy as soon as they are diagnosed with diabetes. Also CPT measurement with the Neurometer has been shown to be clinically valuable in detecting peripheral nerve dysfunction. Applying 5Hz current detected the most patients with diabetic neuropathy compared to the other two frequencies, finding that confirm the well-known fact that diabetes mellitus is a small fiber disease.

Keywords— **diabetes, neuropathy, Neurometer**

I. Introduction

Diabetic neuropathy is one of the most common neuropathy especially in industrialized countries and it is associated with a wide range of clinical manifestations. The vast majority of patients with clinical diabetic neuropathy have a distal symmetrical form of the disorder that progresses following a fiber-length-dependent pattern, with sensory and autonomic manifestations predominating [1]. Due to the fact that diabetic neuropathy is one of the main risk factor for development of diabetic foot ulcers (being associated as a predictive factor for limb loss) and it's also significantly associated with patient's increased rate of morbidity and mortality, it's important to detect peripheral neuropathy early so that diabetic foot care education can be provided and protective measures can be used to avoid devastating complications with the diabetic foot [2, 3, 4].

For diagnosing peripheral neuropathy there is no gold standard available. The San Antonio consensus panel has recommended that at least one measurement should be performed in five different diagnostic categories. These are symptom scoring, physical examination scoring, quantitative sensory testing (QST), cardiovascular autonomic function testing and electro-diagnostic studies (EDS) [5,6].

Novel investigative techniques, such as quantitative sensory testing and subcutaneous pressure perception threshold measurement, have shown much promise, but applicability in the clinical setting remains limited. Among the quantitative methods, measurement of the current perception threshold (CPT) using the Neurometer® (Neurotron Inc., Baltimore, Maryland, USA) has been shown to detect and quantify disorders of peripheral nerve function in several clinical situations [7, 8, 9].

II. Objectives

To study the trend of incidence of sensory neuropathy detected in diabetic patients with different durations of diabetes.

To compare the incidence of neuropathy detected by two different modalities of assessment for sensory neuropathy: Semmes-Weinstein Monofilament Test (SWMT) and Rapid Current Perception Threshold (R-CPT) measurements using the Neurometer.

III. Material and methods

The study involved 60 patients with type 2 diabetes treated at Unirea Medical Center. 38.3% were females and 61.7% were males. Their ages ranged between 21 and 69 years, with the average being 54.63 years. The patients were divided into three groups according to their duration of diabetes: <5 years (Group A), 5-10 years (Group B), >10

S. Vlad and R.V. Ciupa (eds.), *International Conference on Advancements of Medicine and Health Care through Technology*, IFMBE Proceedings 44,
DOI: 10.1007/978-3-319-07653-9_36,

years (group C) [10]. All three groups were assessed for peripheral sensory neuropathy using Semmes-Weinstein Monofilament Testing and Rapid-Current Perception Threshold (R-CPT) measurements using the Neurometer.

A. 5.07 Semmes-Weinstein Monofilament Test

A 5.07 Semmes-Weinstein nylon monofilament was employed to apply a consistent 10 g force on 4 different sites on the plantar surface of the foot as shown in Fig. 1.

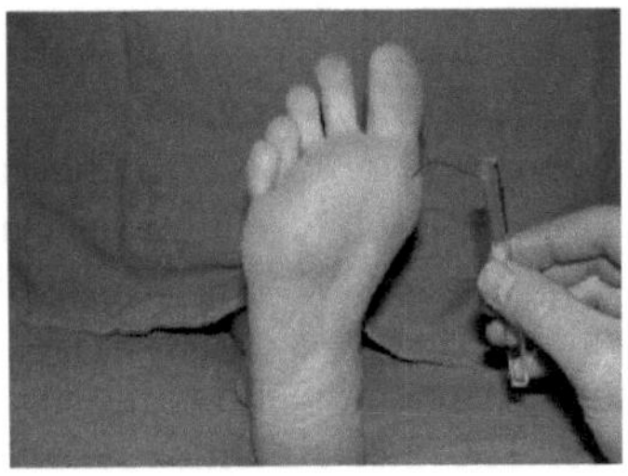

Fig. 1 Applying 5.07 Semmes-Weinstein monofilament

With the patients unable to see their feet, the monofilament was placed on the plantar surface of the foot at right angles to the skin and the pressure increased until the filament buckled. The patients were asked to say when they felt something. Protective sensation is considered to be present if the patient correctly answers two or more of the three applications, one of which was a sham. If the patient correctly answers only one or none of the three applications, the sites will be retest. The patient is considered to have insensate feet if they fail on retesting at just one more sites on either foot [11].

B. Neurometer

The Neurometer generates R-CPT readings based on the minimal strength of alternating current (AC) stimulus that the patient can detect. AC stimulus was applied to hallux (Fig. 2).

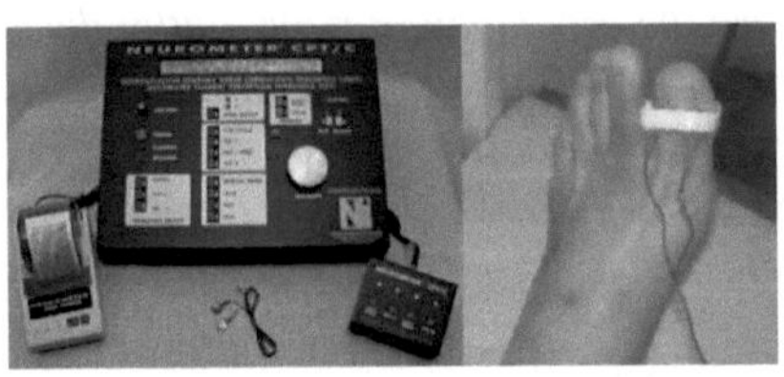

Fig. 2 Neurometer. Applying the electrodes to the big toe

At each test site, three different frequencies of 2000, 250 and 5Hz of AC current were applied to stimulate large myelinated alpha beta fibers, small myelinated alpha delta fibers and small unmyelinated C fibers, respectively (Fig. 3) [12].

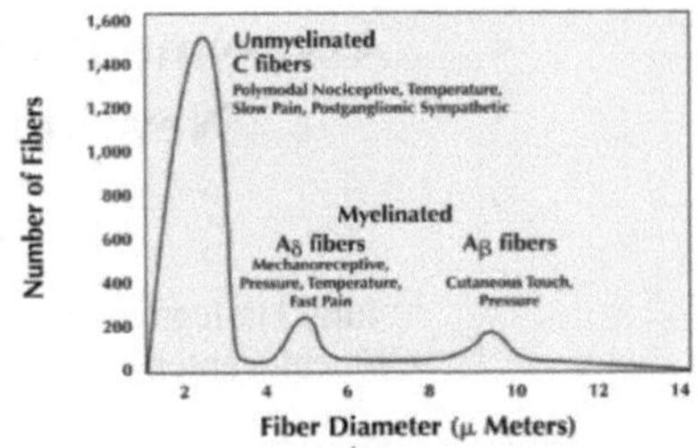

Fig. 3 Sub-population of nerve fibers and the conducted sensations

Alpha beta fibers detect cutaneous pressure; alpha delta fibers detect fast pain and temperature, whereas small diameter C fibers detect slow pain and temperature. At each frequency (2000, 250 and 5Hz), an R-CPT value was generated and ranged from 1 to 25. A value ranging from 6 to 13 was classified as normal, while a value ranging from 1 to 5 showed hyperesthesia (increased sensation). A value between 14 and 25 showed hypoesthesia (decreased sensation). Both hyperesthesia and hypoesthesia indicated the presence of sensory neuropathy (Fig. 4) [13].

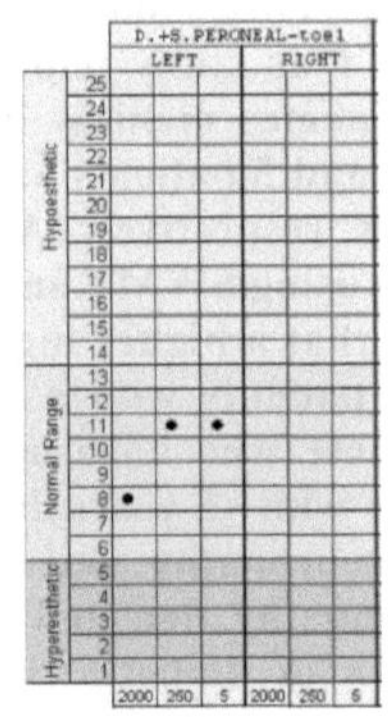

Fig. 4 R-CPT values generated at each frequency

IV. Results

Statistical analysis was performed using SPSS-15.

Group A (less than 5 years duration of diabetes) included 35 patients, group B 15 patients and group C 5 patients.

Incidence of sensory neuropathy with different durations of diabetes:

- The SWMT showed that sensory neuropathy was found in 11.4% for group A, in 26.6% for group B and in 50% for group C. There was significantly higher proportion of patients from group C who had sensory neuropathy as compared to group B.
- When current perception threshold was assessed using Neurometer, for group A, 17.14% of patients showed sensory neuropathy at 2000Hz, 22.85% of patients showed sensory neuropathy at 250Hz and 25.71% of

patients showed sensory neuropathy at 5Hz. For group B, sensory neuropathy was detected in 20% of patients at 2000Hz, 30% of patients at 250Hz and 66.66% of patients at 5Hz. For group C, 20% of patients showed sensory neuropathy at 2000Hz, 30% of patients at 250Hz, and 90% of patients at 5Hz (the difference between 2000Hz and 5Hz is statistical significant p=0.02) (Table 1).

Table 1 Incidence of sensory neuropathy (% of patients)

		Neurometer (hallux site)		
Duration of diabetes (years)	SWMT	2000Hz	250Hz	5Hz
<5	11.4	17.14	22.85	25.71
5-10	26.6	20	30	66.66
>10	50	20	33.33	90
All durations	21.7	21.6	30	46.6

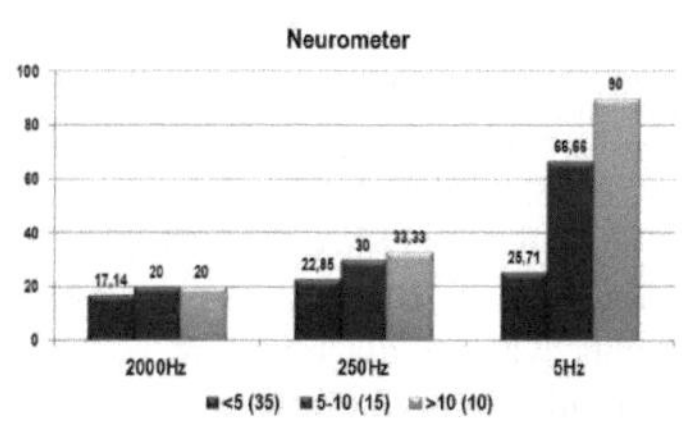

Fig. 5 Incidence of sensory neuropathy with different durations of diabetes

Incidence of sensory neuropathy with different modalities of assessment:

- SWMT detected sensory neuropathy in 21.7% of all patients. R-CPT measurements at the big toe site showed a higher proportion of patients with sensory neuropathy for 250Hz and 5Hz (30% respectively 46.6%) (Fig.6). We also obtain statistical significance between patients with neuropathy when 2000Hz and 5Hz stimulus was applied (p=0.04).

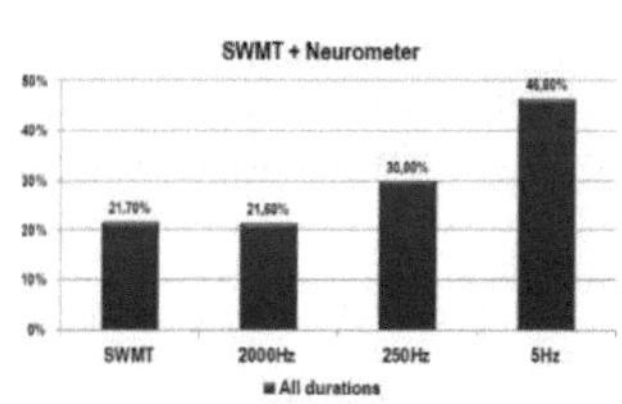

Fig. 6 Incidence of sensory neuropathy with different modalities of assessment

We also performed analysis of lot depending on the stage of nerve damage (hyperesthesia or hypoesthesia). We noticed that the number of patients diagnosed with hyperesthesia is even higher as the duration of diabetes is higher (for group A: 2,85% at 2000Hz, 0% at 250Hz and 8,57 at 5Hz; for group B: 6,66% at 2000Hz, 13,33% at 250Hz and 40% at 5Hz; for group C: 10% at 2000Hz, 20% at 250Hz and 50% at 5Hz) and found that the frequency of 5Hz have the highest incidence of patients with hyperesthesia.

We observed the same trend for patients with hypoesthesia, their number being correlated with duration of diabetes. In this situation also, the routine application of 5Hz frequency identified most patients with hypoesthesia.

Patients also completed a symptom questionnaire (neuropathy symptoms score), a score of 3-4 points highlight mild symptoms, 5-6 points moderate impairment and more than 7 points means severe symptoms [14]. In patients with more than 10 years of diabetes duration were obtained significantly higher scores, severity of symptoms is clearly correlated with duration of diabetes. Thus a score of less than 3 was achieved in 71.4% of patients in group A, 33.3% in group B and 20% in patients group C. A score between 7 and 10 points were obtained 13.3% of group B patients and 60% of patients in group C.

V. Discussions

In our study there was a marked increase in the amount of sensory neuropathy detected in patients with >10 years duration of diabetes using the SWMT and R-CPT measurements by the Neurometer. Our results also showed a statistically higher incidence of sensory neuropathy in patients with >10 years duration of diabetes when compared with those with <5 years duration of diabetes (SWMF: p=0.03, Neurometer 250Hz: p=0.038; 5Hz: p=0.02). These findings are consistent with existing evidence. Sosenko et al. (1999), in their study involving 3638 American Indians, found that marked foot insensitivity detected with the SWMT was uncommon within the first few years of diagnosis of diabetes, and that individuals who had diabetes between 5 and 10 years were twice as likely to have had sensory neuropathy than those who had diabetes for <5 years [15].

The incidence of sensory neuropathy detected by the Neurometer (250Hz: 30%, 5Hz: 46.6%) is significantly higher than that detected by the SWMT (21.7%), statistical significant only for 5Hz (p=0.01). Hence, we find that the Neurometer can be a useful additional tool for the detection of sensory neuropathy, in addition to SWMT. In a similar study done by Cheng et al. (1999) which involved 558 type 2 diabetics, 59 were found to be positive on SWMT, 45 positive on Vibration Perception Threshold and 189 positive on R-CPT measurements by the Neurometer [16]. They found that the Neurometer detected peripheral sensory neuropathy in significantly more patients as compared to SWMT and Vibration Perception Threshold.

Even for patients with <5 years duration of diabetes (Group A), sensory neuropathy was present in 11.4% (SWMT) and 17.4% (big toe site 2000Hz) of the patients. This incidence is considerable. Neuropathy further increased in Group B and Group C.

VI. Conclusions

Our results showed that a higher incidence of sensory neuropathy was found in patients with a longer duration of diabetes, especially in those who have been diagnosed for >5 years. We found a significant incidence of sensory neuropathy in diabetics with less than 5 years duration of diabetes. Therefore, we recommend screening for sensory neuropathy in patients as soon as diabetes is diagnosed.

Also CPT measurement with the Neurometer has been shown to be clinically valuable in detecting peripheral nerve dysfunction. Applying 5Hz current detected the most patients with diabetic neuropathy compared to the other two frequencies, finding that confirm the well- known fact that diabetes mellitus is a small fiber disease. Also, frequency of 5Hz was found to be the most sensitive in detecting patients with hyper and hypoesthesia. This method has the advantages of being able to assess large myelinated, medium-size myelinated and unmyelinated fibres, and to divide patients with diabetic neuropathy into those with normoaesthesia, hyperaesthesia and hypoaesthesia.

However, it does have limitations in terms of its sensitivity and large variability. A combination of conventional methods with CPT should therefore be helpful in elucidating disordered peripheral nerve function in diabetic patients.

Conflict of Interest

The authors declare that they have no conflict of interest.

Statement of Human and Animal Rights

The procedures involving human subjects conducted in this study were in accordance with the ethical standards of the responsible committee on human experimentation (institutional and national) and with the Helsinki Declaration of 1975, as revised in 2000 and 2008.

References

1. Boulton AJ, Vinik AI, Arezzo JC, et al.; American Diabetes Association. Diabetic neuropathies: a statement by the American Diabetes Association. Diabetes Care 2005; 28: 956-962
2. Duby, J. J., Campbell, R. K., Setter, S. M., White, J. R., & Rasmussen, K. A. (2004). Diabetic neuropathy: An intensive review. American Journal of Health-System Pharmacy, 61 (2), 160– 173
3. Rith-Njarian S, Branchaud C, Beaulieu O, Gohdes D, Simonson G,Mazze R. Reducing lower-extremity amputation due to diabetes: application of the staged diabetes management approach in a primary care setting. J Fam Pract 1998; 47: 127-32
4. Nather A, Bee CS, Huak CY, Chew JL, Lin CB, Lin CB, Neo S, et al. Epidemiology of diabetic foot problems and predictive factors for limb loss. J Diabetes Complications. 2008; 22: 77-82
5. American Diabetes Association, American Academy of Neurology: Report and recommendations of the San Antonio Conference on Diabetic Neuropathy (Consensus Statement). Diabetes Care 11:592–597, 1988
6. Solomon Tesfaye, Andrew J.M. Boulton, Peter J. Dyck, et al. on behalf of the Toronto Diabetic Neuropathy Expert Group. Diabetic Neuropathies: Update on Definitions, Diagnostic Criteria, Estimation of Severity, and Treatments. Diabetes Care. 2010; 33(10): 2285–2293
7. Matsutomo, R., Takebayashi, K., & Aso, Y. (2005). Assessment of peripheral neuropathy using measurement of the current perception threshold with the Neurometer in patients with type 2 diabetes mellitus. Journal of International Medical Research, 33 (4), 442– 453
8. Nather, A, Lin WK, Aziz, Z., et al. Assessment of sensory neuropathy in patients with diabetic foot problems. Diabetic Foot & Ankle. 2011; 2: 6367
9. Oh,O.S.H., Sung, J.J., Hong, Y.H., Park, S. H., Lee, K.W., Park, W.S.. The value of measuring current perception threshold in diabetic sensory polyneuropathy with normal routine NCS. European Journal of Anaesthesiology. 2008; 25(43): 1–36
10. Aziz Nather, Shu Hui Neo, Siok Bee Chionh, Stanley C.F. Liew, Eileen Y. Sim, Jocelyn L.L. Chew. Assessment of sensory neuropathy in diabetic patients without diabetic foot problems. Journal of Diabetes and its Complications 22 (2008) 126-131
11. American College of Physicians Clinical Skills Module "Diabetic Foot Ulcers"
12. Masson, E. A., Veves, A., Fernando, D., & Boulton, A. J. (1989). Current perception thresholds: A new, quick and reproducible method for the assessment of peripheral neuropathy in diabetes mellitus. Diabetologia, 32 (10), 724–728.
13. www.neurotron.com
14. Meijer JW, Smit AJ, Sonderen EV, Groothoff JW, Eisma WH, Links TP. Symptom scoring systems to diagnose distal polyneuropathy in diabetes: the Diabetic Neuropathy Symptom score. Diabet Med. 2002;19:962-965
15. Sosenko, J. M., Sparling, Y. H., Hu, D. S.,Welty, T., Howard, B. V., Lee, E., & Robbings, D. C. (1999). Use of the Semmes-Weinstein monofilament in the Strong Heart Study. Diabetes Care, 22, 1715–1721
16. Cheng, W. Y., Jiang, Y. D., Chuang, L. M., Huang, C. N., Heng, L. T., & Wu, H. P. (1999). Quantitative sensory testing and risk factors of diabetic sensory neuropathy. Journal of Neurology, 246, 394– 398.

Author: Georgeta Inceu
Institute: "IULIU HATIEGANU" University of Medicine and Pharmacy
Street: 2-4 Clinicilor Street
City: Cluj-Napoca
Country: Romania
Email: georgetainceu@yahoo.com

An Evolutionary Multi-objective Optimization Approach to Design the Sound Processor of a Hearing Aid

P. Faragó, C. Faragó, S. Hintea, and M. Cîrlugea

Bases of Electronics Department, Technical University of Cluj-Napoca, Faculty of Electronics, Telecommunications and Information Technology, Cluj-Napoca, Romania

Abstract— **Hearing impairment is one of the most common problems nowadays which affects the quality of life in terms of speech understanding and communication abilities. Therefore, untreated hearing loss may negatively impact social life. Mild to moderate hearing loss may be compensated by employing a hearing aid. The hearing aid performs sub-band division of the auditory signal, and then amplifies each sub-band in order to correct the patient's audiogram. Designing the hearing aid sound processor for optimal audiogram correction requires the determination of the number of sub-bands, filter order and sub-band gains respectively. Considering the conflicting nature between solution quality and hardware resources, designing the sound processor is a matter of compromise. This article proposes an evolutionary approach to designing the sound processor, which treats the design as a multi-objective optimization (MOO) problem. Thus, the sub-band number, the sub-band filter order and the audiogram correction function are simultaneously optimized. The determination of the sub-band gains, for a given configuration of sub-band number and filter order, is treated as a single-objective optimization (SOO) problem. Dedicated genetic algorithms (GA) are used to solve both MOO and SOO problems. The MOO was handled with the Pareto frontier method. The functionality of the proposed design algorithm is illustrated on two conclusive design examples for optimal audiogram correction.**

Keywords— **hearing aid, sound processor, genetic algorithms, multi-objective optimization, Pareto frontier.**

I. Introduction

Hearing impairment is one of the most common problems nowadays which affects the quality of life. More than 500 million people worldwide experience a certain degree of hearing loss [1].

Hearing impairment affects speech understanding, and consequently communication abilities. Adults suffering from hearing loss may experience difficulties with respect to employment, education, and general well-being. As far as children are concerned, hearing loss can severely impact learning and development. Thus, untreated hearing loss may negatively impact the social life [2].

The three basic types of hearing loss are classified, depending on the underlying disease, into conductive hearing loss, sensorineural hearing loss, and mixed hearing loss [2]. For a correct assessment of the severity of hearing impairment, hearing loss is characterized in terms of degree of hearing loss and configuration of hearing loss.

The degree of hearing loss provides a quantitative representation in dB of the auditory signal attenuation. Different ranges of the degree of hearing loss are listed in Table 1 [2]. Accordingly, hearing impairment accounts for more than 20 dB hearing loss.

Table 1 Ranges of the degree of hearing loss [2]

Degree of hearing loss	Hearing attenuation in dB
Normal	<15
Slight	16 to 25
Mild	26 to 40
Moderate	41 to 55
Moderately severe	56 to 70
Severe	71 to 90
Profound	> 91

The configuration of the hearing loss provides an assessment of the degree of hearing loss vs. frequency. A graphical representation of the configuration of hearing loss is the audiogram. The shape of the audiogram differs depending on the underlying disease. For example, conductive hearing loss accounts for a flat audiogram. Sensorineural hearing loss, mixed hearing loss and hearing loss caused by noise damage and aging account for a high-frequency hearing loss. Another common type of audiogram describes the reverse sloping hearing loss [3, 4]. While conductive hearing loss can be treated with medical or surgical intervention, sensorineural hearing loss is permanent and must be compensated with some form of auditory prosthesis.

A hearing aid is a battery powered electronic device used to restore hearing to patients with mild to moderate hearing loss. Hearing aids basically consist of a microphone, a sound processor and a miniature speaker, i.e. the receiver. The sound received by the microphone is amplified with certain frequency selectivity within the sound processor and applied by the speaker into the patient's ear.

A typical implementation of the speech processor is illustrated in figure 1 and resembles a multi-channel

DOI: 10.1007/978-3-319-07653-9_37,

processing strategy. An automatic gain control (AGC) compresses the microphone signal into a narrower dynamic range. A bank of bandpass filters (BPF) performs sub-band division of the incoming auditory signal, and then each sub-band is amplified independently. Digital implementations of the sound processor are common nowadays due to numerous advantages, e.g. flexibility, high number of channel filters, high-order BPFs, programmability feature, etc. However, advances in programmable low-power analog electronics have enabled the analog implementation of the AGC [5, 6] and analog filters [7, 8], making analog signal processing an attractive alternative to the digital counterpart.

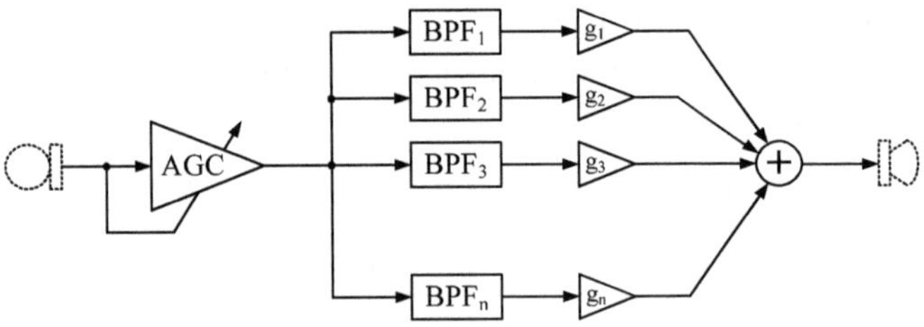

Fig. 1 Block diagram of the multi-channel speech processor

In this article we propose an evolutionary approach to automate the design of the sound processor for optimal audiogram correction. Designing the sound processor for audiogram correction requires two stages: designing the filter-bank for sub-band division and designing the sub-band gains. The novelty of this article stands in the employment of genetic algorithms (GA) to solve the design problem.

This article is organized as follows. Section 2 defines the sound processor design problem. Section 3 describes the evolutionary approach to the sound processor design problem. Finally, some conclusive simulation results are given in Section 4.

II. THE SOUND PROCESSOR DESIGN PROBLEM

The sound processor of a multi-channel hearing aid is defined by a vector

$$[n, H_i \mid i=1\ldots n] \quad (1)$$

where n is the number of sub-bands and H_i is the transfer function of sub-band i processing chain, with i ranging from 1 to n. The transfer function H_i of the ith sub-band processing chain, consisting of a BPF and an amplifier, is defined by a vector:

$$[g, fc, BW, o] \quad (2)$$

where g is the sub-band amplifier gain, fc is the sub-band central frequency, BW is the sub-band bandwidth and o is the filter order.

The sub-band division of the audio bandwidth into n sub-bands is illustrated in figure 2,

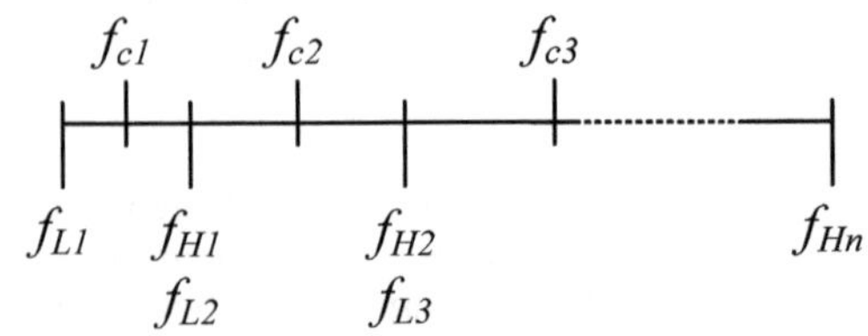

Fig. 2 Division of the audio bandwidth into n sub-bands

where f_{ci}, f_{Li} and f_{Hi}, are the center, lower cutoff and upper cutoff frequencies respectively, and BW_i is the bandwidth of band-pass filter i. A logarithmic sub-band distribution, expressed as

$$\begin{cases} f_{c_{i+1}} = q \cdot f_{c_i} \\ BW_{i+1} = q \cdot BW_i \end{cases} \quad (3)$$

where q is a constant defined as

$$q = \frac{f_{c_{i+1}}}{f_{c_i}} = \frac{f_{H_i}}{f_{L_i}} = \sqrt[n]{\frac{f_{H_n}}{f_{L_1}}} \quad (4)$$

best reproduces the physiology of hearing [9] and is therefore used in the hearing aid sound processor. The central frequency of each BPF is computed using factor q as

$$f_{c_i} = f_{L_1} \cdot q^{i-\frac{1}{2}} \quad (5)$$

which is then used to compute the BPF boundary frequencies [9]

$$\begin{cases} f_{L_i} = \frac{f_{c_i}}{\sqrt{q}} \\ f_{H_i} = f_{c_i} \cdot \sqrt{q} \end{cases} \quad (6)$$

At this point stands the question of the optimal BPF number for sub-band division. A high number of BPFs obviously provides a fine resolution for the approximation of the audiogram correction function. This benefit comes with the cost of increased power consumption. On the other hand, design for a small number of BPFs will reduce the power consumption, but will affect the resolution, and implicitly the quality of the audiogram correction. Similarly, high-order BPFs achieve good sub-band selectivity. High-order filters however require more active elements, which increases the power consumption. In digital implementations, high-order filters will also cause higher signal latency. Therefore, the choice of the BPF number, filter order and filter shape is a matter of compromise.

Once the filter-bank is designed, the next step is to determine the sub-band gains to compensate the auditory signal attenuation in each sub-band respectively.

Therefore, designing the sound processor translates to the complete determination of vector (1).

III. THE PROPOSED EVOLUTIONARY DESIGN APPROACH

In the proposed sound processor design approach, the design problem is defined as a multi-objective optimization (MOO) problem and is solved with genetic algorithms.

Genetic algorithms (GA) are an iterative search method which operate on a population of solution candidates in order to minimize an objective function. A flow diagram of the GA is illustrated in figure 3 and is explained as follows.

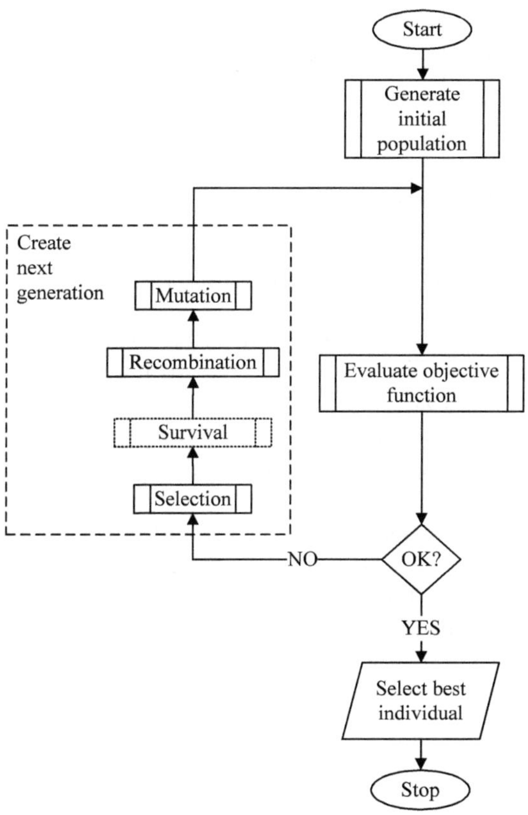

Fig. 3 Block diagram of the Genetic Algorithm [10]

An initial population is randomly created according to a predefined chromosome pattern. The population is then evaluated in order to compute the fitness of each individual and see whether the optimization criteria are met. Should the optimization criteria be met, the algorithm stops. Otherwise, the algorithm enters the evolutionary loop to create a new generation by applying genetic operators inspired from natural evolution: selection, recombination and mutation. Additionally, the GA implementation from figure 3 applies the survival operator which copies the fittest individuals from one generation to the next. The evolutionary loop is repeated until the optimization criteria are finally met. The fittest individual from the final generation is the result of the evolutionary process [10, 11].

The chromosome to represent a solution candidate is defined as a triplet

$$[n,o,G] \quad (7)$$

where G is a vector of n gain values, corresponding to the n sub-bands respectively. Chromosome (7) is decoded as follows. The filter bank is designed with equations (4-6) starting from BPF number n and filter order o. Next, each sub-band is amplified with the corresponding gain value from vector G.

The MOO problem aims to optimize three distinct, yet competing, objectives. The first objective is to optimize the audiogram correction function for an increased hearing experience. This is performed by minimizing an error function which measures the difference between the expected and the instantaneous audiogram correction function respectively. The audiogram correction error is defined as

$$err = \sum_f \left| a^{audiogram}(f) - G^{correction}(f) \right| \quad (8)$$

where $a^{audiogram}$ is the attenuation in the patient's audiogram, $G^{correction}$ is the sub-band amplifier gain and f is the frequency for which the error value is estimated. The error value is computed as the sum of the audiogram correction error values for every frequency in the audiogram.

The next two objectives target the minimization of the BPF number – n, and the filter order – o. The MOO objective function is thus a vector of three elements, standing for the three distinct objectives respectively, each aiming towards minimization:

$$[err, n, o] \quad (9)$$

To be noticed is that, while individual objectives n and o directly appear in the definition of the GA chromosome (7), objective err is computed only after evaluating the current solution candidate. The determination of an optimal vector G to minimizes error function err is treated as a single-objective optimization (SOO) problem, and is solved in a dedicated GA run for each instantaneous value of n and o respectively.

We have chosen the Pareto frontier method to solve the MOO problem, because it is proven to maintain population diversity along the evolutionary process [12]. In Pareto optimization all distinct objectives are considered equally important, and the solution candidates are evaluated in terms of Pareto optimality, i.e. Pareto non-dominance.

Consider two distinct solutions to the MOO problem a_1 and a_2, and multi-objective function OF with k independent objectives OF_i, i=1…k. Solution a_1 dominates solution a_2 if and only if a_1 is not weaker than a_2 in any of the k objectives, but it is better in at least one objective [11, 12]. Dominance is expressed as:

$$a_1 \preccurlyeq a_2 \; iff \begin{cases} OF_i(a_1) \leq OF_i(a_2), \forall i \in \{1 \dots k\} \\ \exists j \in \{1 \dots k\}, OF_j(a_1) < OF_j(a_2) \end{cases} \quad (10)$$

A solution a^* is Pareto optimal, or non-dominated, if and only if it is not dominated by any other solution a. Pareto optimality is expressed as follows:

$$\begin{gathered} a^* \; is \; Pareto \; optimal \; iff \\ \nexists a \; for \; which \; a \preccurlyeq a^* \end{gathered} \quad (11)$$

Considering the conflicting nature of the individual objective, it is clear that any Pareto optimal solution is not unique. The set of Pareto optimal solutions constitutes the Pareto optimal set, i.e. the Pareto frontier. Thus, the solution to the MOO problem in terms of Pareto optimality is the Pareto frontier, rather than a single solution. The difficulty of using the Pareto frontier method to solve the MOO problem stands in the fact that user intervention is needed to choose the preferred solution from the Pareto optimal set.

IV. Simulation Results

The proposed sound processor automatic design algorithm was implemented in Matlab using the Genetic algorithm and Direct Search Toolbox.

The GA to solve MOO problem, in order to optimize the number of sub-channels, the filter order and the audiogram correction function was implemented as follows. The population size was initialized to 30. The GA was implemented with a 80% cross-over rate and 20% mutation rate. Reproduction was implemented with a tournament selection scheme, an intermediate cross-over and a constraint dependent mutation scheme. Mutation was implemented with a Gaussian probabilistic function. The stopping criteria accounts for a maximum GA runtime of 400 generations, or a number of 100 stall generation with an objective function tolerance of 10^{-4}.

For practical reasons, the maximum number of sub-channels was restricted to 16 and the maximum filter order was restricted to 12.

The GA to solve SOO problem, in order to compute the sub-channel gains, was implemented as follows. The population size was initialized to 60. The GA was implemented with a survival of 3 individuals, 70% cross-over rate and 30% mutation rate. Fitness scaling was implemented with a rank-based scaling scheme. Reproduction was implemented with a stochastic uniform selection scheme and a scattered cross-over scheme. Mutation was implemented with a Gaussian probabilistic function. The stopping criteria accounts for a maximum GA runtime of 200 generations, or a number of 10 stall generation with a function tolerance of 10^{-6}.

Two conclusive design examples are presented as follows to illustrate the functionality of the proposed design algorithm.

The first design example presents the correction of an audiogram, resembling a rather flat configuration of a mild hearing loss, figure 4.

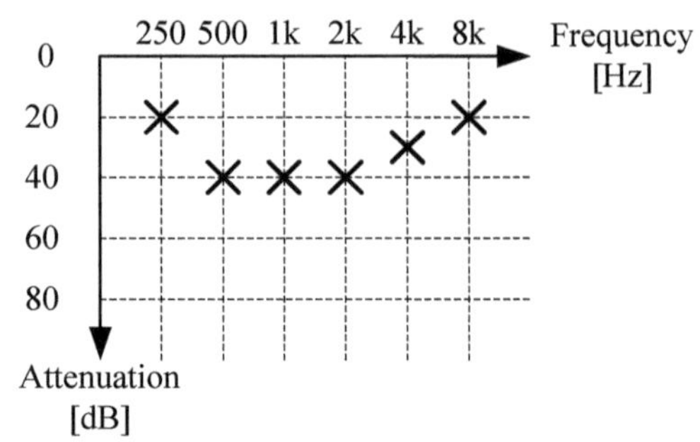

Fig. 4 Audiogram, resembling a flat configuration of a mild hearing loss

The multi-objective GA run lasted for 30 generations. The Euclidian distance d between two individuals i and j, $i \neq j$, expressed as

$$d = \sqrt{(n_i - n_j)^2 + (o_i - o_j)^2 + (G_i - G_j)^2} \quad (12)$$

is used to investigate population diversity along the evolutionary process. The average distance between individuals is plotted in figure 5, demonstrating that population diversity is indeed maintained along the evolutionary process.

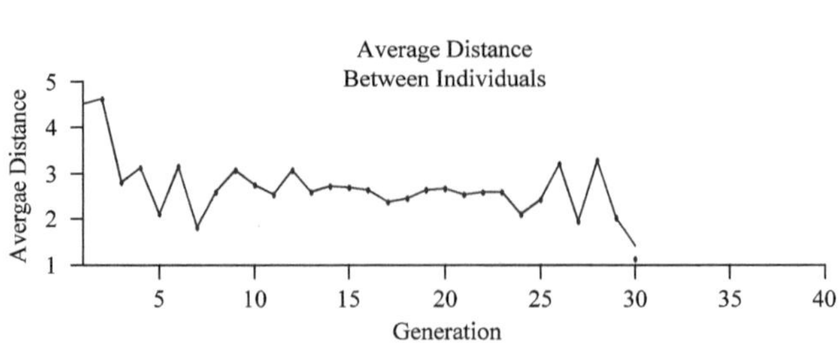

Fig. 5 Average distance between individuals vs. generations

The individuals on the Pareto frontier are listed in table 2. The *n* vs. *err* objectives for the individuals on the Pareto frontier are plotted in figure 6. The *o* vs. *err* objectives for the individuals on the Pareto frontier are plotted in figure 7.

Table 2 The Pareto frontier after the GA run

Individual	err	n	o
1	5.0912	1	2
2	0.7035	4	4
3	0.6921	4	6
4	1.5475	2	2
5	1.5453	2	2
6	1.4759	3	2
7	1.4414	3	4

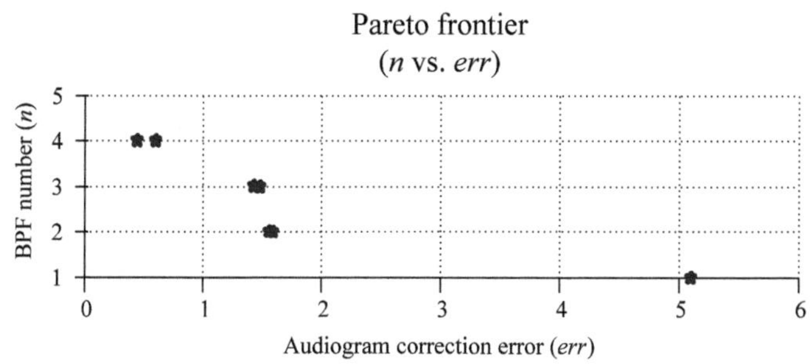

Fig. 6 Pareto frontier *n* vs. *err*

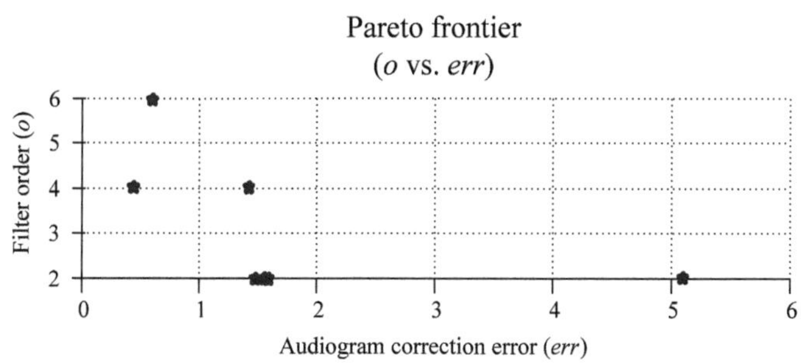

Fig. 7 Pareto frontier *o* vs. *err*

As expected, a high audiogram correction accuracy is achieved for a high number of BPFs in the filter bank. Similarly, a high audiogram accuracy is achieved for high sub-band selectivity, i.e. high filter order.

We have chosen Individual 2 from the Pareto frontier because it is the best compromise between audiogram correction accuracy, number of sub-channels and filter order. For individual 2, the vector of sub-band gains resulting after the SOO GA run is

$$G = [20\ 40\ 30\ 20] \qquad (13)$$

The single-objective GA run lasted for 128 generations. The evolution of the objective function vs. generations is plotted in figure 8, with solid line for the best fitness and dotted line for the mean fitness, illustrating algorithm convergence.

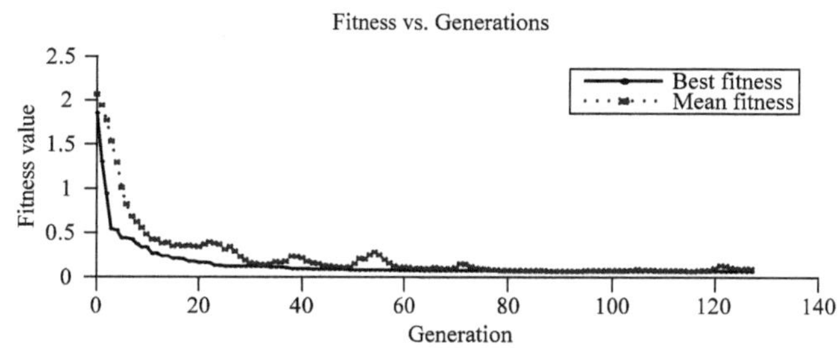

Fig. 8 Evolution of the fitness value vs. generations

The filter-bank with the corresponding sub-band gains for optimal audiogram correction is illustrated in figure 9.

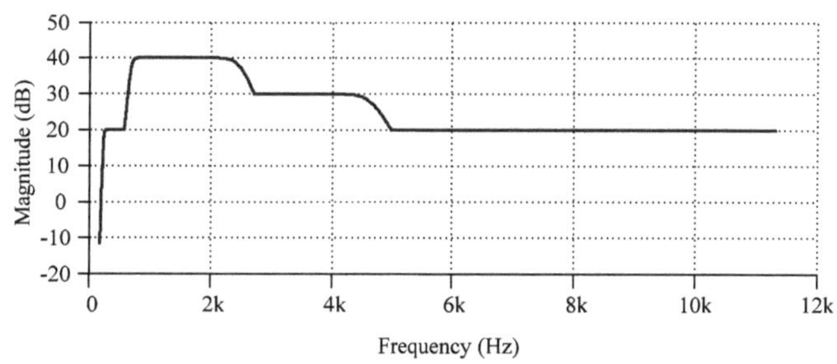

Fig. 9 The audiogram correction characteristics

The second design example presents the correction of an audiogram, resembling a high-frequency severe hearing loss, figure 10.

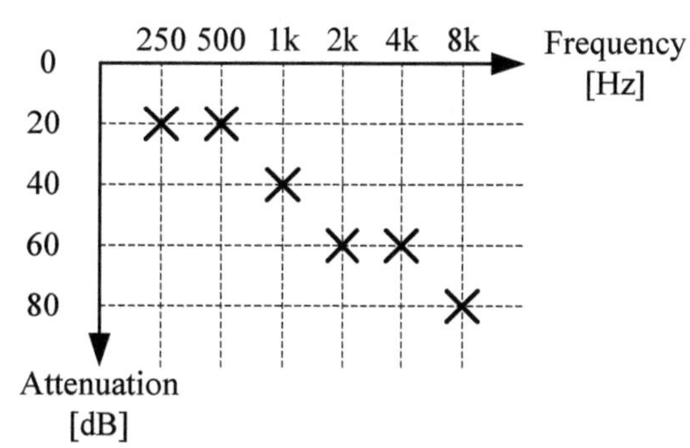

Fig. 10 Audiogram, resembling a severe high-frequency hearing loss

The individuals on the Pareto frontier are listed in table 3. We have chosen Individual 5 from the Pareto frontier because it is the best compromise between audiogram correction accuracy, sub-channel number and filter order. For individual 5, the vector of sub-band gains resulting after the SOO GA run is

$$G = [20\ 40\ 60\ 60\ 80\ 80] \quad (14)$$

Table 3 The Pareto frontier after the GA run

Individual	err	n	o
1	1.8220	12	2
2	2.1810	9	2
3	7.1900	1	2
4	1.4240	3	12
5	0.8480	6	8
6	1.7130	3	6
7	1.7330	4	8

The single-objective GA run lasted for 132 generations. The filter-bank with the corresponding sub-band gains for optimal audiogram correction is illustrated in figure 11.

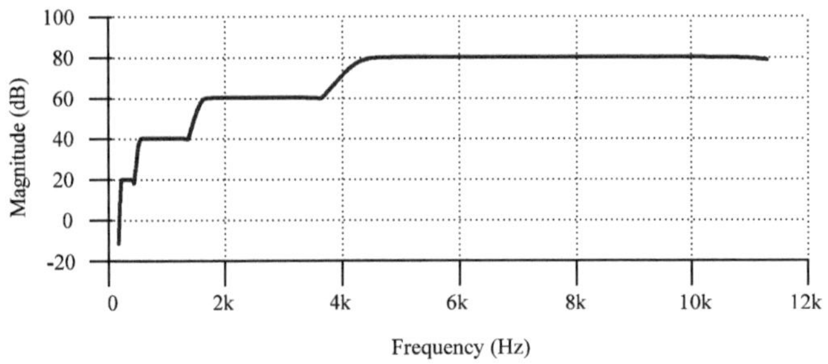

Fig. 11 The audiogram correction characteristics

V. Conclusions

This article illustrated an evolutionary approach to solve the problem of designing a multi-channel sound processor for optimal audiogram correction with hearing aids. The design problem was formulated as a MOO problem and was solved with GAs. The Pareto frontier method was used to handle the multi-objective nature of the optimization problem. The functionality of the proposed design algorithm was illustrated on two specific examples of audiogram correction.

The simulation results illustrate that the specifications for audiogram correction are fully satisfied. However, the recorded design times are rather long, stemming from the imbrication of two distinct GAs. As future work, we propose to shorten the design time by defining a variable length representation of the design problem and solve it in a single evolutionary process.

Conflict of Interest

The authors declare that they have no conflict of interest.

References

1. Unitron at http://unitron.com/unitron/global/en/consumer/your_hearing-c/hearing_loss.html
2. American Speech-Language-Hearing Association at http://www.asha.org/public/hearing/What-is-Hearing-Loss/
3. Auditory Neuroscience at http://auditoryneuroscience.com/
4. Pediatric hearing loss at http://www.utdallas.edu/~thib/rehabinfo/index.html
5. Hintea S, Farago P, Roman M N, Oltean G, Festila L (2011) A Programmable Gain Amplifier for Automated Gain Control in Auditory Prostheses, J. Med. Biol. Eng., Vol. 31. No 3. 2011, pp 185–192.
6. Baker W, Sarpeshkar R (2006) Low-power single-loop and dual-loop AGCs for bionic ears, IEEE J. Solid-St. Circ., 41: 1983-1996, 2006
7. Csipkes G, Festila L, Csipkes D (2006) Modular Design of Current Input-Current Output Filters Based on Passive LC Ladder Prototypes, Communications 2006, 8-10 June, Bucharest, pp 37-40
8. Hintea S, Farago P, Festila L, Soser P (2010) Recon-figurable Filter Design for Implantable Auditory Prosthesis, Electronics and Electrical Engineering No.3(99), 2010, pp.712
9. Gratzl M, Janata J, (1989) Filter banks for power spectrum estimation with a logarithmically uniform frequency resolution, J. Phys. E: Sci. Instrum. 22, 1989, pp. 863-868
10. Hintea S, Csipkes G, Csipkes D et al (2011) Reconfigurable Analog Circuits for Mobile Communications - Variable topology filters and design automation, Editura Casa cărtii de ştiinţa, 2011
11. Zebulum R S, Pacheco M A C, Vellasco M M B R (2002) Evolutionary Electronics - Automatic Design of Electronic Circuits and Systems by Genetic Algorithms, CRC Press
12. Cvetkovic D, Parmee I C (1999) Genetic Algorithm–based Multi–objective Optimisation and Conceptual Engineering Design, Congress on Evolutionary Computation, Washington D.C., USA, 1999.

Author: Paul FARAGÓ
Institute: Technical University of Cluj-Napoca, Faculty of electronics, Telecommunications and Information Technology, Bases of Electronics Department
Street: Baritiu 26-28
City: Cluj-Napoca
Country: Romania
Email: paul.farago@bel.utcluj.ro

Equipment for SEMG Signals Acquisition and Processing

E.P. Vesa and B. Ilie

Computer and Electric Engineering Department, "Lucian Blaga" University Sibiu, Romania

Abstract— **Electromyography is a technique for evaluating the electrical activity of muscles. The EMG signal measurement is useful for the detection and analysis of muscle tissue activity. If the EMG signal is acquired from the surface of the skin, the signal is called Surface EMG or SEMG. The SEMG signal is a small amplitude signal which is strongly affected by noise. SEMG signal processing increases the signal–to-noise ratio (SNR), optimizes the electrode-skin impedance, and cancels the crosstalk of adjacent units. The SNR depends on external electromagnetic disturbances, and also on the quality of the equipment involved in the acquisition of EMG signal, like electrodes, preamplifiers, analogue-to-digital convertors (ADC) and digital processing blocks. This paper presents the development and implementation of a SEMG signal acquisition block. This block amplifies, filtrates, converts and memorizes in digital format for further processing the SEMG signal. The main IC is TI's ADS1298 Low-Power, 8-Channel, 24-Bit analogue front-end for biopotential measurements. Our implementation uses in front of the ADS1298 a set of instrumentation amplifiers, AD620, in order to increase the SNR. The ADS1298 transfers the digital data to a microcontroller via a SPI interface. We intend to use the Xilinx XUPV5 platform to digitally process the signal, so this board is interfaced with the microcontroller via a parallel interface.**

Keywords— **SEMG amplifier, ADS1298, instrumentation amplifier, microcontroller**

I. INTRODUCTION

Electromyography is a technique for evaluating the electrical activity of muscles. [1].

Small electrical currents are generated by muscle fibres prior to the production of muscle force. These currents are generated by the exchange of ions across muscle fibre membranes, as part of the signalling process for the muscle fibres to contract [2]. The EMG signal can be measured by applying electrodes to the skin surface.

The measurement of the SEMG signal is dependent on a series of factors: the timing and intensity of muscle contraction, the distance of the electrode from the active muscle area, the properties of the tissue, the skin – electrode characteristics, the electrodes' and amplifiers' properties. [2]. The SEMG signal processing increases the signal-to-noise ratio (SNR), optimizes the electrode-skin impedance, and cancels the cross talk of adjacent units. The SNR depends on external electromagnetic disturbances, and also on the quality of the equipment involved in the acquisition of the EMG signal, like electrodes, preamplifiers, analogue-to-digital convertors (ADC) and digital processing blocks. The goal in SEMG signal measurements is to maximize the signal-to-noise ratio SNR [2]. The most important noise parameter is the ambient noise generated by electromagnetic devices such as power lines, the AC power supply, especially switching power supply, and any kind of electrical equipment in the vicinity, including computers and cell phones.

Using a bipolar electrodes arrangement, with a differential amplifier input stage, the transducer noise and common signal components can be suppressed [3]. The stability of the skin electrode's impedance and the balance in impedance between the electrodes sites increases the SNR. The electrode-skin interface generates a DC voltage potential, mainly caused by a large increase in impedance from the outermost layer of skin, included dead skin material and oil secretion [2]. The DC potential can be minimized using gelled electrodes, or electrode gel between electrodes and skin. Crosstalk can be avoided by choosing the appropriate size of the electrodes' conductive area and the appropriate inter-electrode distance [2]. Decreasing the inter-electrode distance decreases the effective recording distance and shifts the EMG bandwidth to higher frequencies [4].

II. MATERIALS AND METHODS

The block schematic of the hardware interface is shown in Fig. 1. The main blocks are: the preamplifier units, the front-end IC with 8 channel amplifiers, filters and 24 bit ADC, the microcontroller block and the Xilinx XUPV5 platform.

The preamplifier units were made with low noise, high CMRR, low power AD 620 instrumentation amplifiers. The gain of the preamplifier was set to 75. The schematic is shown in Fig. 2. This block was added after several tests with the electrodes connected directly to ADS1298 front-end IC. In these tests the SNR was very poor, and we decided to introduce this preamplifier. In part III, Experimental Results, we will show that the decision to add this preamplifier brought about improved outcomes.

S. Vlad and R.V. Ciupa (eds.), *International Conference on Advancements of Medicine and Health Care through Technology*, IFMBE Proceedings 44,
DOI: 10.1007/978-3-319-07653-9_38,

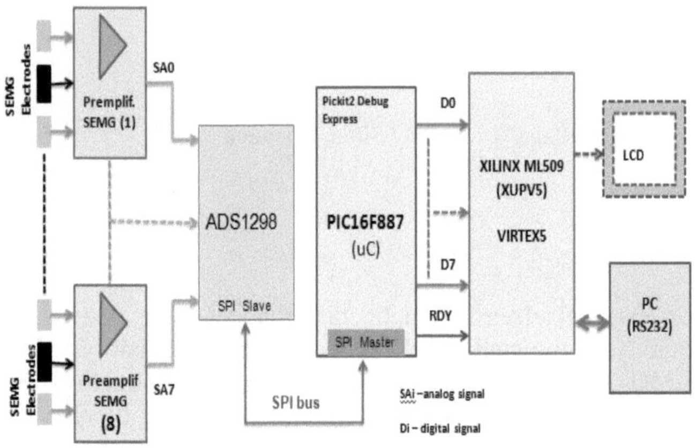

Fig. 1 Block diagram of the surface SEMG processing equipment

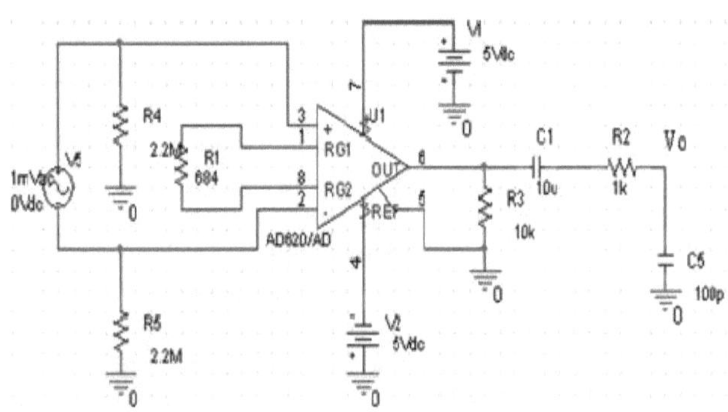

Fig. 2 SEMG signal preamplifier

The electrical parameters of the preamplifier are:

- Gain: 75
- Frequency bandwidth: 0 – 70kHz
- CMRR: 95 dB
- Input impedance: 4.4 MΩ
- Output impedance: 50 Ω
- Slew-rate: 1.2V/us
- Equivalent electrical noise at f=1kHz: $100uV/\sqrt{Hz}$

For SEMG electrodes we used low-cost, auto adhesive ECG electrodes. In this case the optimal values for R4 and R5 resistors (2.2 MΩ) were determined experimentally for minimum noise. The R1 resistor set the gain.

The global frequency characteristics of the SEMG preamplifier, plotted from simulation in ORCAD Pspice v.9.2 environment, are shown in Fig. 3. The characteristic is for a band–pass amplifier with f_{LP}=0.16Hz, f_{HP}=76.5 kHz, and 37dB gain. The C1 capacitor avoids the DC saturation of the ADS1298 due to the skin-electrode offset voltage.

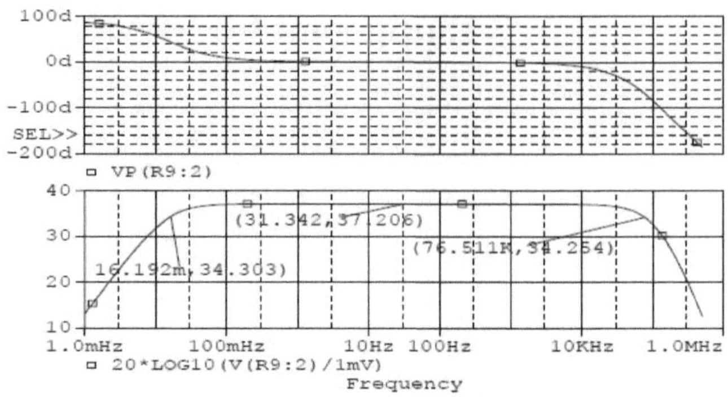

Fig. 3 SEMG preamplifier phase/frequency characteristics

The front–end of this equipment was designed with a powerful IC ADS1298 made by Texas Instruments. The ADS1298 is a multichannel, simultaneous sampling, 24-bit, delta-sigma (ΔΣ) analog-to-digital converters (ADCs) with built-in programmable gain amplifiers (PGAs), internal reference, and an onboard oscillator [10]. The ADS1298 incorporates all of the features that are commonly required in medical applications that involve biological signal measurements, like ECG, EEG or EMG. The internal structure of this IC is very flexible and we use this features in order to develop a specific SEMG signal application.

The ADS1298 is connected to the preamplifiers stages in a single–ended configuration. This configuration is not the best one for noise, but allows us to measure the signal with the oscilloscope.

In the case of SEMG signals, the amplification of the preamplifier unit built in the IC can be set to a maximum 12. This is not enough in SEMG measurement case. The ADS1298 functions are the following:

- Amplify the SEMG signal to the max amplitude $U_{PP}=U_{REF}$=2.4V.
- Simultaneous sampling and 24 bit conversions of 8 channels.
- Act as slave SPI circuit, and transmits the discrete SEMG signal to the microcontroller board.

We use the *ADS1298ECG-FE* board from Texas Instruments.

The microcontroller board, built with PIC16F887 IC, acts as master in SPI communication, configures the ADS1298 via SPI, and converts the digital SEMG data in a parallel structure of 3 words of 8 bits for the Virtex-5 circuit. For the compatibility with the Xilinx XUPV5 board inputs, the PIC16F887 is powered with 3.3V. The schematic for connecting the microcontroller with ADS1298 and Xilinx XUPV5 board is shown in Fig. 4.

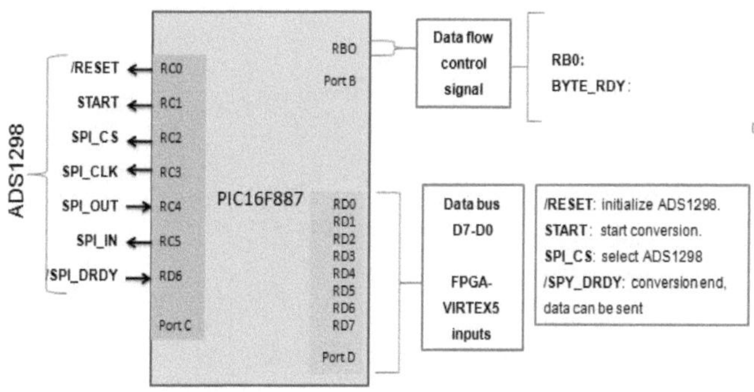

Fig. 4 Microcontroller connections with ADS1298 and Xilinx XUPV5

The data flow diagram is shown in Fig. 5. The total time for 1 channel read at F_{OSC}=20 MHz isT_{C1}=10.4us. For 8 channels the read cycle is: T_{C8}=83.2us.

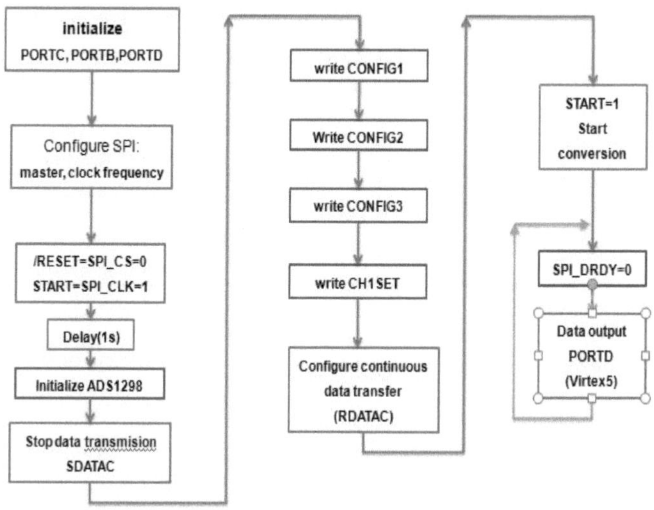

Fig. 5 Microcontroller data flow diagram

The hardware architecture is designed to permit watching the data flow between the component blocks.

For data processing we used the Xilinx XUPV5 board. Virtex-5 FPGAs contain many hard-IP system level blocks, including the powerful 36-Kbit block RAM/FIFOs, second generation 25 x 18 DSP slices, Select IO™ technology with built-in digitally controlled impedance, ChipSync™ source-synchronous interface blocks, system monitor functionality, enhanced clock management tiles with integrated DCM (Digital Clock Managers) and phase-locked-loop (PLL) clock generators, and advanced configuration options [9]. Figure 7 shows circuit internal architecture of Xilinx Virtex-5 used in the trial.

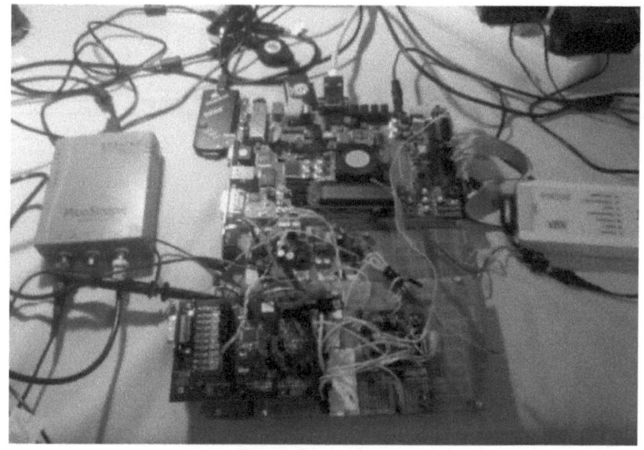

Fig. 6 Connecting Xilinx XUPV5 board to ADS1298 [12]

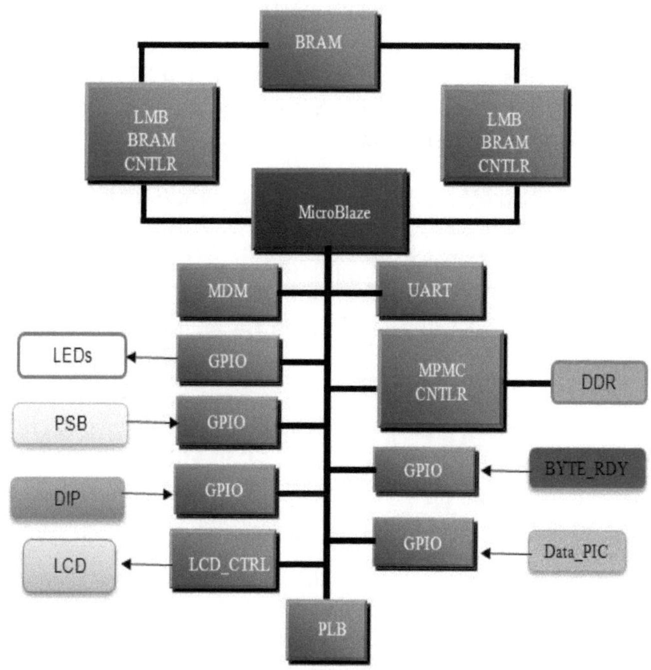

Fig. 7 Xilinx XUPV5 hardware configuration

III. EXPERIMENTAL RESULTS AND DISCUSSION

For reproducibility of the input signal, we use a special feature of the PicoScope 2205 MSO Oscilloscope. This feature permits to record a signal, to select a useful part of this signal as a pattern and generate this pattern at a chosen rate. The input signal is shown in Figure 8.

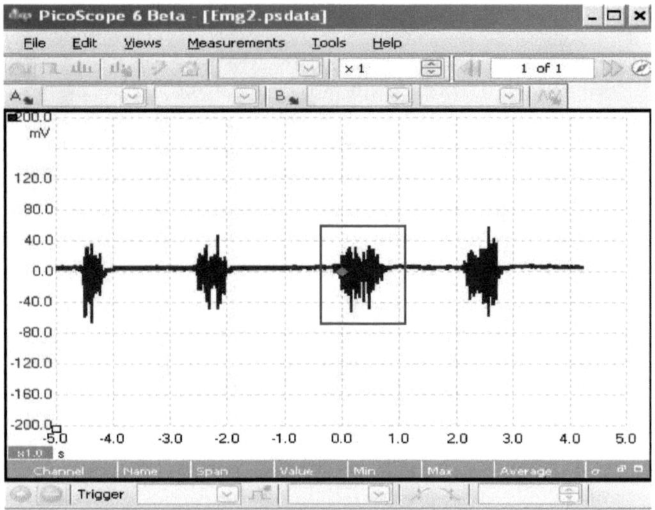

Fig. 8 Original SEMG signal

In the red square is the part of the original SEMG signal that we will use as pattern for test signal. Figure 9 shows the parameters of the test signal.

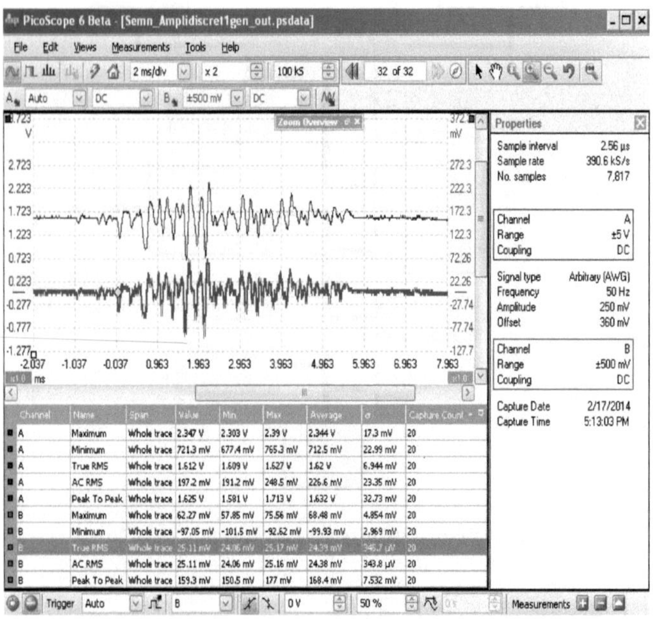

Fig. 9 Recorded SEMG signal by PicoScope 2205 MSO

The SEMG signal used to generate the pattern was sampled with three ECG electrodes, amplified and sampled with a 64.1 kHz frequency. For testing the equipment we used the block schematics depicted in Figure 10.

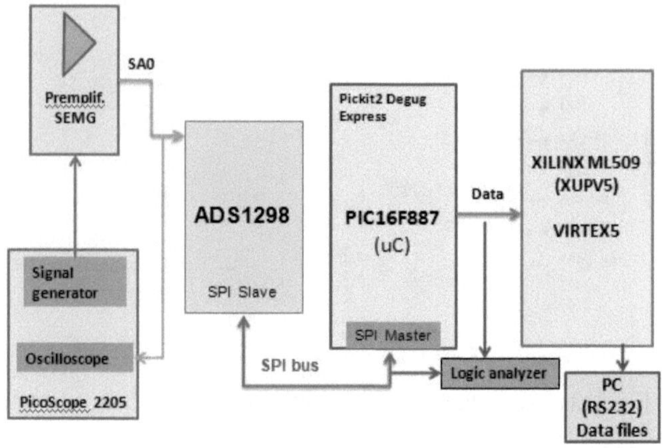

Fig. 10 Block diagram of the experimental setup

The SEMG signal used in the tests is a 20ms repetitive signal of the recorded pattern (Fig.10). The MISO line of the SPI signal between ADS1298 and PIC16F887 content the digital data of the SEMG signal, the data format for each channel data are two's complement ands first, and is depicted in Figure 11.

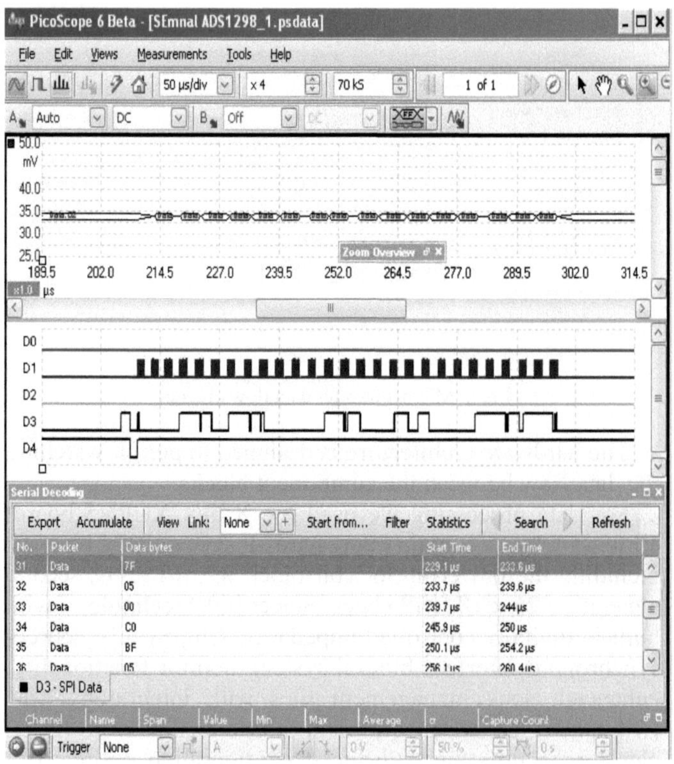

Fig. 11 The data signal on SPI interface between SDA1298 and PIC16F887

We used two logic analysers, first a PicoScope 2205 MSO with PicoScope 6 software, and second a Sigma Logic Analyzer 1.11, in order to exhaustively test the equipment.

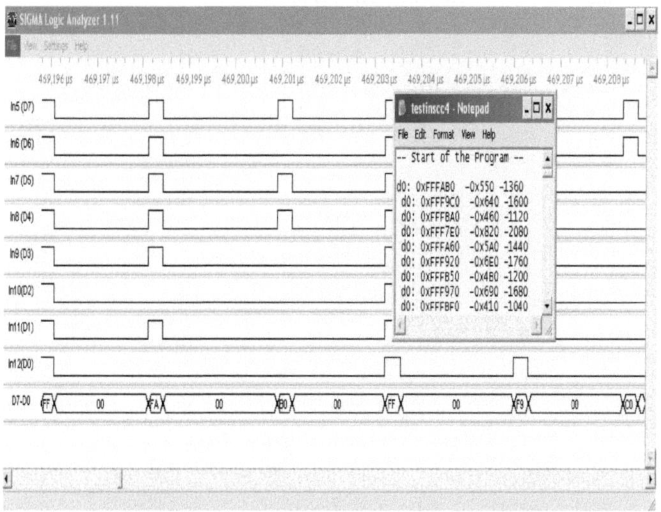

Fig. 12 The data signal on parallel interface between PIC16F887 and J6 connector on Xilinx board

The SEMG recorded in the DDR2 memory on XUPV5 board and converted from bins to voltage, as shown in Figure 13.

For the conversion the following relationship was used:

SEMG (V) =bins*LSB=bins*2.861e-7 (V);

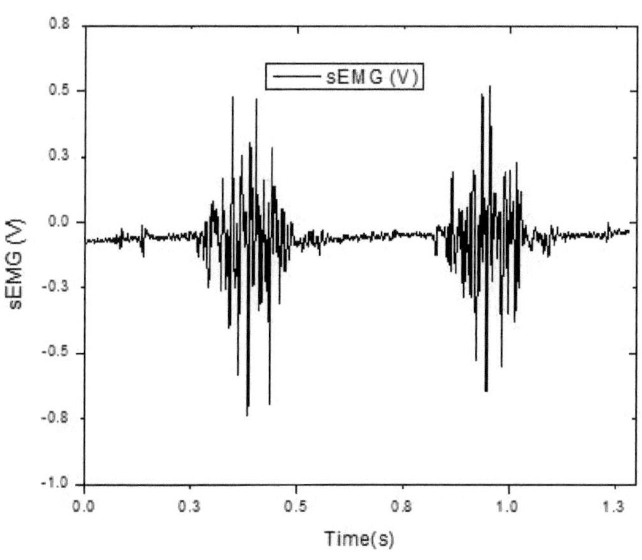

Fig. 13 The recorded signal (time voltage)

IV. Conclusions

In this paper we have developed an original SEMG signal acquisition system. The original part is the analogue-to-digital processing block. The decision to add a preamplifier section in front of the front-end ADS1298 reduced the noise, and increased the CMRR for SEMG signals in the case of the use of regular ECG gel electrodes. The development advantages of this method will be emphasised in future papers.

We have used the PIC16F877 microcontroller as a protocol adapter between the ADS1298 and the Xilinx board. This decision has allowed us to better track the digital signal. In future versions of this equipment the ADS1298 will be directly interfaced via a SPI interface with the Xilinx board.

Using the Xilinx board has allowed us to make on-line and off-line processing of the SEMG signals. The hardware algorithms for processing of the SEMG signal are very fast ones, making this equipment a valued platform for future research.

Conflict of Interest

The authors declare that they have no conflict of interest.

References

1. Merletti R, Parker P A (2004) Electromyography: physiology, engineering, and non-invasive applications, Wiley, New York
2. Malik R, Malik A (2012) Electromyography based hand control signals: a review, IJCSC, vol.3, no.1, January- June 2012, pp 43-45
3. Ahsan M R, Ibrahimy M I, Khalifa O O (2011) Neural network classifier for hand motion detection from EMG signal, IFMBE Proceedings 35, 2011, pp 536-541
4. Hansen J, Borau A et al (2007) Urethral Sphincter EMG as event detector for neurogenic detrusor overactivity, IEEE Transaction on biomedical engineering, vol. 54, no. 7, July 2007, pp 1212-1219
5. Song R, Tonga A Y et al. (2013) Myoelectrically controlled wrist robot for stroke rehabilitation, Journal of NeuroEngineering and Rehabilitation, 10:52, http://www.jneuroengrehab.com/content/10/1/52, DOI: 10.1186 / 1743 - 0003 - 10-52
6. Aditya V S R, Aggarwal R (2013), 2-D robotic arm control EMG signal, IJCA (0975-8887), vol. 72, no. 14, June 2013
7. Orosco E C, Lopez N M, Sciascio F (2013) Bispectrum-based features classification for myoelectric control, Biomedical Signal Processing and Control, vol. 8, issue 2, 2013, pp 153-168
8. Ganesh R N, Sridahar A, Dinesh K (2011) Applications of ICA and fractal dimension in sEMG signal processing for subtle movement analysis: a review, Australas Phys Eng Sci Med. 2011, 34 92):179-193, DOI 10.1007/s13246-011-0066-4

9. Xilinx XUPV5 at http://www.xilinx.com/univ/xupv5-lx110t.htm
10. http://www.ti.com/ADS1298
11. http://www.microchip.com/
12. Vesa E P (2013) Hardware processing of EMG signals, PhD report no. 1, Technical University Cluj-Napoca

Author: Vesa Eugen Petru
Institute: "Lucian Blaga" University Sibiu
Street: Bulevardul Victoriei, 10
City: Sibiu
Country: Romania
Email: eugen.vesa@ulbsibiu.ro

Assessment of Temperature Distribution in Intraperitoneal Chemohyperthermia

C. Lungoci[1], I. Raus[2], T. Oniu[1], D. Moga[3], N. Stroia[3], V. Muntean[1], D. Petreus[3], and I.A. Mironiuc[1]

[1] "Iuliu Haţieganu" University of Medicine and Pharmacy Cluj-Napoca, Romania
[2] "Dr. Constantin Papilian" Military Emergency Hospital of Cluj-Napoca, Romania
[3] Technical University of Cluj-Napoca, Romania

Abstract— **Advanced modeling techniques and multipoint temperature measurement devices are required in order to create a complex intraperitoneal chemohyperthermia physical model. This paper proposes two configurations appropriate for the implementation of a multipoint temperature measurement system. The design constrains were carefully defined considering the overall chemohyperthermia performance expectations and the need to provide thermal data for building a consistent *3D* thermal map of the intra-peritoneal volume.**

Keywords— **chemohyperthermia, peritoneal carcinomatosis, wireless sensor, temperature measurement**

I. INTRODUCTION

Peritoneal Carcinomatosis (PC) together with the hepatic metastases is related to the final stage of the cancer. Most authors consider PC as a systemic disease, featuring a remarkable resistance to standard treatments [1] [2], being considered a surgically incurable pathological state, with diminished response to the systemic chemotherapy.

Sustained research efforts are devoted to the improvement of the treatment of peritoneal carcinomatosis patients with chemohyperthermia equipment [3]. Such equipment can be developed based on a complex intra-peritoneal chemohyperthermia physical model and a *functional model* of the *hyperthermic intra-peritoneal chemotherapy* system (HIPEC).

HIPEC requires intra-peritoneal spread of cytostatic drugs, at high temperatures ($41 - 43°C$), accomplished within 60-120 minutes, during surgical interventions. HIPEC is superior to the intra-peritoneal administration of cytostatic drugs, because the association of hyperthermia has a series of advantages: cytotoxic effect directly on the malignant cells (even more as the tumor vascularization is better), favors the penetration of cytostatic drugs in tumors and the increase of cytotoxicity of certain chemotherapy substances (most important), by acting at DNA level. Although the cytostatic effect is proportional to the increase of the temperature, the human organism is the one to set the limits, as temperatures exceeding $45 - 46°C$ may induce local abdominal injuries and systemic hyperthermia [4]. The currently accepted (closed procedure) requires the usage of an equipment that can assist in maintaining the intra-peritoneal temperature of the cytostatic fluid in the range $42 - 43°C$, as well as in producing an even distribution of the cytostatic fluid flow.

The problems of the commercially available equipment are: ▷ lack appropriate distributed temperature monitoring for providing comprehensive information regarding the intraperitoneal temperature distribution; ▷ uncontrolled flow distribution that favored the existence of multiple areas with a temperature that is lower than the appropriate one, compromises the synergic effect of the cytostatic drug; ▷ lack of the properly quantification of the volumes of the peritoneal cavity before in order to identify optimal cytostatic liquid volume; ▷ lack of advanced control mechanisms implemented in order to achieve homogenous temperature in the peritoneal cavity. These limitations can be surpassed by the development of a complex intra-peritoneal chemohyperthermia model able to provide the basis for the development of high performance HIPEC equipment. The key issues that have to be addressed are: the design of a complex inflow distribution system with multiple nozzles; a multipoint temperature measurement system; smart control algorithms for localized flow and temperature control; advanced perfusion system, based on multiple delivery channels with individually adjustable flow and temperature.

Most devices monitor the intra-peritoneal temperature in several points (2 to 4), which is insufficiently to be sure that the whole peritoneum is exposed to the optimal temperature. In addition, up to the present, there are no criteria to consider for standardization of the location of temperature sensors.

II. ARCHITECTURE OF THE MULTIPOINT TEMPERATURE MEASUREMENT SYSTEM

Maintaining a homogenous temperature of the entire volume of cytostatic solution certainly requires permanent temperature monitoring in multiple points, so one challenge is the design of optimal placement of the sensors able to provide a consistent *3D* thermal map of the intra-peritoneal volume during the whole procedure. The design of a HIPEC *multipoint temperature measurement system* must address the placement, the number, the mobility and transmission method of the temperature sensors, in order to provide an

S. Vlad and R.V. Ciupa (eds.), *International Conference on Advancements of Medicine and Health Care through Technology*, IFMBE Proceedings 44,
DOI: 10.1007/978-3-319-07653-9_39,

architecture able to collect relevant and accurate temperature data. A fully automated system allowing multipoint temperature measurement in HIPEC procedures with minimal exposure of the personnel, would have to address: ▷ a scalable temperature measurement system (8 to 16 input channels) ▷ an accuracy of at least $0.2°C$ and resolution better than $0.1°C$ ▷ appropriate size and geometry of the transducers for reduced inertia and easy placement ▷ hermetically sealed implementation - all the devices have to withstand multiple sterilization cycles ▷ wireless communication and power source (batteries) included in order to avoid cables and connectors ▷ energy efficient hardware/software codesign for assuring operation for the whole duration of the procedure with batteries having small size/capacity.

The above design constraints lead to several important consequences. First of all, the transducers that offer small dimensions and the required accuracy at low cost are the platinum RTDs. This type of resistive transducers is usually available in 1000Ω and 100Ω configuration, so low power operation implies low currents that would produce quite low voltage drops across the transducer. In the case of voltage analog to digital converters (ADC), that are considered in what follows, that would in turn determine an operation of the ADC with voltage levels covering only a small fraction of the input range. Any amplification of the signal would make the system susceptible to further errors and supplementary power consumption. The key elements of the proposed architecture are: a low power microcontroller, a wireless transceiver operating in the $2.4GHz$ industrial, scientific and medical band, some ADC with serial bus interface and 1000Ω platinum RTD transducers.

When selecting the AD converters, the main features considered were the resolution and the current consumption. Both in the first configuration (Fig. 1) and the second configuration (Fig. 2), the use of a ratiometric setup has many advantages, but requires a precision series resistor R_{ref}, to serve as a reference. The low current constrain requires this series resistance to be at least ten times larger than of the transducer ($R_t = 1000\Omega$). As a consequence, less than one tenth of the ADC input range will be used.

A reduction of the useful resolution of the converter with 3 or 4 bits imposes an analysis of the quantization error, since the design has to offer the 0.2 accuracy and $0.1°C$ resolution. The influence of the quantization error (maximum of ± 1 LSB) on the measured temperature value is significant when the resolution is less than 12 bits (Fig. 3). For this reason, although microcontrollers with internal ADC are available, they can be used in our setups only if their resolution is at least 12 + 3 bits (or 12+4 bits, depending on the ratio between R_t and R_{ref}).

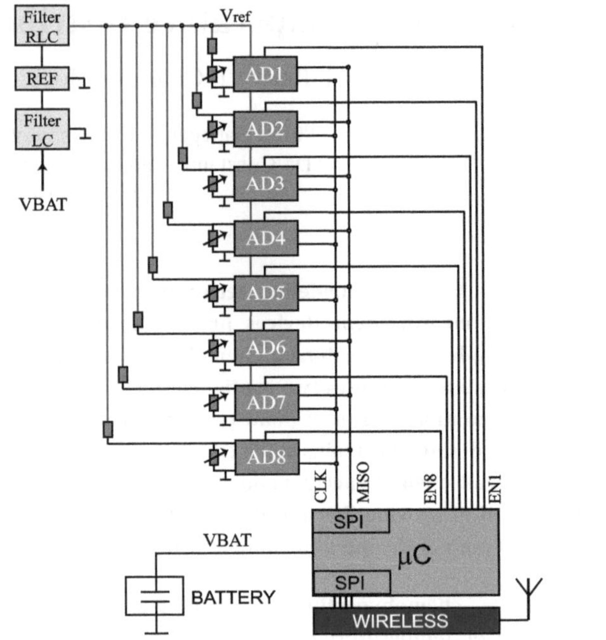

Fig. 1 Setup for a multipoint temperature measurement using individual ADC for each channel

The setups of Fig. 1 and 2 were prototyped using 1000Ω RTDs, $10k\Omega$ high precision wraparound thin film chip resistors with tolerances of $\pm 0.01\%$ and $5ppm/°C$ max. temperature coefficients, $3,6V$ LI-ION rechargeable batteries having a nominal capacity of $2900mAh$, and low cost 8-bit microcontrollers and 2.4 GHz transceivers.

III. Estimation of the Power Consumption

A common approach to reduce the energy consumed by a sensor is *duty-cycling*, which aims to achieve lower average power consumption by setting the device into inactive state whenever possible. The main consumers typically encountered in a wireless sensor are: the processing unit, the sensing unit, and the communication unit. The duty cycle can be defined as [5]:

$$\delta = \frac{T_{act}}{T_{act} + T_{inact}}, \; 0 < \delta < 1 \quad (1)$$

where T_{act} is the period spend by the consumer in active state and T_{inact} is the period in inactive state. The average current consumption obtained by duty-cycling can be written as [5]:

$$I_{\delta} = \frac{I_{act}T_{act} + I_{inact}T_{inact}}{T} = \delta I_{act} + (1-\delta)I_{inact} \quad (2)$$

where $T = T_{act} + T_{inact}$. For a low average current consumption δ should be considerably smaller than 1.

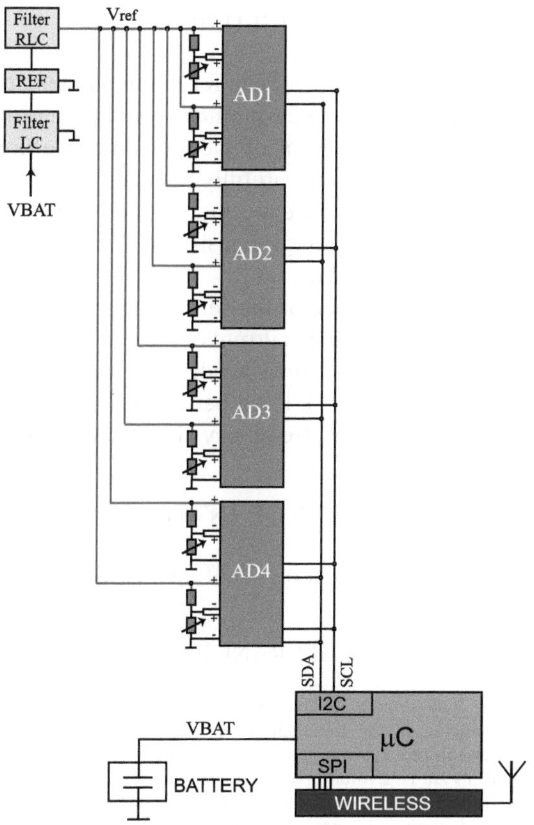

Fig. 2 Setup with four I2C output ADCs for multipoint temperature measurement

Table 1 presents the current consumption and the timing of the active/inactive states for the main components used in our setups. The average current consumption computed by duty-cycling for each of these components is detailed in what follows. A sampling period, T_s, of $2s$ is assumed.

The AD converters considered are low current consumption circuits with differential input channels and two conversion modes: one-shot conversion mode and continuous conversion mode. Since low power consumption is a key requirement for the considered setups, the devices are used in one-shot conversion mode, where a single conversion is performed after which the shutdown mode is automatically entered. The active period, T_{act}, can be expressed as the sum between the start-up time, the conversion time and the serial communication time, thus the duty-cycle and the average current consumption can be expressed as:

$$\delta_{sens} = \frac{T_{sens,startup} + T_{sens,conv} + T_{sens,comm}}{T_{sens,startup} + T_{sens,conv} + T_{sens,comm} + T_{sens,inact}}$$

$$I_{sens,\delta} = \delta_{sens} I_{sens,act} + (1 - \delta_{sens}) I_{sens,inact}$$

For the setup in Fig. 2 (comprising four 16 bits ADCs, each with four differential channels and I2C serial interface), the timing for one converter is expressed as: ▷ When a power-up event occurs, approximately $300\mu s$ are required before a conversion takes place: $T_{sens,startup} = 300\mu s$ ▷ The conversion time for one channel is $66.7ms$, thus $T_{sens,conv} = 66.7ms/channel$ ▷ For reading the conversion results, three bytes are needed for each channel: the read command initiated by the master, followed by two bytes containing the conversion results. Two more bytes are required for changing the active conversion channel (write command followed by the configuration byte). Setting the I2C frequency to $400kHz$, the communication time is $T_{sens,comm} = 117.5\mu s/channel$, resulting that $T_{sens,active} = 267.6ms$, $\delta_{sens} = 0.1338$, $I_{sens,\delta} = 0.0183mA$.

Table 1 Current consumption

Module	State	Time	Current
C8051F930 [6]	Active	$285ms$ / $90ms$	$3.5mA$
	Inactive	$Ts - T_{active}$	$0.85\mu A$
CYRF6936 [7]	Crystal Start-up	$700\mu s$	$1mA$
	Synthesize	$100\mu s$	$8mA$
	Active TX	$458\mu s$	$26mA$
	Active RX	$228\mu s$	$21.2mA$
	Inactive	$Ts - 1.5ms$	$0.8\mu A$
MCP3551 [8]	Active	$73.1ms$	$120\mu A$
	Inactive	$Ts - 73.1ms$	$1\mu A$
MCP3428 [9]	Active	$267.6ms$	$135\mu A$
	Inactive	$Ts - 267.6ms$	$0.3\mu A$
RTD transducer ($V_{ref} = 2.048V$)	Active	T_s	$1.5mA$

For the setup in Fig. 1 (comprising eight 22 bits ADCs, each with one differential input channel and SPI serial interface), the timing for one converter is: ▷ $T_{sens,startup} = 300\mu s$ ▷ $T_{sens,conv} = 72.73ms$ ▷ For reading the conversion results (three bytes) at a frequency of $500kHz$, $T_{sens,comm}$ is $48\mu s$, resulting that $T_{sens,active} = 73.1ms$, $\delta_{sens} = 0.0365$, $I_{sens,\delta} = 0.0053mA$.

The active period of the wireless communication unit takes into account the crystal start-up time, the settling time of the frequency synthesizer and the transmit/receive timings [7], thus the duty-cycle and the average current consumption are:

$$\delta_w = \frac{T_{w,osc_{start}} + T_{w,synth} + T_{w,RX} + T_{w,TX}}{T_{w,osc_{start}} + T_{w,synth} + T_{w,RX} + T_{w,TX} + T_{w,inact}},$$

$$I_{w,\delta} = \frac{I_{w,osc_{start}} T_{w,osc_{start}} + I_{w,RX} T_{w,RX}}{T_w} + \frac{I_{w,TX} T_{w,TX} + I_{w,inact} T_{w,inact}}{T_w}$$

resulting in the following values: $\delta_w = 0.0007$, $I_w = 0.0099mA$.

The duty-cycle and the average current consumption for the microcontroller is:

$$\delta_{\mu C} = \frac{T_{\mu C,act}}{T_{\mu C,act} + T_{\mu C,inact}}$$

$$I_{\mu C,\delta} = \delta_{\mu C} I_{\mu C,act} + (1 - \delta_{\mu C}) I_{\mu C,inact}$$

resulting the values $\delta_{\mu C} = 0.1425$ and $I_{\mu C} = 0.4995mA$ for $T_{\mu C,act} = 285ms$ and the values $\delta_{\mu C} = 0.0431$ and $I_{\mu C} = 0.1516mA$ for $T_{\mu C,act} = 90ms$.

Table 2 and 3 summarizes the duty-cycle and the average current consumption computed for a sampling period of 2 seconds for the setups in Fig. 1 and Fig. 2, respectively. The estimated consumptions for the two setups are presented in Fig. 4 for $T_s = 2s$, $T_s = 4s$ and $T_s = 6s$.

Table 2 Average current consumption by dutycycling for the setup in Fig.1

Module	Duty-cycle	Average-Current[mA]
C8051F930	0.0431	0.1516
CYRF6936	0.0007	0.0099
MCP3551	0.0365	0.0053
RTD transducer	1	1.5

Table 3 Average current consumption by dutycycling for the setup in Fig. 2

Module	Duty-cycle	Average-Current[mA]
C8051F930	0.1248	0.4376
CYRF6936	0.0007	0.0099
MCP3428	0.1338	0.0183
RTD transducer	1	1.5

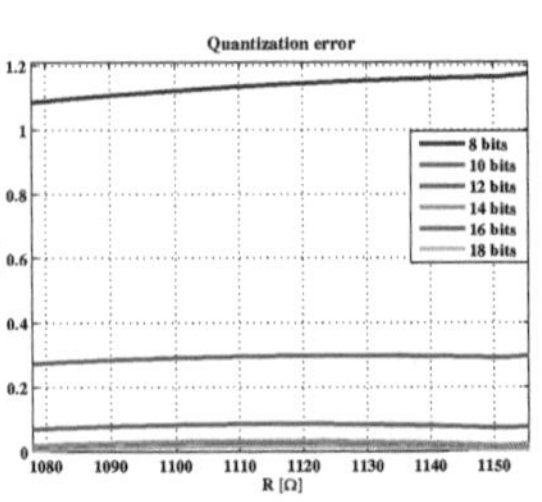

Fig. 3 Quantization error

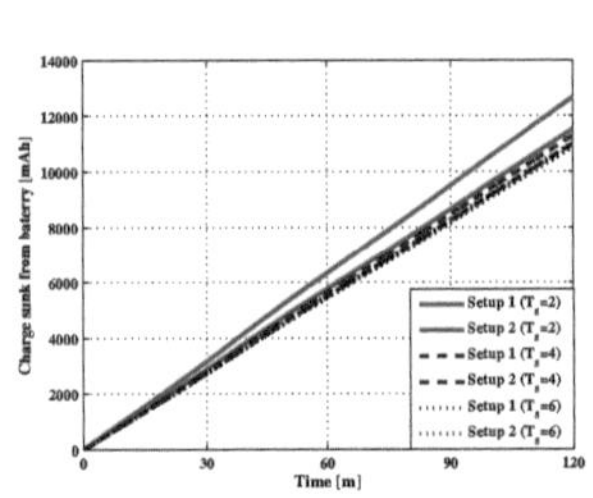

Fig. 4 Estimated consumptions

The active period of the microcontroller was set to be greater than the ADC's conversion time. Further improvements can be made by setting the microcontroller in sleep mode during the conversion period, in order to lower the current consumption.

IV. CONCLUSION

Two configurations appropriate for the implementation of a multipoint temperature measurement system are proposed and analyzed from the point of view of energy efficiency. The design constrains were carefully defined considering the overall HIPEC performance expectations and the need to provide thermal data for building a consistent $3D$ thermal map of the intra-peritoneal volume.

The better performance of the setup described in (Fig. 1) is mainly due to the reduced current of the converter in active mode and to the reduced time needed for transferring data from the converter (Fig. 2). Even better figures could be obtained with a higher clock frequency (1MHz or 2MHz).

CONFLICT OF INTEREST

The authors declare that they have no conflict of interest.

REFERENCES

1. Nissan A, Stojadinovic A, Garofalo A, Esquivel J, Piso P. Evidence-based medicine in the treatment of peritoneal carcinomatosis: Past, present, and future. *Journal of surgical oncology.* 2009;15:335–344.
2. Sugarbaker Paul H. Evolution of cytoreductive surgery and perioperative intraperitoneal chemotherapy for peritoneal carcinomatosis: are there treatment alternatives? *American journal of surgery.* 2011;201:157–9.
3. Roviello Franco, Caruso Stefano, Marrelli Daniele, et al. Treatment of peritoneal carcinomatosis with cytoreductive surgery and hyperthermic intraperitoneal chemotherapy: state of the art and future developments. *Surgical oncology.* 2011;20:e38–54.
4. González-Moreno Santiago, González-Bayón Luis a, Ortega-Pérez Gloria. Hyperthermic intraperitoneal chemotherapy: Rationale and technique. *World journal of gastrointestinal oncology.* 2010;2:68–75.
5. Bader Sebastian. *Enabling Autonomous Environmental Measurement Systems with Low-Power Wireless Sensor Networks.* PhD thesisMid Sweden University 2011.
6. Silicon Laboratories*C8051F93x-C8051F92x* 2013. Data Sheet.
7. Shone Tran, Cypress Semiconductor . Clearing the Confusion on Battery Life and Range for 2.4-GHz Low Power RF *RF Design Line.* 2009. (http://www.rfdesignline.com/howto/lowpowerrf/212900777).
8. Microchip Technology Inc.*MCP3551/3 - Low-Power, Single-Channel 22-Bit Delta-Sigma ADCs* 2005. Data Sheet.
9. Microchip Technology Inc.*MCP3426/7/8 - 16-Bit, Multi-Channel Delta Sigma Analog-to-Digital Converter with I2C Interface and On-Board Reference* 2009. Data Sheet.

Capacitive Monitoring of a Tubular Layered Substance Delivery System

B. Ţebrean, S. Crişan, V.D. Zaharia and T.E. Crisan

Electrical Engineering and Measurements Department, Technical University of Cluj-Napoca, Cluj-Napoca, Romania

Abstract— **The aim of this paper is to present the modeling results obtained when a liquid flows through a tubular device which contains a solid soluble substance isolated from the fluid flux by a porous membrane. For monitoring the delivery process, a capacitor was built in the protective layer of the tubular structure, the variation of concentrations being revealed by electrical relative permittivity change. The presented device can be easily adaptable to various fields of applications used in medicine, engineering, chemistry, biology, food processing and in water supply systems.**

Keywords— **capacitive monitoring, porous membrane, substance delivery, transport phenomena**

I. Introduction

In various fields of science, the controlled delivery of a substance is a concern of researchers. In medicine, the studies are focused on drug delivery capsules or implants, in engineering, on devices that can lubricate or clean moving parts, in chemistry on adding components in slow process reaction.

This paper presents a solution for the modeling of a tubular device that contains a solid soluble substance which is delivered into a liquid. The substance is isolated from the fluid flux by a porous membrane.

In order to monitor the delivery process of the substance into a fluid flux, a capacitor was built in the protective layer of the tubular structure. The variation of concentrations is revealed by electrical relative permittivity change.

The modeling was performed using the COMSOL Multiphysics® software. The modules used involve predefined equations describing the laminar flow, the transport of the solutions in variable saturated porous media and the electrostatics laws.

II. Modelling condition

A. Device Configuration and Working Principles of the Analyzed Model

The device that is subject to the present study has the structure presented in figure 1.

The main components are: the porous membrane (1), the substance (2), the capacitor's armatures (3), the protective layer (4).

A 15 mm exterior diameter was chosen for the tubular device, together with a length of 25 mm. Those dimensions ware randomly chosen, any subsequently change can be easily processed by the used software to adapt the model for any given application.

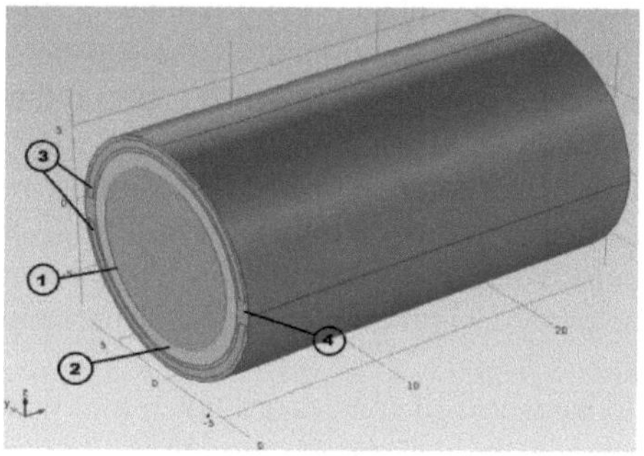

Fig. 1 The tubular device structure

The porous membrane can be made from a large variety of materials with different porosity, the permeability of the membrane being one of the most important properties in the substance delivery process. The internal diameter of the porous membrane is 11 mm, the thickness being 0.1 mm.

The tubular substance layer has an external diameter of 13 mm, the thickness being 0.9 mm. In the analyzed case we had considered a solid, soluble and porous substance in order to solve the model, but a liquid solution may also be taken into account. Another variant is that the substance included in the capsule can be uniformly distributed in a solid matrix support which is insolvable in the liquid that flows through the device.

The protective layer, 1 mm thick, has to keep the substance in the tubular structure so it has to be made from an impermeable material. This layer must avoid evaporation, dissolution, volatilization or any other chemical or physical process that can damage or modify substance properties.

The capacitor used for concentration detection has two armatures with a thickness of 0.5mm. It is built in the protective layer being electrically insulated from the rest of the components.

A liquid will flow inside the tubular structure and it will pass to the substance through the porous membrane. The substance will be dissolved and carried into the fluid flux outside the device.

S. Vlad and R.V. Ciupa (eds.), *International Conference on Advancements of Medicine and Health Care through Technology*, IFMBE Proceedings 44,
DOI: 10.1007/978-3-319-07653-9_40, © Springer International Publishing Switzerland 2014

During the delivery process, the electrical permittivity of the mixture created inside will vary, so the role of the capacitor is to measure the amount of the substance present in the tubular structure.

B. Theoretical Approach and Simulation Conditions

The modules of the COMSOL Multiphysics® software involve predefined equations describing the laminar flow, the transport of the solutions in variable saturated porous media and the electrostatics laws.

The process we studied is considered to include absorption, diffusion and dispersion process. The following assumptions have been made: there are no chemical reaction phenomena throughout the entire process; there are no volatile components or gas absorption phenomena; there are no cavitation phenomena; the volume of the substance domain remains constant throughout the entire process; the temperature is constant and considered T=37°C.

In order to impose the simulation conditions, we have to choose the appropriate equations to avoid the overcharging of the model involved. For this reason, the three main phenomena are treated simultaneously, but separately on each subdomain.

Flow and transport of species are taken into account only in the substance, in the porous membrane and inside the cylindrical subdomain created within the porous membrane. Because the protective layer is impermeable, there is no reason to include it and the capacitor's armatures in fluid transport computation.

The capacitance evaluation is made involving all the components of the device, because the variation of the electrical relative permittivity is a function of the changing of concentration.

All the above problems are solved simultaneously. The software imposes that the initial hypothesis and conditions, the variables and solving restrictions are to be performed at two levels: domain and boundary level.

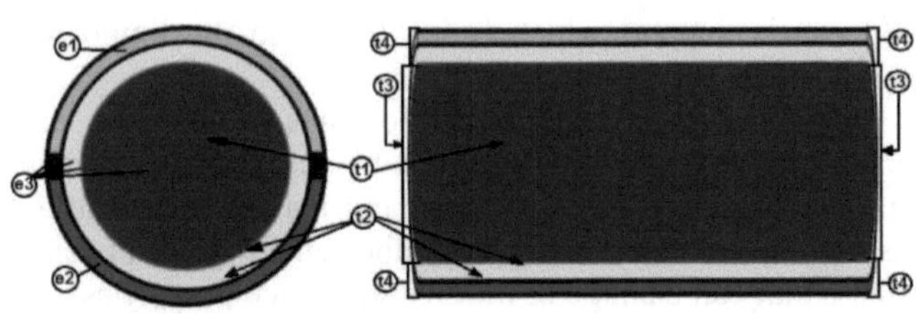

Fig. 2 Simple sketch of the computational domain

The equations that are used for the present model are derived from the general equation of transport of species in porous and nonporous media.

Inside the cylindrical subdomain, created by the porous membrane, the transport phenomenon is achieved just by the free flow of the liquid. An equation based on [1] [2] [3] is used to solve the free flow phenomenon:

$$\frac{\partial c}{\partial t} - D_{Fll} \cdot \nabla c + u_x \cdot \nabla c = 0 \qquad (1)$$

where:
-c - the concentration of the liquid which flows inside the tubular structure;
-D_{Fll} - the fluid phase self-diffusion coefficient of the liquid;
-u_x - the velocity field on x axis of the liquid at the entrance.

When the transport phenomena are analyzed in the porous membrane and in the substance, the porosities of those media are involved, so the equation used in this case is similar for both situations [1] [2] [3] [4] [5]:

$$(e_m + \rho_{bm} \cdot \frac{k_{Lm} \cdot c_{p\max.m}}{1 + k_{Lm} \cdot c}) + (c - c_{p.m} \frac{\rho_{bm}}{1 - e_m}) \frac{\partial e_m}{\partial t} - (D_{Dm} + D_{Fm}) \nabla c + \nabla (u_m \cdot c) = 0 \qquad (2)$$

where:
-e_m - the porosity of the medium;
-ρ_{bm} - the bulk density of the medium's material;
-k_{Lm} - the Langmuir constant in the medium;
-$c_{pmax.m}$ - the maximum amount adsorbed in solid particles of the medium;
-$c_{p.m}$ - the amount of the liquid adsorbed in solid particles of the medium;
- D_{Dm} - the dispersion in the porous material of the medium;
- D_{Fm} - the fluid phase diffusion coefficient in the medium;
-u_m - the flow velocity in the medium.

The capacitance is computed for all the domains. We have considered two terminals, one placed to a positive potential and other to ground. When the discretization of the model take place, the device will be transformed in a "n" terminals system, where at least one must be grounded. The global capacitance is computed using the superposition method. The capacitance of the system is given by:

$$C_{ii} = \frac{2}{V_i^2} \int_\Omega W_e d\Omega$$
$$C_{ij} = \frac{1}{V_i V_j} \int_\Omega W_e d\Omega - \frac{1}{2}\left(\frac{V_i}{V_j} C_{ii} + \frac{V_j}{V_i} C_{jj} \right) \qquad (3)$$

where: V_i is the electrical potential of the i element, $W_e$is the energy and Ω is the integration volume, C_{ii} and C_{ij} are the own capacitance of the i element and the capacitance between the i and j element respectively. [6]

The system's capacitance variation is directly related to the relative electrical permittivity. This permittivity is constant in the protective layer, but variable in respect to the liquid's concentration in the substance and in the fluid tube computational domains.

Considering that inside the tubular structure, after the transport phenomena are taking place, the medium starts to be anisotropic, it is very difficult to approximate the precise value of the electrical relative permittivity with simple analytical equations.

Usually, practical determinations are used for these approximations. Some bibliographical references [7] [8] [9] [10] suggests several solutions for the correlation between concentration and relative permittivity. The following relation has been chosen for the proposed model:

$$\varepsilon_{r.mean}(c) = \varepsilon_{rl} + \frac{3c}{c_{li}} \cdot \frac{\varepsilon_{rl} - \varepsilon_{rs}}{\varepsilon_{rl} + 2 \cdot \varepsilon_{rs} - \frac{c}{c_{li}} \cdot (\varepsilon_{rl} - \varepsilon_{rs})} \quad (4)$$

where:

- c_{li} - the initial concentration of the liquid at the entrance of the tubular structure;
- ε_{rl} - the relative permittivity of the liquid;
- ε_{rs} - the relative permittivity of the substance.

At the domain level the conditions imposed for fluid flow and species transport are:

- *free flow* – (t1 Figure 2) - for the laminar flow inside the cylindrical subdomain created inside the porous membrane;
- *mobile fluid/immobile solid* – (t2 Figure2) - for the porous membrane and the substance subdomain.

The additional boundary conditions are:

- *inflow* and *outflow* – (t3 Figure2) - for the ends of the flow channel;
- *no flow/no flux* – (t4 Figure2) - for the ends of the porous membrane tube, the substance tube and also for the border between substance and the protective layer.

With these conditions we can predict how the liquid passes through the porous membrane and enters in the substance matrix, dissolving it. The membrane also acts as a safety layer, in case bulk parts of the substance should enter the fluid flux.

For the electrostatic evaluation, the domain level conditions are:

- *electric potential* – (e1 Figure2) - for the capacitor's voltage terminal;
- *zero voltage* – (e2 Figure2) - for the capacitor's ground terminal;
- *charge conservation* – (e3 Figure2) - for the rest of the domains.

The boundary conditions are kept the same as the domain condition for the terminal borders, continuity for all the remaining interior borders and charge conservation for the exterior ones.

C. The Tubular Device's Mesh

The configuration of the mesh was chosen in respect with the modeling conditions, considering that two modules are used for simulation: one for the species transport in porous media and one for electrostatic simulation.

The structure was meshed differently for each component starting from one lateral surface.

The domain's edges have been divided differently in order to obtain a finer mesh in the most important areas and a coarser one in less significant regions.

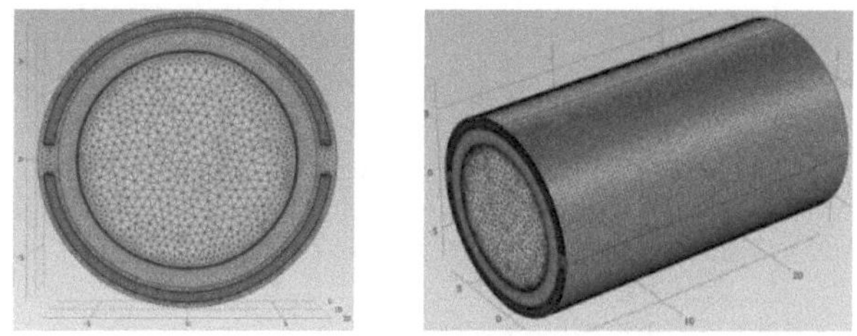

a) b)

Fig. 3 The domains of the capsular structure (a), 3D view of the model's mesh (b)

Based on the edges distribution, a triangular mesh was applied to obtain the 2D mesh of the chosen area.

For the 3D mesh, a sweeping method was applied, starting from the source face along the domain to the opposite destination face. This kind of mesh was preferred because it is adapted to the fluid dynamics solving algorithms.

III. Modeling results

In order to simulate the behavior of the tubular structure. initial values necessary to compute the concentrations and respectively the electrical relative permittivity variation during the process have been imposed.

The substance used has properties closely related to NaCl in solid form. The bulk density is ρ_s=1154[kg/m^3], the porosity e_s=0.5 and the relative permittivity ε_{rs}=40. The initial concentration of the substance is c_{is}=37000[mol/m^3].

The liquid that flows through the tubular structure has the properties of distilled water. The initial concentration of the liquid is c_{il}= 55555[mol/m^3], the bulk density is ρ_s=1000[kg/m^3] and the relative permittivity is ε_{rl}=80. The velocity field on the *x* axis of the liquid at the entrance of the tubes is u_x=0.005 [m/s];

The porous membrane is made of ethylene-vinyl acetate in solid form, with a concentration of vinyl acetate of 28%. The bulk density of the considered material is ρ_{bm}=957[kg/m^3], the porosity: e_m=0.5 and the relative permittivity: ε_{rm}=35;[11]

The protective layer is made of nylon. The porosity is e_t=0 (impermeable) and the relative permittivity is ε_{rt} =40;

The capacitor's terminals are made of copper, with a relative permittivity of ε_{rc}=1.

Regarding the diffusion coefficients, the imposed fluid phase diffusion coefficient of the liquid in the porous membrane is D_{Flm}=6.88e-13[m^2/s]. The fluid phase diffusion coefficient of the solution in the porous membrane is D_{Fsm}=8.75e-13[m^2/s]. The fluid phase diffusion coefficient of the liquid in the substance is D_{Fls}=4e 13[m^2/s].

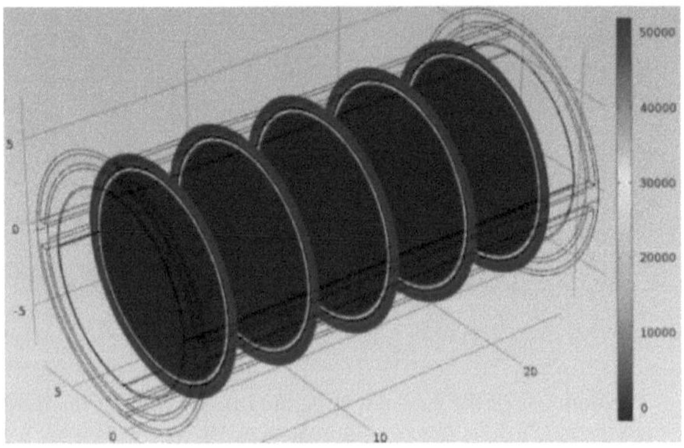

Fig. 4 3D view of the initial liquid concentration

The period of time for the process was set to 30 days, with a 1h time step. The variation of liquid concentration in the tubular structure is presented in figures 4 and 5. In order to illustrate the gradual penetration of the liquid inside the substance layer, four different time values were chosen: initial, after first, second and third week.

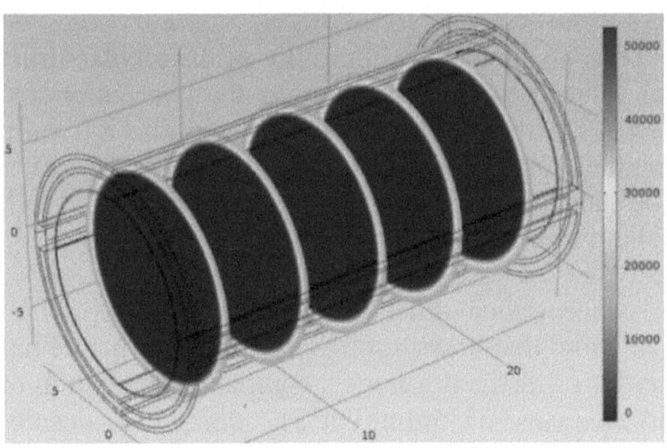

Fig. 5 3D view of the liquid's concentration after the third week

As seen in the previous figures, the liquid gradually enters the substance layer, the modeling results predicting how the phenomena take place. For other desired geometries of the substance layer or some embedded porous tubes in a substance block, the computing algorithm may remain the same, the main idea of the modeling being to provide a uniform dissolution and implicitly leading to a more effective action of the device.

For the purpose of emphasizing the variation of concentration in time with respect to some imposed changes of material properties, a specific probe point was chosen. This point is placed in the median part of the tubular structure, in the middle of the substance tube, half way between the protective layer and the porous membrane.

The most important parameters that can influence the behavior of the present device are the porosity of the components and the diffusion coefficients of the liquid in different types of materials that can be used to build them.

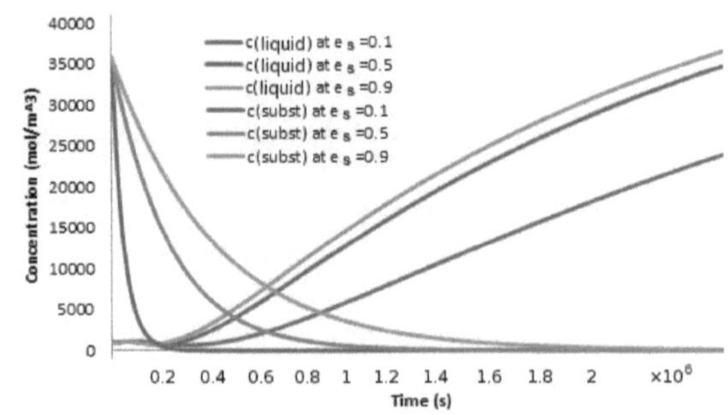

Fig. 6 The substance's and the liquid's concentration variation at different porosities of the substance

For three different porosities of the substance, the values of concentration of the liquid and the substance in probe point are presented in figure 6: e_{s1}=0.1, e_{s2}=0.5 and e_{s3}=0.9. The results show the way that the porosity of the substance can influence the delivery process. Any adjustment of the porosity gives the possibility to modify the time dependent parameters of the process.

Another important factor is the porosity of the membrane. Three different values of the porosity of the membrane: e_{m1}=0.3, e_{m2}=0.5 and e_{m3}=0.7, were chosen.

Figure 7 illustrates the degree up to which this parameter can be used for controlling the rate the device acts.

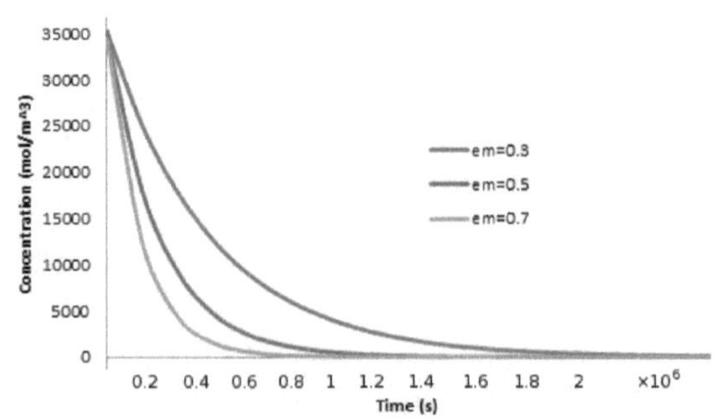

Fig. 7 The substance's concentration variation at different porosities of the porous membrane

The diffusion coefficients of the liquid in different types of materials can also influence the behavior of the presented tubular device.

The delivery time can be influenced by the variation of the fluid phase diffusion coefficient of the liquid in the porous membrane. Three values were used: D_{Flm1}=6.88e-11[m^2/s], D_{Flm2}=6.88e-13[m^2/s] and D_{Flm3}=6.88e-15[m^2/s].

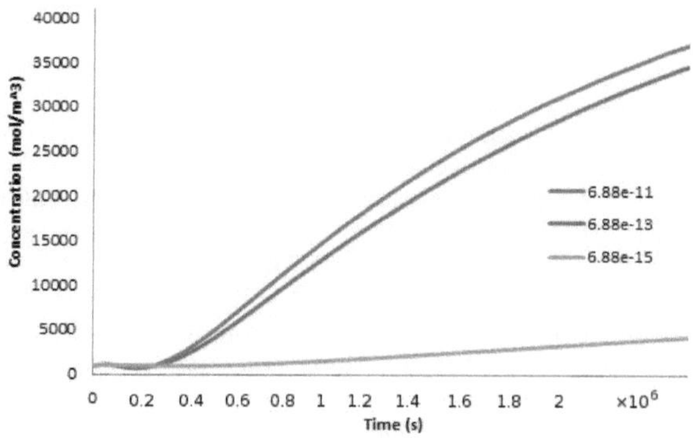

Fig. 8 The liquid's concentration variation at different diffusion coefficients of the liquid in the porous membrane

The liquid concentration variation at three different diffusion coefficients of the liquid in substance is represented in figure 9, using D_{FIs1}=4e-11[m^2/s], D_{FIs2}=4e-12[m^2/s] and D_{FIs3}=4e-13[m^2/s]. In this context the choice of materials for the membrane also appears essential.

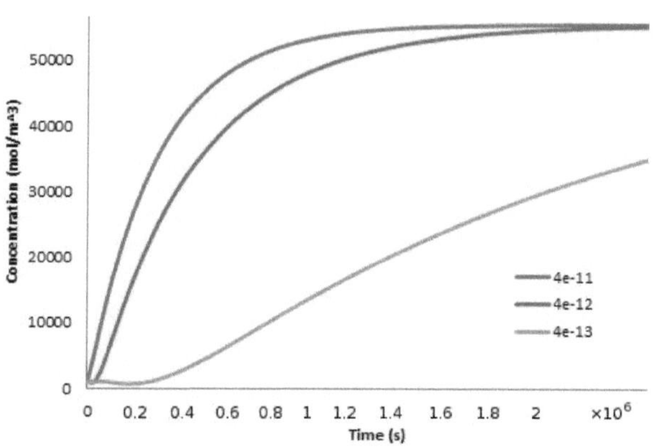

Fig. 9 The liquid's concentration variation at different diffusion coefficients of the liquid in substance

In any of the previous given situations, the second step of the modeling has to determine the capacitance variation due to the change of the electrical relative permittivity of the mixture inside the analyzed device.

The capacitor has two armatures, on one a voltage is imposed, the second armature being the ground terminal.

Figure 10 presents the voltage and the normalized electric field:

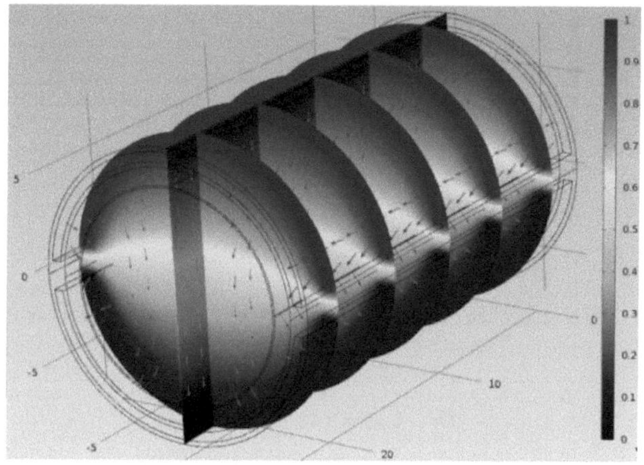

Fig. 10 The voltage and the electric field in the tubular structure

As it was previously discussed, several properties of the components of the tubular structure or of the liquid which flows through it can influence the transport phenomena.

Two significant situations were chosen to show where the computed capacitance varies when an initial parameter is changed.

Figure 11 shows the variation of the capacitance for five different values of the porosity of the substance, $e_{m=}$0.1…0.9.

The concentration of the liquid is bigger when the porosity increases at a certain time value. The capacitance is growing proportionally to the porosity of the tubes.

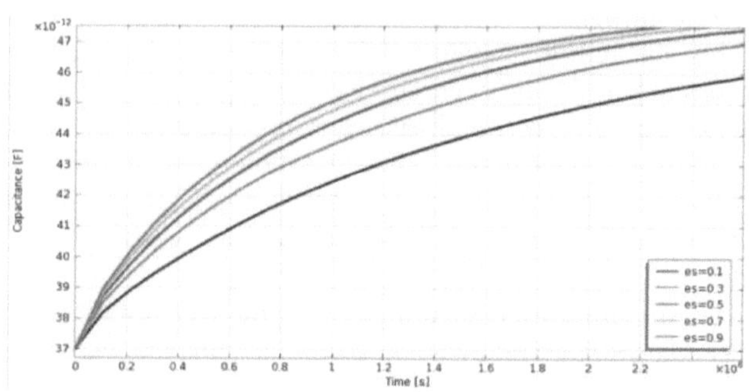

Fig. 11 The capacitance variation at different porosities of the substance

The electrical permittivity of the substance is also an important aspect which has to be considered when computing the capacitance variation. Figure 12 shows that the variation of the capacitance in time is significantly changed for different values of ε_{rs}. If the electrical relative permittivity of the substance has the same value as the liquid, the capacitance remains constant all the time, and the current method cannot be used.

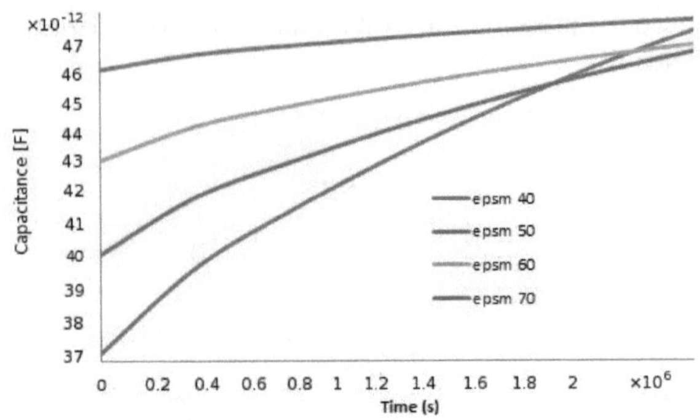

Fig. 12 The capacitance variation at different electrical permittivity of the substance

IV. Conclusions

This paper has described the modeling of the behavior of a tubular device that contains a solid soluble substance when a fluid flows through it. The delivery of the substance in a fluid flux process is monitored with a capacitor built in the protective layer of the tubular structure. Different aspects of correlation between concentrations variation and electrical relative permittivity were analyzed.

The present model is easily modifiable and adaptable for other desired geometries or various other situations/conditions, the computation algorithm remaining the same.

The numerical values that was presented here, to show how the variation of components' properties (e.g. diffusion coefficients, porosity, electrical permittivity, flow velocity), can radically change the delivery process (time of delivery, realized substance - mass or concentrations).

The capacitive method for monitoring the delivery process is simple and accurate. Even if apparently the variations of capacitance obtained are relatively small (order of pF), those are measurable values, avoiding all interferences and there are already several common applications: fingerprint readers, certain touch-screen devices, capacitive humidity sensors.

The modeling was performed using the COMSOL Multiphysics® software and was based on the capacitance definition equation and on the equation describing the transport of the species in variable saturated porous media respectively.

The applicability of such structure can be found in various fields of applications - medicine, engineering, chemistry, biology, food processing and in water supply systems.

Conflict of Interest

The authors declare that they have no conflict of interest.

References

1. Bear J. (1991)Introduction to Modeling of Transport Phenomena in Porous Media, Springer, ISBN 978-0792311065
2. Bear J.(1978) Dynamics of Fluids in Porous Media, American Elsevier Publishing Company, ISBN 798-0-486- 65675-5.
3. Bird B.R., et al.(2002) Transport Phenomena - 2nd edition, John Wiley & Sons, ISBN 0-471-41077-2
4. Vasquez J. L.(2006) The Porous Medium Equation- Mathematical Theory, Oxford University Press, ISBN: 978-0198569039.
5. Warsi Z. (2005) Fluid Dynamics: Theoretical and Computa-tional Approaches, Third Edition, Taylor and Francis, ISBN-13: 978-0849333972.
6. Jianming Jin (2002) "The Finite Element Method in Electromagnetics, 2nd ed.", Wiley-IEEE Press. ISBN: 978-0-471-43818-2.
7. Carpi F.,et al.(2008) Dielectric Elastomers as Electromechanical Transducers, Elsevier Science, ISBN 978-0080474885
8. Cherepanov D.A., et al.(2003) Low Dielectric Permittivity of Water at the Membrane Interface: Effect on the Energy Coupling Mechanism in Biological Membranes, Biophysical Journal, 85, pp. 1307–1316.
9. Teschke O., et al.(2001) "Interfacial Water Dielectric-Permittivity-Profile Measurement Using Atomic Force Microscopy", Physical Review E, 64.
10. Wang P., Anderco A.(2001) Computation of Dielectric Constants of Solvent Mixtures and Electrolyte Solution, Fluid Phase Equilibria, 186, pp. 103-122.
11. ***, "Ethylene Vinyl Acetate - EVA 12% VA - Data Sheet" at http://www.azom.com/article.aspx?ArticleID=410.

Author: Bogdan TEBREAN
Institute: Technical University of Cluj-Napoca
Street: Memorandumuluino.28
City: Cluj-Napoca
Country: Romania
Email: bogdan.tebrean@ethm.utcluj.ro

Potential Distribution and Nerve Fiber Responses in Transcutaneous Lumbosacral Spinal Cord Stimulation

S.M. Danner[1,2], U.S. Hofstoetter[1], M. Krenn[1], W. Mayr[1], F. Rattay[2], and K. Minassian[1]

[1] Center for Medical Physics and Biomedical Engineering, Medical University of Vienna, Vienna, Austria
[2] Institute for Analysis and Scientific Computing, Vienna University of Technology, Vienna, Austria

Abstract—**Transcutaneous electrical spinal cord stimulation is a non-invasive method to stimulate afferent structures connected to the human spinal cord. Here, computer simulations are presented that aim at shedding light on why distant skin electrodes selectively activate specific groups of afferent fibers localized in the spinal canal and whether other neural structures are concomitantly stimulated.**

The simulation was conducted in two steps: i) A finite element model of the human trunk was applied to calculate the electric potential generated by electrodes placed over the paravertebral skin and the abdomen. ii) The electric potential evaluated along the trajectories of target neural structures was used as the input for nerve fiber models and to calculate activating functions. Due to the electrophysiological findings, the responses of large diameter myelinated fibers in the posterior root (PR), anterior root (AR) and posterior column (Pcol) of the lumbar spinal cord were simulated.

The activating functions revealed sites of strong depolarization at the entrance of the PR fibers into the spinal cord and at the entrances/exits of the PR and AR fibers into/from the spinal canal. The nerve fiber model confirmed that action potentials were initiated at these low threshold sites. No such 'hot-spots' were found for the Pcol fibers. Activation thresholds for the most preferentially located fibers of each class were 14.1 V, 22.6 V and 45.4 V for the PRs, ARs and Pcols, respectively.

'Hot-spots' for extrecellular stimulation appear at axon bends and at transitions through media with different conductivities. PRs are the preferential targets, while direct coactivation of Pcol fibers is improbable.

Keywords—**Spinal cord stimulation, posterior root-muscle reflexes, computer simulation, activating function**

I. INTRODUCTION

Stimulation of nervous tissue of and close to the spinal cord has neuromodulatory benefits in upper motor neuron disorders, like reduction of spasticity [1, 2, 3] and modification of gait [4, 5]. Further, evoked spinal reflexes can be used in electrophysiological studies [6, 7, 8]. Magnetic or electrical stimulation are methods to induce electrical fields around the nerve structures of interest. Both can be applied non-invasively at the skin over the spine. Paraspinal magnetic stimulation, following the principles of electromagnetic induction, induces circular ionic current flows. The restriction of a coils placement dorsal to the lumber spinal cord predominantly induces currents oriented parallel to the frontal plane [9]. The common muscle responses are due to stimulation of efferent fibers to the muscles, but afferents in the spinal roots can be stimulated as well [10, 11, 12]. Transcutaneous electrical stimulation produces a potential difference between the skin electrodes and current flows from the anode to the cathode, passing the intermediate anatomical structures. Thus, transcutaneous electrical stimulation enables more freedom of steering the current flow than magnetic stimulation and specifically allows for current flows perpendicular to the frontal plan [9]. This is achieved by placing electrodes paraspinally and the centrally over the abdominal surface or the iliac crest [7, 13, 14, 15], e.g. two round 5 cm diameter electrodes placed paraspinally at the level between the T11–T12 spinous processes and two larger rectangular electrodes centrally over the abdominal surface. Electrophysiological investigations showed that with such electrode setup, reflexes can be elicited in the lower limb muscles [7]. These reflexes can be modified by vibration, by applying double stimuli paradigms [7], by performing volitional motor tasks [7, 13, 8] and by the stimulation of peripheral nerves [16]. They were shown to be similar to those elicited by epidural spinal cord stimulation [6] and dubbed as posterior root-muscle (PRM) reflexes, according to their initiation and recording sites [7]. Therefore and also due to the latencies of the recorded compound motor action potentials (CMAPs), it could be deduced that Ia afferents are among the stimulated structures. Yet, with differences in the stimulation setup, including body posture, electrode positions, and polarity of the stimulation, it is possible to co-activate efferent fibers. Yet, it is not clear from the electrophysiological studies whether other fiber types are co-activated. Computer simulations that addressed these questions [17, 18, 19] are reviewed here in detail. Furthermore, their results are extended by a comparison of two widely used mammalian nerve fiber models.

II. METHODS

To simulate the effect of electrical stimulation on neural tissue located deeply inside the body, it is customary to

S. Vlad and R.V. Ciupa (eds.), *International Conference on Advancements of Medicine and Health Care through Technology*, IFMBE Proceedings 44,
DOI: 10.1007/978-3-319-07653-9_41,

apply two simulation steps. First, the generated electrical potential in the volume conductor, here the human torso, is simulated by numerically solving partial differential equations using the finite element method [20, 19, 21]. This calculation of the electrical potential Φ is based on a reduced form of Maxwell's equation and depends from the conductivity σ the medium:

$$\nabla \cdot (\sigma \nabla \Phi) = 0.$$

The second step involves using the solution of the previous step, the generated potential of the electrical stimulation, along the target nerve fibers, as the input to compartment models of neurons, especially axons, or for the activating function [22] in order to assess the effectiveness of the electrical field in activating these neurons [21]. In the first step, the excitable neural structures are not part of the simulation. The activation function [22] is given by

$$f_n = \frac{d\Delta x}{4\rho_i Lc} \frac{V_{e,n-1} - 2V_{e,n} + V_{e,n+1}}{\Delta x^2},$$

where d is the fiber diameter, Δx the node-to-node distance, L the node length, ρ_i the axomplasmatic resistivity, c the capacity, V_e the extracellular potential and n the compartment index. Positive values of f_n indicate de- and negative values hyperpolarization. Note that if $L = \Delta x$ and $\Delta x \to 0$ then f_n becomes proportional to the second order, spatial derivative of the extracellular potential along the fiber.

In the simulation of transcutaneous spinal cord stimulation the target structures are located deeply inside the body, surrounded by various anatomical structures that possibly induce electrical inhomogeneities and anisotropies, which in turn influence the generated electric potential at the regions of interest. Thus, the simulations [17, 18] included a detailed, yet, stereotypical, model of the gray and white matter of the spinal cord, the cerebrospinal fluid, the vertebrae, paraspinal muscles, body fat and skin as well as a rough representation of the torso (see figure 1). The electrical parameters of the distinct tissues were selected from the literature and measurements (see [17, 18]). Neumann boundary conditions were used for the external surface of the skin, the midsagittal symmetry plane, thus reducing the complexity of the model by half, and the bottom and top surfaces of the model. For the electrodes, Dirichlet boundary conditions were used, where the paraspinal electrodes acted as the active and the abdominal electrodes as the reference electrode. The steady-state solutions were calculated using COMSOL.

The solution of the finite element model was evaluated along fibers in the posterior roots (PR), the anterior roots (AR) and the posterior columns (Pcol). They present myelinated nerve fibers with the largest diameters, outside as well as inside the spinal cord. Since myelinated fibers are easier to excite electrically than unmyelinated ones and thicker fibers have lower thresholds [23], these fiber classes are the prime candidates for the simulation and only if all three classes would be easily excitable, additional fiber classes would be necessary to consider. Fibers in the PRs and ARs entering and exiting the spinal cord at different segmental levels (see figure 1a,e,f) and Pcol fibers with different depth and mediolateral positions in the white matter were simulated using the activating function [22] and two nerve fiber models, the McIntrye-Richardson-Grill (MRG) [24] and the Chiu-Ritchie-Rogart-Stagg-Sweeney (CRRSS) [25, 26] models. Anodic and cathodic monophasic stimulation pulses with 1 ms width were applied. Activation thresholds and sites were calculated for different fiber diameters, depending on

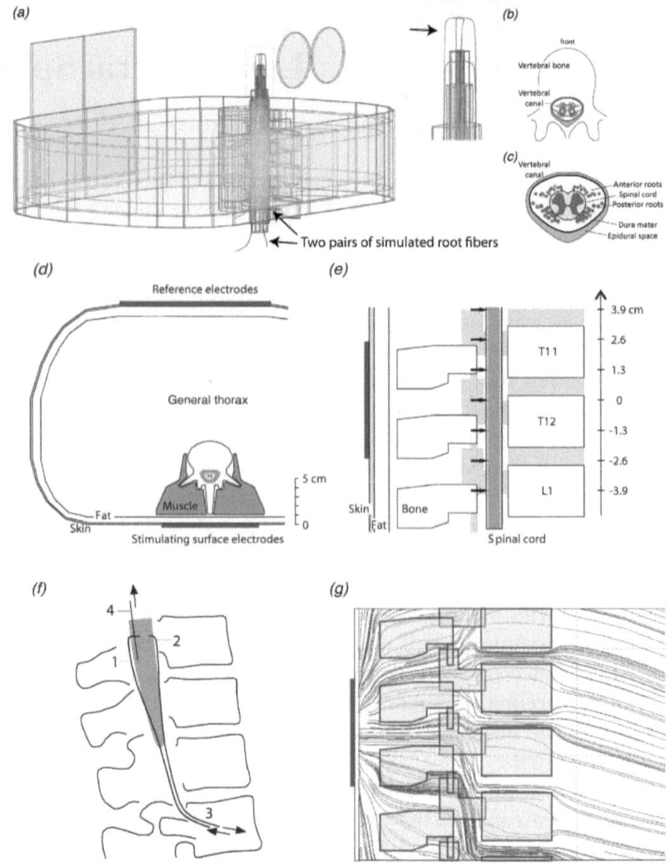

Fig. 1 Representation of the model geometry **(a)** and the paths of the simulated axons (marked by arrowheads). **(b-c)** Sketches of spinal canal cross sections. **(d)** Cross section of the volume conductor model. **(e)** Midsagittal section showing the relation between the spine, spinal cord, intervertebral discs and the transcutaneous paravertebral electrode. Model fiber entry and exit levels into the spinal cord are marked with arrows. **(f)** Sketch of posterior (1) and anterior root fibers (2), joining together at the intervertebral foramina (3), and of the posterior columns (4) in relation to the spinal geometry. **(g)** Computer simulated current flow within a 2 mm layer at the midsagittal plane. The electrodes are illustrated in red (adapted from [17, 18]).

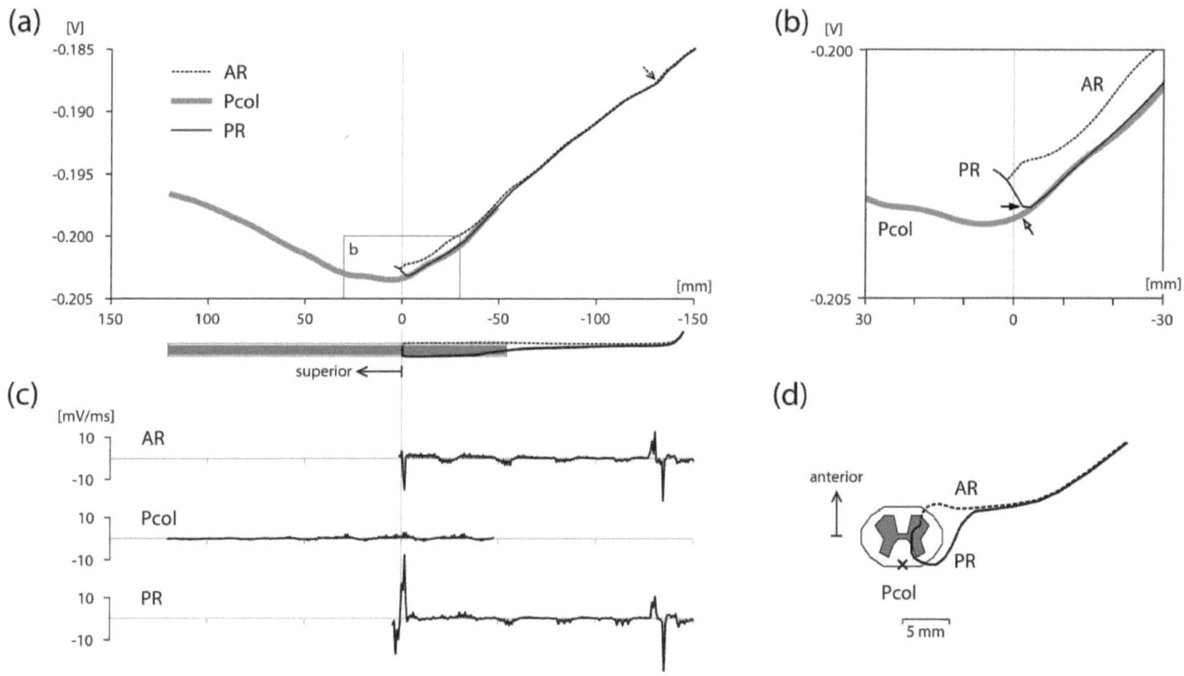

Fig. 2 Stimulation effect evaluated along exemplary target nerve structures. **(a)** Extracellular potential along the three fiber types studied. The posterior root (PR) and the anterior root (AR) fibers enter and exit the spinal cord, respectively, at the level of the stimulating electrode. The posterior column fiber is located medially and superficially in the posterior white matter. **(b)** Enlarged view of the box in **(a)**. **(c)** Activating functions corresponding to **(a)**. **(d)** Topview of the fiber trajectories and the spinal cord. The excitation thresholds for these fibers calculated by the MRG model were 17.6 V, 51.7 V and 67.4 V for the PR, AR and Pcol, respectively. (adapted from [18]).

the fiber classes (10.5 μm for Pcol, 14 μm for AR and 16 μm for PR) [27, 28, 29, 18].

III. RESULTS

The electrical field produced by transcutaneous stimulation with –1 V along selected target nerve structures is illustrated in figure 2a and b and the simulated current flow can be seen in figure 1g. The corresponding activating functions are depicted in figure 2c and the geometrical relations in figure 2d. Along the most preferentially located (medial and superficial) Pcol fiber, there are few inhomogeneities of the potential and also the activating function showed the lowest deviations from 0. The fibers in the PR and AR on the other hand had strong discontinuities in the potential along the fiber, specifically at the locations where the fibers entered/exited the spinal cord and canal. At these points, also the activating functions showed strong deviations from 0. The strongest depolarization—as suggested by a positive peak of the activating function (cf. figure 2c)—of the PR fiber occurred at its entrance into the spinal cord. At the exit of the AR fiber from the spinal cord it was mainly hyperpolarized. At the exits of both fibers from the spinal canal, they were comparably excitable. Fittingly, the sites of action potential initiation of the fiber in the PR was at the node of Ranvier closest to its entrance into the spinal cord and the one of the AR fiber closest to its exit from the spinal canal. The fiber in the Pcol was activated at the node of Ranvier closest to the stimulation electrode.

The activation thresholds of PR and AR fibers with different positions entering and exiting the spinal cord are depicted in table 1. The thresholds were lower for the PR than the AR fibers. Cathodic stimulation was more efficient to stimulate PR fibers. To stimulate AR fibers, anodic and cathodic stimulation were both similarly effective, with a slight advantage for the anodic case. Furthermore, the stimulation was more effective for PR fibers caudal to the stimulation electrode. For the AR fibers, the opposite was evident.

Cathodic and anodic excitation thresholds of PR and AR fibers were computed using the MRG and CRRSS model. The MRG model resulted in considerably lower thresholds for any of the calculated target fibers and both stimulation modes (table 1) as compared to the CRRSS model. The thresholds were 23.2% $\pm$ 4.6% (mean $\pm$ SD) of the values derived by the CRRSS model. The range varied from 15.9% to 38.6%. The straight Pcol fiber that had a threshold of 67.4 V according to the MRG model, and an excitation threshold of even 611 V when evaluated with the CRRSS model.

Table 1 Excitation threshold (in V) of root fibers

	posterior root				anterior root			
	cathodic		anodic		cathodic		anodic	
d[1]	MRG[2]	S[3]	MRG	S	MRG	S	MRG	S
3.9	20.1	97	50.0	272	23.2	110	**22.6**	105
2.6	26.1	101	51.5	324	28.9	103	37.1	161
1.3	29.5	129	49.5	230	37.1	147	51.4	224
0	17.6	76	65.0	224	51.7	222	67.9	176
-1.3	21.5	99	87.1	307	72.2	333	68.5	356
-2.6	**14.1**	69	110.9	405	82.4	433	67.6	238
-3.9	14.4	65	114.1	482	33.9	174	70.9	401

[1] *d* (in cm) denotes the vertical distance of the entry point of the root fibre into the spinal cord from the centre of the stimulation electrode. The lowest excitation thresholds are written in bold.
[2] MRG: **M**cIntyre-**R**ichardson-**G**rill model,
[3] S: Chiu-Ritchie-Rogart-Stagg-Sweeney (CRRSS) model.

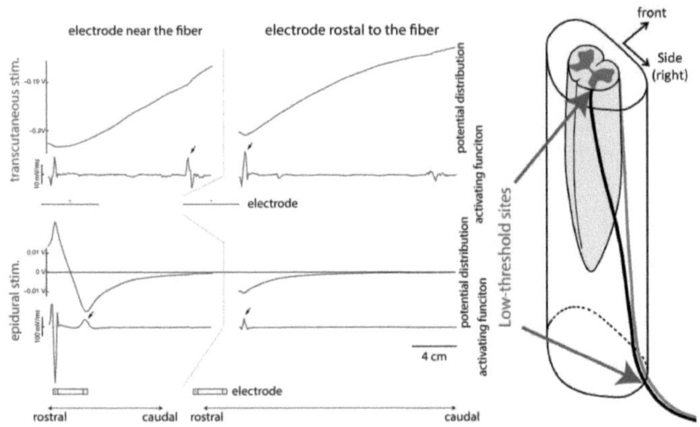

Fig. 3 Stimulation effect of transcutaneous and epidural electrodes located at levels of and rostral to the posterior root fibers (**left**). The two low-threshold sites can be seen in case of transcutaneous stimulation. Depending on the distance of the electrode to these sites, either one is the site of action potential initiation. In case of epidural stimulation, the electrode placed near the fiber introduced strong, local deflections of the potential distribution and the activating function at the level of the contacts of the electrode. Whereas, the electrode located rostral to the fiber introduced an electric potential and activating function along the fiber similar to those in case of transcutaneous stimulation. Arrows indicate the site where the spikes were initiated at the threshold intensity. **Right**: Sketch of anatomically determined low-threshold sites ('hot-spots'; adapted from [19]).

Pcol fibers were easiest excitable at their most medial and superficial location in the white matter (67.4 V). This is also the location where the fiber was closest to the paraspinal electrodes and the potential was highest. The influence of an increase in fibre diameter for the medially and most superficial located fibre was also investigated. With the diameter increased to 16 μm, same as assumed for the posterior root fibers, the excitation threshold of the posterior column fibre decreased to 40.1 V. The activation threshold was also decreased by introducing collaterals. A single collateral, attached to the node of Ranvier that was the action potential initiation site reduced the threshold to 59.6 V. Additional nine collaterals attached to the neighboring nodes above and below reduced the activating threshold to 45.4 V, which is still approx. 3 times the threshold of the most excitable PR fiber.

Transcutaneous was compared to epidural stimulation (see figure 3). With former stimulation the root fibers were always activated at either one of the 'hot-spot' sites, i.e. their points of entry/exit into/from the spinal cord and canal, while in the case of epidural stimulation, action potentials were initiated usually close to the cathode. Yet, if the cathode of the epidural electrode was located rostral to the target fibers, the action potential initiation sites were at the entrances of the PR fibers into the spinal cord.

IV. Discussion

The reviewed modeling studies elaborated the direct effects of transcutaneous spinal cord stimulation on sensory structures and motor fibers within lumbar spinal roots as well as fibers within the posterior white matter of the human lumbar spinal cord. The MRG model was applied to calculate realistic, relatively low excitation thresholds. In fact, the thresholds were about four times lower than the results computed by the CRRSS model. Large diameter posterior root afferent fibers had the lowest excitation threshold followed by anterior root efferent fibers. Excitation thresholds of fibers in the posterior columns were relatively high even when calculated with the MRG model. For the most preferential position (superficial and medial) and features (large diameters and presence of collaterals), their thresholds were still three times higher than the thresholds of posterior root fibers.

'Hot-spots', sites with low activation thresholds, were identified at the entry point of posterior rootlets into the spinal cord, at the entry/exit point of the posterior and anterior roots into/from the spinal canal and at the branching points of the collaterals from the posterior column fibers. These 'hot-spots' were given rise to by the electrical properties of the surrounding tissues and the trajectory of the nerve fibers, thus caused by the anatomy [17, 19]. Transitions of nerve fibers, as seen from the cathodic electrode, between a highly conducting (here the cerebrospinal fluid) into a relatively lower conducting medium (here the white matter) cause a large positive peak of the second-order spatial derivative of the potential along the nerve fiber [22]. Thus, the threshold is significantly lowered. Depending on the electrode position relative to the nerve fiber one of the 'hot-spots' has the lowest threshold (cf. figure 3). The anterior root fibers only have one 'hot-spot' at their exit from the spinal canal, and thus more rostrally located fibers have lower thresholds, since for those fibers, the 'hot-spot' is closer to the stimulation electrodes. This is also corroborated by preliminary experimental results, where M-wave components in the recorded CMAPs were more often identified in quadriceps than in triceps surae [14, 30].

Stimulation of fibers in the posterior columns can be expected only at relatively high stimulation intensities, around three times the threshold of posterior root fibers. This is due to the relatively few inhomogeneities introduced into the electrical field surrounding the posterior column fibers, which would influence the excitability of the nerve fibers [22, 21]. By contrast, the electrical field produced by epidural stimulation is focused on its own, producing large values in the activating function, even in straight fibers inside a medium with homogenous electrical properties. Thus, direct stimulation of fibers in the posterior column is more likely with epidural than with transcutaneous stimulation [31, 32].

The thresholds calculated by the CRRSS model were reported to be 2–3 times higher than the thresholds of the corresponding clinical effects [33, 34]. Independently, the MRG model has been shown to reproduce threshold values of transcutaneous electrical stimulation more realistically [35]. Indeed, threshold values reported by Ladenbauer et al. [17] were overestimated and could be reduced here by applying the MRG model (see table 1) on average to about a fourth of the CRRSS model. Applying the MRG model, thresholds of posterior root afferents are now closer to the thresholds of reflex responses to transcutaneous spinal cord stimulation in lower limb muscles. These PRM reflexes were elicited simultaneously in the key muscles of thighs and lower legs at a common threshold of 28.6 ± 6.3 V in a group of eight individuals with an intact nervous system [7]. The seemingly underestimation (14 V threshold for posterior root activation here) can be explained by differences between the threshold of activating the lowest threshold Ia afferents and generating appropriate temporal and spatial synaptic summation for eliciting a reflex. A synchronous volley of action potentials is needed to activate a motoneuron. Also note that the relationship between the excitation thresholds calculated by the CRRSS and the MRG model is not trivial and cannot be approximated with a common constant factor.

Only the steady-state solution was calculated with the finite element model, neglecting capacitive, which might cause a depth dependent filtering of the applied electrical signal, thus altering the pulse shapes acting on the nerve fibers. Since the pulse shapes strongly influence the effectiveness of the stimulation, specifically if the pulse duration is relatively long [36], the thresholds and their relationships might be affected. Furthermore, the stereotyped and simplified geometry is not sufficient for the investigation of more complex phenomena, like the influence of the body or (rostro-caudal) electrode positions on the activation thresholds. A more detailed model including the sacrum and properties of the individual vertebrae including their relative positions would be necessary. These shortcomings will be addressed in future work.

V. Conclusion

The computer simulations demonstrated that the activation of specific neural structures by transcutaneous spinal cord stimulation is predominantly due to the electrical properties of the anatomy that introduce inhomogeneities into the electrical field, which otherwise would be rather diffuse. The simulation results support that posterior root fibers have the lowest thresholds followed by anterior root fibers. Thresholds of posterior column fibers are still not effectively reduced by the introduction of multiple collaterals, their direct activation is unlikely. The finding of the rather high thresholds of posterior column fibers grants important information for the potential of direct stimulation of other intraspinal neural structures. Posterior column fibers superficially located within the white matter with large diameters and multiple collaterals can be assumed to be the intraspinal neural structures with the lowest thresholds. Thus, excitation of other white matter tracts would require even higher stimulus intensities and direct electrical activation of grey matter structures can be excluded with applicable stimulus intensities.

Conflict of Interest

The authors declare that they have no conflict of interest.

Acknowledgements

Wings for Life Spinal Cord Research Foundation, WFL-AT-007/11; Vienna Science and Technology Fund, LS11-057.

References

1. Pinter MM, Gerstenbrand F, Dimitrijevic MR. Epidural electrical stimulation of posterior structures of the human lumbosacral cord: 3. Control of spasticity *Spinal Cord.* 2000;38:524-531.
2. Danner SM, Dimitrijevic MR. Spasticity: Pathophysiology and Neural Control in *3rd Asia-Oceanian Conference of Physical and Rehabilitation Medicine in Conjunction with XI Annual Scientific of Indonesian Association of Physical Medicine and Rehabilitation* (Kusumastuti P, Tulaar ABM. eds.):9–15 2012.
3. Hofstoetter US, McKay WB, Tansey KE, Mayr W, Kern H, Minassian K. Modification of spasticity by transcutaneous spinal cord stimulation in individuals with incomplete spinal cord injury *J Spinal Cord Med.* 2013;doi: 10.1179/2045772313Y.0000000149.
4. Hofstoetter US, Hofer C., Kern H, et al. Effects of transcutaneous spinal cord stimulation on voluntary locomotor activity in an incomplete spinal cord injured individual *Biomed Tech (Berl).* 2013;doi: 10.1515/bmt-2013-4014.

5. Minassian K., Hofstoetter U. S., Tansey K. E., Mayr W.. Neuromodulation of lower limb motor control in restorative neurology *Clin Neurol and Neurosur.* 2012;114:489-497.
6. Minassian K., Jilge B., Rattay F., et al. Stepping-like movements in humans with complete spinal cord injury induced by epidural stimulation of the lumbar cord: electromyographic study of compound muscle action potentials. *Spinal Cord.* 2004;42:401–416.
7. Minassian K, Persy I, Rattay F, Dimitrijevic MR, Hofer C, Kern H. Posterior root-muscle reflexes elicited by transcutaneous stimulation of the human lumbosacral cord *Muscle Nerve.* 2007;35:327-336.
8. Hofstoetter US, Minassian K, Hofer C, Mayr W, Rattay F, Dimitrijevic MR. Modification of reflex responses to lumbar posterior root stimulation by motor tasks in healthy subjects *Artif Organs.* 2008;32:644-8.
9. Hofstoetter US, Danner SM, Minassian K. Paraspinal magnetic and transcutaneous electrical stimulation in *Encyclopedia of Computational Neuroscience: SpringerReference* (Jaeger D, Jung R. eds.)Berlin, Heidelberg: Springer-Verlag. doi: 10.1007/978-1-4614-7320-6_603-4 2013.
10. Ugawa Y, Rothwell JC, Day BL, Thompson PD, Marsden CD. Magnetic stimulation over the spinal enlargements *J Neurol Neurosurg Psychiatry.* 1989;52:1025-32.
11. Cretu M, Ciupa RV, Darabant L. Evaluation of spinal cord response during magnetic stimulation of the lumbar area *Biomed Tech (Berl).* 2013;doi: 10.1515/bmt-2013-4009.
12. Knikou M. Neurophysiological characteristics of human leg muscle action potentials evoked by transcutaneous magnetic stimulation of the spine *Bioelectromagnetics.* 2013;34:200-10.
13. Courtine G, Harkema SJ, Dy CJ, Gerasimenko YP, Dyhre-Poulsen P. Modulation of multisegmental monosynaptic responses in a variety of leg muscles during walking and running in humans *J Physiol.* 2007;582:1125-39.
14. Roy FD, Gibson G, Stein RB. Effect of percutaneous stimulation at different spinal levels on the activation of sensory and motor roots *Exp Brain Res.* 2012;223:281-9.
15. Knikou M. Neurophysiological characterization of transpinal evoked potentials in human leg muscles *Bioelectromagnetics.* 2013;34:630-40.
16. Mayr W, Danner SM, Sarabon N, et al. Effect of functional electrical stimulation on the central state of excitability of the spinal cord in *World Congress on Medical Physics and Biomedical Engineering May 26-31, 2012, Beijing, China* (Long Mian. ed.);39 of *IFMBE Proceedings*:2240-2243Springer Berlin Heidelberg 2013.
17. Ladenbauer J, Minassian K, Hofstoetter US, Dimitrijevic MR, Rattay F. Stimulation of the human lumbar spinal cord with implanted and surface electrodes: a computer simulation study *IEEE Trans Neural Syst Rehabil Eng.* 2010;18:637-45.
18. Danner SM, Hofstoetter US, Ladenbauer J, Rattay F, Minassian K. Can the human lumbar posterior columns be stimulated by transcutaneous spinal cord stimulation? A modeling study *Artif Organs.* 2011;35:257-262.
19. Danner SM, Hofstoetter US, Minassian K. Finite element models of transcutaneous spinal cord stimulation in *Encyclopedia of Computational Neuroscience: SpringerReference* (Jaeger D, Jung R. eds.)Berlin, Heidelberg: Springer-Verlag. doi: 10.1007/SpringerReference_348669 2013.
20. Holsheimer J. Computer modelling of spinal cord stimulation and its contribution to therapeutic efficacy *Spinal Cord.* 1998;36:531-40.
21. Rattay F, Danner SM, Hofstoetter US, Minassian K. Finite element modeling for extracellular stimulation in *Encyclopedia of Computational Neuroscience: SpringerReference* (Jaeger D, Jung R. eds.)Berlin, Heidelberg: Springer-Verlag. doi: 10.1007/SpringerReference_348658 2013.
22. Rattay F. The basic mechanism for the electrical stimulation of the nervous system *Neuroscience.* 1999;89:335-46.
23. Ranck JB. Which elements are excited in electrical stimulation of mammalian central nervous system: a review *Brain Res.* 1975;98:417-40.
24. McIntyre CC, Richardson AG, Grill WM. Modeling the excitability of mammalian nerve fibers: influence of afterpotentials on the recovery cycle *J Neurophysiol.* 2002;87:995-1006.
25. Chiu SY, Ritchi JM, Rogart RB, Stagg D. A quantitative description of membrane current in rabbit myelinated nerves *J Physiol.* 1979;292:149–166.
26. Sweeney JD, Mortimer JT, Durand D. Modeling of mammalian myelinated nerve for functional neuromuscular electrostimulation *Proceedings of the 97h Annual Conference IEEE EMBS.* 1987:1577–1578.
27. Lloyd DCP. Neuron patterns controlling transmission of ipsilateral hind limb reflexes in cat *J Neurophysiol.* 1943;6:293–315.
28. Brodal P, Rinvik E. The somatic afferent pathways in *Neurological anatomy in Relation to Clinical Medicine* (Brodal A. ed.)ch. 2, :46–147New York: Oxford University Press 1981.
29. Feirabend HKP, Choufoer H, Ploeger S, Holseimer J, Gool JD. Morphometry of human superficial dorsal and dorsolateral column fibers: Siginificance to spinal cord stimulation *Brain.* 2002;125:1137–1149.
30. Krenn M, Toth A, Danner SM, Hofstoetter US, Minassian K, Mayr W. Selectivity of transcutaneous stimulation of lumbar posterior roots at different spinal levels in humans *Biomed Tech (Berl).* 2013;doi: 10.1515/bmt-2013-4010.
31. Struijk JJ, Holsheimer J, Heide FG, Boom HBK. Recruitment of dorsal column fibers in spinal cord stimulation: influence of collateral branching *IEEE Transactions on Biomedical Engineering.* 1992;39:903–912.
32. Holsheimer J. Which neuronal elements are activated directly by spinal cord stimulation *Neuromodulation.* 2002;5:25–31.
33. Struijk JJ, Holsheimer J, Barolat G, He J, Boom HBK. Paresthesia thresholds in spinal cord stimulation: A comparison of theoretical results with clinical data *IEEE T Rehabil Eng.* 1993;1:101–108.
34. Wesselink WA, Holsheimer J, Boom HBK. A model for the electrical behaviour of myelinated sensory nerve fibres based on human data *Med Biol Eng Comput.* 1999;37:228–235.
35. Kuhn A, Keller T, Lawrence M, Morari M. A model for transcutaneous current stimulation: Simulations and experiments *Med Biol Eng Comput.* 2009;47.
36. Krouchev NI, Danner SM, Vinet A, Rattay F, Sawan M. Energy-optimal electrical-stimulation pulses shaped by the least-action principle *PLoS One.* 2014;9:e90480.

Corresponding author: Simon M. Danner
Institute: Medical University of Vienna
Street: Währinger Gürtel 18-20/4L
City: 1090 Vienna
Country: Austria
Email: simon.danner@meduniwien.ac.at

Influence of the Electrical Parameters Variation of the Membrane Cell over the Nerve Fiber Activation

M. Crețu and R.V. Ciupa

Technical University of Cluj-Napoca, Electrotechnics and Measurements Department, Cluj-Napoca, Romania

Abstract— **The neuronal structures ca be modeled in the form of a cable, which contains active Hodgkin-Huxley elements. The membrane response can be computed by solving the cable equation, describing the transmembrane potential, in the presence of an electric field. The electric field is induced in the tissue by magnetic stimulation technique. In the active model of the nervous fiber (Hodgkin-Huxley model), the properties of the membrane cell are uniform along the fiber. The paper considered possible non-homogeneities of the nerve's electrical properties; and we assess their influence on the activation of the nerve fiber.**

Keywords— **Magnetic stimulation, non-homogeneous Hodgkin-Huxley model, action potential**

I. Introduction

Modeling the behavior of the nervous cell is very important, especially in the study of the nervous fibers response to stimulation [1]. The stimulation of the nerve fiber can occur on the electric or magnetic ways and it determines an action potential in the excitable cells. So, a current, flowing along the membrane, determines the ions loaded with electrical charges to pass the cellular membrane. In this way, depolarization of a part of the cellular membrane occurs. When the current has an adequate intensity and orientation, an action potential appears.

In the Hodgkin-Huxley model, the membrane behavior was modeled using an electric circuit with constant parameters along the entire length of the nervous axon [1], [2]. This paper considers possible non-homogeneous points of the membrane, by taking into account the variation of fiber parameters along the length of the nerve. The response of the nervous fiber (the action potential) for this case will be compared with the transmembrane potential computed for invariable membrane parameters. Also, these possible non-homogeneities of the nervous fiber parameters will lead to considerable changes of the activation threshold of the nervous cell and of the latency period.

The paper starts by emphasizing theoretical background of fiber excitation by magnetic stimulation (computation of induced electric field, the description of the stimulating circuit and the behavior of the nerve fiber – active cable model). Then, the parameters variation of the cellular membrane and their influences over the response of the nervous fiber (the action potential) will be studied.

At the end of the paper, some important aspects and conclusions will be drawn.

II. Theoretical considerations

A. Mechanism of Fibers Excitation by Magnetic Stimulation

Fibers excitation by magnetic stimulation is a painless method for cortical stimulation or for the activation of deep lying peripheral nerves. The magnetic stimulation is based on Faraday's law and is referred to induce an electric field in nervous tissue by an alternating current, flowing through a coil, placed near the fiber to be stimulated. According to the electromagnetic field theory, the electric field inside the tissue can be computed by means of the scalar electric potential and the vector magnetic potential:

$$\overline{E} = \underbrace{-\frac{\partial \overline{A}}{\partial t}}_{\overline{E}_A} \underbrace{- gradV}_{\overline{E}_V} \tag{1}$$

The first term of the electric field $\overline{E_A}$, is due directly to the electromagnetic induction phenomenon, while the second term $\overline{E_V}$, is due to charge accumulation on the tissue-air boundary. The mathematical model for computations of $\overline{E}_A$, for coils of non- or traditional shapes is fully described in [3].

A common application of magnetic stimulation is to excite peripheral nerves [4]. We assume that we stimulate the forearm, which can be modeled as a cylindrical volume conductor. The $\overline{E}_V$ component of the electric field depends on the geometry of the tissue-air interface, considered a cylindrical surface, and it is computed using the algorithm from [3].

For the operating frequency of magnetic stimulation, the electrical and magnetic properties of the medium are assumed to be σ=1S/m and μ=μ0.

B. Stimulating Circuit

The coil current *I(t)* is predicted by a series RLC model of the current stimulator. The circuit works in transient state. Considering the medical application [5], the overdamped case is used for single pulse magnetic stimulation, the underdamped oscillatory regime is more suitable for

S. Vlad and R.V. Ciupa (eds.), *International Conference on Advancements of Medicine and Health Care through Technology*, IFMBE Proceedings 44,
DOI: 10.1007/978-3-319-07653-9_42, © Springer International Publishing Switzerland 2014

repetitive stimulation, while the third transient regime, the critically damped, is not used, because is difficult to achieve it experimentally.

Considering the overdamped state, the condition to be fulfilled is: $\left(\frac{R}{2L}\right)^2 > \frac{1}{LC}$. If the inequality is reversed, the circuit works in an underdamped transient state. The oscillation frequency is: $f = 1/2\pi \cdot \sqrt{LC}$.

The current waveforms for both these regimes are predicted in [3].

The coil's inductance is evaluated by taking the line integral of the vector potential around the coil for unit current: $L = \oint \overline{A} \cdot \overline{dl}$ (This formula permits the computation of inductances of the special coils) [6].

The coil is part of a magnetic stimulator that also comprises a capacitance, C=200μF. The resistance from the circuit is evaluated using the analytical formula:

$$R = \frac{\rho_{Cu} 2\pi r N}{\pi r_w^{\ 2}} \tag{2}$$

where ρ_{Cu} - copper resistivity; r – radius of the coil; N – number of turns; r_w - radius of the wire conductor.

If the total resistance (including the coil and wires resistances) is considered to be 1.75Ω, for a larger value of the total resistance (R=3Ω), the above inequality is reversed and the transient regime is overdamped.

C. Hodgkin-Huxley Model

Neuronal structures can be modeled in the form of a cable and the membrane response can be computed by solving the equations describing the transmembrane potential across the membrane of the cable in the presence of induced electric fields [1]. The relation between the transmembrane potential along an infinitely long nerve fiber (placed along the z axis) in the presence of induced electric fields is given by the passive cable model [1], [2]:

$$\tau \frac{\partial V_m}{\partial t} + V_m - \lambda^2 \frac{\partial^2 V_m}{\partial z^2} = \underbrace{-\lambda^2 \frac{\partial E_z}{\partial z}}_{=f(z)}, \tag{3}$$

where V_m is the transmembrane voltage, E_z the axial component of the induced electric field, λ the space constant of the cable and τ the time constant.

The term on the right of equation (3) represents the activation function of the neuronal structures, equal to the spatial derivative of the electric field induced along the nerve fiber.

While the passive cable model provides the way of the interaction between the induced electric field and the nerve, it does not completely describe the dynamics of nerve stimulation. In order to study the stimulation and propagation of action potentials, we must consider an active membrane model. We use the Hodgkin-Huxley model to represent the nerve membrane (Figure 1). To implement this model, we modify the initial passive cable model. The extracellular potential produced by the fiber's own activity is negligible. This assumption is valid because the extracellular potential produced by an action potential propagating along a single nerve axon lying in a large extracellular volume conductor is less than 1 mV [1].

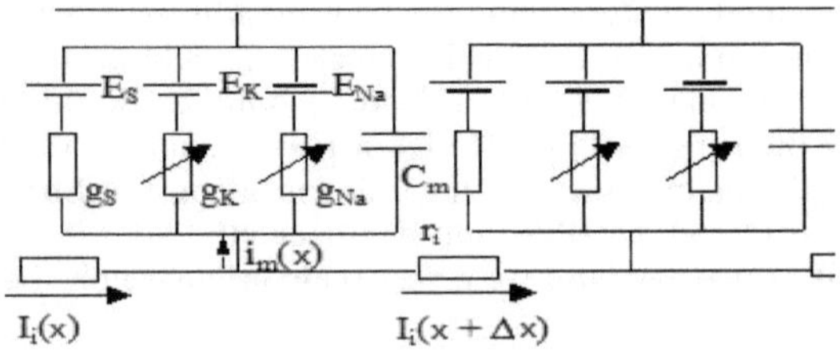

Fig. 1 Hodgkin-Huxley model of the active cellular membrane [1]

The resistance per unit length of the fiber r_i can be expressed in terms of the fiber radius a and the resistivity of the axoplasm R_i, as: $r_i = R_i/\pi a^2$. The membrane current per unit length i_m is related to the membrane current density J_m by the expression: $i_m = 2\pi a J_m$; similarly the membrane capacitance per unit length c_m is related to the capacitance per unit area C_m by: $c_m = 2\pi a C_m$. Finally we replace the membrane resistance per unit length r_m by an active model of time and voltage dependent sodium, potassium and leakage channels. With these changes, the cable equation becomes [1]:

$$\frac{a}{2R_i}\frac{\partial^2 V_m}{\partial z^2} - \left(g_{Na} m^3 h(V_m - E_{Na}) + g_K n^4 (V_m - E_K) + g_S (V_m - E_S)\right) = C_m \frac{\partial V_m}{\partial t} + \frac{a}{2R_i}\frac{\partial E_z}{\partial z}(z,t) \tag{4}$$

where g_{Na}, g_K and g_S are the peak sodium, potassium and leakage membrane conductances per unit area, and E_{Na}, E_K and E_S are the sodium, potassium and leakage Nerst potentials. The gating variables m, n, h are dimensionless functions of time and voltage which vary between zero and one:

$$\frac{\partial m}{\partial t} = \alpha_m (1 - m) - \beta_m m \tag{5}$$

$$\frac{\partial h}{\partial t} = \alpha_h (1 - h) - \beta_h h \tag{6}$$

$$\frac{\partial n}{\partial t} = \alpha_n (1 - n) - \beta_n n \tag{7}$$

where α and β are voltage dependent rate constants, determined from the voltage clamp measurements [7].

We assumed that the resting potential is -65mV, V_m is measured in mV, α and β in ms^{-1}. Equations describing the Hodgkin-Huxley model of the cellular membrane ((4) - (7), including the equations describing α and β from the voltage clamp measurements [7]) constitute a system of four, nonlinear, coupled partial differential equations.

The values of model parameters used in our computations are given in Table 1 [1]:

Table 1

E_{Na}	Sodium Nerst potential	50 mV
E_K	Potassium Nerst potential	-77 mV
E_S	Leakage Nerst potential	-54.387 mV
g_{Na}	Sodium conductance	120 mΩ/ cm^2
g_K	Potassium conductance	36 mΩ/ cm^2
g_S	Leakage conductance	0.3 mΩ/ cm^2
C_m	Membrane capacitance	1 μF/ cm^2
R_i	Resistivity of axoplasm	0.0354 kΩ·cm
a	Fiber radius	0.0238 cm

III. Results and Discussions

Figure 2 shows the geometry of the problem: the coil from the excitation circuit, used to magnetic stimulation of the nervous fiber, is placed parallel with the tissue, but with 25mm displacement with respect to the cylinder axis.

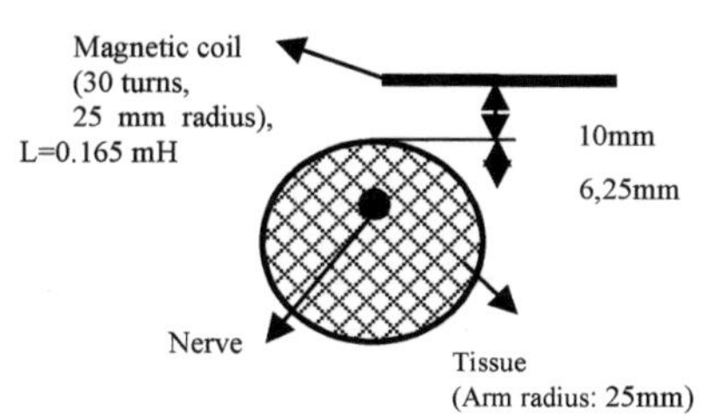

Fig. 2 Geometry of the problem

In order to obtain the response of the fiber to stimulation (the action potential) as a function of distance and time, first we modulate the electric field gradient in time ($\frac{\partial E_z(z,t)}{\partial z}$). The electric field gradient represents the activation function [8] and is calculated along the cylinder (the forearm) – Oz axis, on a line with y=0mm and z= 25–6.25 = 18.75mm, that is on a depth of 6.25mm inside the tissue, below the edge of the coil. For simulation purposes, the initial voltage on the circuit's capacitor is set to U_0=30V (the minimum value for the initial voltage on the circuit's capacitor, required to produce fiber activation) and Figure 3 shows the induced electric field gradient as a function of time and distance along the fiber.

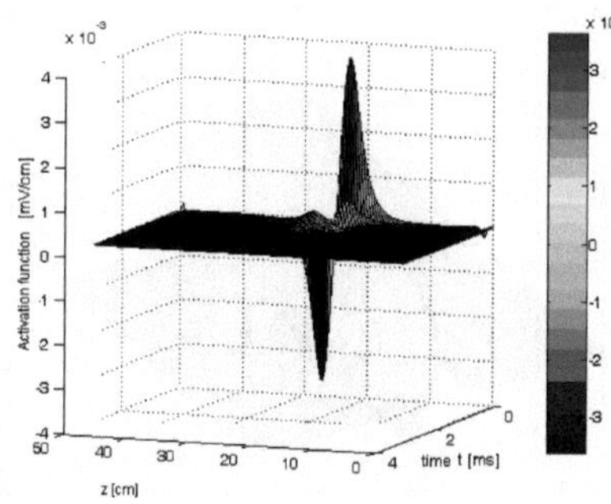

Fig. 3 The activation function evaluated along the length of the nerve fiber

Then, we implemented the algorithm of the problem using Matlab, and the transmembrane potential $V_m(z,t)$ and the three gating parameters $m(z,t)$, $n(z,t)$ and $h(z,t)$ are computed using the method of finite differences, implemented with an iterative algorithm [9] (we compute the value of each parameter knowing its value for the previous time step - 0.1ms). The space discretization uses a step of 5mm.

It is assumed that the membrane is initially at rest:

$$\frac{\partial V_m}{\partial t} = \frac{\partial m}{\partial t} = \frac{\partial h}{\partial t} = \frac{\partial n}{\partial t} = 0 \quad for\, t = 0 \tag{8}$$

The transmembrane voltage is taken to be its resting value and the initially m, n and h each are evaluated at the resting potential -65mV.

The boundary conditions of the problem, applied for $z = \pm L$, far from the region where the stimulus strength is large, are that the axial gradients in the transmembrane potential and the three gating parameters vanish.

$$\frac{\partial V_m}{\partial z} = \frac{\partial m}{\partial z} = \frac{\partial h}{\partial z} = \frac{\partial n}{\partial z} = 0 \tag{9}$$

The proposed model is used to determine the behavior of the nervous fiber to magnetic stimulation, the action potential (Figure 4).

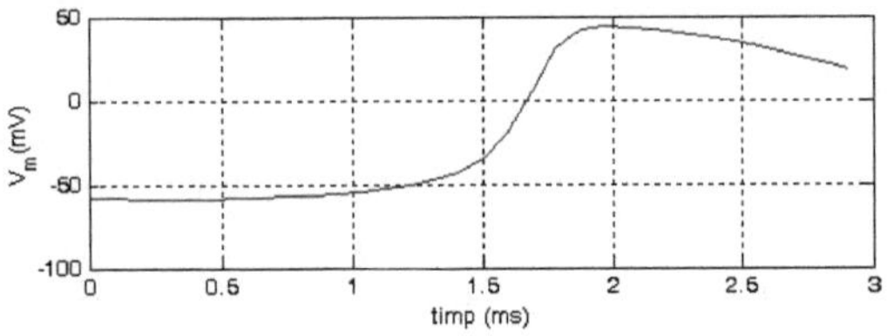

a)

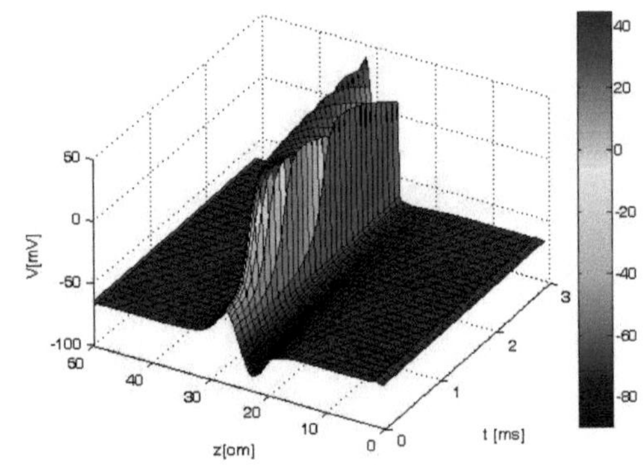

b)

Fig. 4 The response of the nerve fiber to magnetic stimulation for U_0=30V a) 2D representation; b) A three-dimensional plot. (The vertical axis is the action potential, and the horizontal axes represents the distance along the fiber x and the time after capacitor is discharged, t.)

The action potential rises rapidly to the value of about 50V, after a latency period of 1.2ms. The three – dimensional plot (Figure 4(a)) shows the depolarized portion of the nerve has been stimulated, while the hyperpolarized portion is not.

In most of the publications the electrical properties of the membrane are considered uniform along the fiber, even in the original model, elaborated by Hodgkin and Huxley [1], [2], [10]. This assumption may not always be true, considering the fact that the human tissue is, always, a very non-homogenous area. Nerve fiber models with parameter variability within the fiber were investigated in [11], [12] resulting in a change of the excitation threshold up to 20% compared to the standard model, when varying only a parameter.

Unlike the existing publications, we assume that the electric parameters of the membrane vary within a range of 10% from the generally assumed value and they have a sinusoidal variation along the nerve fiber. The electrical parameters we changed are: g_{Na} – Sodium conductance; g_K – Potassium conductance and C_m – Membrane capacitance. We assumed that:

$$\begin{cases} g_{Na} = 120 + 12 \cdot \sin(j \cdot 2\pi / 10)\, m\Omega / cm^2 \\ g_K = 36 + 3.6 \cdot \sin(j \cdot 2\pi / 10)\, m\Omega / cm^2 \\ C_m = 1 + 0.1 \cdot \sin(j \cdot 2\pi / 10)\, \mu F / cm^2 \end{cases} \quad (10)$$

The variation of the electrical parameters of the membrane does not influence the excitation threshold of the nervous fiber, the activation occurs for the same initial voltage on the circuit's capacitor (U_0=30V) as in the model with constant parameters.

Next, our work consisted in assessing the influence of every parameter's variation on the transmembrane potential.

Changing the sodium conductance, will lead to the transmembrane potential decrease of about 20% from its initial value (with constant parameters) – Figure 5 (a). Instead, changing the potassium conductance, one can see that very little increase of V compared to $V_{initial}$, from 38mV to 45mV – Figura 5 (b).

When the membrane capacitance varies with 10% compared to Hodgkin-Huxley model, there is an increasing of the action potential from 38mV to 40mV – Figura 5 (c).

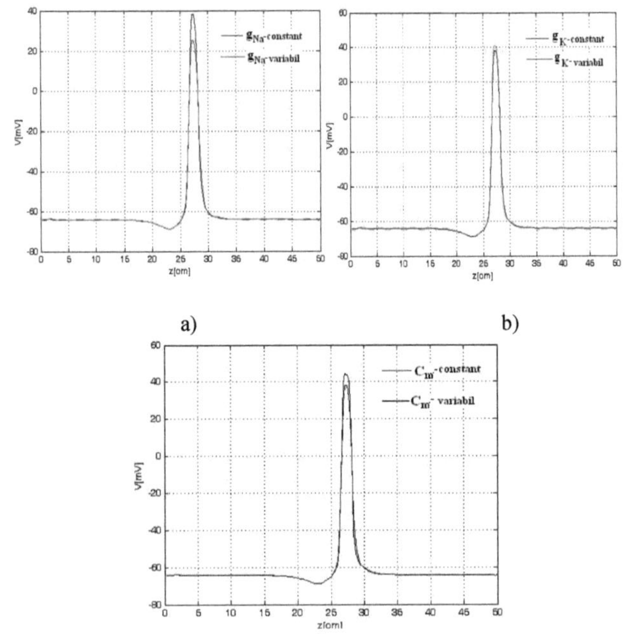

a) b)

c)

Fig. 5 Variation of the action potential at the variation of the electrical parameters of the cellular membrane along the nervous fiber. a) g_{Na} – varies; b) g_K – varies; c) C_m – varies.

Figure 5 shows that the modification of only one parameter from the nervous cell model, leads to significant changes of the action potential, by up to 20% for sodium conductance, but the excitability threshold or the latency period in stimulation do not change.

When is it apply a stimulus with a higher intensity (the initial voltage on the capacitor is set to U_0= 200 [V]), one can see a change in the pulse shape of the action potential (Figure 6).

Further, we vary every electric parameter of the membrane cell for U_0=200V (Figure 7).

Figure 7 shows that the most significant change is recorded for the variation of g_{Na}, where the value of the action potential for the model with variable parameters decreases compared with the model for constant parameters, while in the case of g_K variation, the action potential increases compared with the model with constant parameters. When the membrane capacitance is changed, one can see that for a slightly larger intensity of the stimulus, there is no notice of any remarkable changes.

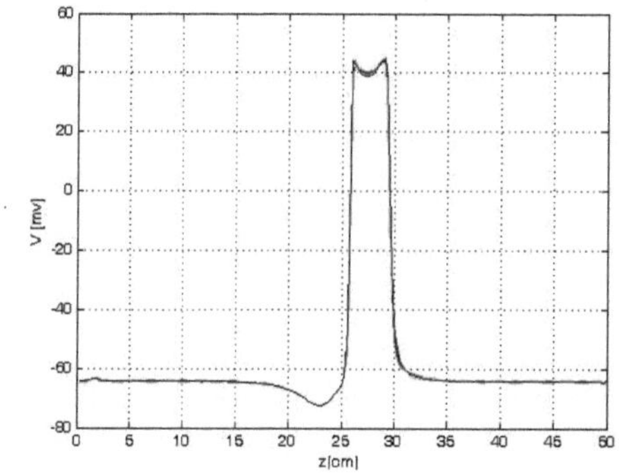

Fig. 6 Variation of the action potential in time, when the initial voltage on the circuit's capacitor is increased U_0=200V

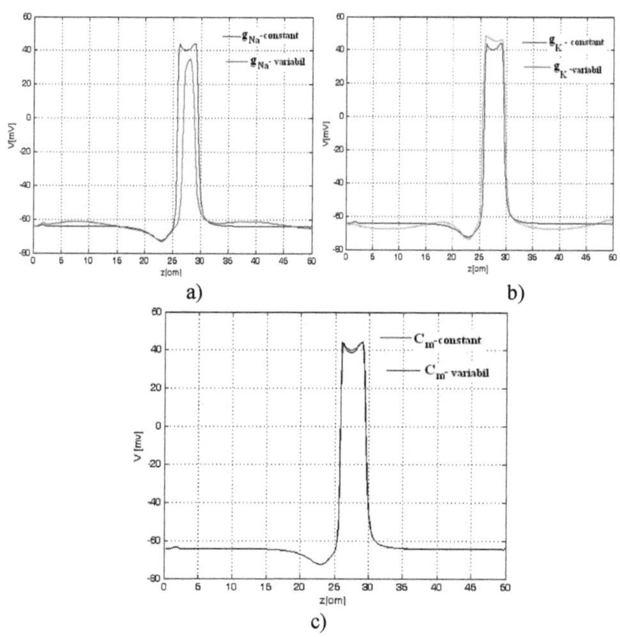

Fig. 7 Variation of the action potential at the variation of the electrical parameters of the cellular membrane along the nervous fiber for U_0=200V. a) g_{Na} – varies; b) g_K – varies; c) C_m – varies.

When all parameters vary simultaneously, the value of the action potential is always higher than the one for constant parameters (Figure 8).

The variation of the electrical parameters of the membrane with 10%, does not influence the excitation threshold of the nervous fiber, instead, if we vary the electrical parameters with more than 10% (20%) the initial voltage on the capacitor and the latency period (the moment when the stimulation appears) is changing. For the case when the parameters vary with 10% the initial voltage on the capacitor's circuit that we considered is U_0=35V, and when the parameters vary with 20% the initial voltage to achieve fiber activation is 50V. Figure 9 also illustrated the latency period; this is about 2ms for the model with constant parameters and 2.5ms, when the parameters change.

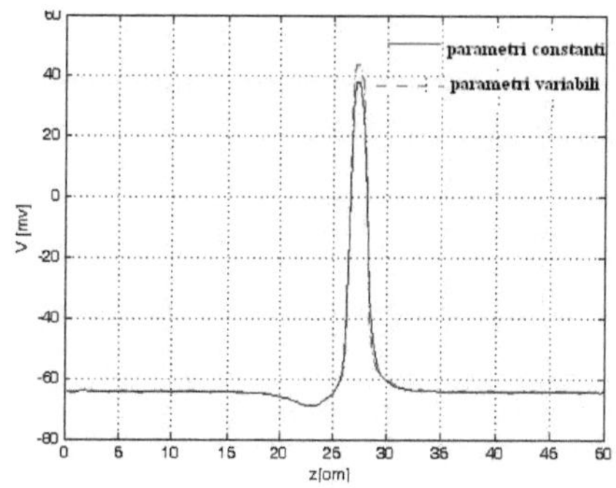

Fig. 8 The action potential at the simultaneous variation of the three parameters of the membrane cell – comparison with the action potential determined from the model with constant parameters of the membrane cell

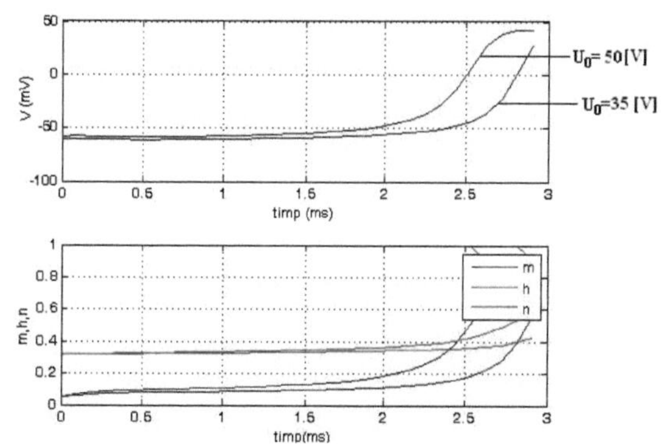

Fig. 9 Variation of the action potential and the three gating parameters in time, at the variation of the electrical parameters of the membrane cell, with 10% and 20% respectively, from their initial values.

IV. Conclusions

In our paper we have computed the response of the nerve fiber to magnetic stimulation, especially taking into consideration possible non-homogeneities of the nervous fiber.

Three aspects are considered together in one model: the current pulse shape, the spatial and temporal distribution of the induced electric field and the interaction of the electric field with the nerve.

The analysis of the neuronal responses during magnetic stimulation requires the solving of the cable equation associated with the active model for every nervous fiber.

The active Hodgkin-Huxley model was solved, using the Method of Finite Differences, the action potential was determined, and was highlighted the moment when the stimulation occurs.

In this paper we investigated the influence of the membrane electric parameter variability upon the response of the nerve fiber to stimulation.

The variation of the sodium conductance with 10% from the initial value, determines an increasing of the action potential with up to 20% compared with the value calculated for constant parameters, without any significant changes of the excitation threshold.

V. Conflict of Interest

The authors declare that they have no conflict of interest.

References

1. Nagarajan S., Durand D., Warman E. (1993) Effects of Induced Electric Fields on Finite Neuronal Structures: A Stimulation Study. IEEE Transactions on Biomedical Engineering, vol. 40, no. 11
2. Roth B.J., Basser P.J. (1990) A Model of the Stimulation of a Nerve Fiber by Electromagnetic Induction. IEEE Transactions on Biomedical Engineering, vol. 37, no. 6
3. Cretu M., Dărăbant L., Ciupa R. V., Nicu A. I., Curta C. (2009) Matlab Modelling of Nerve Fiber Activation by Magnetic Stimulation, MEDITECH 2009, 24-26 Septembrie, Cluj-Napoca, Romania, ISBN 978-3-642-04291-1, ISSN 1680-0737, Springer Verlag Berlin, pp. 327-332
4. Ruohonen J., Ravazzani P., Nilsson J., Panizza M., Grandori F., Tognola G. (1996) A volume-conduction analysis of magnetic stimulation of peripheral nerves. IEEE Trans. Biomed. Eng. Jul;43(7):669-78
5. Aciu C., Cobarzan N., Bumaru M., (2011), An Innovative Training Tool for Accesible Built Environment, IFBME Proceedings, Vol. 36, ISSN 1680 – 0737, pp. 1-4
6. Cret O., Trestian I., De Dinechin F., Darabant L., et all. (2007) Accelerating The Computation of The Physical Parameters Involved in Transcranial Magnetic Stimulation Using FPGA Devices, Romanian Journal of Information Science and Technology, Vol. 10, No. 4, pp. 361-379
7. Rafiroiu D., (2001) Bioelectromagnetism, Casa Cărții de Știință, Cluj-Napoca6
8. Rattay F., (1989), Analysis of Models for Extracellular Fiber Stimulation, IEEE Trans. On Biomed. Eng., Vol. 37, No. 7, pp. 676-682.
9. Darabant A. S., Darabant L., (2011) Clustering methods in data fragmentation, Romanian Journal of Information Science and Technology, Vol. 14, No. 1, pp. 81–97
10. Hodgkin A. L., Huxley A. F., (1952) A Quantitative Description of Membrane Current and its Application to Conduction and Excitation in Nerve, Journal of Physiology, Vol. 117, pp. 500-544
11. Krasteva V.T., Papazov S.P., Daskalov I.K. (2003) Peripheral nerve magnetic stimulation: influence of tissue non-homogeneity. Biomed. Eng. Online. 2003 Dec 23;2:19
12. Struijk J. J., Schnabel V., (2000) Influence of Parameter Variability on Stimulus Thresholds in Nerve Fiber Models, Proceedings of the 5th conf. of the IFESS, pp. 245-248

Application of Virtual Instrumentation for Transmitting and Processing ECG Signals

M. Munteanu[1], P. Bechet[2], C. Rusu[3], D.D. Micu[1], R.A. Munteanu[1], R. Moga[4], and C. Amza[5]

[1] Electrical Engineering Faculty, Technical University of Cluj-Napoca, Romania
[2] "Nicolae Balcescu" Land Forces Academy, Sibiu, Romania
[3] Faculty of Electronics, Telecommunications and Information Technology, Technical University of Cluj-Napoca, Romania
[4] Faculty of Automation and Computer Science, Technical University of Cluj-Napoca, Romania
[5] Department of Material Technology and Welding, "Politechnica" University of Bucharest, Romania

Abstract— **The paper aims to emphasize the possibilities offered by Virtual Instrumentation (LabVIEW) in the field of biomedical engineering. Thus, it proposes a low cost and flexible wireless transmission (between two equipments) and ECG signals processing architecture. Since during acquisition the signal may be corrupted by noise, in the first stage of the application the signal is filtered by implementing a designed mean averaged filter, followed by a Butterworth filter. The second stage of the application is represented by the infrared transmission of the signal between two infrared "in range" compatible devices. Finally, for an accurate R-peak detection, the Pan-Tomkins algorithm was implemented.**

Keywords— **LabVIEW programming, infrared transmission, ECG filtering, R-peak detection, Pan-Tompkins algorithm**

I. INTRODUCTION

In the last two decades, the use of wireless communication technologies through the new concept of telemedicine and remote monitoring has demonstrated the potential to improve the quality and the efficiency of patients' health care process [1], [2].

One positive aspect concerning the use of wireless techniques is the elimination of cables; the decrease of the number of connections and cables decreases the risk of accidental disjunction of the equipments [3]. Moreover, using the virtual instrumentation concept (LabVIEW), the system becomes more flexible, offering better maintenance; also, the transfer is performed in real time, which is the key issue when dealing with biomedical signals [4].

II. METHODS AND RESULTS

The application was developed according with the block-diagram presented in figure 1. The biomedical signal transferred and processed by this LabVIEW application is a *"ante finem"* real ECG signal, obtained through a holter recording from a patient (male, 80 years old, sinusal rhythm) that died because of a sudden heart failure [5]; during the acquisition process, the signal was contaminated by Gaussian white noise.

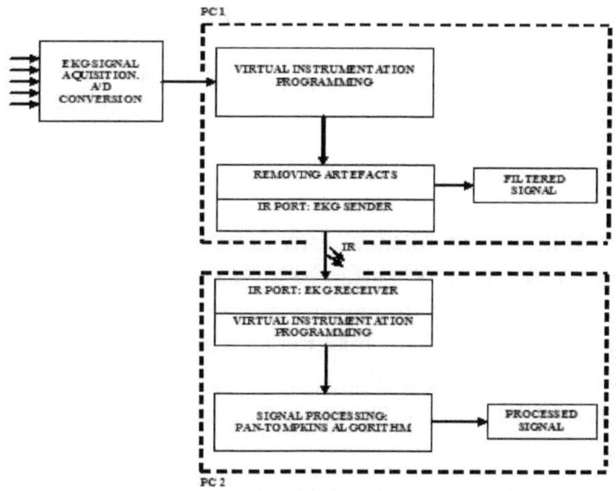

Fig. 1 The block-diagram of the application

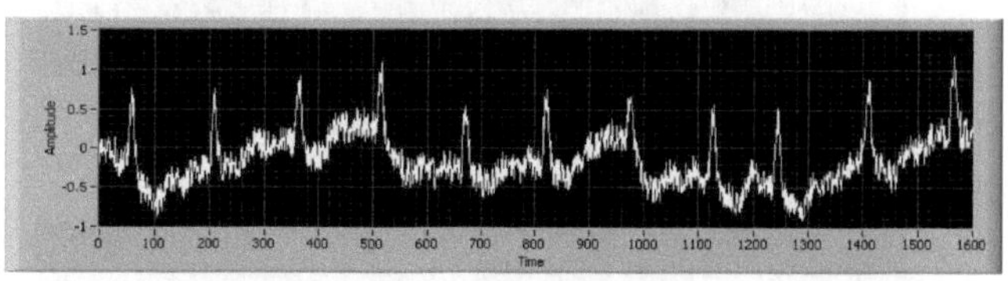

Fig. 2 ECG signal, after acquisition, contaminated by white noise

This setup was chosen for experimenting a two stage application: first, a preprocessing is performed on PC 1 (that will later be replaced by an embedded board with limited processing capabilities); than, the more complex algorithms are performed on PC 2.

Thus, as presented in figure 1, first of all the ECG is filtered, in order to provide a "clean" signal to the medical staff, from which the useful information can be extracted. Then, it is transmitted by using a wireless technology (infrared) from the module 1 of the equipment (PC 1) to the module 2 (PC 2).

S. Vlad and R.V. Ciupa (eds.), *International Conference on Advancements of Medicine and Health Care through Technology*, IFMBE Proceedings 44,
DOI: 10.1007/978-3-319-07653-9_43,

A. Signal Processing – Removing the Artifact

First of all, the transmitted signal (contaminated by Gaussian white noise) has to be filtered, in order to obtain a clean signal. The white noise is an infinite band noise [6], [7], [8], [9]; thus, the proposed filtering solution consists in a mean average filter, followed by a Butterworth filter (Band pass configuration). The mean averaged filter is a 7 taps low-pass FIR filter, characterized by a linear phase (the cutoff frequency is f_l=85 Hz). Mathematically, it is described by the following equation:

$$y(n)=\frac{1}{7}\left[x(n)+x(n-1)+....+x(n-6)\right] \qquad (1)$$

Its transfer function is given by:

$$H(\omega)=\frac{1}{7}(1+e^{-j\omega}+...+e^{-j6\omega})=\begin{cases}1, \omega=0\\ \frac{1}{7}e^{-j3\omega}\dfrac{\sin\left(\frac{7\omega}{2}\right)}{\sin\left(\frac{\omega}{2}\right)}\end{cases} \qquad (2)$$

The Butterworth filter, already defined in the LabVIEW libraries [10], is a 6th order band pass configuration IIR filter, with the cutoff frequencies at f_l=6 Hz and f_h=270 Hz. It provides sharper edges than the FIR filters, less computational effort for prescribed characteristics and an abrupt roll-off. The results of the filtering are presented in figure 3.

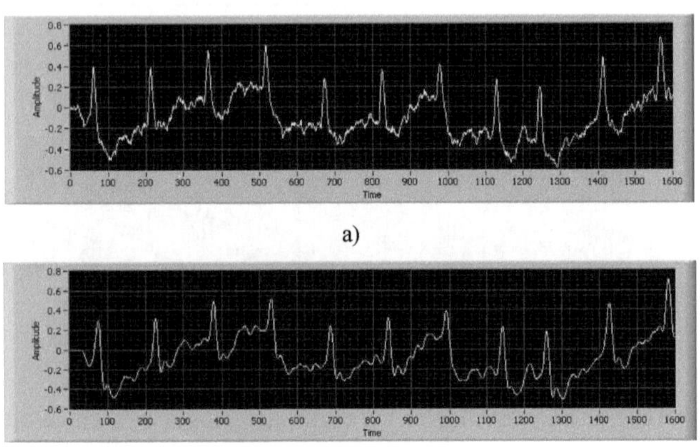

a)

b)

Fig. 3: a) Mean average filtering of the ECG signal;
b) „Clean" signal, after Butterworth filtering

Once filtered, the ECG signal is ready for the infrared transfer to another device/part of the equipment, where - in order to extract useful information - further signal processing operations will be performed.

B. Infrared Transfer of the ECG Signal

Wireless transfer of biomedical signals was performed also in the last years; but the infrared technology available at that moment was the so called *Slow speed Infrared*, providing slow speed, up to 115kbit/s [11], [12].

The latest versions of the infrared technology provide high speed data transfer (MIr – *Medium speed Infrared* with transfer rate up to 1,15 Mbps and FIr – *Fast speed Infrared* with transfer rate up to 4 Mbps) [13]. Therefore, we thought it useful to implement the FIr standard in LabVIEW and use it for biomedical signal transmission.

In order to transmit the ECG signal, the Client-Server application (developed in LabVIEW) [10] requires the following hardware: two computers (on both running LabVIEW) and two FIr-USB adaptors.

The Server detects the „in range" compatible device, identifying its name and ID. Then, the ECG is converted in string format, in order to be written to the infrared port.

The Client identifies the server by its ID and then receives the sent data. Finally, in order to be displayed, the ECG signal is reconverted from the string format (the format used by the infrared transmission) to numeric. The result of the transmission is presented in figure 4.

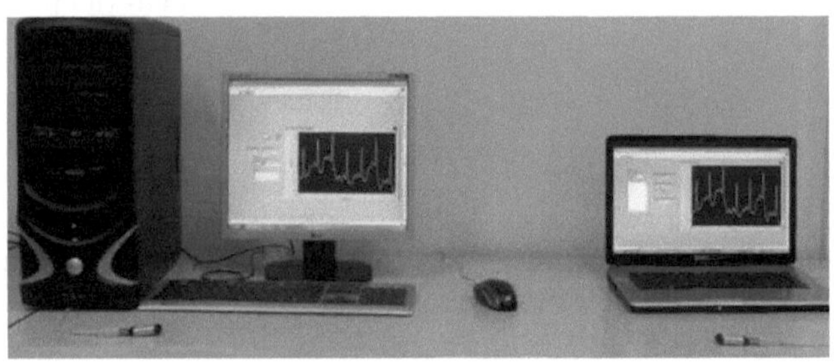

Fig. 4 ECG transmission using FIr technology

C. Signal Processing – Pan-Tompkins Algorithm

The most important element when calculating the pulse of the patient is the R-peak detection. For ideal, simulated signals [14], this is not a difficult task, as it can be reached by simply defining a threshold reference: any part of the signal exceeding the established threshold is labeled as R peak; thus, the pulse can be calculated easily (figure 5).

But in clinical situations, due to different reasons (technical and biological interferences), there are signals presenting a strong ascending or descending drift of the baseline.

When dealing with such signals, R-peak detection by setting a threshold limit is not working properly, as it can „miss" R-peaks, or it can false detect P or T wave as R-peaks (as presented in figure 6).

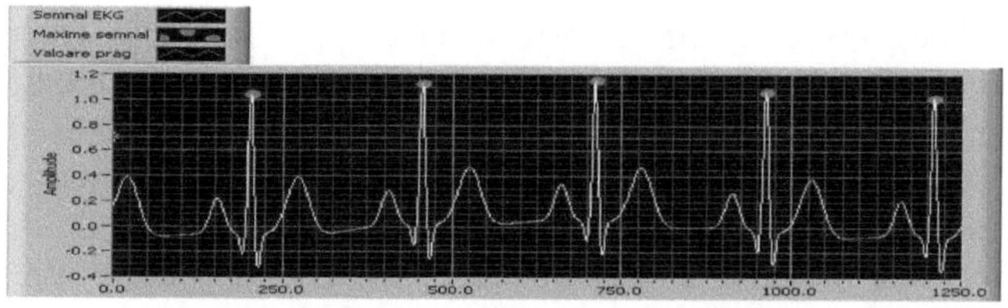

Fig. 5 Treshold R peak detection for a simulated signal

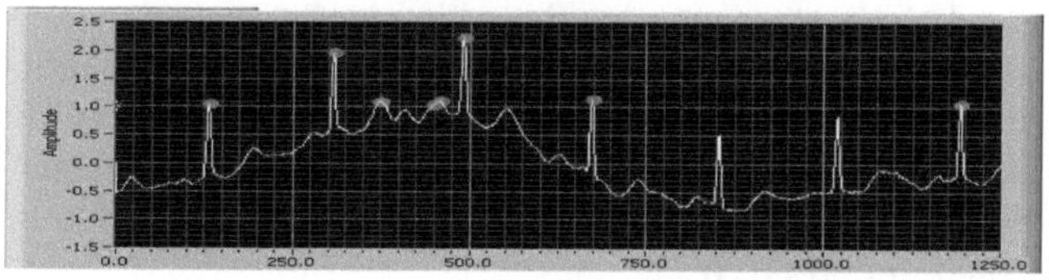

Fig. 6 False R detection – missing real R-peaks and misdetection of P or T wave as R-peaks

Although in the last years, there are studies recommending R-peak detection (or high amplitude varying parts of a medical signal) by the mean of wavelet analysis, the method used in our study implemented the Pan-Tompkins algorithm, that implies three different steps, as follows [8], [15]:

- Linear transformations that highlights the important information: filtering (two cascaded filters, low-pass and high-pass for removing different artifacts) and differentiation (to emphasize the QRS steep slopes in the signal, eliminating the components for P and T wave);
- Non-linear transformation: squaring (in order to amplify the high frequencies contained by the QRS);
- Moving average integrator.

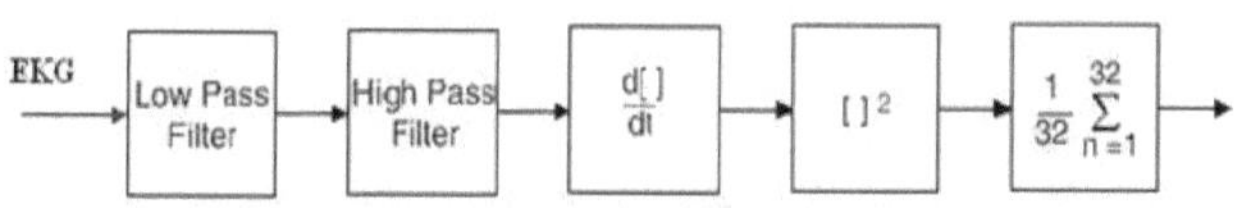

Fig. 7 Steps included in Pan-Tompkins algorithm [15]

Finally, the algorithm implies also a decisional stage, establishing adaptive threshold values (upper and lower), computed based on running estimates on signal/noise peak [15]. At the beginning, the signal and noise peaks are filtered using IIR low-pass filters; then, the output of IIR low-pass filters are weighted to get the superior threshold. The lower threshold is set half of the upper threshold [15].

The Pan-Tompkins algorithm was implemented in LabVIEW [10] and the results of each step are presented below:

a) Filtering

The two cascaded filters (low-pass and high-pass) are IIR filters, that will pass frequencies between 5-15 Hz, band which will highlight the energy of the QRS complexes [15], [16].

The low-pass filter is successfully used to reject the power supply interferences. Mathematically, is described by the following equation [8]:

$$y(n) = \frac{1}{32}\left[2y(n-1) - y(n-2) + x(n) - 2x(n-6) + x(n-12)\right] \quad (3)$$

The high-pass filter is implemented as an "all-pas" filter minus a first order "low pass" filter. The result is presented in figure 8.

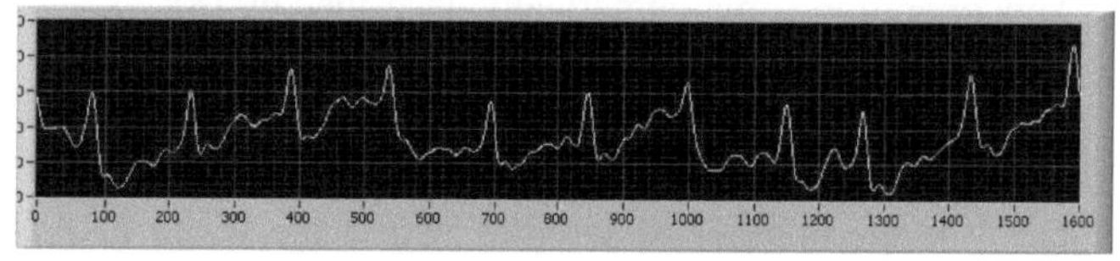

Fig. 8 Filtering of the ECG signal

b) Differentiation

This operation is mathematically described by [8]:

$$y(n) = \frac{1}{8}\left[2x(n) + x(n-1) - x(n-3) - 2x(n-4)\right] \quad (4)$$

The result of differentiation is presented in figure 9.

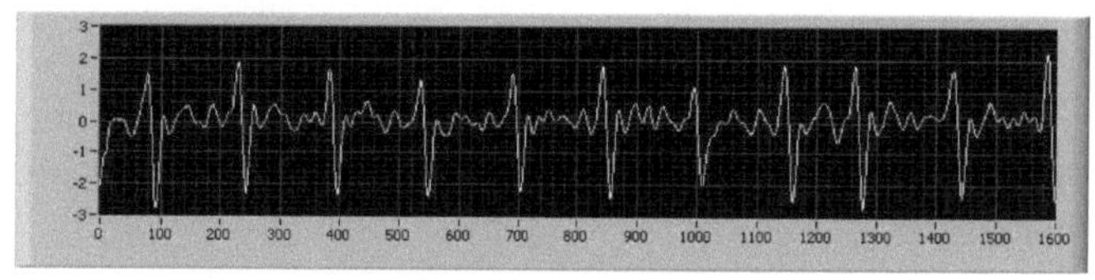

Fig. 9 Differentiation of the ECG signal

c) Squaring

The samples of the waveform obtained after differentiation are squared, point by point, according to [8]:

$$y(n) = [x(n)]^2 \quad (5)$$

This transformation aims to convert the signal to positive values, before integration; thus, it highlights only the high frequency components, obtained after the differentiation stage. The result of squaring is presented in figure 10.

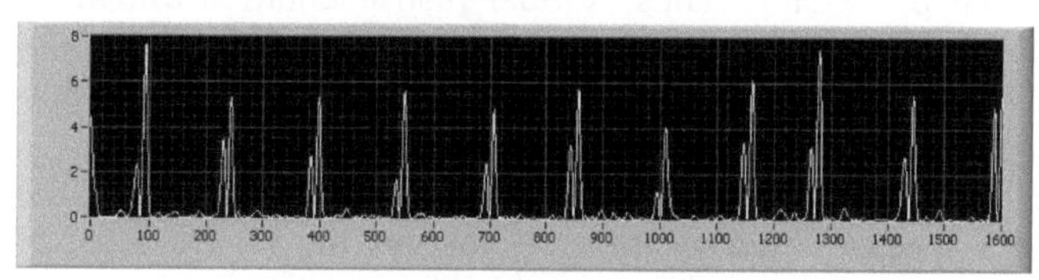

Fig. 10 Squaring the ECG signal

d) Moving Average Integrator

The slope of the QRS complex cannot be used as a singular method for detecting the R peak (there are abnormal QRS complexes, characterized by high amplitude and time-duration, but also by a not very steep slope); then, after the squaring operation, there are more peaks within the same QRS complex. For overcoming these situations, at this stage the signal is smoothened with a moving averaging integrator filter [8], [15].

The width of the window must be small enough to cover only one event (QRS complex, without overlapping the following T wave) and wide enough to cover an abnormal QRS complex.

This operation is mathematically described by [8]:

$$y(n) = \frac{1}{N}\left[x(n-(N-1)) + x(n-(N-2)) + \ldots x(n))\right] \quad (6)$$

where N is the number of samples within the width of the window, N=32. The result of the moving average integrator is presented in figure 11.

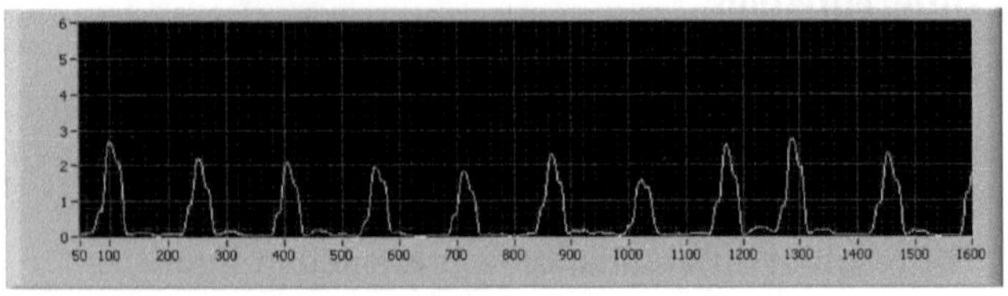

Fig. 11 Signal obtained after applying the moving average integrator

The events corresponding to R-peaks can then be represented, counted and used for calculating the pulse of the patient.

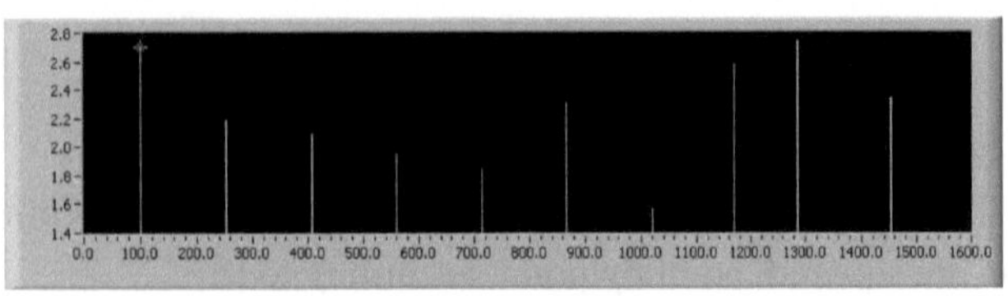

Fig. 12 Events corresponding to R-peaks

III. Conclusions

The paper presents the importance of LabVIEW in designing equipments used in biomedical signal transfer and signal processing. Thus, Virtual Instrumentation allows to develop flexible architectures, that can transfer and process data in real time – a key problem when dealing with humans' medical signals.

The Infrared transfer was reconsidered because of the high speed offered by its latest version, the FIr (so most of medical signals can be transmitted in real time). Moreover, being a wireless transmission, it decreases the number of cables in the already crowded space of hospital environment. Although it has these advantages, the infrared technique has a limited range and is influenced by light conditions (natural or artificial); for this reason is recommended for a short range transfer (between different modules of one equipment). For longer range transmission, Bluetooth or RF transmission would perform better.

The versatility of LabVIEW is emphasized also when processing the medical signals: the filters are easy to reconfigure, depending on the type of noise and the signal used. Then, the complex Pan-Tompkins algorithm is implemented rapidly, providing very good results in detecting R-peak, for any type of ECG signal. Also, the simulation possibilities offered by Virtual Instrumentation would help to understand the best way to reject noises or how to react in critical situations, before experimenting them "in vivo".

Further work will focus on detecting the limits of infrared transmission, the range in constant light and how the transmission range is influenced by varying the light intensity; also, more signal processing operations will be implemented in LabVIEW.

Conflict of Interest

The authors declare that they have no conflict of interest.

References

1. Balas, E. A., Jakovidis I. - Distance technologies for patient monitoring, BMJ, 1999
2. Webster, John W. (Editor) – Medical Instrumentation: Application and Design, third edition, John Wiley&Sons, 1998
3. Munteanu, M., Rusu, C., Rafiroiu, D., Chindris, G., Munteanu, R. A., Moga, R. – A hierarchical implementation of medical data transmission, in 2008 IEEE International Conference on Automation, Quality and Testing, Robotics AQTR 2008, ISBN 978-1-4244-2576-1, Cluj-Napoca, Romania, 2008, p. 77-80
4. Munteanu, M., Moga, D., Munteanu, R., I., Ciupa, R., Rafiroiu,D., Roman, M. - Interfacing Solutions for PC Based Medical Instruments, Proceedings of the 2nd Flemish-Romanian Workshop ANCME 2003, Gent, Belgium, 2003
5. www.physionet.org
6. Akay, M. - Biomedical Signal Processing, Acad. Press, 1994
7. Ifeachor, E., Jervis B. - Digital Signal Processing, A practical approach, Addison-Wesley, Ltd. 1993
8. Rangayyan, M. Rangaraj - A case-study approach to solve problems in Biomedical Signal Analysis, draft of the book to be published by the IEEE Press, Piscataway, NJ, march 13, 2000
9. Rusu, C.- Prelucrări digitale de semnale, Editura Mediamira, 2000
10. Clark, C. L. – LabVIEW Digital Signal Processing and Digital Communications, 2005
11. Hyder, D. - Infrared Sensing and Data Transmission Fundamentals, Motorola Semiconductor Application Note
12. Brief Introduction of the Infrared Transmission (www.zeroplus.com.tw)
13. http://www.authorstream.com/Presentation/dabhiDON-935369-infrared-system/
14. McSharry Patrick E., Clifford Gari, Tarassenko Lionel, Smith Leonard A. - A dynamical model for generating synthetic electrocardiogram signals. IEEE Transactions on Biomedical Engineering 50 (3), p. 289-294, march, 2003
15. Suri J. S., Acharya U. R., Spaan J. A. E., Krishnan S. M. (Editors) - Advances in Cardiac Signal Processing, Springer, 2007
16. Tompkins, W. - Biomedical Digital Signal Processing, Prentice Hall, 1993

Approximation Method of the Temperature Propagation Parameters in Biological Media

N.M. Roman[1], H.A. Colosi[2], D.C. Colosi[3], and V. Mureşan[4]

[1] Technical University of Cluj-Napoca, Electrotechnics and Measurements Department, Cluj-Napoca, Romania
[2] Iuliu Hatieganu University of Medicine and Pharmacy, Medical Informatics Department, Cluj-Napoca, Romania
[3] State University of New York, School of Dental Medicine, Prosthodontics and Digital Technology Department, New York, USA
[4] Technical University of Cluj-Napoca, Automation Department, Cluj-Napoca, Romania

Abstract— **The paper defines the following temperature propagation parameters in biological media:**

a) **Time constants (T_1) and (T_2), for example in seconds [s].**
b) **Space constants (S_1) and (S_2), for example in [mm].**

The objective is the approximation of these structure parameters from measurements of expert type. For the data we obtained we elaborated and used a dedicated program CTISP01(02). This program is based on numerical solving of two transcendental equations, in relation to both the propagation time (t) and space (s); it assures a large diversity of results for (T_1, T_2, S_1, S_2), with controlled approximation errors.
As propagation media we considered representative samples made of skin, fat, muscle, bone, tooth and steel.

Keywords— **Heating source, thermal propagation in biological media, analogical modeling, partial differential equations, numerical simulation**

I. INTRODUCTION

The source (J) is considered that generates the thermal energy u(t), oriented to the biological medium (Z) [1], with uniform and compact structure, from Fig. 1.

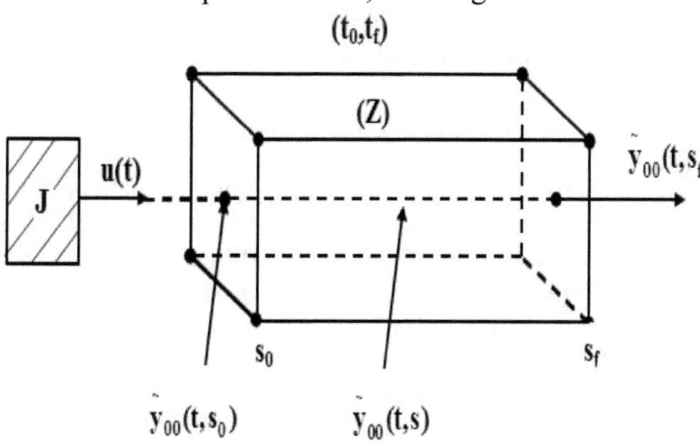

Fig. 1 The heating source and the biological medium

The notations (s_0) and (s_f) are used for initial, respectively final lengths of this zone (Z), and (t_0), respectively (t_f) correspond to the initial, respectively the final moments of the transitory heating regime. The temperature $\tilde{y}_{00}(t,s)$ is considered that is axially propagated [2], at the middle of this zone (Z), from $\tilde{y}_{00}(t,s_0)$ at the input, until to $\tilde{y}_{00}(t,s_f)$ at the output. The parallelepiped form of this zone, can be replaced with other forms too, of lengths (s_f – s_0) and with other sections, for example circular, elliptical. The lateral surfaces of these zones are considered thermally isolated. Being a propagation phenomenon through absorption [3], the $\tilde{y}_{00}(t,s)$ temperature progressively decreases with the increasing of depth getting through (s), as it is formally exemplified in Fig. 2, for the temperature in steady state regime $\tilde{y}_{00}(t_f,s)$.

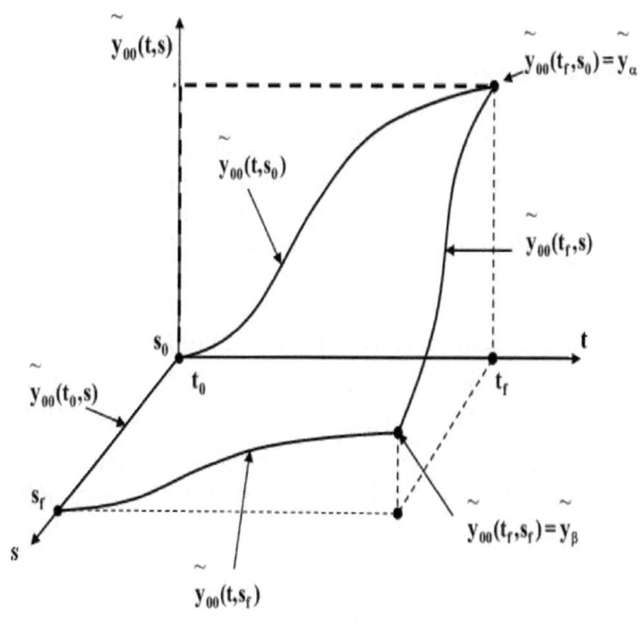

Fig. 2 The evolution in time and space of the thermal propagation phenomenon

DOI: 10.1007/978-3-319-07653-9_44, © Springer International Publishing Switzerland 2014

The temperature $\tilde{y}_{00}(t,s)$ increases in relation to time (t), so that the $\tilde{y}_{00}(t,s_0)$ temperature increases much more at the input (s_0) than at the output (s_f), where the temperature increase $\tilde{y}_{00}(t,s_f)$ presents a more damped evolution.

II. Analogical Modeling

The increasing or the decreasing evolutions of the temperature, can be usually expressed, through exponential functions in relation with time (t), respectively with the propagation depth (s) [4,5,6,7,8], so that the final solution will be approximated through:

$$\begin{aligned}\tilde{y}_{00}(t,s) &= \tilde{y}_{00}(t,s_0)\cdot\tilde{y}_{00}(t_f,s)\cdot u(t) = \\ &= K_y\cdot F_{0T}(t,s_0)\cdot F_{0S}(t_f,s)\cdot u(t)\end{aligned}, \quad (1)$$

where

$$F_{0T}(t,s_0) = 1 - \frac{T_1}{T_1 - T_2}\cdot e^{-\frac{t}{T_1}} - \frac{T_2}{T_2 - T_1}\cdot e^{-\frac{t}{T_2}}, \quad (2)$$

$$F_{0S}(t_f,s) = \frac{S_1}{S_1 - S_2}\cdot e^{-\frac{s}{S_1}} + \frac{S_2}{S_2 - S_1}\cdot e^{-\frac{s}{S_2}}. \quad (3)$$

The signals $\tilde{y}_{00}(t,s_0)$ and $\tilde{y}_{00}(t_f,s)$ are real signals, measured (or approximated through measurements), and $F_{0T}(t,s_0)$, respectively $F_{0S}(t_f,s)$ correspond to some rated signals, with values between the limits (0) and (1). The step of thermal energy applied at the input is notated with u(t), and (K_y) is a proportionality coefficient.

The structure parameters [9] are the time constants (T_1) and (T_2), for example in seconds [s], and the space constants for the depth propagation are notated with (S_1) and (S_2), for example in [mm].

Stretching the terminology, it can be considered that the increasing evolution $F_{0T}(t,s_0)$ from (2) represents the time characteristic (or dynamical, from the input s_0), and the decreasing evolution $F_{0S}(t_f,s)$ from (3) represents the space characteristic (or statical, at the final moments t_f). From (2) and (3) can be remarked that the two slopes $[\frac{dF_{0T}(t)}{dt}]_{t\to t_f} \to 0$ and $[\frac{dF_{0S}(s)}{ds}]_{s\to s_f} \to 0$.

III. Numerical Simulation

For the numerical simulation [10], the following two dedicated programs are used:

3.1. For the approximation of the structure parameters (T_1, T_2, S_1, S_2) and of the inflection points (t_i, s_i), it is operated with the dedicated program CTISP01(02). For the start of the calculations the following values are declared in the program: s_f [the length of the sample, in (mm)], t_f [the final time, necessary to assure the steady state regime, in (s)], and $\tilde{y}_\alpha = \tilde{y}_{00}(t_f,s_0)$ and $\tilde{y}_\beta = \tilde{y}_{00}(t_f,s_f)$ from Fig. 2 which represent the over-temperatures (in relation to the ambient medium), in the steady state regime at the input (s_0), respectively at the output (s_f), both in (^{0}C).

With these four data, respectively (s_f, t_f, $\tilde{y}_\alpha$ and $\tilde{y}_\beta$), the program calculates: (T_1, T_2, S_1, S_2), as well as the inflexion points (t_i, s_i), with the values $\tilde{y}_{00}(t_i,s_0)$, respectively $\tilde{y}_{00}(t_f,s_i)$, associated to these inflexions. The program permits also the graphical representations of these curves $\tilde{y}_{00}(t,s_0)$ and $\tilde{y}_{00}(t_f,s)$, in order to verify the correctness of the results $\tilde{y}_\alpha = \tilde{y}_{00}(t_f,s_0)$ and $\tilde{y}_\beta = \tilde{y}_{00}(t_f,s_f)$.

3.2. In order to represent the families of the curves $\tilde{y}_{00}(t,s_j)$, which represent the temperature propagation in the depth of the sample, [or successively in some different samples (biological media), existing contact surfaces between them] [1], the dedicated program ZPROP01(02) is used. The numerical integration is operated in relation to time (t), from (t_0) to (t_f), for (s) considered constant, where (Δs) is the advance step [10] (from s = s_0, progressively until to s = s_f) which is chosen small enough in order to assure a sufficiently compact “mesh”.

IV. Experimental Examples

For each from the six biological media [1] (or zones Z), respectively skin, fat, muscle, bone, tooth and steel, it is accomplished a sample of appropriate dimensions. On it the thermal energy source u(t) is applied as it is schematically shown in Fig. 3. The over-temperatures (in relation to the ambient temperature) $\tilde{y}_\alpha = \tilde{y}_{00}(t_f,s_0)$ and $\tilde{y}_\beta = \tilde{y}_{00}(t_f,s_f)$, associated to the two edges (s_0), respectively (s_f) are measured in steady state regime (t = t_f). These data, respectively ($\tilde{y}_\alpha$, $\tilde{y}_\beta$, $s_f - s_0$ and $t_f - t_0$) represent the initial conditions, necessary to the dedicated program

CTISP01(02), in order to obtain the specifications from the paragraph 3.1.

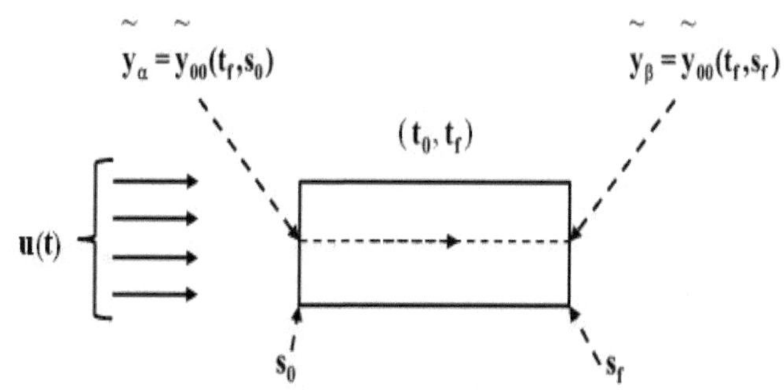

Fig. 3 The heating source applied to the biological medium

In Table 1, the ideal behaviours [11] of the heat insulating and of the thermo-conductive zones are qualitatively anticipated, with the obvious remark that between the sums (T_1+T_2) and (S_1+S_2) there are reverse relations.

Table 1 The ideal behaviours of the heat insulating, respectively thermo-conductive zones

Regime\Data	$\tilde{y}_\beta / \tilde{y}_\alpha$	$T_1 + T_2$	$S_1 + S_2$
Heat insulating	→0	big	Small
Thermo-conductive	→1	small	big

The measurements results (experimentally obtained), associated to Fig. 3, respectively $(s_f - s_0)$, $(t_f - t_0)$, $\tilde{y}_\alpha$ and $\tilde{y}_\beta$ are presented in Tables 2 and 3.

Table 2 The measurements results

Zone/ Data	$s_f - s_0$ [mm]	$t_f - t_0$ [s]	$\tilde{y}_\alpha$ [°C]	$\tilde{y}_\beta$ [°C]	y_α	y_β
A Skin	1	5	50	40	0.9892996	0.7914341
B Fat	2	6	50	30	0.9892929	0.5935757
C Muscles	3	4	50	35	0.9892918	0.6925
D Tooth	4	8	50	30	0.9892918	0.4946459
E Metal	5	3	50	45	0.9892929	0.8903635

Table 3 The measurements results

Zone/ Data	K_y	T_1	T_2	S_1	S_2	$\frac{t_i}{F_{Ti}}$	$\frac{s_i}{F_{Si}}$
A Skin	50.54	0.587	0.881	0.984	1.477	$\frac{0.711}{0.259}$	$\frac{1.197}{0.740}$
B Fat	50.54	0.705	1.057	1.175	1.763	$\frac{0.857}{0.259}$	$\frac{1.429}{0.740}$
C Muscles	50.54	0.470	0.705	2.215	3.323	$\frac{0.571}{0.259}$	$\frac{2.695}{0.740}$
D Tooth	50.54	0.940	1.410	2.404	3.607	$\frac{1.143}{0.259}$	$\frac{2.925}{0.740}$
E Metal	50.54	0.352	0.528	6.118	9.178	$\frac{0.428}{0.259}$	$\frac{7.443}{0.740}$

The data from Tables 2 and 3 are correlated with the notations from Fig. 2, for propagation depths $(s_f - s_0)$ in [mm], respectively propagation duration $(t_f - t_0)$ in [s].

On the entire duration $(t_f - t_0)$the same experimental step $\tilde{y}_\alpha = \tilde{y}_{00}(t_f, s_0) = 50\,^0\mathrm{C}$ was applied for the over-temperature considered at the input (s_0), and was followed the evolution $\tilde{y}_{00}(t, s_f)$ at the edge (s_f), until when this gets steady, resulting $\tilde{y}_\beta = \tilde{y}_{00}(t_f, s_f)$, with different values for the five samples (A, B, C, D, E).

The initial conditions of the program CTISP01(02) contain: the final values (t_f) and (s_f), the over-temperatures $(\tilde{y}_\alpha)$ and $(\tilde{y}_\beta)$, $\lambda_T = \frac{T_2}{T_1}$, $\lambda_S = \frac{S_2}{S_1}$, the following iterative advance steps [10] $\Delta T_1 = 10^{-4} \cdot t_f$ and $\Delta S_1 = 10^{-4} \cdot s_f$.

The differences are calculated

$$\mathrm{DIF}(T_1) = \tilde{y}_\alpha - F_{0T}(T_1) \cdot 1.01 \cdot \tilde{y}_\alpha, \tag{4}$$

$$\mathrm{DIF}(T_1 + \Delta T_1) = \tilde{y}_\alpha - F_{0T}(T_1 + \Delta T_1) \cdot 1.01 \cdot \tilde{y}_\alpha, \tag{5}$$

$$\mathrm{DIF}(S_1) = \tilde{y}_{\beta} - F_{0S}(S_1)\cdot \tilde{y}_{\alpha}\,, \qquad (6)$$

$$\mathrm{DIF}(S_1 + \Delta S_1) = \tilde{y}_{\beta} - F_{0S}(S_1 + \Delta S_1)\cdot \tilde{y}_{\alpha}\,, \qquad (7)$$

until

$$\mathrm{DIF}(T_1)\cdot \mathrm{DIF}(T_1 + \Delta T_1) < 0\,, \qquad (8)$$

and

$$\mathrm{DIF}(S_1)\cdot \mathrm{DIF}(S_1 + \Delta S_1) < 0\,, \qquad (9)$$

conditions for which results (T_1) and $T_2 = \lambda_T \cdot T_1$, respectively (S_1) and $S_2 = \lambda_S \cdot S_1$.

Because the iterative advance steps (ΔT_1) and (ΔS_1) are very small, the numerical solving errors of those two transcendental equations become negligible.

In Fig. 4 the significance of the notations can be easy followed, as example: $\tilde{y}_{\alpha} = 50^0 C$; $\tilde{y}_{\beta} = 40^0 C$; $y_{\alpha} = F_{0T}(t_f) = 0.989$; $y_{\beta} = F_{0S}(s_f) = 0.80$, and the proportionality coefficient in steady state regime from (1) resulted $K_y = 50.54$.

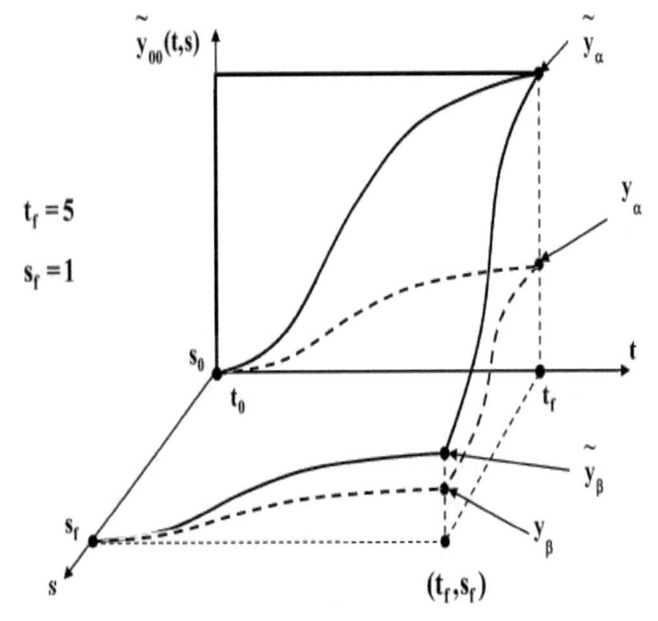

Fig. 4. The thermal propagation phenomenon, at the two edges of the biological medium

V. Conclusions

a) The approximation of the temperature propagation parameters in biological media, is based on the evolution in time, through (T_1) and (T_2), respectively on an evolution in space, through (S_1) and (S_2), that enters in the structure of the solution $\tilde{y}_{00}(t,s)$ from relation (1).

b) Through the determination, in steady state regime, of a minimum number of data, respectively (t_f), (s_f), ($\tilde{y}_{\alpha}$) and ($\tilde{y}_{\beta}$) (data resulted through the experiment schematically presented in Fig. 3), the dedicated program CTISP01(02) could have been initialized, for the numerical solving of the two transcendental equations, finally obtaining (T_1), (T_2), respectively (S_1), (S_2), as it was presented in Tables 2 and 3.

c) Using these structure parameters, respectively the time constants (T_1,T_2) and space constants (S_1,S_2), can be approached unitary and systemized stages of analysis and synthesis of the propagation phenomena using the numerical integration of some categories of partial differential equations, linear or non-linear.

Conflict of Interest

The authors declare that they have no conflict of interest.

References

1. Colosi H., Achimaş A., Roman N. M. (2011) Evaluarea Biomecanicii Ortodontice prin Modelare şi Simulare. Galaxia Gutenberg, Cluj-Napoca
2. Abrudean, M. 1998 Systems theory and automatic regulation. Mediamira, Cluj-Napoca
3. Coloşi T., Abrudean M., Ungureşan M.-L., Mureşan V. (2013) Examples of numerical Simulation for systems with distributed and lumped parameters through the Mpdx method with approximating solutions. UTPRESS, Cluj-Napoca
4. Li H.-X., Qi C. (2011) Spatio-Temporal Modeling of Nonlinear Distributed Parameter Systems: A Time/Space Separation Based Approach. Springer
5. Krstic M. (2006) Systematization of approaches to adaptive boundary control of PDEs. Int. J. of Robust and Nonlinear Control, 16: 801-818
6. Morris K. A. (2010) The Control Theory Handbook, Control of Systems Governed by Partial Diferential Equations. ed. W. S. Levine, CRC Press
7. Frihauf P., Krstic M. (2011) Leader-enabled deployment into planar curves: A PDE-based approach. IEEE Trans. on Automatic Control, 56: 1791-1806
8. Curtain R.F., Morris K.A. (2009) Transfer Functions of Distributed Parameter Systems. Automatica, 45, 5: 1101-1116
9. Inoan I. (2010) Movement control of an unloading machine from a rotary furnace, Proc. of AQTR 2010, THETA 17th edition, Cluj-Napoca, România, 2010, pp. 131-134
10. Coloşi T., Abrudean M., Ungureşan M.-L., Mureşan V. (2013) Numerical simulation of distributed parameter processes. Springer
11. Ungureşan M.-L., Niac G. (2011) Pre-equilibrium Kinetics. Modeling and Simulation. Russian J. of Physical Chemistry, 85, 4: 549-556

PID Control of a Distributed Parameter Biological Process

V. Mureşan[1], D.C. Colosi[2], H.A. Colosi[3], and N.M. Roman[4]

[1] Technical University of Cluj-Napoca, Automation Department, Cluj-Napoca, Romania
[2] State University of New York, School of Dental Medicine, Prosthodontics and Digital Technology Department, New York, USA
[3] Iuliu Hatieganu University of Medicine and Pharmacy, Medical Informatics Department, Cluj-Napoca, Romania
[4] Technical University of Cluj-Napoca, Electrotechnics and Measurements Department, Cluj-Napoca, Romania

Abstract— **For the analogical modeling and the numerical simulation of a simple PID control diagram, containing a biological distributed parameter process, the method of Partial Derivatives Matrix of the State Vector (Mpdx) is used, associated with approximating solutions. Through the present example, the unitary and systemized character of this method is highlighted, considered known from [1]. A numerical simulation program was elaborated for the entire PID control scheme, the results permitting a more complete phenomenological interpretation of the results and of the obtained performances.**

Keywords— **Ordinary differential equations, Partial differential equations, State vector, Initial conditions, Approximating solutions, Taylor series, PID control**

I. INTRODUCTION

The control diagram [1] from Fig. 1 is considered and the elements (ODE1), (ODE2) and (ODE3) are modeled through ordinary differential equations, and the (PDE) element is modeled through a partial differential equation of II order, with two independent variables (t) and (s).

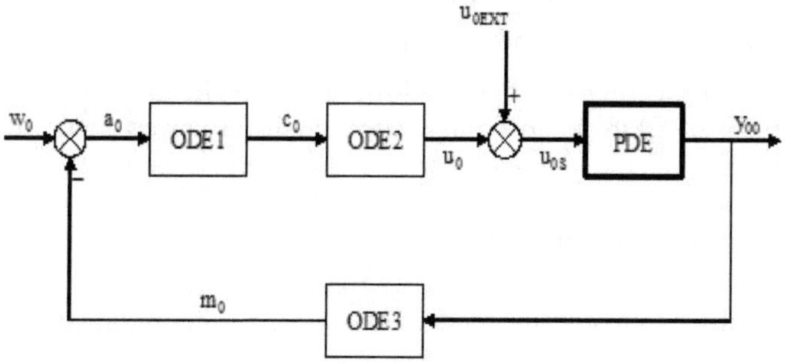

Fig. 1 The control structure

The signals from the control structure, can have either a single index, corresponding to the differentiation order with respect to time (t), or two indexes, the first corresponding to the differentiation order with respect to time (t), and the second corresponding to the differentiation order with respect to the spatial parameter (s). For example $c_n = \frac{d^n c}{dt^n}$, and $y_{nm} = \frac{\partial^{n+m} y}{\partial t^n \cdot \partial s^m}$, where n=0,1,2,..., respectively m=0,1,2,....

The element (ODE1) is a PID controller modelled through

$$c_1 + T_R \cdot c_2 = K_{PR} \cdot a_1 + K_{IR} \cdot a_0 + K_{DR} \cdot a_2, \qquad (1)$$

where (K_{PR}), (K_{IR}) and (K_{DR}) are weighting coefficients of the proportional, integrative respectively derivative effects, with respect to time, and (T_R) represents the time constant of the controller. With

$$a_0 = w_0 - m_0 \qquad (2)$$

is notated the control error, where (w_0) and (m_0) correspond to the reference signal, respectively feedback (measurement).

The element (ODE2) is the actuator that adapts the control signal (c_0), resulting the actuating signal (u_0). This element is modelled through

$$u_0 + T_V \cdot u_1 = K_V \cdot c_0, \qquad (3)$$

where (K_V) and (T_V) correspond to the proportionality coefficient in steady state regime, respectively to the time constant. An external disturbance signal (u_{0EXT}) can operate on the actuating signal (u_0), resulting

$$u_{0S} = u_0 - u_{0EXT}. \qquad (4)$$

The (PDE) element is considered the technological (biological) process [2] that is going to be controlled, modeled through a partial differential equation [3,4,5] of second order with respect to the (t) and (s) variables, respectively

$$a_{00} \cdot y_{00} + a_{10} \cdot y_{10} + a_{01} \cdot y_{01} + a_{20} \cdot y_{20} + a_{11} \cdot y_{11} + \\ + a_{02} \cdot y_{02} = K_y \cdot (\varphi_{0.00} \cdot u_{0S} + \varphi_{1.00} \cdot u_{1S} + \varphi_{2.00} \cdot u_{2S}), \qquad (5)$$

where: $y_{..}(t,s)$, $\varphi_{0.00}(t,s)$, $\varphi_{1.00}(t,s)$, $\varphi_{2.00}(t,s)$, $K_y = 1$, $u_{1S} = \frac{\partial u_{0S}}{\partial t}$, and $u_{2S} = \frac{\partial^2 u_{0S}}{\partial t^2}$. The (a...)

DOI: 10.1007/978-3-319-07653-9_45, © Springer International Publishing Switzerland 2014

coefficients are considered constant, but can present the next significances too: $a_{00}=1$, $a_{10}=T_1+T_2$, $a_{20}=T_1\cdot T_2$, $a_{01}=S_1+S_2$, $a_{02}=S_1\cdot S_2$ and $a_{11}=(T_1+T_2)\cdot(S_1+S_2)$. The notations ($T_1$) and ($T_2$) are the time constants, respectively (S_1) and (S_2) are space constants (for example length or depth) and represent an analogy with the second order transfer functions, from the classical theory of the linear control systems. The element (ODE3) is the feedback (measurement) transducer, that transforms the controlled signal $y_{00}(t,s)$, in the feedback signal $m_0(t)$, of the same nature and comparable with the reference signal $w_0(t)$. This element is modelled through

$$m_0+T_M\cdot m_1=K_M\cdot y_{00}, \tag{6}$$

where (K_M) and (T_M) correspond to the proportionality coefficient in steady state regime (amplification-damping), respectively to the time constant.

II. The Elaboration of the Matrix of Partial Derivatives of the State Vector (Mpdx)

To establish the (**Mpdx**) of the entire control system from Fig. 1, it is proceeded at the next preliminary grouping of the component signals, in order to result, all, successively, from the known initial conditions, respectively:

$$\left.\begin{array}{l} m_0 \\ m_1=\dfrac{1}{T_M}\cdot(K_M\cdot y_{00}-m_0) \\ m_2=\dfrac{1}{T_M}\cdot(K_M\cdot y_{10}-m_1) \end{array}\right\} \tag{7}$$

$$\left.\begin{array}{l} c_0 \\ c_1=\dfrac{1}{T_R}\cdot[K_{PR}\cdot(w_0-m_0)+K_{DR}\cdot(w_1-m_1)-c_0] \\ c_2=\dfrac{1}{T_R}\cdot[K_{PR}\cdot(w_1-m_1)+K_{IR}\cdot(w_0-m_0)+ \\ \quad +K_{DR}\cdot(w_2-m_2)-c_1] \end{array}\right\} \tag{8}$$

$$\left.\begin{array}{l} u_0 \\ u_1=\dfrac{1}{T_V}\cdot(K_V\cdot c_0-u_0) \\ u_2=\dfrac{1}{T_V}\cdot(K_V\cdot c_1-u_1) \end{array}\right\} \tag{9}$$

$$\left.\begin{array}{l} u_{0S}=u_0+u_{0EXT} \\ u_{1S}=u_1+u_{1EXT} \\ u_{2S}=u_2+u_{2EXT} \end{array}\right\} \tag{10}$$

$$\left.\begin{array}{l} y_{00} \\ y_{10} \\ y_{20}=\dfrac{1}{a_{20}}\cdot[K_y\cdot(\varphi_{0.00}\cdot u_{0S}+\varphi_{1.00}\cdot u_{1S}+\varphi_{2.00}\cdot u_{2S})- \\ -(a_{00}\cdot y_{00}+a_{10}\cdot y_{10}+a_{01}\cdot y_{01}+a_{11}\cdot y_{11}+a_{02}\cdot y_{02})] \end{array}\right\}. \tag{11}$$

The groups of signals from above correspond to: (7) for ODE3, (8) for ODE1, (9) for ODE2, (10) for the adder of the disturbances and (11) for PDE.

For the structure parameters the next values are chosen: $T_M=0.055$; $K_M=1$; $T_R=0.05$; $T_V=0.06$; $K_V=1$, with the remark that if the control loop is considered open, respectively (PDE) isolated, then $K_M=0$ and $K_V=0$. The controller tuning (ODE1) from (8) becomes an open problem, because the process considered for the control, is modeled through PDE (5), respectively (11). However, it was operated with the next approximations, for the weighting coefficients, of the proportional, integrative, respectively derivative effects: $K_{PR}=\dfrac{T_1+T_2}{2\cdot T_\Sigma\cdot K_{EX}}$, $K_{IR}=\dfrac{1}{2\cdot T_\Sigma\cdot K_{EX}}$ and $K_{DR}=\dfrac{T_1\cdot T_2}{2\cdot T_\Sigma\cdot K_{EX}}$, where $T_\Sigma=T_M+T_R+T_V$. The choice of the (K_{EX}) is made iterative, for each case until the indicial response of the stabilization control from the examples from chapter IV are enclosed in an overshoot of (3-6)%.For the time constants: $T_1=0.1\cdot t_f$, $T_2=0.15\cdot t_f$ and the space (length) constants are considered $S_1=0.1\cdot s_f$ and $S_2=0.15\cdot s_f$, where the final time $t_f=2$ and $s_f=4$.

Respecting the signals flow, from (ODE3) to (ODE1), then to (ODE2) and finally, after the disturbances adder, to (PDE), all the signals presented above result from the elements previously passed through. It is possible, hence, to determine that the state vector (**x**) is made up of eight elements ($m_0, m_1, c_0, c_1, u_0, u_1, y_{00}\cdot y_{10}$) as shown in (12). In order to assure the start of calculations, the initial conditions (IC) need to be known at $t=t_0$, for $\mathbf{x}(t_0)=\mathbf{x}_{IC}$.

Through the repeated differentiation of (x) with respect to time, ($\mathbf{x}_T$) is obtained, bounded in (12) up to the order six, with the remark that for each stage of differentiation with respect to (t), the number of elements is bounded to four. Because the signals (m..., c...., and u....) are functions only depending on time, all the lines of the ($\mathbf{x}_S$) and ($\mathbf{x}_{TS}$) matrices corresponding to these signals become null, and the associated lines to the partial derivatives for the signals (y_{00}, y_{10}, y_{20} ,..., y_{60}) will be null. Finally, the ($\mathbf{M}_{\mathbf{pdx}}$)

dimensions for the control system from Fig. 1, result from: $\mathbf{x}(8\times1)$, $\mathbf{x}_T$ (20×1), $\mathbf{x}_S$ (8×6) and $\mathbf{x}_{TS}$ (20×6), so that $\mathbf{M}_{pdx}(28\times7)$.

$$\mathbf{M}_{pdx} = \begin{bmatrix} \mathbf{x} & \mathbf{x}_S \\ \mathbf{x}_T & \mathbf{x}_{TS} \end{bmatrix} =$$

m_0	0	0	....	0
m_1	0	0	....	0
c_0	0	0	....	0
c_1	0	0	....	0
u_0	0	0	....	0
u_1	0	0	....	0
y_{00}	y_{01}	y_{02}	....	y_{06}
y_{10}	y_{11}	y_{12}	....	y_{16}
m_2	0	0	....	0
c_2	0	0	....	0
u_2	0	0	....	0
y_{20}	y_{21}	y_{22}	....	y_{26}
m_3	0	0	....	0
c_3	0	0	....	0
u_3	0	0	....	0
y_{30}	y_{31}	y_{32}	....	y_{36}
⋮	⋮	⋮	....	⋮
m_6	0	0	....	0
c_6	0	0	....	0
u_6	0	0	....	0
y_{60}	y_{61}	y_{62}	....	y_{66}

(12)

To assure the start of the calculations, 20 initial conditions are imposed to be known, from that a number of eight belong to the state vector $x = \mathbf{x}_{IC}$, respectively $(m_0, m_1, c_0, c_1, u_0, u_1, y_{00}, y_{10})_{IC}$ and a number of 12 belong to those two non-null lines from the structure of the $\mathbf{x}_S = \mathbf{x}_{S,IC}$, respectively $(y_{01}, y_{02}, ..., y_{06})_{IC}$ and $(y_{11}, y_{12}, ..., y_{16})$. These initial conditions (in general, null values) are considered at the sequence (k-1). Reductively, the stages (7), (8), (9), (10) and (11) represent the analogical modeling for the determination of (**Mpdx**) from (12) forward necessary, for the numerical simulation of the control scheme from Fig. 1.

III. The Numerical Simulation through (Mpdx) Associated with Approximating Solutions and Taylor Series

Reconsidering the (**Mpdx**) from (12), the next three major stages are necessary, that assure the calculations advance, from the sequence (k-1) associated to the moment $t_{k-1} = (k-1)\cdot\Delta t$, to the sequence (k), associated to the moment $t_k = k\cdot\Delta t$, where the advance or integration step Δt is considered small enough [1].

Stage 1:

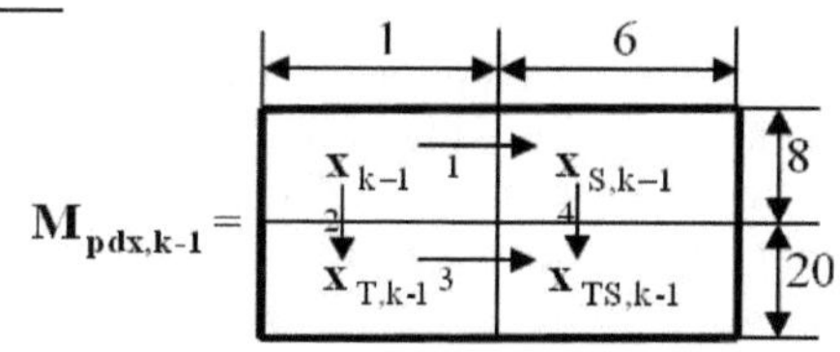

(13)

$(\mathbf{x}_{k-1})$ is known, inclusively at the start of the program for the initial conditions (IC), from which are calculated $(\mathbf{x}_{S,k-1})$, (arrow 1), then $(\mathbf{x}_{T,k-1})$ (arrow 2) and finally $(\mathbf{x}_{TS,k-1})$ (arrows 3 and 4).

Stage 2:

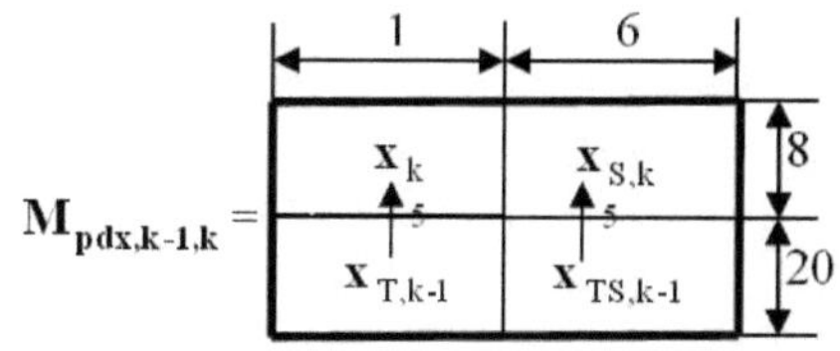

(14)

From $(\mathbf{x}_{T,k-1})$ and $(\mathbf{x}_{TS,k-1})$, $(\mathbf{x}_k)$ and $(\mathbf{x}_{S,k})$ are approximated through Taylor series (arrows 5).

Stage 3:

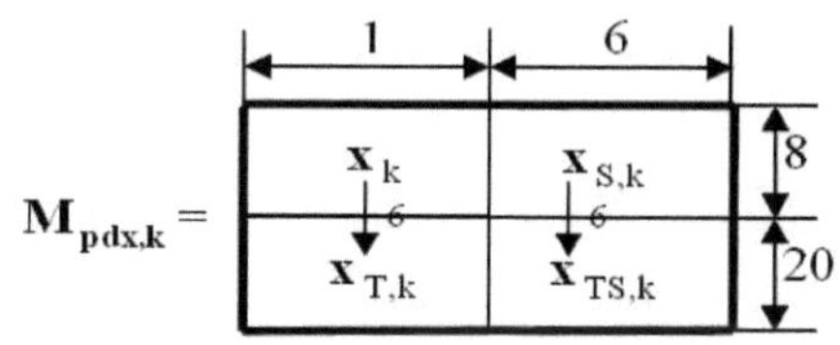

(15)

From the elements disposed on the over lines of the $(\mathbf{x}_k)$ and $(\mathbf{x}_{S,k})$, result the elements at the sequence (k) for $(\mathbf{x}_{T,k})$ and $(\mathbf{x}_{TS,k})$ (arrows 6). Reductively, for each advance, from the sequence (k-1) to the sequence (k), the stages (13), (14) and (15) are successively passed through, hence resulting the numerical simulation through (**Mpdx**) from (12), of the control diagram from Fig. 1. The advance of the state vector (**x**) and of the $(\mathbf{x}_S)$ matrix, from the sequence (k-1) to the sequence (k), is based on the Taylor series, formally exposed through

$$\mathbf{x}_k = \mathbf{x}_{k-1} + \sum_{T=1}^{\omega} \frac{\Delta t^T}{T!} \cdot \mathbf{x}_{T,k-1}, \qquad (16)$$

respectively

$$\mathbf{x}_{S,k} = \mathbf{x}_{S,k-1} + \sum_{T=1}^{\omega} \frac{\Delta t^T}{T!} \cdot \mathbf{x}_{TS,k-1}, \qquad (17)$$

where (ω) represents the maximum order of the partial derivatives with respect to time (t), that is commonly enclosed between the limits $4 \le \omega \le 8$.

IV. EXAMPLES RUN ON THE COMPUTER

All the simulations are made using some dedicated programs implemented by the authors in MATLAB [5] environment. The next two examples of numerical simulation through (**Mpdx**) with approximating solutions are presented, run on the computer and associated to the control diagram from Fig. 1:

4.1) The $y_{00}(t,s)$ response at the step signal of the (PDE) element considered isolated, for the input signal $u_{0EXT} = u_{0EXTA} = 1000$. It is also considered: $t_f = 2$; $s_f = 4$; $T_1 = 0.1 \cdot t_f$; $T_2 = 0.15 \cdot t_f$; $S_1 = 0.1 \cdot s_f$; $S_2 = 0.15 \cdot s_f$; $K_y = 1$; $K_M = 0$; $K_V = 0$; $\Delta t = 10^{-3}$.

4.2) The $y_{00}(t,s)$ response for the complete control scheme, in stabilization regime, for: $u_{0EXTA} = 0$; $u_{0EXTB} = 0$; $T_1 = 0.2$; $T_2 = 0.3$; $t_f = 2$; $S_1 = 0.4$; $S_2 = 0.6$; $s_f = 4$; $\Delta t = 10^{-3}$; $K_y = 1$; $K_M = 1$; $K_V = 1$.

The next stabilization regimes were considered:

4.2.1) At the depth of s = 1, successively for the reference signals: $w_0 = 150$; $w_0 = 200$; $w_0 = 300$.

4.2.2) At the depth of s = 2, successively for the reference signals: $w_0 = 60$; $w_0 = 90$; $w_0 = 120$.

4.2.3) At the depth of s = 3, successively for the reference signals: $w_0 = 5$; $w_0 = 10$; $w_0 = 15$.

In all the above variants, the approximating solution for PDE isolated from Fig. 1, is considered of the following form

$$y_{00}(t,s) = K_y \cdot F_{0T}(t) \cdot F_{0S}(s) \cdot u_0(t), \quad (18)$$

where (K_y) is a proportionality coefficient, that can be unitary or non-unitary, and:

$$F_{0T}(t) = 1 - \frac{T_1}{T_1 - T_2} \cdot e^{-\frac{t}{T_1}} - \frac{T_2}{T_2 - T_1} \cdot e^{-\frac{t}{T_2}} \quad (19)$$

respectively

$$F_{0S}(s) = \frac{S_1}{S_1 - S_2} \cdot e^{-\frac{s}{S_1}} + \frac{S_2}{S_2 - S_1} \cdot e^{-\frac{s}{S_2}}. \quad (20)$$

The functions from (19), (20) are formally exemplified in Figs. (2) and (3), where for the final values (t_f) and (s_f) result $F_{0T}(t_f) \to 1$, respectively $F_{0S}(s_f) \to 0$. The approximating solution $y_{00}(t,s)$ from (18) is also exemplified formally, in Fig. 4, for the depths (s_0), (s_1), (s_2), (s_f), with the remark that $F_{0T}(t) \cong y_{00}(t,s_0)$ and $F_{0S}(s) \cong y_{00}(t_f,s)$, also $y_{00}(t_0,s) = 0$, respectively $y_{00}(t,s_f) \to 0$.

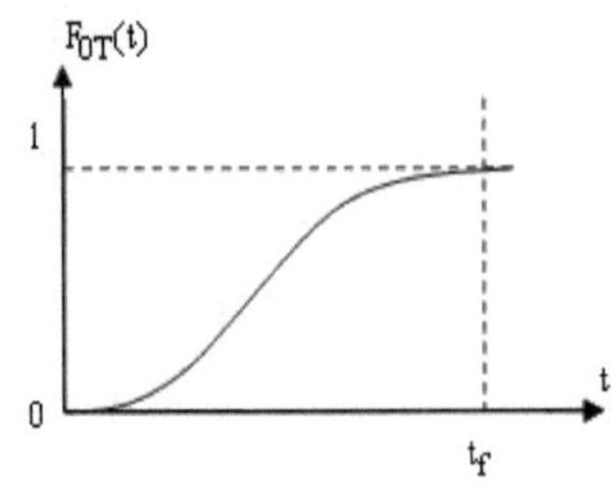

Fig. 2 The $F_{0T}(t)$ function

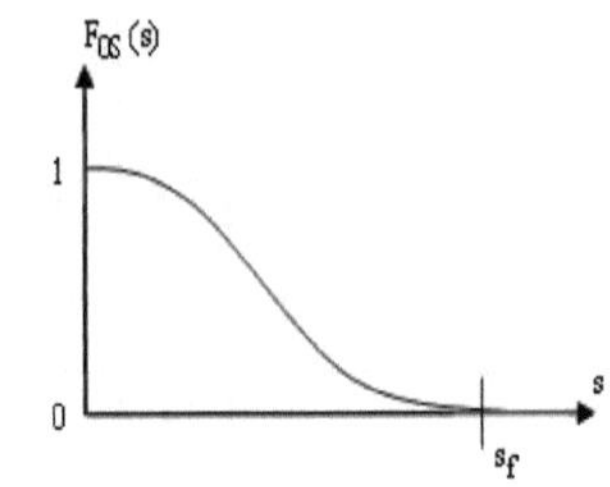

Fig. 3 The $F_{0S}(s)$ function

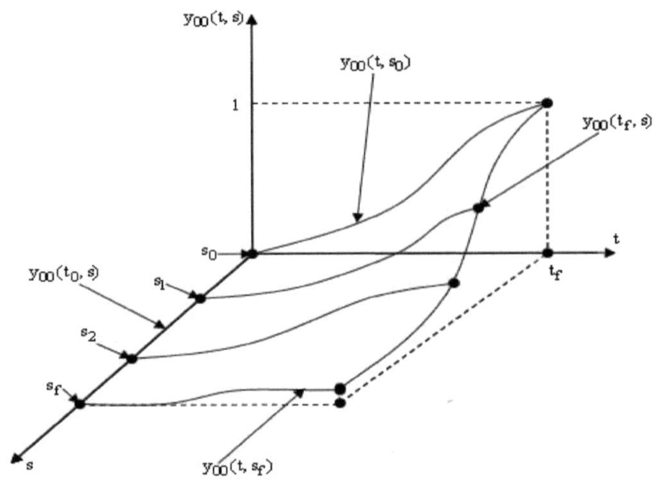

Fig. 4 The approximating solution $y_{00}(t,s)$

The choice of the approximating solutions is an open problem. These can be determined through different procedures of expert type, and their diversity, respectively their complexity can be sometimes very high [6]. Even for this simple example, the determination of the time constants (T_1) and (T_2), respectively of the space constant (S_1) and (S_2), can become laborious enough.

Example 4.1: $y_{00}(t,s)$, for (PDE) isolated with the step input signal: $u_0 = u_{0EXT} = 1000$. In Fig. 5, the results of the numerical simulation with respect to time (t) are presented, for five depth (s) samples. It can be remarked the increasing exponential evolution for $y_{00}(t,s)$ with respect to time and the decreasing exponential evolution for the solution $y_{00}(t,s)$ with respect to the depth (s).

<u>Examples 4.2</u> correspond for three stabilization regimes, grouped at the depths $s=1$; $s=2$ and $s=3$.

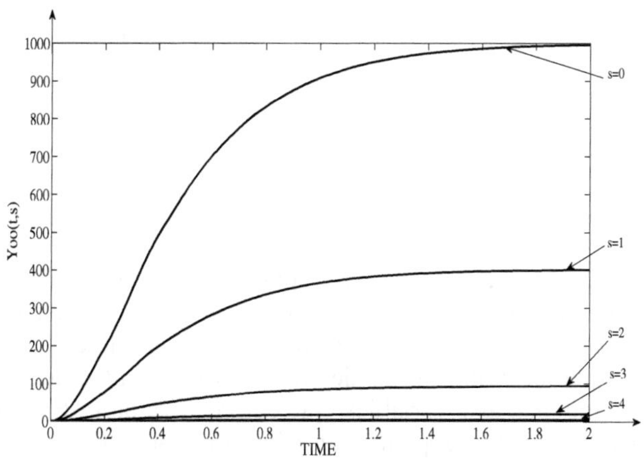

Fig. 5 The open loop process step signal response

In Figs. 6-11, the signals $y_{00}(t,s)$ and the corresponding signals $c_0(t)$ are presented, localized at the depths $s=1$; $s=2$ and $s=3$ for three variants of the reference signal (w), respectively $w=150;200;300$ at the depth $s=1$, then $w=60;90;120$ at the depth $s=2$ and finally $w=5;10;15$ at the depth $s=3$. At all these control regimes with stabilization, an overshoot was assured for $y_{00}(t,s)$ of (3~6%). In Fig. 12 can be noticed that the three signals considered to the stabilization, $y_{00}(t,1)$, $y_{00}(t,2)$ and $y_{00}(t,3)$ corresponding to the depths $s=1$; $s=2$ respectively $s=3$.

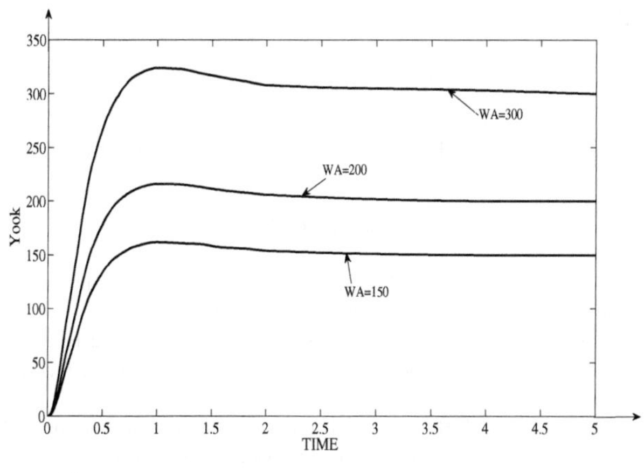

Fig. 6 The controlled signal $y_{00}(t,s)$ for the case s=1

In Table 1 it can be noticed that at the progressive increasing of the depth (s), the weighting coefficients of the proportional, integrative and derivative effect increase (K_{PR}), (K_{IR}) respectively (K_{DR}), hence increasing the control effort, main highlighted through the control signal (c_{0k}).

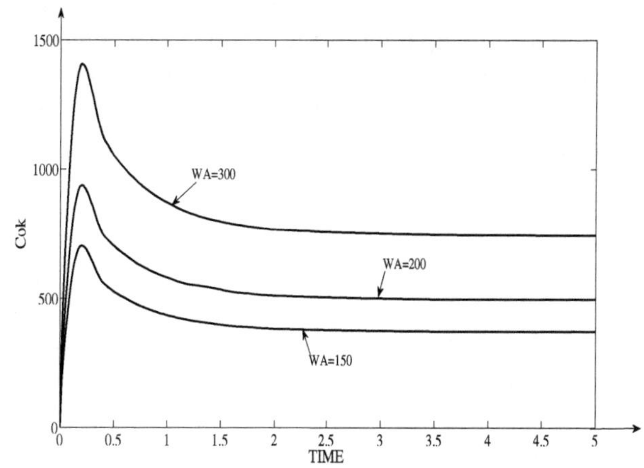

Fig. 7 The control signal $c_0(t)$ for the case s=1

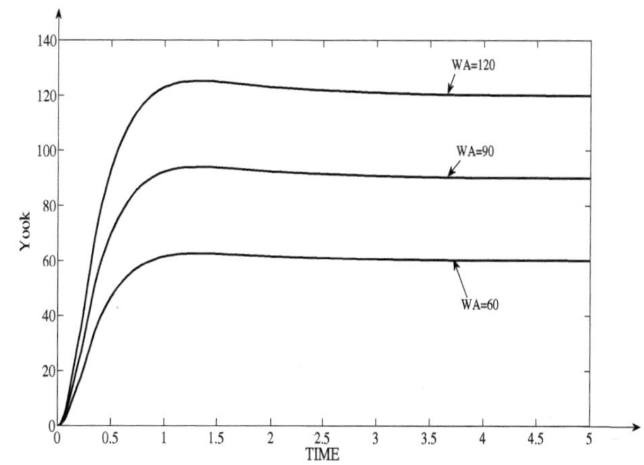

Fig. 8 The controlled signal $y_{00}(t,s)$ for the case s=2

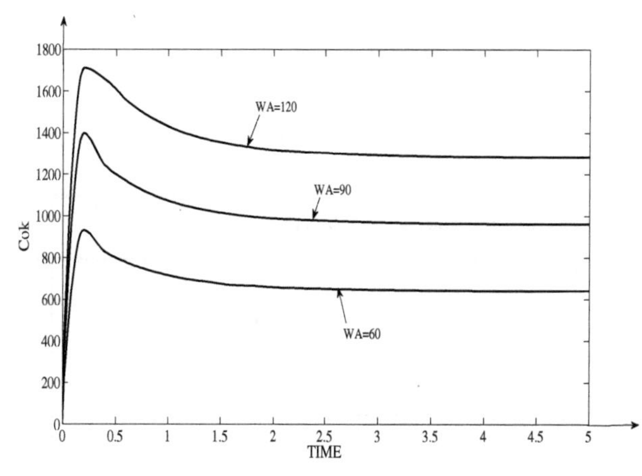

Fig. 9 The control signal $c_0(t)$ for the case s=2

Comparing the corresponding results at the depths $s=1$; $s=2$ respectively $s=3$, from Fig 5. and Figs. 6-11, can be noticed that y(t,s) presents more rapid increasing evolutions in Figs. 6,8,10 comparing to Fig. 5, due to the stabilization control associated with big value of the control signal (c_{0k}), that forces the more rapid dynamics of the stabilization regime.

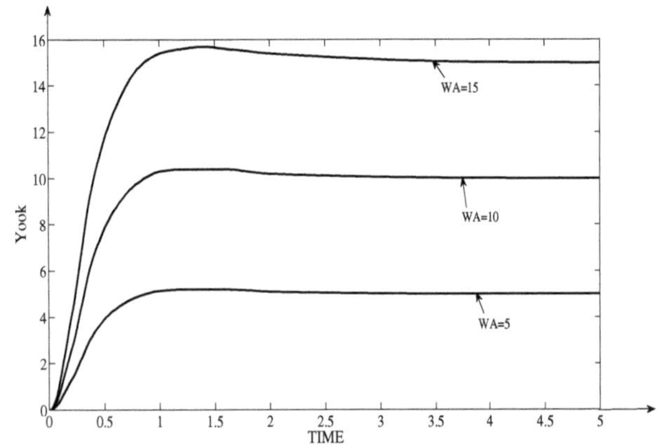

Fig. 10 The controlled signal $y_{00}(t,s)$ for the case s=3

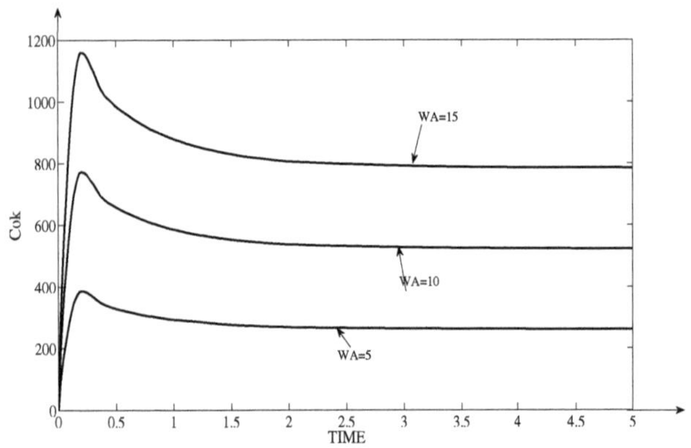

Fig. 11 The control signal $c_0(t)$ for the case s=3

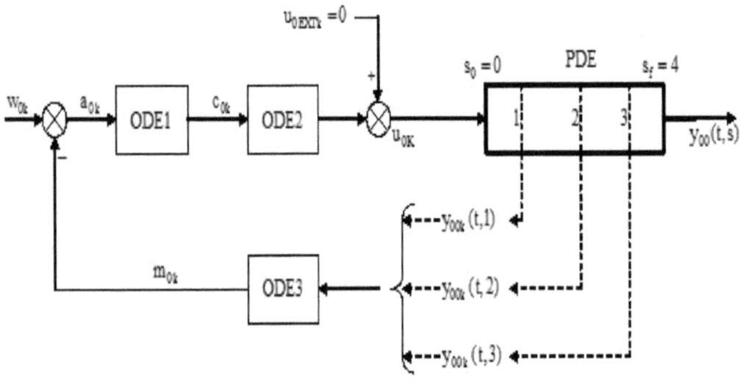

Fig. 12 The detailed control structure

Table 1 The controller's parameters

S	$w=w_A$	K_{PR}	K_{IR}	K_{DR}
1	150; 200; 300	5.05	10.1	0.606
2	60; 90; 120	15.15	30.3	1.82
3	5; 10; 15	76	151.5	9.09

V. Conclusions

The (**Mpdx**) method with approximating solutions, considered to be known from [1], was oriented, in this paper, in an example of the inclusion of a process, modeled through an equation with partial derivatives of second order, with two independent variables, [a temporal variable (t) and a spatial variable (s)], in a classical diagram of control, in stabilization regime. The presented example leads to a unitary and systemized study, based on this method.

The approximating solution is necessary to assure the start of the calculations and eventually to verify the results correctness. In this circumstance, it was operated with a performance indicator defined through the "cumulated relative error in percentage" (CREP y_{00K}), that for all examples from the paper, didn't exceed $10^{-2}\%$. To simplify the presentation, the independent variables were enclosed from $t_0=0$; $s_0=0$, up to $t_f=2$ and $s_f=4$, and the measurement units were avoided. The (**Mpdx**) method with approximating solutions has been used in many engineering applications and the general approach presented in this paper can be singularized, being valid for the case of the biological processes control, having many applications in medicine.

Conflict of Interest

The authors declare that they have no conflict of interest.

References

1. Coloşi T., Abrudean M., Ungureşan M. et al. (2013) Numerical simulation of distributed parameter processes. Springer
2. Colosi H., Achimaş A., Roman N. M. (2011) Evaluarea Biomecanicii Ortodontice prin Modelare şi Simulare. Galaxia Gutenberg, Cluj-Napoca
3. Li H.-X., Qi C. (2011) Spatio-Temporal Modeling of Nonlinear Distributed Parameter Systems: A Time/Space Separation Based Approach. Springer
4. Krstic M. (2006) Systematization of approaches to adaptive boundary control of PDEs. Int. J. of Robust and Nonlinear Control, 16: 801-818
5. User Guide, Matlab 7.5.0 (R2007b)
6. Morris K. A. (2010) The Control Theory Handbook, Control of Systems Governed by Partial Differential Equations. ed. W. S. Levine, CRC Press

Wavelet Based HRV Analysis

Z. Germán-Salló, A. Gligor, and H.S. Grif

"PetruMaior" University, Electrical Engineering and Computer Department, TirguMures, Romania

Abstract— **Filtering time series is an important task in many domains as biomedical signal processing. The Heart Rate Variability (HRV) is the analysis of the RR time series obtained as intervals between heart beats. Usually the RR time series obtained are non-stationary and are present ectopic beats, which prevents extraction of useful information, therefore must often be filtered in order to emphasize different characteristics or properties. This paper presents a method to filter R-R time series, using wavelet shrinkage techniquein order to have a new and more adapted visualization of the HRV's graphical interpretation as Lorenz plot.**

Keywords— **heart rate variability, non-linear filtering, Lorenz plot, wavelet shrinkage**

I. INTRODUCTION

Heart rate variability (HRV) is a recognized parameter of the autonomous nervous system activity. In a long term electrocardiographic (ECG) record, each heartbeat(QRS complex) is detected, and the so-called normal-to-normal (NN) intervals (that is all intervals between adjacent QRS complexes resulting from sinus node de-polarizations), or the instantaneous heart rate is determined[3]. Heart rate variability analysis has been shown to provide an effective evaluation of cardiac disease such as different stages in the atrial fibrillation [1]. There are several methods to analyze HRV, in time domain, frequency domain and other geometrical and graphical tools. Fourier transform, the most commonly used method to analyze variability in a frequency domain, does not offer an easy assessment of its dynamics because of limitations inherent in its stationary hypothesis[5]. The wavelet transform allows analysis of non-stationary signals, offering a time localization of different frequency components[7].

The so-called "Lorenz plots" (or Poincaré plots) are scatterplots that show the R-R interval as a function of the previous R-R interval.These plots might be used for visualization of the variability of the heart rate and the results can be obtained fasterand they might be superior to conventional measures of HRV. Proper filtering of these plots helps extract important (and maybe interesting) information from the data and filtering as a preprocessing task can lead to a more accurate parameter extraction.

II. THEHEART RATE VARIABILITY

A. *Interpretation*

Heart rate is usually estimated as the number of R-wave events (heartbeats) per unit time on the electrocardiogram (figure 1) or as the average of the R-R interval reciprocals within a specified time window. Several approaches are used to characterize heart rate variability: statistical measures [5], spectral analysis of heart rate or R-R interval time series [1], deterministic dynamical systems assessments of heart rate signal properties [8,], and approximate entropy measures of R-R interval regularity [4].Non-linear phenomena are certainly involved in the genesis of HRV. They are determined by complex interactions of hemodynamic,electrophysiological and humeral variables, as well as byautonomic and central nervous regulations. It has been told that analysis of HRV based onthe methods of non-linear dynamics might elicit valuable information for the physiologicalinterpretation of HRV and for the assessment of the risk of sudden death.The parameters whichhave been used to measure non-linear properties of HRV include 1/f scaling of Fourier spectra, H scaling exponent, and Coarse Graining Spectral Analysis (CGSA) [8].

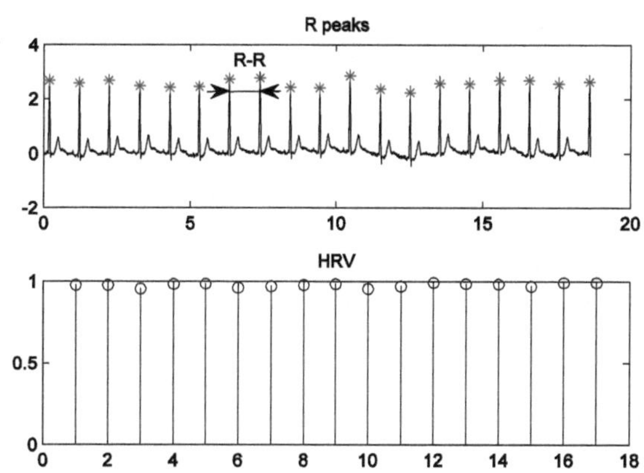

Fig. 1 Heart rate variability

S. Vlad and R.V. Ciupa (eds.), *International Conference on Advancements of Medicine and Health Care through Technology*, IFMBE Proceedings 44,
DOI: 10.1007/978-3-319-07653-9_46, © Springer International Publishing Switzerland 2014

B. Measuring Methods

Variations in heart rate may be evaluated by a number of methods. Perhaps the simplest to perform are the time domain measures. With these methods either the heart rate at any point in time or the intervals between successive normal complexes are determined. The series of NN intervals can also be converted into a geometric pattern, such as the sample density distribution of NN interval durations, sample density distribution of differences between adjacent NN intervals, Lorenz plot of NN or RR intervals, etc., and a simple formula is used which judges the variability based on the geometric and/or graphic properties of the resulting pattern.Simple time–domain variables that can be calculated include the mean NN interval, the mean heart rate, the difference between the longest and shortest NN interval, the difference between night and day heart rate, etc.

The simplest variable to calculate is the standard deviation of the NN interval (SDNN), i.e. thesquare root of variance. Since variance is mathematically equal to total power of spectral analysis,SDNN reflects all the cyclic components responsible for variability in the period of recording. Inmany studies, SDNN is calculated over a 24-h period and thus encompasses both short-term highfrequency variations, as well as the lowest frequency components seen in a 24-h period. As theperiod of monitoring decreases, SDNN estimates shorter and shorter cycle lengths. It should alsobe noted that the total variance of HRV increases with the length of analysed recording [7].

In frequency domain, power spectral density (PSD) analysis provides the basic information of how power distributes as a function of frequency. Independent of the method employed, only anestimate of the true PSD of the signals can be obtained by proper mathematical algorithms.Methods for the calculation of PSD may be generally classified as non-parametric andparametric.In most instances, both methods provide comparable results. The advantages of the non-parametric methods are the simplicity of the algorithm employed (Fast Fourier Transform— FFT — in most of the cases) and the high processing speed, whilst the advantages of parametric methods are smoother spectral components which can be distinguishedindependently of preselected frequency bands, easy post-processing of the spectrum with anautomatic calculation of low and high frequency power components and easy identification of thecentral frequency of each component, and an accurate estimation of PSD even on a smallnumber of samples on which the signal is supposed to be stationary. Theseanalyticaltechniquesare complementaryin that they are different mathematicalanalysesof the same phenomenon.Thereforecertain time and frequencydomainvariablescorrelates stronglywitheach other[11].

III. The Discrete Wavelet Transform

A. Definition

The wavelet transform analysis is an alternative tool for analysis of non-stationary signals whose spectral characteristics change over time. The design and implementation includes a specially adapted decomposition-reconstruction filter bank for the frequency bands of interest.The wavelet transform (WT) of signal *x(t)* is defined as combination of a set of basis functions, obtained by means of dilation a and translation b of a mother wavelet [1].

$$W_a x(b) = \frac{1}{\sqrt{|a|}} \int_{-\infty}^{+\infty} x(t)\,\psi\left(\frac{t-b}{a}\right)dt \tag{1}$$

The Discrete Wavelet Transform (DWT) is defined as a discretized dilations and translations of the mother function, (or analyzing wavelet). The main idea is the same as it is in the CWT. A time-scale representation of a digital signal is obtained using digital filtering techniques. Recall that the CWT is a correlation between a wavelet at different scales and the signal with the scale (or the frequency) being used as a measure of similarity. The continuous wavelet transform was computed by changing the scale of the analysis window, shifting the window in time, multiplying by the signal, and integrating over all times. In the discrete case, filters of different cut-off frequencies are used to analyze the signal at different scales. The signal is passed through a series of high pass filters to analyze the high frequencies, and it is passed through a series of low pass filters to analyze the low frequencies. In its most common form, the DWT employs a dyadic grid (integer power of two scaling in *a*and*b*) and orthonormal wavelet basis functions and exhibits zero redundancy.

$$\psi_{(s,l)}(x) = 2^{-\frac{s}{2}}\psi(2^{-s}x - l) \tag{2}$$

The variables s and l are integers that scale and dilate the mother function ψ to generate wavelets (analyzing functions). The scale index s indicates the wavelet's width, and the location index l gives its position. The mother wavelets are rescaled, or "dilated" by powers of two, and translated by integers, in this case we have a dyadic decomposition structure. The Discrete Wavelet Transform decomposition of the signal into different frequency bands (according to Mallat's algorithm [2]) can be obtained by successive high-pass and low-pass filtering (digital FIR filter structures) of the time domain followed by downsamplig to eliminate the redundancy, as shown in Fig. 2.

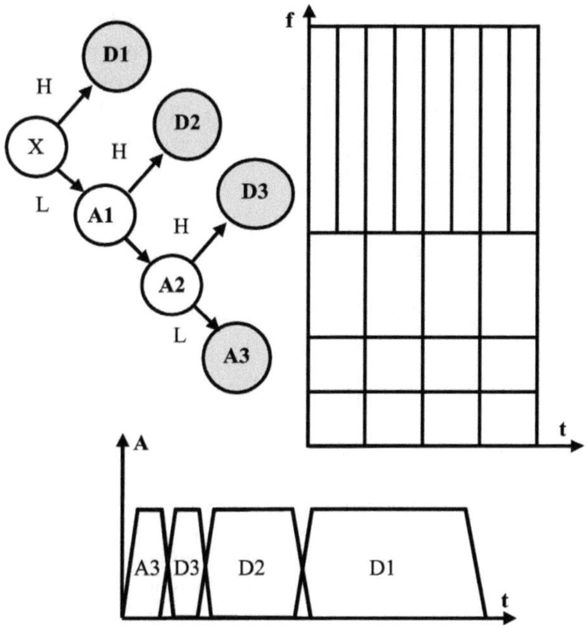

Fig. 2 The DWT based decomposition

IV. THE PROPOSED METHOD

The proposed procedure is presented on Fig. 3. The HRV signal is decomposed (as time series) through Discrete Wavelet Transform algorithm, the detail coefficients are filtered and the signal is reconstructed from these modified components. The main idea is to remove non-characteristic intervals which aren't specific for analysis, using DWT decomposition based nonlinear filtering. That means detail coefficient shrinkage (all components which are smaller than a previewed threshold will be erased) and a reconstruction with the new components [3]. Only the detail coefficients [Di] are thresholded, the average components [Ai] (output from the low pass filters) are conserved. Usually the noise is attributed to the high frequency components of the signal which correspond to small detail sizes when performing wavelet analysis.

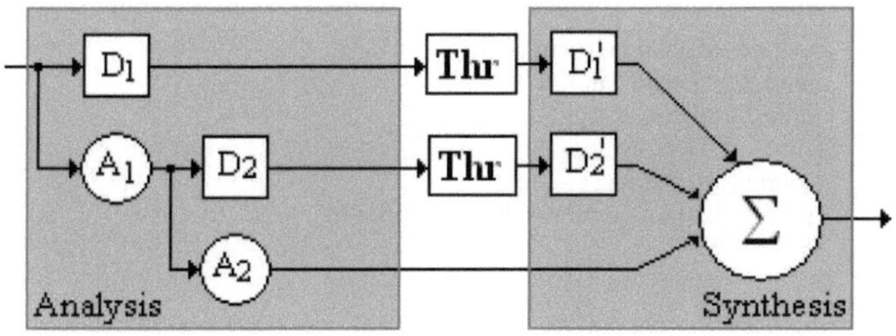

Fig. 3 The proposed procedure

Therefore the idea is to remove high frequency (small detail) components such that underlying signal structures are preserved and will emerge from the denoising process. After filtering, the new Lorenz plots could be more significantly presented in order to compute the demanded parametersusing the usual threshold value [5].

V. RESULTS

The study was performed on signal 14046 from MIT-BIH Long Term ECG Data Base (obtained from http://www.physionet.org).The DWT based filtering and reconstruction procedures were performed in Matlab environment using specific toolboxes. The nonlinear filtering is performed through hard thresholding (this sets any coefficient less than or equal to the threshold to zero), the used wavelet function is db4 type.One of the most important task is choosing the right threshold. In this study the chosen value was the universal threshold level (VisuShrink) proposed by Donoho and Johnstone(1994) equal to $\sigma\sqrt{2logM}$, where σ is the noise variance and M is the number of samples in the signal. The Lorentz plot of the analyzed signal is shown in Fig. 4.

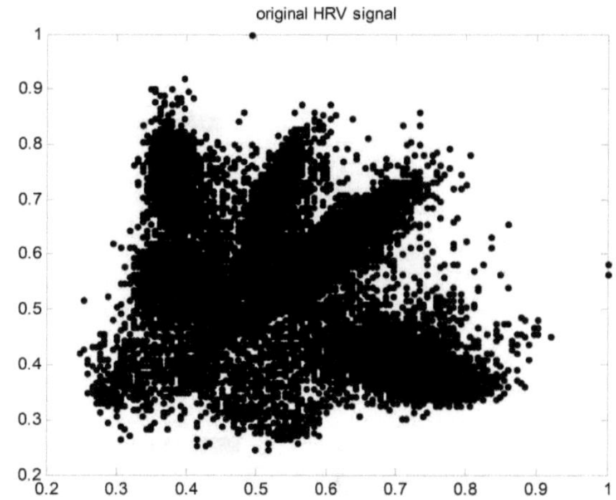

Fig. 4 The Lorenz plot of the original signal

The first order DWT decomposition based filtered HRV signal and the detail coefficients based one are presented on Fig. 5. The first it seems to be a normal heartbeat's correspondent Lorenz plot. The details coefficients based Lorenz plot contains the fast changes and also the noise based relations, but can be important if fast variations are searched.

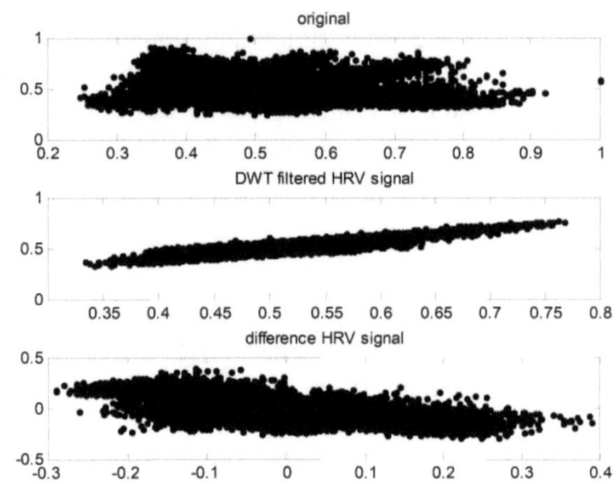

Fig. 5 First order filtered HRV versus original

As it can be seen, the average components trend to emphasize the normal part of HRV signal, preserving the average and the detail coefficient based representation contains the higher frequency components as fast changes in HRV or noise. Figure 6 presents the corresponding histograms for the original, for the filtered and the difference signal, which with the Lorentz plots together give a fast and accurate interpretation for specialists.

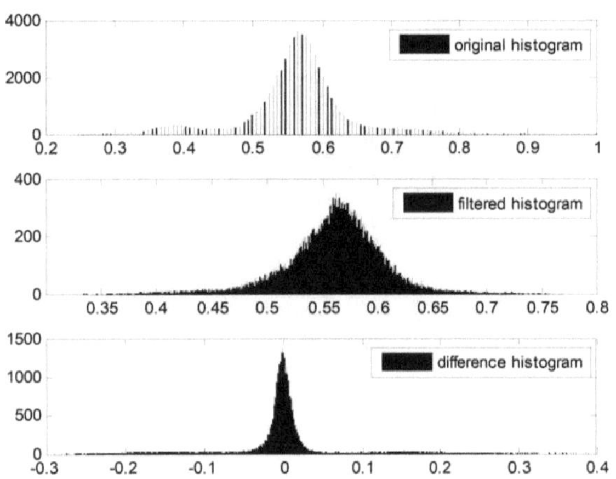

Fig. 6 The Lorenz plot of the original signal

VI. Concluding Remarks

This work shows the importance of the Lorenz plots, as a simple and efficient method for visualization the behavior of complex phenomena as HRV. The results demonstrate the importance of filtering as preprocessing.

A detailed analysis of Lorenz plots is feasible and could be more clinically useful than the conventional measures of HRV. For further work, there could be more other methods applied, as wavelet packet transform based filtering for a more accurate frequency component analysis or wavelet transform based prediction.

Conflict of Interest

The authors declare that they have no conflict of interest.

References

1. Heart rate variability. Standards of measurement, physiological interpretation, and clinical use. Task for of the European Society of Cardiology and the North American Society of Pacing and Electrophysiology. European Heart Journal 1996; 17:354–81.
2. Sameni, R. ,Shamsollahi, M. B.,Jutten, C. Clifford, G. D. A nonlinear Bayesian filtering framework for ECG denoising, IEEE Transactions on Biomedical Engineering, vol. 54, pp.2172 -2185 2007.
3. Donoho, D.L.; I.M. Johnstone (1994), Ideal spatial adaptation by wavelet shrinkage, Biometrika, vol 81, pp. 425-455 Engineering in Medicine and Biology 27th Annual Conference Shanghai, China, September 1-4, 2005
4. Han, M., Liu, H., Xi, J. H. Guo, W.Noise smoothing for nonlinear time series using wavelet soft threshold, IEEE Signal Processing Letters, vol. 14, pp.62 -65 2007.
5. Gao, J., Sultan, H., Hu, J., Tung, W.,Denoising Nonlinear Time Series by Adaptive Filtering and Wavelets Shrinkage: A comparison, IEEE Signal Processing Letters , Vol. 17, No. 3. March 2010.
6. Gao, J. B. Detecting nonstationarity and state transitions in a time series", Phys. Rev. E, vol. 63, pp.066202-1 -066202-8 2001.
7. Yamamoto, Y., Hughson, R., L., Coarse-graining spectral analysis: new method for studying heart rate variability. Journal of Applied Physiology, 1991 Sep;71(3):1143-50
8. Piskorski, J., Guzik, P. Filtering Poincaré plots. Computational Methods in Science and Technology 11(1), pag. 39-48, 2005
9. Burri, H., Chevalier, P.,Arzi, M.,Rubel, P.,Kirkorian, G., Touboul,P.,Wavelet transform for analysis of heart rate variability precedingventricular arrhythmias in patients with ischemic heart disease,International Journal of Cardiology 109, pp 101 – 107, (2003)
10. Constantino A. García, Abraham Otero, Xosé Vila, David G. Márquez, Biomedical Signal Processing and Control, Volume 8, Issue 6, November 2013, Pages 542–550

Author: Zoltan German-Sallo
Institute: "PetruMaior" University
Street: NicolaeIorga Street nr 1
City: Tirgu-Mures
Country: Romania
Email: zoltan.german-sallo@ing.upm.ro

Evaluation of ZigBee Technology for a Low-Cost Video Surveillance System

E. Lupu[1], A. Tigauan[2], G.P. Pop[1], and R. Arsinte[1]

[1] Technical University of Cluj-Napoca, Communications Dept., Cluj-Napoca, Romania
[2] EBS, Software Dept., Cluj-Napoca, Romania

Abstract— **IEEE 802.15.4/ZigBee wireless sensor networks (WSNs) have proved their value as an alternative to cabled systems for patient monitoring. The low power and small size ZigBee devices are able to form self-configuring networks which are expendable such that they can cover an entire hospital area. The current paper presents a low cost video system for patients or elderly persons, also finding applications in security surveillance. The low data rate protocols provided by IEEE 802.15.4 are met by several challenges, due to its protocols having been designed to primarily operate in low traffic load scenarios. Yet, a large volume of data may be generated by some video cameras or vital signs sensors. The system is based on a BeagleBoard –XM platform connected to a video camera (or to other sensors) and a Zigbee module so as to send images or data to the collector station. In the current implementation only the images are acquired and sent to the collector when a movement is detected.**

Keywords— **wireless sensor networks, Zigbee, BeagleBoard, video surveillance, open source**

I. Introduction

In order to serve more specialized goals such as networking battery-powered sensing devices in healthcare, low-power wireless network technologies were introduced. This technology allows short-distance communication, which justifies the Wireless Personal Area Network (WPAN) name for this technology, which has received increasing interest in the last few years, such that enhanced mobility and comfort are made possible for patients while being monitored. The three common types of wireless network technologies employed are Bluetooth, ZigBee and Wi-Fi. Some of the main features for these technologies can be found in table 1 [1] [2] [8].

Zigbee is a Personal Area Network (PAN) technology based on the IEEE 802.15.4 standard. Zigbee devices are able to form a mesh network between nodes, unlike Bluetooth or wireless USB devices, meshing being a type of daisy chaining from one device to another. This allows the short range of an individual node to be expanded and multiplied, this leading to much larger area coverage.

Our approach aims at designing a system which is capable of monitoring by using video techniques patients/elderly persons or safety-monitored areas using a wireless Zigbee network. Its main advantage consists of being a low-cost survey system solution used to monitor a larger area using a certain number of cameras.

Table 1 Main features of Bluetooth, ZigBee and Wi-Fi

Technology	Bluetooth	Zig-Bee		Wi-Fi
IEEE Specifications	802.15.1	802.15.4		802.11g
Frequency Band	2.4 GHz	868/915 MHz	2.4 GHz	2.4GHz
Supported data rate	1 Mb/s	250 Kb/s		54 Mb/s
Range (Indoor)	2-10 m	10-30m		38m
Support Communication	data/voice	data		mainly for data
Typical transmit power in mW	10	0.01-3.2		32-100
Size of stack	250kbits	4-32kbits		n/a
Basic cell	Piconet	Star		BSS
Max number of cell nodes	8/piconet	< 65535		32/access point
Complexity	Very complex	Simple		Complex
Power consumption	Low	Very low		Medium

II. Surveillance System Overview

The video surveillance system consists of the acquisition part and the centralizing data part, fig.1. In the acquisition part the images are obtained using the video camera connected to the BeagleBoard XM platform via USB. An XBee-Pro module is also connected to the platform through an USB-serial adapter. Images are transmitted using XBee-Pro radio modules that implement the Zigbee communication protocol. Radio communication is done to the frequency of 2.4 GHz and the modules use a 10 dBm transmission power (equivalent to 10mW). In the data centralization part we employ a laptop/PC where the images arrive from several acquisition systems. The computer is also connected to an XBee-Pro module to participate in radio communication, to receive the image frames.

A. Hardware

BeagleBoard XM is a single board computer built for the Open Source community.

S. Vlad and R.V. Ciupa (eds.), *International Conference on Advancements of Medicine and Health Care through Technology*,
IFMBE Proceedings 44,
DOI: 10.1007/978-3-319-07653-9_47, © Springer International Publishing Switzerland 2014

Dual-core DM3730 based Embedded System

- DM3730(Texas Instruments) found in new generation smart-phones is a dual-core (ARM+DSP) Digital Media Processor, which is compatible with OMAP™3 architecture and has the following prominent features [4]:
- The processor core is ARM Cortex A8 - 1 GHz
- TMS320C64x DSP (800 MHz able of processing HD video stream at 720p and 30 fps)
- Imagination Technologies PowerVR SGX 2D/3D graphics processor that supports two independent displays
- 512 MB RAM LPDDR
- 4 GB capacity micro SD card supplied with the BeagleBoard-XM.

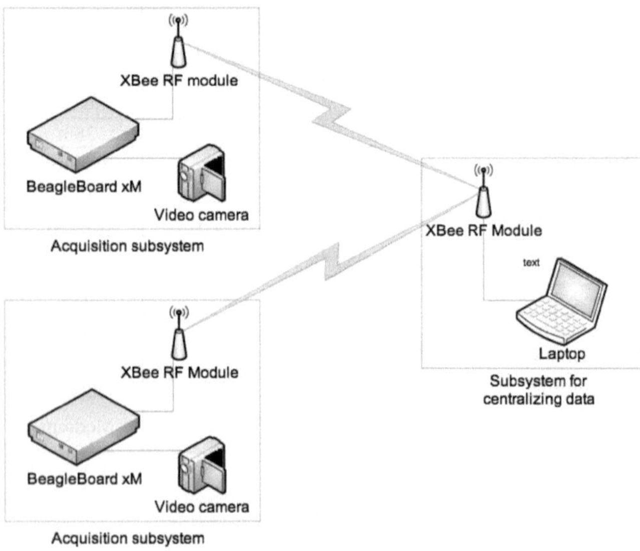

Fig. 1 Overall scheme of the system

The USB-powered Beagle-Board XM (beagleboard.org) shown in Fig. 2 is a DM3730 based development board and comprises of all needed components in order to access the peripherals such as mouse, keyboard, monitor, speakers, microphone, memory cards/sticks, internet, USB, WLAN adaptor etc. [5]. Attaching peripherals can be done by using any of the following ports and connections:

- DVI-D (HDMI connector chosen for size - maximum resolution is 1400x1050)
- S-Video
- USB OTG (mini-AB)
- 4 USB ports
- Ethernet Port
- Card slot for Micro SD / MMC
- Stereo input and output
- RS-232 port
- JTAG connector
- Expansion port (for adding new functionalities).

A user-friendly Linux distribution "Angstrom"for the BeagleBoard XM is available on a mini SD card [3]. The Angstrom is a distribution with a highly portable and reconfigurable core, built using the OpenEmbedded build system with special attention to embedded devices [3].

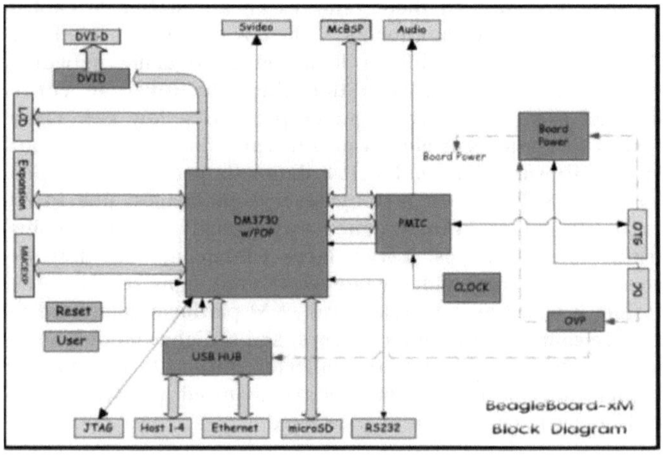

Fig. 2 The Beagle Board–XM architecture [5]

XBee-Pro PRO RF Module (Radio frequency) was designed to meet the specifications of IEEE 802.15.4 and to support the needs of a low-cost and low power wireless network. The module requires less power and provides reliable data transfer between devices. The module operates in the ISM band (Industrial, Scientific and Medical) of 2.4 GHz. Some of the key features of the module are presented hereinafter.

While communicating, data integrity is preserved under the following conditions: transmission distance in an enclosed space (indoor) or in urban areas is less than 60 m and transmission distance is no more than 750 m in open field. Transmission power is at most 10 mW (10 dBm) but can be changed by software and receiver sensitivity is -100 dBm. RF data rate is a fixed 250 kbps. The data rate on the serial interface of the software can be selected and can be from 1200 bps to 250 kbps. One can also select non-standard data rates. The power consumption is relatively low compared with other wireless modules: the peak current consumption at transmission is of 150 mA (3.3 V); the current during reception or idle state is 55 mA (3.3 V) and power-down current consumption of less than 10 μA.

The module supports the following network topologies: point-to-point, point-to-multipoint and peer-to-peer. 12 channels using direct sequence can be used and the channel number can selectable by software. Addressing modules is done either by using the PAN identifier, the channel number or the source and destination addresses.

The XBee-Pro Module interfaces with a host device through a digital-level asynchronous serial port. Using this serial port, the module can communicate with any device equipped with UART (universal asynchronous receiver / transmitter [6].

XBee-Pro USB Explorer (Sparkfun) is an adapter board from USB to serial line for the XBee-Pro modules. XBee-Pro module must be connected to XBee-Pro Explorer and then by a mini USB cable to the host. It will get direct access to serial communication terminals and programming pins of the XBee-Pro unit [7].

B. Software

The X-CTU software is an application based on Windows (not compatible with the Linux Operating system) provided for free by MaxStream Digi. This program was designed to interact with the firmware files found on Digi RF products and to provide an easy to use graphical interface. This software can be used to configure and test Digi radio modules. This application has the following features:

- Support for all Digi-MaxStream RF products;
- Integrated terminal interface – for configuring the modules manually;
- Easy to use loopback test range;
- Display indictor for the Receive Signal Strength (RSSI);
- Remote firmware upgrade for RF modules;
- Save and retrieve frequently used module configurations
- Automatically detect the type of RF module;
- Restore the factory settings;
- Easily modify each radio parameter from the graphical interface;
- Integration with LabVIEW and other software production test through command line interface.

The software is easy to use and allows customers to test the radio modems in the actual environment with just a computer and a few extra items included with the radio modems. X-CTU is used for configuring baud-rate, addresses and transmission power level, but can also be used for restoring the firmware on the XBee-Pro modules.

Other terminal programs such as **HyperTerminal** and **Minicom** can be used for configuring the modules.

OpenCV (Open-Source Computer Vision Library) is a library developed in C++ mostly designed for use with real-time image processing and artificial vision. The library was developed by Intel. It can be used for free under the open source BSD license. If the library finds Intel's Integrated Performance Primitives on the system, it uses these proprietary optimized routines to accelerate the software.

Improved and new algorithms are now developed for OpenCV in the C++ interface. It should be mentioned that the functions in this library are optimized to work with Intel architecture and will therefore have poor results on the BeagleBoard which uses ARM v7 architecture.

The library can be used for capturing images from the video camera but they have very poor performance. That is why images are retrieved from the video camera driver using the GStreamer framework. OpenCV will be used strictly for image processing.

III. Experiments and Results

The low data rate protocols provided by IEEE 802.15.4 are met by several challenges, due to its protocols having been designed to primarily operate in low traffic load scenarios. Yet, a large volume of data may be generated by some video cameras or vital signs sensors.

In order to protect the system from overload, it could be considered to have a priority sensor and video system. For instance, when motion is detected in a patient it should gain priority to images in the waiting room. Images are captured periodically and are compared to detect tracking changes. The decision whether motion has been detected or not is taken based on the differences between consecutive images. If motion is detected, frames will be sent more often.

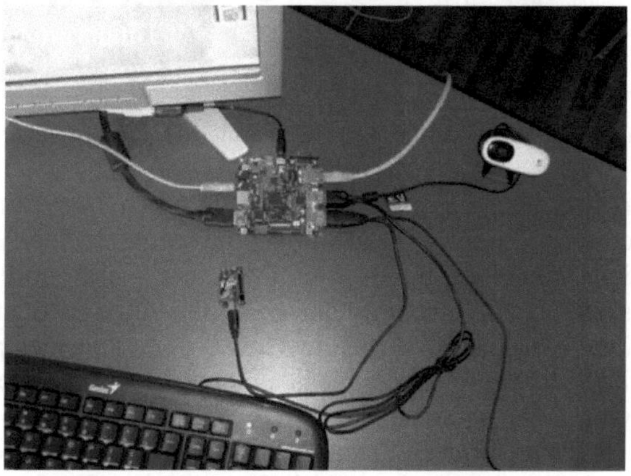

Fig. 3 The acquisition system based on BeagleBoard–XM

XBee-Pro module configuration may be done by employing AT commands or more simply by the X-CTU application. The steps followed by the system in order to transmit an image start with video camera initialization.

For retrieving an image from the video camera the following command is used, which saves the image in JPEG format.

```
gst-launch v4l2src ! ffmpegcolorspace ! video/x-raw-yuv ! jpegenc ! filesink location=test.jpg
```

Gst-launch is a tool that builds and runs streams. It is based on integrating different plug-ins for reading and writing in certain file formats and also for converting between different formats. In this case a JPEG encoder is used for converting from video format to JPEG format. Image processing is necessary for performing motion detection. The motion detection algorithm uses OpenCV functions.

Frames captured from the video camera are in color mode but for faster processing they are converted to grayscale. The figure below contains four images used in motion detection.

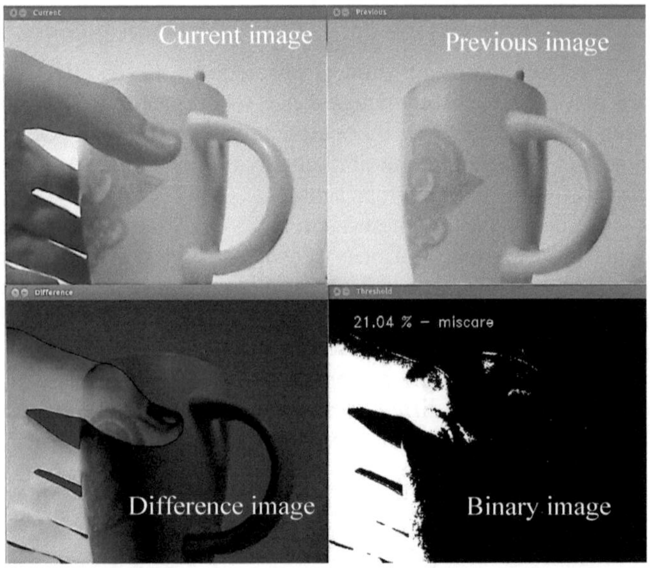

Fig. 4 The motion detection algorithm is illustrated on these figures

The first image is the current frame taken from camera and converted into grayscale mode; the second picture is the previous frame captured from the camera and stored in grayscale mode. The third image is the difference image obtained by subtracting the gray levels of two images pixel by pixel and the fourth image is a binary image obtained by applying a threshold to the difference image. If important differences are noticed in consecutive frames then motion is detected. Two images have to differ more than 2% from the total number of pixels for the frame to be considered in motion. This threshold may be selected by the user.

Duration for an image acquisition consists of three steps:

- image capture and processing time (delay in transmission)
- image transmission time via radio link
- duration of the reception processing (delay at reception).

The delays introduced in the transmission chain from source to the collector depend on the image resolution and the baud rate. In table 2 may be observed these delays for a 640x480 video cam resolution (an average of 40kB for the file size).

Table 2 Image acquisition delay (for 640x480 image resolution)

Data rate (bps)	Transmission Delay (s)	Total Delay (s)
1200	273.33	275.73
2400	136.67	139.07
4800	68.33	70.73
9600	34.17	36.57
19200	17.08	19.48
38400	8.54	10.94
57600	5.69	8.09

IV. Conclusions

In our work we proposed and evaluated the use of the ZigBee technology for the implementation of low-cost video surveillance systems, which can be useful for the monitoring of patients or elderly persons or for security purposes. The delay introduced by the system processing chain and the limited data rate transmission achieve reasonable values to account for the usefulness of the system. Some improvements may be introduced by using moving sensors, different network topologies, video and image formats. For more complex systems some physiological sensors (ECG, blood pressure or glucose, respiration, body temperature) may be connected to the acquisition subsystem (BeagleBoard XM) to be transmitted via the ZigBee network.

Conflict of Interest

The authors declare that they have no conflict of interest.

References

1. Wang Q , Balasingham I Wireless Sensor Networks - An Introduction, Wireless Sensor Networks: Application Centric Design, 2010, ISBN: 978-953-307-321-7
2. Liu Y, Wireless Remote Patient Monitoring on General Hospital Wards, Doctor of philosophy thesis, sept. 2010
3. Ångström- Distributions. http://linuxtogo.org/gowiki/ Angstrom Oct. 2009. Web 28 Jun. 2013
4. DM3730 datasheet: Texas Instruments. Digital Media Processors. July. 2011. Literature Number : SPRS685D.
5. BeagleBoard XM System Reference Manual, Revision C3.0, May 2009.
6. XBee®/XBee-PRO® RF Modules, Product Manual http://www.sparkfun.com/datasheets/Wireless/Zigbee/XBee-Datasheet.pdf
7. XBee Explorer Serial https://www.sparkfun.com/products/9111
8. ZigBee.Alliance, *ZigBee Alliance Document 053474r17,ZigBee Specification, v. 1.0 r17*, Z. Alliance, Editor. 2007.

Pathological Voice Assessment Using TESPAR Analysis

G.P. Pop[1], E. Lupu[1], and E. Onaca[2]

[1] Comm. Dept., Technical University of Cluj-Napoca, Romania
[2] "Iuliu Hatieganu" Medicine and Pharmacy University/Family Medicine Dept., Cluj-Napoca, Romania

Abstract— **Voice disorders have experienced significant growth in recent years mainly due to unhealthy social habits and voice abuse, and therefore, there is an increased interest in their early diagnosis. Acoustic analysis can be helpful in diagnosing these diseases, being a noninvasive tool and providing an objective diagnosis. In this paper we suggest the use of TESPAR analysis for detection of voice with disorders. Our experiments shows that TESPAR A-matrix can be used to discriminate between normal and pathological voices.**

Keywords— **voice disorders, voice assessment, acoustic analysis, time domain analysis, TESPAR analysis**

I. INTRODUCTION

It is widely recognized that voice diseases do not necessarily cause changes in voice quality as perceived by another listener. A lot of studies have focused on identifying acoustic measures that highly correlate with pathological voice qualities (also referred to as voice alterations or voice disorders). Acoustic analysis seeks objective assessment, in a noninvasive way, for the degree of voice alterations.

Pathologies that affect vocal folds usually modify their morphology and, consequently, abnormal vibration patterns and increased turbulent airflow at the level of the glottis may appear [1]. Acoustic analysis is usually performed by the extraction of acoustic parameters from voice signal using digital signal processing techniques. These parameters are then analyzed to determine particular characteristics of the voice.

One approach in acoustic analysis allows to estimate of long-term acoustic parameters such as: the pitch, jitter, shimmer, Amplitude Perturbation Quotient (APQ), Harmonics to Noise Ratio (HNR), Pitch Perturbation Quotient (PPQ), Voice Turbulence Index (VTI), Normalized Noise energy (NNE), Frequency Amplitude Tremor (FATR), Soft Phonation Index (SPI), Glottal to Noise Excitation (GNE) [2]. However, their reliable estimation is based on an accurate measurement of the fundamental frequency which is not a trivial task in the case of certain vocal pathologies. Another approach is short-time analysis of the speech which use a non-parametric approach able of modelling the effects of pathologies on both the excitation (vocal folds) and the system (vocal tract). Short-term Mel frequency cepstral coefficients (MFCCs) features together with other features (fundamental frequency, energy, noise features), can be reliably employed for assessment of normal and pathological voices [3].

Correlation of the various suggested features and representations with voice pathology is evaluated using techniques like linear multiple regression analysis [3], or likelihood scores using Gaussian Mixture Models and Hidden Markov Models [4]. Also neural networks and Support Vector Machine classifiers have been suggested [4].

In this work, we suggest the use of TESPAR matrices for detection of voice with disorders.

II. TESPAR METHOD BACKGROUND

TESPAR (Time Encoded Signal Processing and Recognition) is a technique which classifies time domain signals according to certain shape parameters. The method is based on the approximations to the locations of the real and complex zeroes, derived from the analysis of a band limited signal. The real zeroes correspond to the zero crossings of the signal while the complex zeroes are associated with local maxima, minima, points of inflexion etc. The real zeroes of a function and some complex zeroes can be detected by visual inspection (Fig. 1), but the detection of all complex zeroes is a complex task. The overcome this drawback, the following procedure may be used:

- the waveform is segmented between successive real zeroes, resulting a number of *epochs* with a certain lengths;
- this duration information is combined with simple approximations of the shape between these two locations.

In this way an important subset of complex zeroes may be identified by examining the features of the wave shape between its successive real zeroes.

In the simplest implementation of the TESPAR method [5], two descriptors are associated with every segment or epoch of the waveform:

- the *duration* (D) between successive real zeroes;
- the *shape* (S) between two successive real zeroes (as number of minima).

Most signals can be expressed as a series of discrete numerical descriptors based on TESPAR symbol alphabets. The standard TESPAR alphabet consists of 28 symbols, as shown in Table 1, and this has proven sufficient to represent most signal waveforms to an acceptable approximation [5].

S. Vlad and R.V. Ciupa (eds.), *International Conference on Advancements of Medicine and Health Care through Technology*, IFMBE Proceedings 44,
DOI: 10.1007/978-3-319-07653-9_48, © Springer International Publishing Switzerland 2014

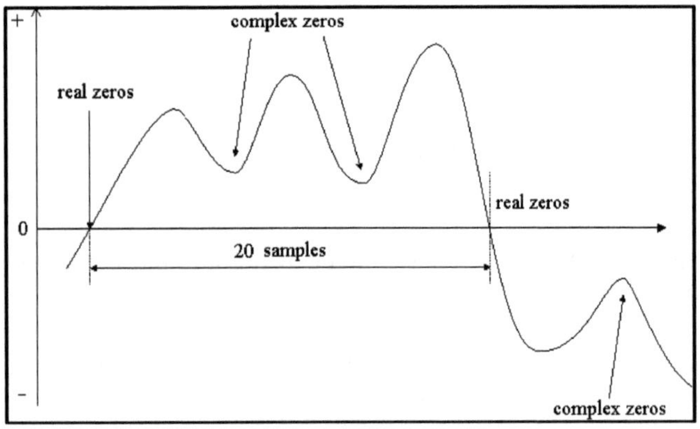

Fig. 1 TESPAR waveform analysis

Table 1. TESPAR alphabet

D	S 0	1	2	3	4	5
1	1	1	1	1	1	1
2	2	2	2	2	2	2
3	3	3	3	3	3	3
4	4	4	4	4	4	4
5	5	5	5	5	5	5
6	6	6	6	6	6	6
7	6	6	6	6	6	6
8	7	8	8	8	8	8
9	7	8	8	8	8	8
10	7	8	8	8	8	8
11	9	10	10	10	10	10
12	9	10	10	10	10	10
13	9	10	10	10	10	10
14	11	12	13	13	13	13
15	11	12	13	13	13	13
16	11	12	13	13	13	13
17	11	12	13	13	13	13
18	11	12	13	13	13	13
19	14	15	16	17	17	17
....						
34	23	24	25	26	27	28
35	23	24	25	26	27	28
36	23	24	25	26	27	28
37	23	24	25	26	27	28

The standard alphabet can be used to convert the sequence of epochs into an equivalent TESPAR symbol stream. The TESPAR coding process is presented in Fig.2, using an alphabet to map the duration/shape (D/S) attributes of each epoch to a single descriptor or symbol.

Another approach involves using an additionally descriptor A, for each epoch, usually epoch maximum amplitude. In this case, the coding is based on a comparison of two successive epochs (for each descriptor D, S, A), as shown in Fig. 3. Now we have 27 symbols, but the number of a symbol has nothing to do with the duration or complexity of an epoch. This alphabet is called TESPAR DZ alphabet [6].

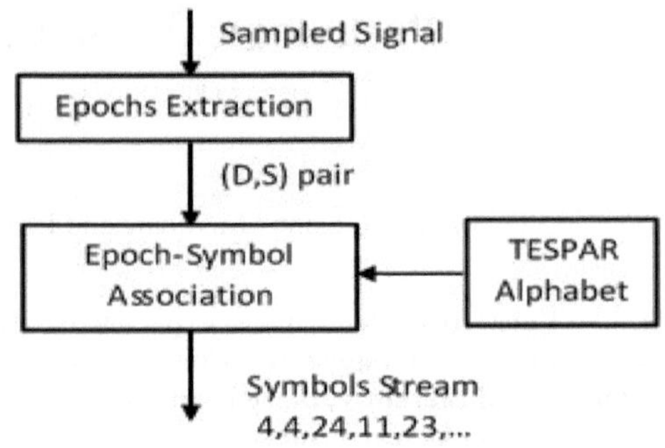

Fig. 2 TESPAR coding process

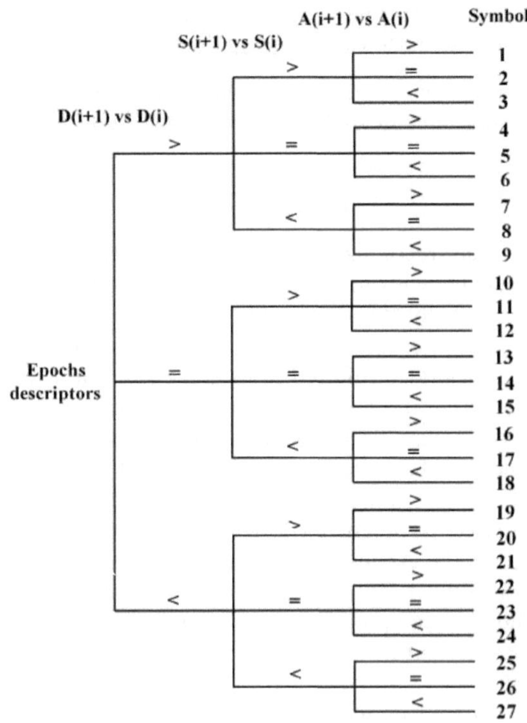

Fig. 3 TESPAR DZ symbols assignation

The TESPAR symbols string may be converted into a variety of fixed-dimension matrices [6]. The *S*-matrix is presented as a histogram of TESPAR symbols. Given a stream *s(i)* of codes *Ti*, the elements of S can be expressed as:

$$S_n = \frac{1}{N}\sum_{i=0}^{M} T_i, \quad 1 \le n \le N \tag{1}$$

where: $T_i = \begin{cases} 1\ if\ s(i) = n \\ 0,\ otherwise \end{cases}$

The contribution of each symbol can be weighted by the value of the A descriptor.

Another option is the A-matrix, which is a two dimensional $N \times N$ matrix that contains the number of times each pair of symbols appears, with a possible lag of L symbols:

$$A_{mn} = \frac{1}{N}\sum_{i=1+L}^{M} T_i, \quad 1 \le m,n \le N \tag{2}$$

where: $$T_i = \begin{cases} 1 \; if \; s(i) = m \; and \; s(i-L) = n \\ 0, \; otherwise \end{cases}$$

The contribution of each pair of symbols can be weighted with a value that implies values of A descriptor from each associated epoch.

III. Experiments and Results

For this study, a dedicated application was designed that allows:

- TESPAR analysis of a speech signal or a derivative (for example, the Teager energy), with the possibility to vizualize the epochs.
- Generating symbol stream (coding) specifying the alphabet used (standard or DZ), the type of additional epoch descriptor (maximum amplitude, average energy).
- Generate and vizualize TESPAR matrices, S and A (for different values of the lag parameter L), with the possibility of applying a weight to each symbol or pair of symbols.

As a case study, we used utterances from subjects with normal voice and the utterances from subjects with voices affected by various pathologies (Unilateral vocal fold paralysis, Bilateral vocal fold paralysis, Presbylaryngis, Adductor spasmodic dysphonia, Abductor spasmodic dysphonia, Muscle tension disorder, Dysphonia plica ventricularis, Paradoxical vocal fold dysfunction) [7]. For all utterances, we used16-bit mono audio recordings, at 22,050 KHz sampling frequency.

We performed several experiments using our application directly on the speech signal or on Teager energy from the voice signal, using as additional descriptor maximum amplitude or square energy for each epoch.

At this stage, we used visual comparison of matrices S and A. We found that the A-matrix is much better suited to differentiate between the normal and the pathological voice. The best results were obtained using the voice signal itself, with square energy as additional descriptor, and $L=1$ for lag. Figures Fig.4-7 shows TESPAR A-matrices for a normal voice while figures Fig.8-11 shows same matrices for a pathological voice.

As can be seen, in the case of a normal voice, when using the standard alphabet, the A-matrix values have a wider distribution, in the central area (Fig. 4, Fig. 5) while for

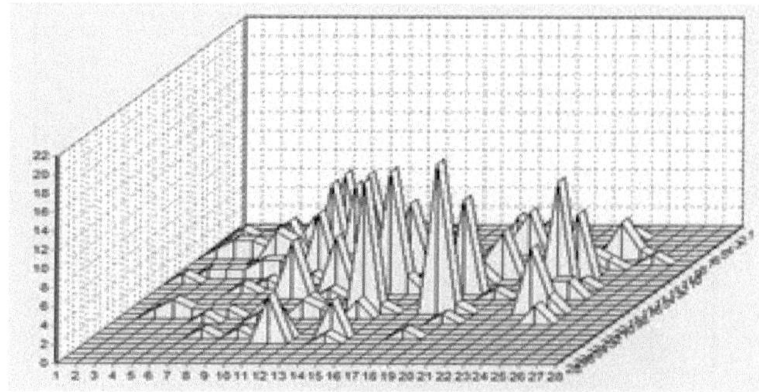

Fig. 4 TESPAR A matrix, normal voice, standard alphabet, no weight

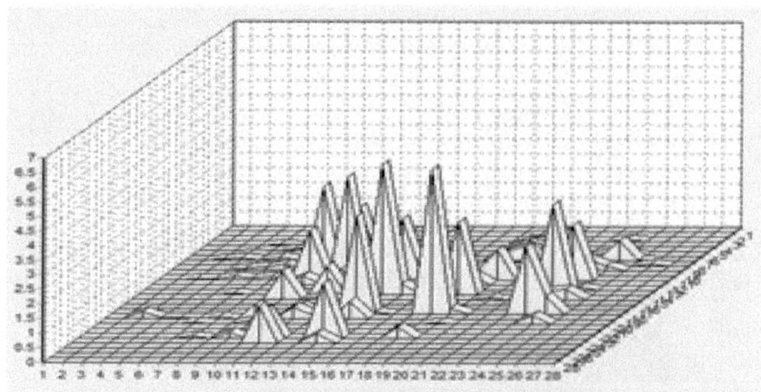

Fig. 5 TESPAR A matrix, normal voice, standard alphabet, weighted

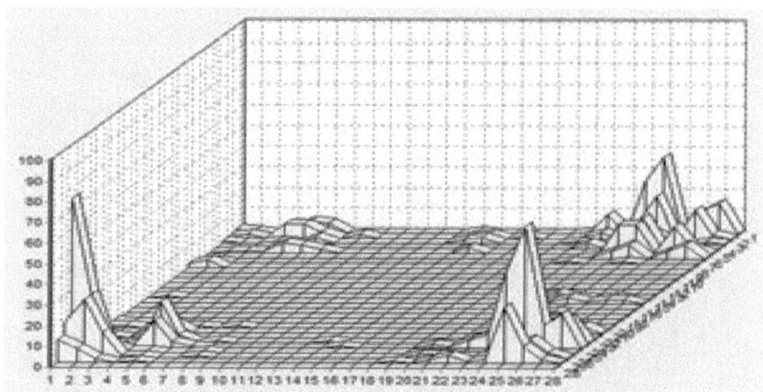

Fig. 6 TESPAR DZ A matrix, normal voice, no weight

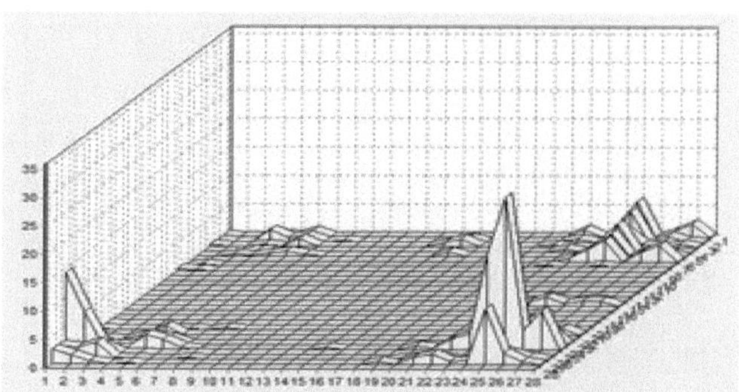

Fig. 7 TESPAR DZ A matrix, normal voice, weighted

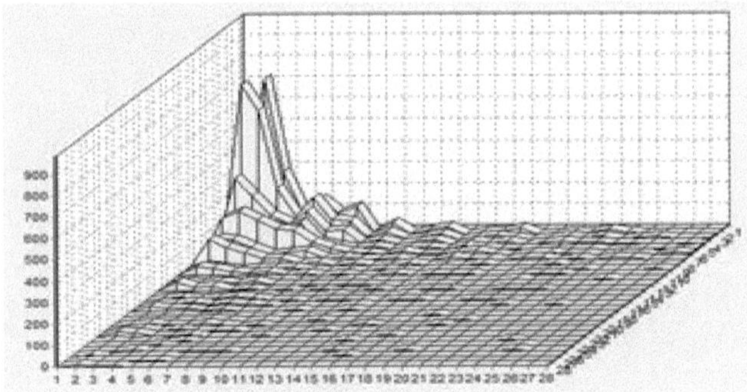

Fig. 8 TESPAR A matrix, pathological voice, standard alphabet, no weight

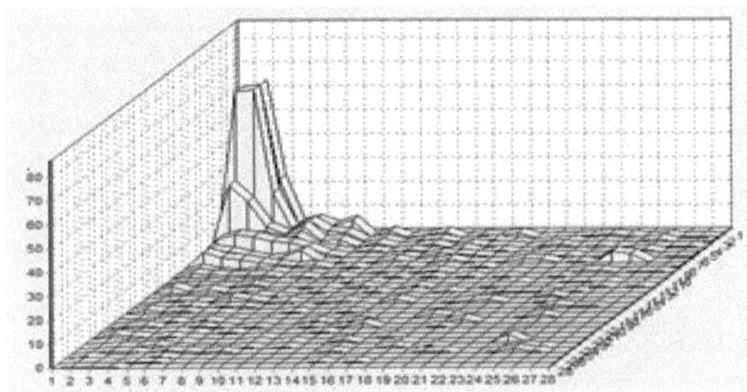

Fig. 9 TESPAR A matrix, pathological voice, standard alphabet, weighted

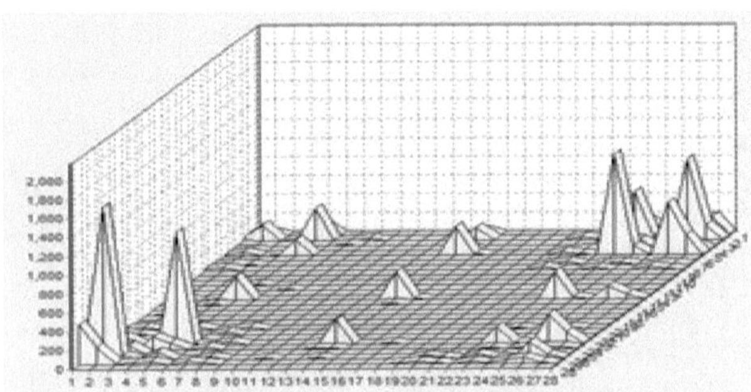

Fig. 10 TESPAR DZ A matrix, pathological voice, no weight

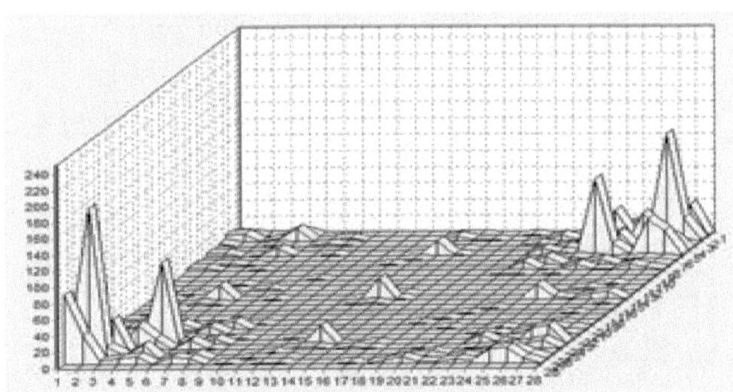

Fig. 11 TESPAR DZ A matrix, pathological voice, weighted

the TESPAR DZ alphabet values of matrix *A* have a restricted distribution in the periphery (Fig. 6, Fig. 7).

In the case of a disordered voice, when using the standard alphabet, the values of the matrix *A* have a more restricted distribution in the first corner (Fig. 8, Fig. 9) while for TESPAR DZ alphabet, the *A*-matrix values have a restricted distribution, only two corners (Fig. 10, Fig. 11). In all cases, the use of weighting lead to greater differences between the two types of voices.

IV. Conclusions

In this work, we suggest the use of TESPAR *A*-matrices to discriminate between normal and pathological voices. First results show that the *A*-matrices can be successfully used for this purpose. Weighting the contribution of each symbol provide better results. More experiments on a database with pathological voices are needed, using a classifier for evaluating the results.

Conflict of Interest

The authors declare that they have no conflict of interest.

References

1. Maria E. Markaki, Y. Stylianou (2011) Voice Pathology Detection and Discrimination Based on Modulation Spectral Features, IEEE Trans. on Audio, Speech & Language Processing 19(7): 1938-1948
2. V. Parsa, D. Jamieson (2000) Identification of pathological voices using glottal noise measures, J. Speech, Language, Hearing Res., 43(2): 469–485
3. M. Little, P. McSharry, S. Roberts, D. Costello, I.M.Moroz (2007) Exploiting nonlinear recurrence and fractal scaling properties for voice disorder detection, BioMedical Engineering, Published online, doi:10.1186/1475-925X-6-23
4. A.A.Dibazar, T.W.Berger, S.S.Narayanan (2006) Pathological voice asessment, IEEE, 28th Eng. in Med. and Biol. Soc., NY, USA, pp. 1669–1673
5. R.A. King , T.C. Phipps (1998) Shannon, TESPAR And Approximation Strategies, ICSPAT 98, Vol. 2, pp. 1204-1212, Toronto, Canada
6. E. Lupu, S. Emerich, F. Beaufort (2009) On-line signature recognition using a global features fusion approach, Acta Tehnica Napocensis, Electronics and Telecomunications, *50(3):* 13-20
7. Texas Voice Center at: http://www.texasvoicecenter.com/diseases.html

Author: Petre G. Pop
Institute: Comm.Dept., Technical University of Cluj-Napoca
Street: G.Baritiu, 26-28
City: Cluj-Napoca
Country: Romania
Email: petre.pop@com.utcluj.ro

A Histogram Method for Detecting Useful Surface Electromyogram Signals

E.P. Vesa and B. Ilie

Computer and Electric Engineering Department, "Lucian Blaga" University Sibiu, Romania

Abstract— **SEMG (Surface Electromyogram) is a common noninvasive method of measuring the electrical activity in muscle tissue. The SEMG signal is used in various applications, from clinical research to application prostheses and human-computer interfaces. The SEMG signal is a small amplitude signal and strongly affected by noise. The aim of this study is to design and implement a hardware method of signal extraction in the time domain, without affecting useful SEMG amplitude and phase characteristics, so with minimal distortion. This approach allows isolating a segment in the time domain of the SEMG signal, based on the statistical histogram method. The selection criterion relies on choosing a signal area with a maximum number of samples that exceed the threshold in the required histogram. The imposed threshold depends on the signal-to-noise ratio of the acquired SEMG signal. We have designed and built equipment for SEMG signal amplification, conversion, and processing. A SEMG signal selection algorithm has been hardware implemented using a Xilinx XUPV5 development board with Virtex-5 FPGA. Experimental results suggest that this algorithm is simple, fast, and easy to implement as a hardware solution. The algorithm reduces the number of SEMG signal samples processed and thus the computation time.**

Keywords— **SEMG, Histogram, Hardware signal processing, Mean value**

I. INTRODUCTION

Skeletal muscles generate EMG signals. Muscular contraction is initiated by pressing the depolarization in a nerve engine with the origin in the brain or the spinal cord [1]. These signals are detected by placing electrodes on the surface of the skin onto the muscle tissues [3], in a procedure known as Surface Electromyogram (SEMG). SEMG signal is important in various fields, from clinical research to application prosthesis, robotics, and human-computer interfaces [7]. The detection, processing, and analysis of EMG signal have become a major research area in the biomedical field. The aim of our study is to design and implement a hardware method of signal extraction in the time domain, without affecting useful SEMG amplitude and phase characteristics, so with minimal distortion [4], [5], [6], [8]. The SEMG signal is strongly affected by noise [2], [7].Sources of noise are the electrical inherent noise in electronics equipment, ambient noise, motion artifact, ECG signal, and the inherent instability of SEMG signal by its random nature [3]. The acquisition of the SEMG signal can be performed using FPGA circuits [9]. The SEMG signal selection method minimizes the influence of noise on the SEMG signal using the histogram method. We have designed and built equipment for EMG signal amplification, conversion, and processing. A SEMG signal selection algorithm has been implemented using a Xilinx XUPV5 development board [9], [10], [11].

II. MATERIALS AND METHODS

A. The EMG Measurement System

Figure 1 shows the block diagram of the SEMG signal processing system. The analog signal captured by electrodes is amplified, filtered, and converted to digital format. Digital signal processing is carried out in a Virtex-5 FPGA development board and the results are sent to the computer and displayed on the monitor.

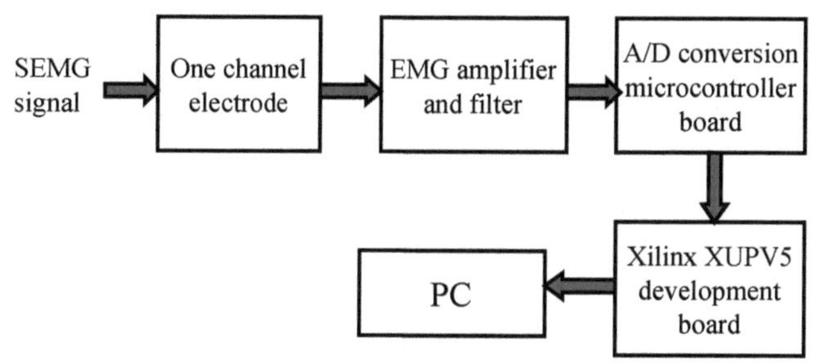

Fig. 1 Block diagram of one channel SEMG system acquisition and processing

The SEMG amplifier structure is shown in Figure 2. The overall amplification factor is 1500, the bandwidth is limited in the range of 5Hz - 5.6 kHz and CMMR factor = 95 dB. A notch filter (hum filter) eliminates the disturbing signal with frequency of 50 Hz. The output stage provides a 1.65V gap in DC voltage. The microcontroller is powered by 3.3V, and the maximal SEMG signal amplitude at the microcontroller input is 3.3 Vpp.

The SEMG amplifier output signal is converted from analog to digital signal by the PIC16F887 microcontroller. Sample value n, is given by (1):

S. Vlad and R.V. Ciupa (eds.), *International Conference on Advancements of Medicine and Health Care through Technology*, IFMBE Proceedings 44,
DOI: 10.1007/978-3-319-07653-9_49, © Springer International Publishing Switzerland 2014

$$Uin = n \times 3.128e - 3\ (V) \quad (1)$$

The A/D converter has a resolution of 10 bits and the sampling frequency is 64.1 kHz. The microcontroller transmits digital data to the FPGAVirtex-5 circuit, J6 connector on Xilinx XUPV5 development board.

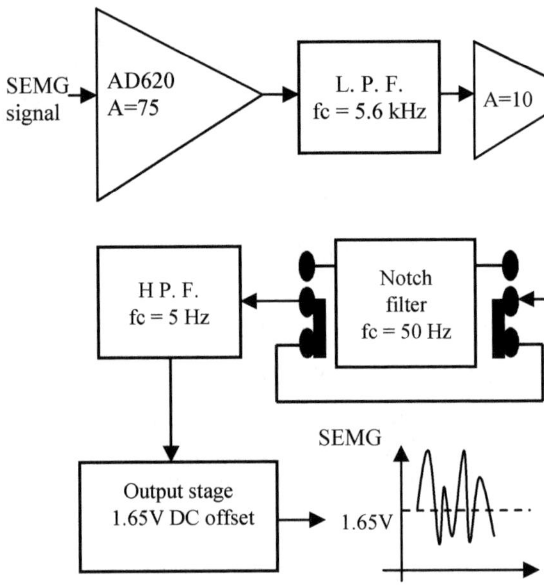

Fig. 2 Block diagram of SEMG amplifier

Figure 3 depicts a schematic diagram for the interconnection between the PIC16F887 microcontroller and the Xilinx XUPV5 development board [11].

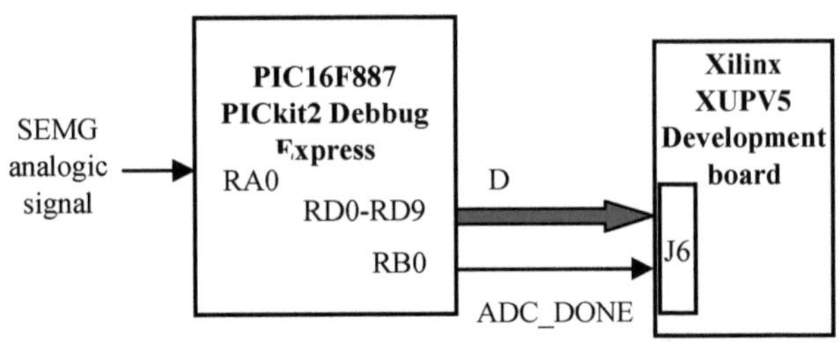

Fig. 3 Connection between Xilinx XUPV5development board and PIC16F887

The ADC_DONE signal acts as the data transmission-timing signal between the microcontroller and the Virtex-5 circuit. D is the data signal and is collected when the signal ADC_DONE=1.

A diagram of the signals recorded with the ASIX Sigma logic analyzer is presented in Figure 4.

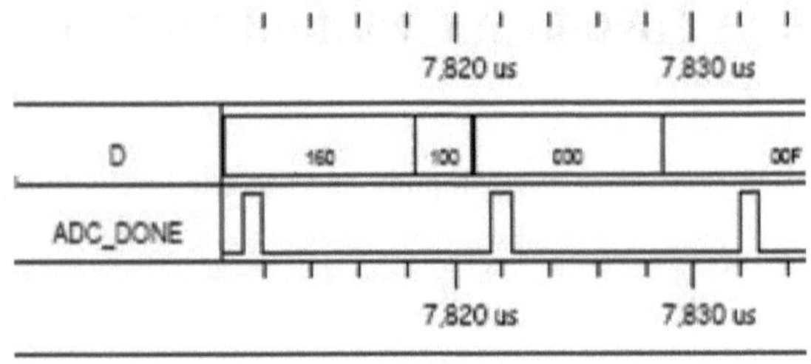

Fig. 4 Data signal timing between Xilinx XUPV5development board and PIC16F887

Sampled EMG signal is stored in DDR2 SDRAM memory of Xilinx XUPV5 development board [9].

The histogram algorithm is designed and implemented in C language programming. The Xilinx Embedded Development Kit (EDK) tool is used to generate and implement the MicroBlaze soft-core processor on the Virtex-5 FPGA, Xilinx XUPV5 [9].The algorithm was designed as separate blocks.

The software for microcontroller was written in MPLAB IDE with the C language compiler.

B. The EMG Signal Histogram Extracting Method

Extraction of useful EMG signal involves the following eight steps:

1) Baseline settings:
   - *Dim_hist*: the histogram size (number of samples in the histogram)
   - *Thr_hist*: the threshold for the minimum value of the histogram;
   - Min_hist: the minimum value of the histogram

   These values are determined experimentally by the recorded SEMG signal quality.

2) Calibration: measuring the noise parameters of the signal in the absence of a SEMG signal with electrodes positioned on the skin:
   - the maximum value of the noise signal U_{maxn}
   - the minimum value of the noise signal U_{minn}
   - the average value of the noise signal U_{medn}

3) Acquired SEMG signal (U_{in}) and samples are stored in DDR2 memory. Figure 5 presents a representation of a DDR2 memory map. The number of samples is NRSAMPLES.

4) Calculate the maximum value of input noise *Max_n_hist* relative to the mean signal noise U_{medn} on the signal line; this value will be used as a parameter in creating the histogram:

```
if (Umaxn-Umedn)>(Umedn-Uminn)
        Max_n_hist=Umaxn-Umedn;
else    Max_n_hist=Umedn-Uminn;
```

5) Calculate the module of the difference (2) of input SEMG signal U_{in} relative to the mean signal noise U_{medn} and store its value in DDR2 memory:

$$modul\_dif\_n=|U_{in} - U_{medn}| \qquad (2)$$

6) Signal samples $|U_{in}-U_{medn}|$ are grouped of *Dim_hist* samples. The histogram value *Hist* of the signal modul_dif_nis determined by the formula:

```
if(Uin-Umedn)>(Max_n_hist+Thr_hist)
        Hist=Hist+1;
else    Hist=Hist;
```

The histogram values *Hist*are stored in DDR2 memory. The number of histograms is (3):

$$NR_{hist} = NRSAMPLES \div Dim\_hist \qquad (3)$$

The noise level imposed is *Max_n_hist+Thr_hist.*

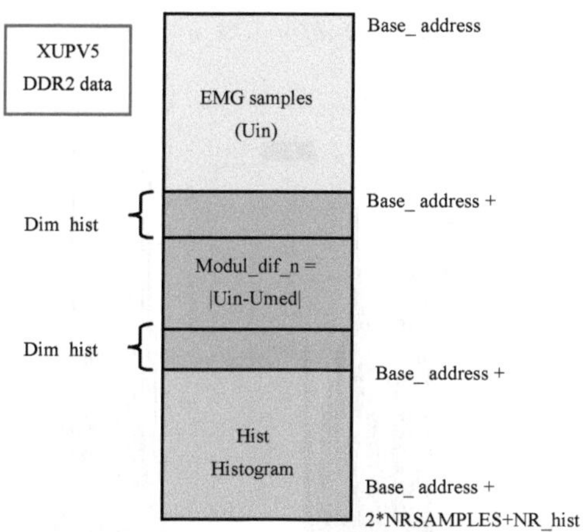

Fig. 5 Xilinx XUPV5 DDR2 data memory

7) Determine the maximum of the histograms *Max_hist* and histogram index *Kmax*. *Max_hist* represents the value histogram with the highest number of samples that exceed the noise level imposed. *Kmax* is the number of histogram with the largest value *Max_hist.*

8) Determine the boundaries of the DDR2 memory in which the useful SEMG signal is stored.
The lower limit of DDR2 memory is done by the first histogram, at the left of Kmax that meet the condition (4).

The upper limit of DDR2 memory is done by the first histogram, at the right of Kmax that meet the condition (4).

$$Hist<Min\_hist \qquad (4)$$

Figure 6 presents the method for the selection of these values. The imposed limits of variation of the index *K* histogram data relationship (5) are:

$$(Nr\_hist)/4 < K < (Nr\_hist)*3/4 \qquad (5)$$

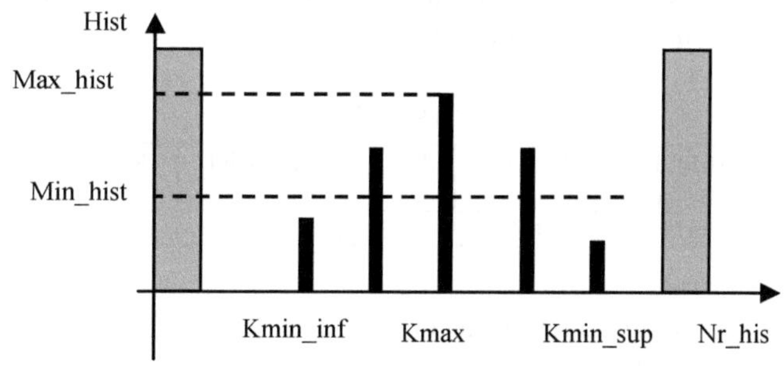

Fig. 6 Determination of *Kmin_inf* and *Kmin_sup* index

Figure 7 shows the calculation of the memory limits of the stored SEMG signal considered useful.

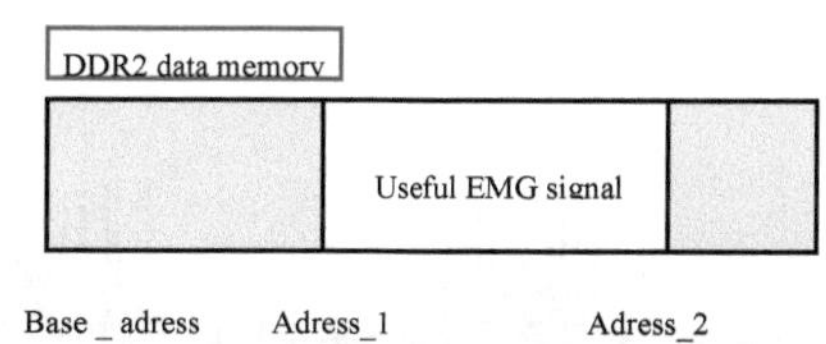

Fig. 7 Calculation of the DDR2 memory limits of the useful EMG signal.

$$Address\_1 = Base\_address + K\min\_inf \times Dim\_hist$$
$$Address\_2 = Base\_address + K\min\_sup \times Dim\_hist$$

III. Experimental Results

The SEMG signal was collected with a set of three electrodes. It was amplified, sampled, and processed on a XILINX XUPV5 development board. Calculation results are recorded in the data file. We applied the algorithm described above, using the following particular settings:

1) In the calibration phase, the noise parameters of the signal line were measured: U_{max}, U_{min}, and U_{medn}. The

program processed a number of samples *NRSAMPLES* = 49062. The results are presented in Table 1:

Table 1 Noise signal parameters on signal line

	Umax	*Umin*	*Umedn*
n-(sample value)	547	494	518
$n \times 3.128$ (*V*)	1.711	1.545	1.62

2) The equipment acquired a number of samples *NRSAMPLES* = 197973 (duration 3s). The size of a histogram is *Dim_hist* = 1000,*Thr_hist* = 10 and *Min_hist* = 5. The results of applying the method on SEMG signal detection are summarized in Table 2. Duration of the digital signal processing is under 1s.

Table 2 Experimental values

NRSAMPLE of SEMG signal	NR_hist	Kmax	Kmin_inf	Kmin_sup
197973	197	135	129	167

The memory area used for recorded SEMG signal is between the limits:

$$Base\_address + 129000 \div Base\_address + 167000$$

The graphical representations in Figures 8 to 11 illustrate the algorithm for processing the SEMG signal in order to extract the useful signal.

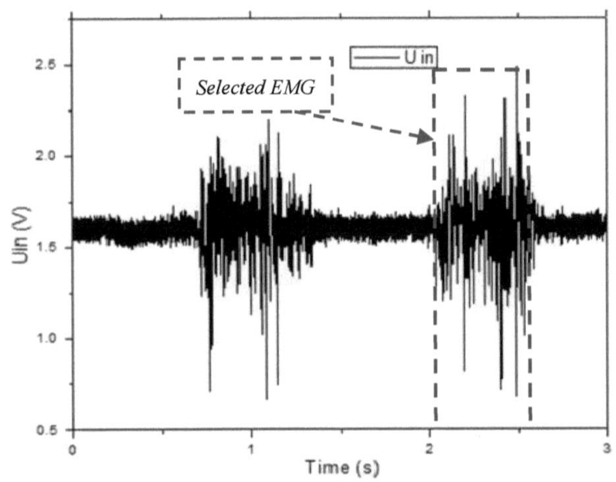

Fig. 8 SEMG analog input signal in microcontroller PIC16F887

From the original signal shown in Figure 8, we want to select the part of the signal in the red area. After the acquisition with the equipment described above, the signal at the input of the PIC16F887 microcontroller board matches Figure 8.

For this signal, we apply the algorithm described in section II.B. First, we calculate the module of the difference of the input sampled signal relative to the mean SEMG signal noise in Figure 9, and calculate the histogram of the module, as per Figure 10. The noise threshold signal is evident in Figure 9 (*Max_n_hist* + *Thr_hist)* and all samples below this threshold are ignored.

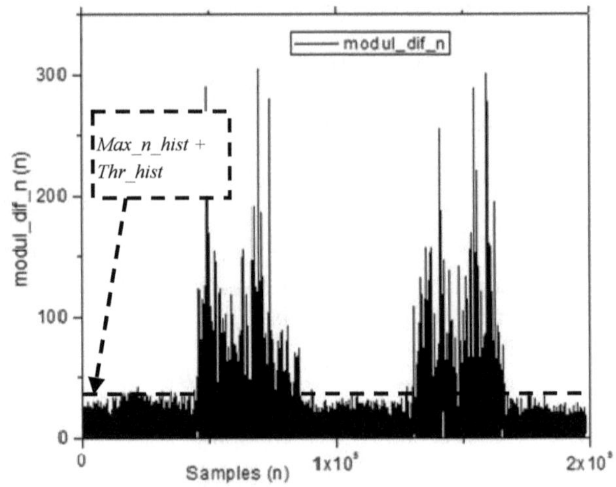

Fig. 9 *modul_dif_n*=|*Uin_n* – *Umed*|

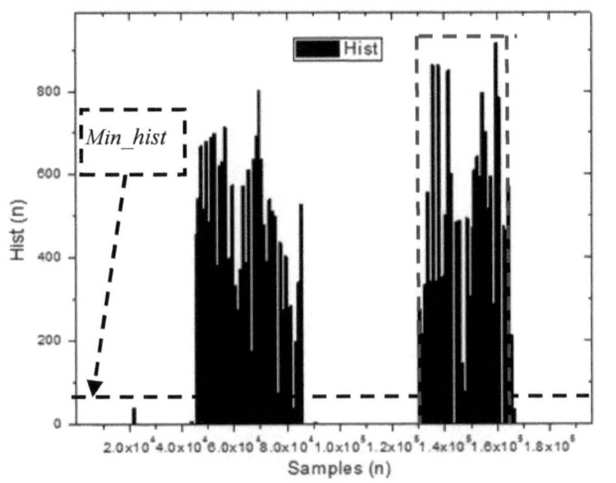

Fig. 10 Histogram of *modul_dif_n*=| *Uin_n* – *Umed*|

Those calculations determine the segment in the original SEMG signal that has the maximum signal–to-noise ratio. With the boundaries calculated from the signal stored, as above, the signal can be segmented like in Figure 11 and the signal between the boundaries, represents the useful signal for further processing.

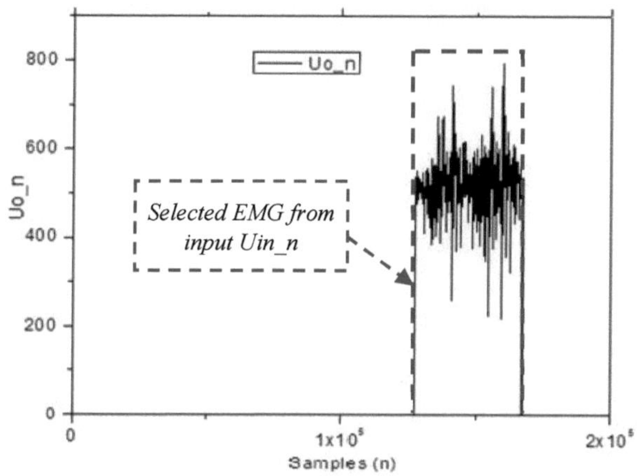

Fig. 11 Output signal Uo_n (selected SEMG from input signal *Uin_n*)

The use of the processor on the Xilinx board is presented in Table 3.

Table 3 Implementation results

Device utilization summary:	system implementation		
Selected Device : 5vlx110tff1136-1,	speed grade -1		
Slice logic utilization	**Used**	**Available**	**Utilization**
Number of Slice Registers:	5448	69120	7%
Number of Slice LUTs:	4370	69120	6%
Number used as Logic:	4160	69120	6%
Number used as Memory:	200	17920	1%
Number of occupied slices	2833	17280	16%
Number of bonded IOBs:	170	640	26%
Number of Block RAM/FIFO:	17	148	11%
Total memory used (kB)	612	5328	11%
Number of DSP48Es:	3	64	4%
Maximum Frequency:	185.587MHz		

IV. Discussion

This signal acquisition equipment for SEMG signals was designed with discrete components, especially in the preamplifier section. The digital-to-analog converter was a built-in microcontroller 10-bit accuracy. A better solution would be to use an integrated front end IC with amplifier and minimum 16 bit A/D converter, like the ADS1298 IC from Texas Instruments [11]. Even in this case, with a lower A/D converter resolution, the original algorithm described in this paper is a useful application.

Unlike other methods used in SEMG signal preprocessing (FFT, filtering, etc) [2], [3], [7], this one possesses the particularity of reducing the samples that must be processed, and does not distorts the signal. It can said that this method (algorithm) does not modify the original signal, but in fact, separates the signal segments with a better signal to noise ratio. This is an important and noteworthy advantage.

In this paper we use a fixed noise threshold determined experimentally, using the rest signal as reference. This approach cannot be useful in daily SEMG measurements. A better way is to determine the noise threshold with an adaptive algorithm, using the measured signals. In this case, the algorithm can be implemented as "real time" measurements. This remains an issue to be addressed by further work.

V. Conclusions

In this paper, we have presented aSEMG signal acquisition system, utilizing an original approach to:

- The block diagram of SEMG amplifier;
- The analog-t-digital processing block of the SEMG signal, using thePIC16F877 8-bit microcontroller. It carries out the ADC conversion (10-bit) and sends the data to the Xilinx board;
- The hardware processing of the SEMG signal with a Xilinx XUPV5 development board
- The histogram method algorithm implemented on the board, as described above.

For the algorithm we used as selection a statistical method based on signal histogram calculation. The optimal SEMG signal is considered to be in area with the highest number of samples that exceed a threshold value that depends on the noise. The threshold constant can be adjusted experimentally.

Experimental results confirm the effectiveness of the method.

Advantages of the method are:

- The EMG signal is not distorted after the DSP
- Reducing the number of sample needed to be processed
- Short time computation

Conflict of Interest

The authors declare that they have no conflict of interest.

References

1. Merletti R, Parker P A (2004) Electromyography: physiology, engineering and non-invasive applications, Wiley, New York
2. Norali A N, Som MH(2009) Surface electromyography signal processing and application: A Review, Proceedings of the International Conference on Man-Machine Systems (ICoMMS) 11–13 October 2009, Batu Ferringhi, Penang, MALAYSIA

3. Hardeep S R, Arora A S, Agarwal R (2010) Interpretations of wrist/ grip operations from SEMG signals at different locations on arm, IEEE Transactions on biomedical circuits and systems, vol.4,no. 2, April 2010, pp 101-111
4. Huang H, Kuiken T A, Lipschutz R D (2007) A strategy for identifying locomotion modes using surface electromyography, IEEE Transaction on biomedical engineering, vol.56, no.1, pp 65-74
5. Shobhitha A J, Jegan R, Melwin A (2013) OWI-535 EDGE Robotic arm control using electromyogram (EMG) signals, IJITEE, vol.2, issue 6, May 2013, pp 282-286
6. Panagiotis K A, Kostas J K (2010)EMG-based control of a robot arm using low-dimensional embeddings, IEEE Transaction on robotics, vol.26, no. 2, April 2010
7. Chowdhury R H, Mamun B I R et al. (2013) Surface electromyography signals processing and classification techniques. Sensors 13:12431-12466,DOI 10.3390/s130912431
8. Takizawa N, Wakita Y, Nagata K, Kazushige M (2009) A development of the equipment control system using SEMG, ICMBE, Proc. 23, 2009, pp 923-926
9. Mou P A, Chang H C, Sio H P et al. (2009) General purpose adaptive acquisition system combining FPGA and FPAA, ICMBE 2008, Proc. 23, 2009,pp 31-34
10. Xilinx XUPV5 documentation at http://www.xilinx.com/univ/xupv5-lx110t.htm
11. Vesa E P (2013) Hardware processing of EMG signals, PhD report no.1, Technical University Cluj-Napoca

Corresponding author:

Author:	Vesa Eugen Petru
Institute:	“Lucian Blaga” University Sibiu
Street:	BulevardulVictoriei ,10
City:	Sibiu
Country:	Romania
Email:	eugen.vesa@ulbsibiu.ro

Preliminary EEG Based Analysis of Few Acupoints Used in the Chronic Low Back Pain Treatment

D.D. Lucache[1], B. Lucache[2], D. Irimia[1] and M. Poboroniuc[1]

[1] Faculty of Electrical Engineering, "Gheorghe Asachi" Technical University, Iasi, Romania
[2] Faculty of Medicine, "Grigore T.Popa" University of Medicine and Pharmacy, Iasi, Romania

Abstract— **In order to uncover the acupuncture mechanism in the pain removal, the paper's aim is to reveal specific changes in the EEG brain response to the acupuncture stimulation in three points (ST36, UB25 and DU3) specific to the chronic low back pain (CLBP) treatment.**

Seven young, right handed and acupuncture naïve subjects have been tested with a 64-ch EEG equipment. The data have been off line processed and statistically analyzed.

The comparison between the results for different testing periods was statistically significant (p<0.05) and led to the conclusion that acupuncture stimulation in the selected acupoints generates an increased power of all spectral bands, especially for ST36 and DU3.

This preliminary study has to be extended on a wider subjects population, allowing comparing results with the ones get from a sham-acupuncture control group.

Keywords— **Acupuncture, Chronic low back pain, EEG, Spectral analysis.**

I. Introduction

The chronic low back pain (CLBP) is a very frequent rheumatic disease that represents a major health problem with high social impact, being not only a source of pain but also of important costs and economics losses [1]. In the industrialized countries, back pain affects between 15% and 30% of the population and generates high costs due to the ambulatory care visits [2].

In the last decades, complementary and alternative medicine (CAM) became an accepted treatment alternative and for the rheumatic diseases acupuncture is considered one of the most efficient. The health care policy makers from many countries have included acupuncture between the recommended procedures for the treatment of incipient chronic rheumatic diseases [3].

Despite the multitude of studies and practical evidences, the effectiveness of the CAM therapies give rise often to disputes and polemics. The first efforts to explain acupuncture in terms of Western medicine have been oriented towards the biologic, electric and tissular proprieties of the acupuncture points (acupoints) or the energy or electricity propagation trough the acupuncture meridians.

Literature suggests that acupuncture influences a diverse set of bodily organs and functions, including brain processing and autonomic nervous system activity [4]. However, the acupuncture mechanism of action is not completely understood and nowadays modern exploration and imagistic techniques are used to reveal the relation between acupuncture stimulation and brain activity.

Multi-channels electroencephalogram (EEG) represents a powerful tool for investigating cortical responses to various stimuli and has an advantage over imaging modalities in that it can provide temporal information on the activity in addition to its location [5].

Based on a literature review, the standard widely accepted acupoints for CLBP mainly belong to three meridians (stomach ST, urinary bladder UB and governor vessel DU) and are: in the lumbar region UB25 and DU3, on lower extremity ST44 and on upper extremity LI4 and TF5 (meridians liver LI and three focus TF). Also, common used points are: ST36 (analgesic point), UB17, UB40, UB62, DU20 and auricular points: Shenmen and Lombar spine.

The aim of this paper is to assess the pain removal potential of three from the mentioned points: two local points UB25 and DU3, as well the wide used analgesic point ST36. The present study was conducted, therefore, to detect the temporal behavior of acupoint stimuli-produced cortical activities using EEG.

II. Materials and methods

A. Participants

In this preliminary study, the subjects were 7 young male healthy university volunteers, Caucasian adult having the age between 21 and 26 years, selected right-handed and acupuncture naive, who have been informed on the purposes of the study, the experimental protocol and the potential risks involved, consigning their written informed consent. The study was approved by the Ethics Committee of the "Gr.T.Popa" University of Medicine and Pharmacy of Iasi.

B. Experimental Design

The subjects were comfortably seated in a lit, quiet and ventilated room. The experiments began after complete disappearance of the willies. For an interval of minimum 6 minutes, control data have been preliminarily recorded. When the experiment started, three needles were inserted in the mentioned acupoints. Acupuncture needling was

S. Vlad and R.V. Ciupa (eds.), *International Conference on Advancements of Medicine and Health Care through Technology*, IFMBE Proceedings 44,
DOI: 10.1007/978-3-319-07653-9_50,

performed by a single experienced acupuncturist under aseptic conditions and performing identical stimulating manipulations. The data were continuously recorded following the paradigm depicted in Fig.1.

The present study involved verum manual acupuncture in three specific acupoint for CLBP: ST36, UB25 and DU3. Standard acupuncture stainless steel needles (0,2mm x 40mm, Seirin Co.Ltd) were inserted (to a depth of 20mm) into the muscle. At certain moments, the three acupoints of each subject were stimulated, in a random order. The stimulation consisted in the bidirectional needle twirling, with amplitudes near to 180°, at a rate of one cycle per second.

The blood pressure (BP) and heart rate (HR) have been monitored before and after the experiment using the digital device Microlife BP A80. At the end, all the subject were questioned about the sensations that they had felt and asked to assess their pain sensation for the three stimulation periods by means of the visual analogical scale (VAS) that ranges from 0 (no pain) to 10 (worst possible pain).

C. EEG Recording and Offline Processing

EEG recordings were performed during an eyes open passive condition. The subjects were told to relax, to think of nothing and to fix calmly a point across the room. They were informed that acupuncture was to be performed at different sites, but not the order in which the acupoints would be stimulated.

A compact active electrode system, gSCARABEO, developed by g.tech medical engineering GmbH (Austria) for high-density EEG and multi-purpose application, has been used. This contains 64 active electrodes which were mounted on the subject's scalps according to the 10-20 International System. The 64-ch montage is depicted in Fig. 2.

All the EEG channels were recorded in an averaged reference and online bandpass - filtered between 0.5 to 100 Hz. The 50Hz perturbation has been removed by a Notch filter.

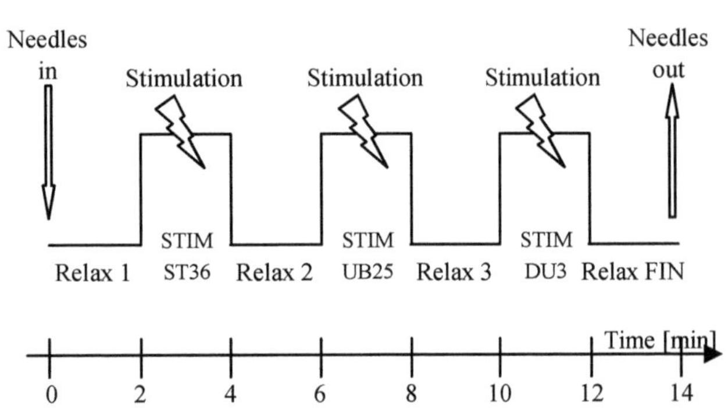

Fig. 1 The experimental paradigm. The order of the 2-minutes stimulated points was pseudo-randomized across patients and each experiments starts with a 6 minutes rest run.

The data have been processed with gBSanalyze software provided by g.tech medical engineering GmbH. In the offline preprocessing phase, the EEG channels were re-referenced through the LAR (Local Average Reference) technique, calculated according to the following equation (1), where i is the channel number and S_i the subset of surrounding electrodes for channel i, meaning that the average of the surrounding electrodes is subtracted it from the active electrode value. The electrodes are weighted according to the distance from the active electrode through the factor $g_{i,j}$.

$$V_{LARi} = V_i - \sum_{j \in S_i} g_{i,j} V_j \quad (1)$$

Afterwards the data were off-line filtered between 0.5 to 70 Hz (bandpass 5th-order Butterwoth filter) and were subjected to epoching (2 s each). After a linear-detrend the preprocessing phase ended with the artifact rejection that consisted in exclusion of the epochs with large amplitude (over ±80 μV) and artifacts caused by eye-blinking.

Finally, each set of EEG data (2-s epoch) was subjected to Fast-Fourier Transform (FFT) analysis to obtain the absolute EEG band power (μV^2) at each electrode in the following 7 bands: Delta (0.5–3.5 Hz), theta (4–7 Hz), Alpha-1 (7.5–10.5 Hz), Alpha-2 (11–14 Hz), Beta-1 (14.5–23.5 Hz), Beta-2 (24–35 Hz) and Gamma (35–45 Hz), defined according to the conventional IFCN guideline [6].

III. Results

All the resulted data have been statistically analyzed using Excel. Statistical comparisons were performed by

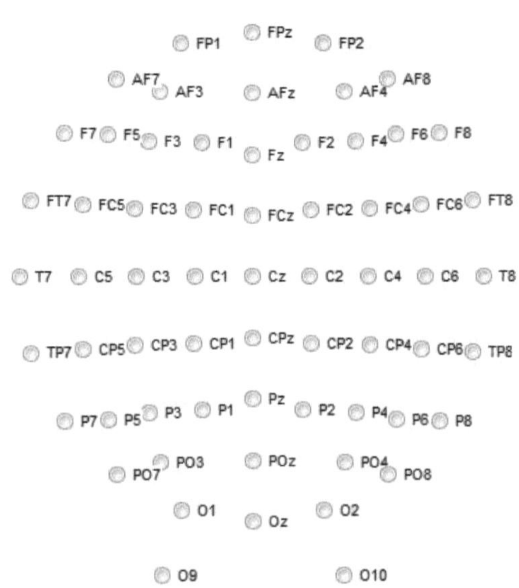

Fig. 2 Map of the 64-ch EEG montage

ANOVA for repeated measures (seven subjects), where the two parameters were the electrodes (columns) and testing period (samples). The ANOVA analysis with $\alpha=0.05$ was performed for every of the considered spectral-band and the results are synthetically given in Table 1. These indicate in all the bands the significant differences related to the testing period and to the electrode ($p<0.05$), while no significant interaction between parameters testing period and electrode can be found ($p>0.05$). A separate ANOVA analysis applied only to the three stimulation periods revealed no statistically significant differences ($p>0.05$) among them. We conclude that the statistically significant differences signaled in Table 1 refer to differences between the stimulation periods and relaxing periods, meaning that EEG signals are changed by acupuncture stimulation.

The mean power of each electrode and broad band was averaged for the three stimulation periods in order to compare the recorded "intensity of stimulation" with the subjective intensity of pain that was estimated by the subjects using the VAS. In order to have a visual comparison, the results have been normalized and represented in Fig. 3. The behavior of the two parameters is quite similar, the main difference being related to DU3 stimulation that appears in the subjective assessment as the main pain source while the most intense recorded stimulation is of ST36.

The mean power in the Delta and Theta broad bands are represented in Fig.4. The similar charts for the rest of the broad-bands look very similar with the one of Theta and

Table 1 Results of 2-way ANOVA analysis of spectral bands

	Source of Variation	SS	DF	MS	F	p-value	F crit
δ	Sample	4349	6	725	2.4	0.030	2.116
	Columns	79845	18	4436	14.4	0.000	1.623
	Interaction	16465	108	152	0.5	1.000	1.265
θ	Sample	73032	6	12172	16.6	0.000	2.116
	Columns	216322	18	12018	16.4	0.000	1.623
	Interaction	31171	108	289	0.4	1.000	1.265
α1	Sample	75600	6	12600	17.3	0.000	2.116
	Columns	223802	18	12433	17.0	0.000	1.623
	Interaction	31468	108	291	0.4	1.000	1.265
α2	Sample	75802	6	12634	17.4	0.000	2.116
	Columns	226690	18	12594	17.4	0.000	1.623
	Interaction	31494	108	292	0.4	1.000	1.265
β1	Sample	74657	6	12443	18.5	0.000	2.116
	Columns	197882	18	10993	16.4	0.000	1.623
	Interaction	30290	108	280	0.4	1.000	1.265
β2	Sample	75321	6	12554	19.3	0.000	2.116
	Columns	175436	18	9746	15.0	0.000	1.623
	Interaction	29692	108	275	0.4	1.000	1.265
γ	Sample	73106	6	12184	18.7	0.000	2.116
	Columns	183268	18	10182	15.7	0.000	1.623
	Interaction	27672	108	256	0.4	1.000	1.265

have not been represented due to the limited length of the paper. A correlation test taking the broad band as parameter shows a very high correlation (the correlation coefficient $r > 0.9$) among the all broad-bands except Delta, for that the correlation is only good for a coefficient of about 0.5. One notes in both pictures from Fig.4 that, for all the electrodes, the highest bars belong to the stimulation periods.

The data related to BP and HR show a low decreasing in both parameters (in average with 7.5% for the systolic BP, 11.2% for the diastolic BP, and 8.1% for the HR) but it can be explained through the subjects' emotional state and initial anxiety attenuation during the experiment.

IV. Discussion

This preliminary study is particular due to the selected acupoints (specific for the treatment of CLBP) and the experimental paradigm. The results are similar with the findings reported by other studies regarding no interaction effect between acupuncture points when a group of points were tested [7] and differ from the other studies conclusions because the main effects of electrodes and of testing period are significant for all the broad-bands not only for few of them [8].

The ST36 and secondly DU3 stimulation showed the most important brain responses, while UB25 stimulation led to moderate to low response. One explanation can be related to the acupuncture-specific subjective De-qi sensation that is considered essential to induce a therapeutic effect [9]. The less pain intensity assessed by VAS for UB25 could be explained with the lack of the De-qi sensation following the

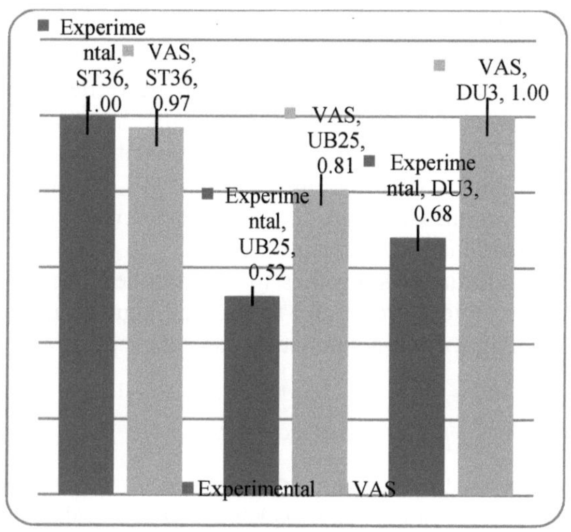

Fig. 3 Comparison between the recorded "stimulation intensity" and the pain intensity assessed using VAS in the three acupoints ST36, UB25 and DU3

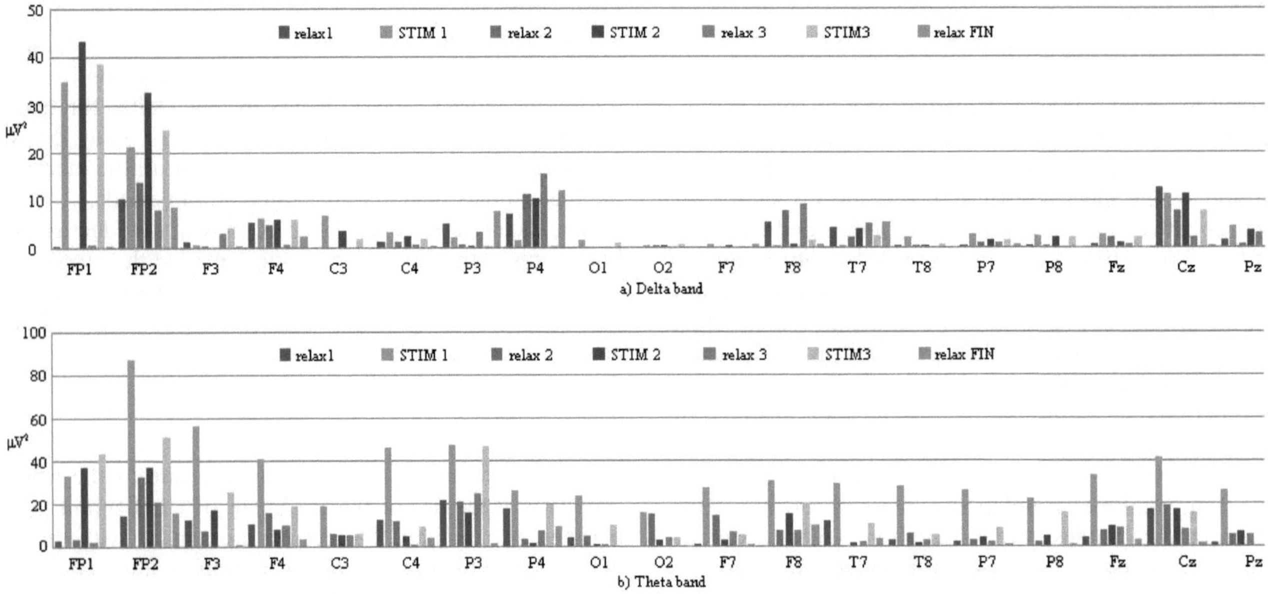

Fig. 4 Changes in the Delta and Theta band power of EEGs during the seven periods of the experimental paradigm depicted in Fig.1

UB25 stimulation and so a low EEG response to this one.

The main study limitation consists in the lack of a control group, following the same experimental paradigm but replacing the real acupuncture with sham acupuncture stimulation (usually in non acupuncture points). In further research we intend to apply different methods for the EEG signals analysis (STFT or Wavelet).

V. Conclusions

The relation between acupuncture stimulation of three specific acupoints for the CLBP treatment and EEG changes has been investigated. The results suggest the increased brain response for two of the tested acupoints, and a moderate low response for the third. The conclusions done by statistical analysis are partially similar with the findings of other studies but which are the broad-bands with significant activity need further research.

This preliminary study has to be extended over a more consistent subject group and to provide significant validation by using a sham-acupuncture control group.

References

1. Chenot JF, Becker A, Leonhardt C, Keller S, et al. (2007) Use of complementary alternative medicine for low back pain consulting in general practice: a cohort study. BMC Complementary and Alternative Medicine; 7(42)
2. Kanodia A (2010) Perceived Benefit of Complementary and Alternative Medicine (CAM) for Back Pain: A National Survey, J. Am. Board Fam. Med.; 23:354 –362
3. Chou R, Huffman LH (2007) Nonpharmacologic therapies for acute and chronic low back pain: a review of the evidence for an American Pain Society/American College of Physicians clinical practice guideline. Ann Intern Med.; 147(7):492-504
4. Dhond RP et al. (2008) Acupuncture modulates resting state connectivity in default and sensorimotor brain networks. Pain 136(3):407-18. doi: 10.1016/j.pain.2008.01.011
5. Zeng Y et al. (2006) Electroacupuncture modulates cortical activities evoked by noxious somatosensory stimulations in human. Brain Res. 1097(1):90-100
6. Chen ACN et al. (2008) EEG default mode network in the human brain: Spectral regional field powers. NeuroImage 41(2): 561-74
7. Huang W et al. (2012) Characterizing acupuncture stimuli using brain imaging with fMRI- a systematic review and meta-analysis of the literature. PLoS ONE 7(4):e32960. DOI: 10.1371/journal.pone.0032960
8. Sakai S et al. (2007) Specific acupuncture sensation correlates with EEGs and autonomic changes in human subjects. Autonomic Neuroscience: Basic and Clinical 133(2): 158–169
9. Zhu S-P et al. (2013) Acupuncture De-qi: from characterization to underlying mechanism. Evid Based Complement Alternat Med. 2013;2013:518784.

Author: Lucache Beatrice
Institute: "Grigore T.Popa" University of Medicine and Pharmacy
Street: 16 Universitatii
City: Iasi
Country: Romania
Email: beatrice.lucache@gmail.com

Optical Coherence Tomography in the Diagnosis, Monitoring and Treatment of Macular Disorders

S.D. Nicoară

"Iuliu Haţieganu" University of Medicine and Pharmacy/Ophthalmology, Faculty of Medicine, Cluj-Napoca, Romania

Abstract— **Optical coherence tomography (OCT) has revolutionized the way we look at the retina, by being able to offer cross-sectional images of the retinal layers, comparable to the histological specimens, in a non-invasive manner. OCT technology is based on the principle of low coherence interferometry. The new spectral domain OCT devices have axial resolution of 2 µm - 5 µm, scanning speed of 27 000 - 100 000 scans per second, perform large, dense raster scans and display three-dimensional data of the target tissue. The practical impact of these capabilities is translated by: better image quality, less artifacts associated with eye motion and the obtaining of detailed surfaces of the retinal layers over large areas resulting in segmentation maps. The most important quantitative parameter measured by OCT, that cannot be precisely evaluated by any other method, is the macular thickness. With the help of this information, surface maps of the internal limiting membrane and retinal pigment epithelium and retinal thickness maps are generated. Registering these maps over time is very useful in identifying and monitoring the dynamics of disease progression and response to therapy. The macular diseases that benefited the most from the development of the OCT technology are: age-related macular degeneration, diabetic macular edema, vitreo-macular interface disorders (vitreo-macular traction, epiretinal membranes, macular hole). The purpose of this paper is to present the principle of OCT technology and its impact on the diagnosis, monitoring and treatment of the macular disorders. Our personal cases are presented in order to illustrate the impact of OCT in the clinical practice.**

Keywords— **optical coherence tomography, age related macular degeneration, diabetic macular edema, macular hole, epiretinal membrane**

I. Introduction

Optical coherence tomography (OCT) has revolutionized patient care by being able to image detailed ocular structures in a simple, fast, precise and noninvasive way. The diagnosis, monitoring and treatment of macular diseases became unthinkable in the absence of OCT examination, during the past two decades [1]. OCT also brought a significant contribution in elucidating the pathogenesis of the macular conditions, by visualizing the retinal layers like a true live biopsy [2, 3]. Current technical considerations and future directions in the development of OCT technology are presented and sustained by our case studies.

II. Technical considerations on OCT

A. Principle

OCT technology is based on the principle of low coherence interferometry where a low coherence light is directed towards the target tissue. The scattered back-reflected light is combined with a reference beam which was split off from the original light beam. An axial A-scan results from the interference patterns, representing the scattering properties of the tissue along the beam path. Many A-scans are generated by moving the light beam linearly, from different incidences, along the tissue. Thus, a cross-sectional two-dimensional image of the target tissue is reconstructed, known as a B-scan. The wavelength of the light source is within the infrared range (840 nm) [1, 2, 3].

B. Qualitative Parameters

The axial resolution depends on the bandwidth of the light source and it varies between 2 µm - 5 µm in the latest commercially available OCT instruments [2, 3]. The lateral resolution is limited by the diffraction caused by the pupil and is about 20 µm. The acquisition time depends on the patient's ability to avoid eye movements and in the typical patients is less than 2 seconds. The crucial parameter that determines the amount of data available for a single OCT dataset is the scanning speed (number of A-scans per second) [1, 2, 3]. The first generation OCT instruments were time-domain (TD-OCT). With TD-OCT, an A-scan was created by moving a mirror to modify the optical path of the reference beam in order to match different axial depths in the target tissue. In this setup, the scanning speed is limited to a few thousand A-scans per second. A newer technique, known as spectral domain OCT (SD-OCT), Fourier domain OCT (FD-OCT), or high definition OCT (HD-OCT) uses an array of detectors instead of multiple reference beams from a moving mirror. This allows to obtain scanning rates of approximately 27 000 - 100 000 scans per second, about 200 times higher than with TD-OCT [1, 2, 3]. With TD-OCT instruments, the scanning pattern consists in six radial, concentric, 6-mm-long B scans centered on the fovea. The recent high speed SD-OCT systems allowed the development of new imaging strategies, based on three-dimensional acquiring of data and B-scan

S. Vlad and R.V. Ciupa (eds.), *International Conference on Advancements of Medicine and Health Care through Technology*, IFMBE Proceedings 44,
DOI: 10.1007/978-3-319-07653-9_51, © Springer International Publishing Switzerland 2014

averaging [1, 3]. The three-dimensional data are obtained by using a two-dimensional dense raster array over a large retinal region. In addition, the OCT datasets allow to obtain frontal images of the retina that permit the spatial colocalization of retinal features between the frontal and the cross-sectional images. A very powerful solution to implement the frontal registration and B-scan averaging is the use of a built-in-laser eye tracking system [1].

C. Quantitative Parameters

The quantitative parameter with the highest clinical usefulness derived from the OCT examinations is the retinal thickness, obtained by segmenting the internal limiting membrane (ILM) and a boundary represented by the retinal pigment epithelium (RPE). With the help of this information, surface maps of the ILM and RPE and retinal thickness maps are generated. Registering these maps over time is very useful in identifying and monitoring the dynamics of disease progression and response to therapy [1, 2, 3]. The definition of the outer retinal boundary differs from one OCT instrument to another and therefore, differences between measurements occur. Foveal macular thickness varies between 180 - 230 μm [1].

Other quantitative parameters revealed by OCT are: thickness of the ganglion cell layer, of the photoreceptors' outer segments, dimension of an area of geographic atrophy, drusen area and volume [1].

III. SD-OCT IN MACULAR DISORDERS

In order to illustrate the clinical impact of OCT, we use the most relevant cases in our own practice. This study was carried out in accordance with the standards of the Ethical Committee of "Iuliu Hațieganu" University of Medicine and Pharmacy and with the Helsinki Declaration of 1975, as revised in 2000 and 2008.

A. Normal Macular Anatomy

The OCT image has been referred to as a live biopsy, because it closely approximates the macular histology [3]. By convention, the tissues with the highest reflectivity are represented in red, the layers with medium reflectivity, in green and the low reflective structures, in blue (Fig. 1). The layers with the highest reflectivity are the RPE (horizontal arrow) and the ILM. The retinal vessels can sometimes be seen on OCT images as round hyperreflective structures located in the inner retina, with a vertical shadow extending in the deeper layers (vertical arrow).

SD-OCT uses a wavelength of 840 nm that results in the light scattering at the level of the RPE and a lower signal from the deep choroidal tissue. Despite this, it is possible to image the choroid and extract quantitative data with the help of high-penetration OCT that uses a light source with a wavelength of 1050 nm [1, 4].

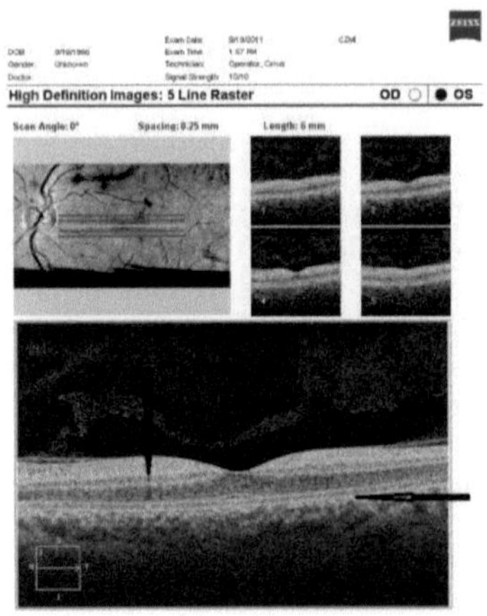

Fig. 1 Normal OCT image

B. Vitreo-Macular Interface Disorders

The vitreo-macular interface disorders include: vitreomacular traction (VMT), epiretinal membrane (ERM) and macular hole (MH). VMT results from persistent vitreomacular adhesions after a partial posterior vitreous detachment (PVD). These adhesions transmit tractional forces to the retina, with the following effects on the macula: deformation, constitution of foveal cavities, cystoid macular edema (CME), limited macular detachment, MH. In some cases, the VMT resolves spontaneously, but in most instances, it persists and requires vitrectomy. OCT is very useful in assisting the decision-making process, by identifying subtle changes at the level of the vitreo-macular interface [1, 3] . On OCT, an ERM appears as a highly reflective band on the inner surface of the retina (Fig. 2).

OCT helps in differentiating a true macular hole from a pseudohole which is a defect in a sheet of an ERM [1, 5]. Generally, MHs are accompanied by the accumulation of a variable amount of fluid as cysts within the retina and under the retina, at the edge of the hole [1, 5] (Fig. 3).

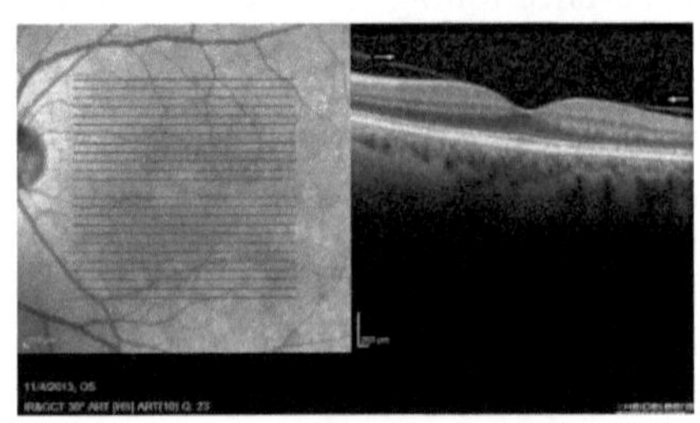

Fig. 2 Epiretinal membrane

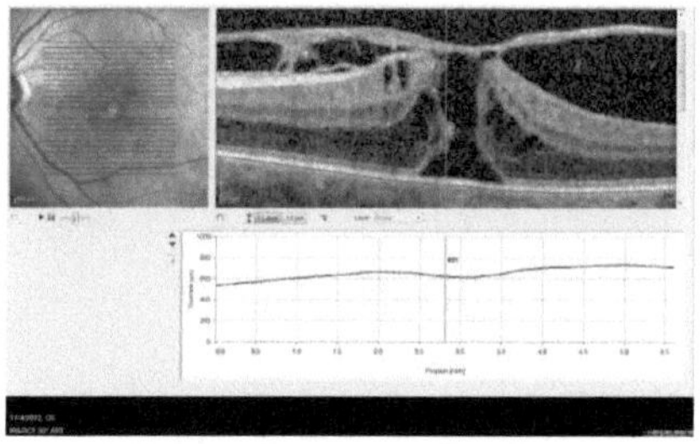

Fig. 3 MH with fluid within and under the retina

The standard treatment of MHs is vitrectomy, with success rates of 85 - 100% [5]. OCT is used to reveal the evolution of the MH after surgery: restoration of the normal foveal contour (Fig. 4), or the persistence of retinal abnormalities.

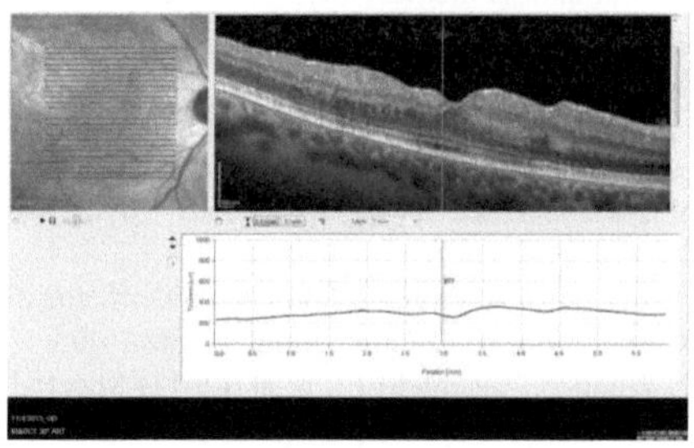

Fig. 4 Closed MH after vitrectomy with normal foveal contour

C. Age-related Macular Degeneration (AMD)

AMD is the most common cause of visual loss in the elderly worldwide [6]. It is classified in two forms: non-neovascular (dry) and neovascular (wet or exudative).

The retinal modifications in *non-neovascular AMD* are early (drusen and pigmentary changes) and late (geografic atrophy). Drusen are seen on OCT as RPE elevations with variable reflectivity depending on the composition of the underlying material (Fig. 5).

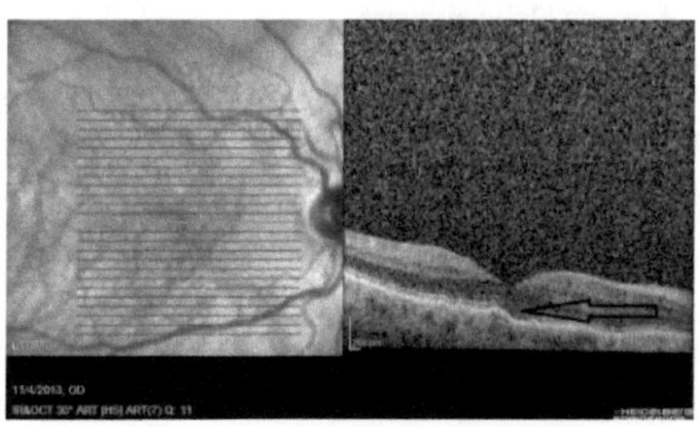

Fig. 5 Drusen

A novel algorithm is able to measure the drusen area and volume [2, 3, 8]. The algorithm compares the patient's map with a normal RPE map and monitors the natural history of AMD [8]. GA is a progressive condition that leads to the loss of vision over many years. The enhanced depth imaging (EDI) of SD-OCT has made it possible to visualize the structure of the choroid in greater detail [4, 9].

Autofluorescence (Fig. 7) is an important feature that predicts the extension risk of a GA lesion [10].

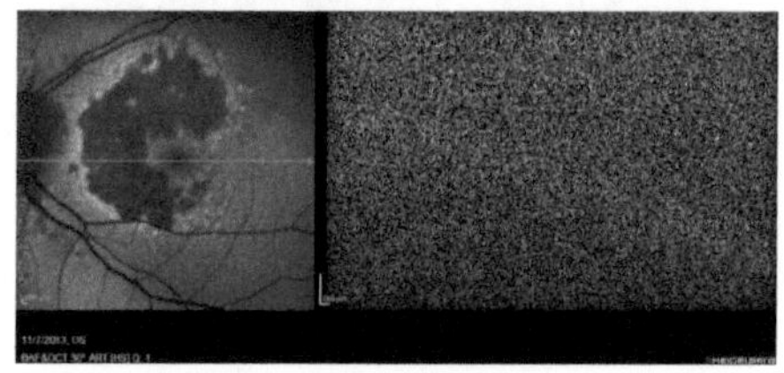

Fig. 6 Autofluorescence

Neovascular AMD is characterized by the growth of abnormal vessels in the macular region that can arise either from the choroidal circulation, or from the retinal vessels. The presence of fluid within or under the retina is the consequence of leakage from the new vessels. The fluid may accumulate between the RPE and the neurosensory retina appearing on the OCT images as homogenous and hyporeflective, if it is serous (Fig. 7), or separated by fibrinous membranes, when protein exudation is present [1].

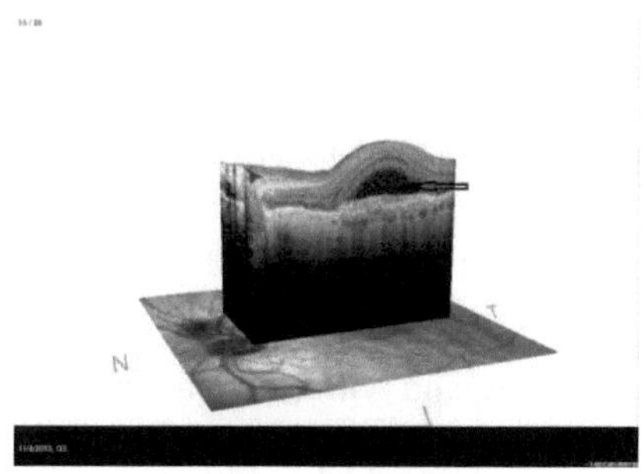

Fig. 7 Neovascular AMD

Currently, OCT-guided strategies are used for the anti-VEGF (Vascular Endothelial Growth Factor) treatment of neovascular AMD. The effect of anti-VEGF therapy is assessed qualitatively, by the evaluation of the amount of macular fluid on the B-scans, and quantitatively, by examining the changes in the retinal thickness maps [1, 2, 3, 6].

D. Diabetic Macular Edema (DME)

The role of OCT in DME is very important for diagnosing and monitoring the response to various therapies [2, 3, 11]. However, OCT cannot provide information on overall retinopathy severity, for which color photographs remain the goldstandard [11]. Serous retinal detachment appears on OCT as a focal elevation of the neurosensory retina overlying a hyporeflective, dome-shaped space (Fig. 8). Small intraretinal hyperreflective dots are identified, corresponding to retinal exudates (Fig. 9).

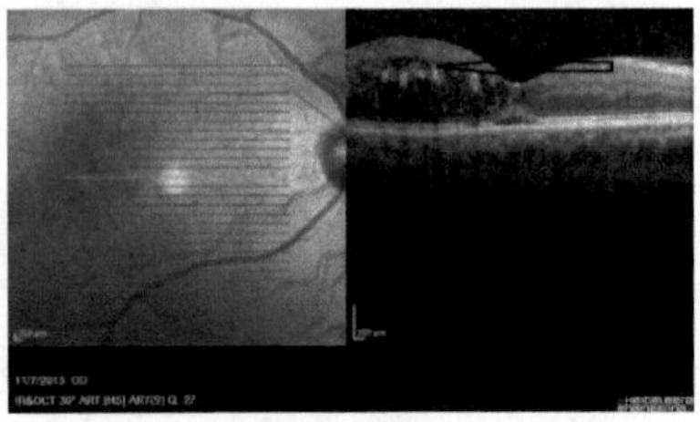

Fig. 8 Diabetic macular edema

Quantitative retinal thickness maps (Fig. 9) are used to direct laser therapy and are better than biomicroscopy alone. In the era of pharmacotherapy, OCT is a valuable tool in monitoring the response of DME to intravitreal injections [2, 3, 11].

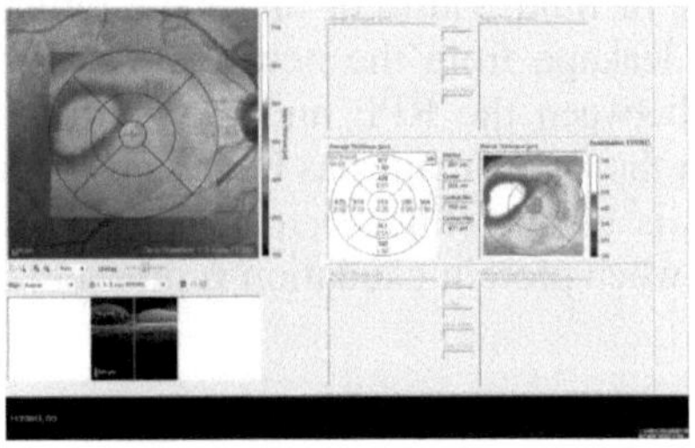

Fig. 9 Retinal thickness map in a patient with DME

IV. Conclusion

Currently, OCT is the most useful tool to investigate the retina. AMD, DME and vitreo-retinal interface disorders benefited the most from the progress in OCT technology. OCT is the only method which is able to measure precisely the macular thickness and therefore it is used to monitor the progression and the response to treatment of the above-mentioned diseases. OCT is very useful in assisting the decision-making process, by identifying subtle changes at the level of the vitreo-macular interface. A novel algorithm is able to measure the drusen area and volume and thus monitor the natural evolution of AMD. The capability to show autofluorescence is an important feature that predicts the extension risk of a GA lesion. The OCT technical features hold the promise for an unprecedented capability to describe and monitor the changes in retinal geometry.

Conflict of Interest

The authors declare that they have no conflict of interest.

References

1. Filho CA, Yehoshua Z, Gregori G, Puliafito CA, Rosenfeld PJ (2013) Optical Coherence Tomography in Retina. Elsevier, Amsterdam
2. Talu SD (2013) Optical Coherence Tomography in the Diagnosis and Monitoring of Retinal Diseases. ISRN Biomedical Imaging 1: 1-13 DOI 10.1155/2013/910641
3. Talu SD (2013) New Insights into the Optical Coherence Tomography –Assessement and Follow-Up of Age-Related Macular Degeneration in Age-Related Macular Degeneration - Etiology, Diagnosis and Management. In Tech, Rijeka
4. Ikuno Y, Maruko I, Yasuno Y, et al. (2011) Reproducibility of retinal and choroidal thickness measurements in enhanced depth imaging and high-penetration optical coherence tomography. Invest Ophthalmol Vis Sci 52:5536–540.
5. Bottoni F, De Angelis S, Luccarelli S, et al. (2011) The dynamic healing process of idiopathic macular holes after surgical repair: a spectral-domain optical coherence tomography study. Invest Ophthalmol Vis Sci 52:4439–4446.
6. Klein R, Peto T, Bird A, et al. (2004) The epidemiology of age-related macular degeneration. Am J Ophthalmol 137:486–495.
7. Gregori G, Wang F, Rosenfeld PJ, et al. (2011) Spectral domain optical coherence tomography imaging of drusen in nonexudative age-related macular degeneration. Ophthalmology 118:1373–1379.
8. Lee SY, Stetson PF, Ruiz-Garcia H, et al. (2012) Automated characterization of pigment epithelial detachment using optical coherence tomography. Invest Ophthalmol Vis Sci 53:164–170.
9. Yehoshua Z, Rosenfeld PJ, Gregori G, et al. (2011) Progression of geographic atrophy in age-related macular degeneration imaged with spectral domain optical coherence tomography. Ophthalmology 118:679–686.
10. Bearelly S, Chau FY, Koreishi A, et al. (2009) Spectral domain optical coherence tomography imaging of geographic atrophy margins. Ophthalmology 116:1762–1769.
11. Al-latayfeh MM, Sun JK, Aiello LP. (2010) Ocular coherence tomography and diabetic eye disease. Semin Ophthalmol 25:192–197.

Author: Simona Delia Nicoară
Institute: "Iuliu Haţieganu" University of Medicine and Pharmacy
Street: V. Babeş City: Cluj-Napoca Country: Romania Email: simonanicoara1@gmail.com

Ultrasound Image Enhancement for Visualization Using Spatially Variant Morphological Filters

I. Jivet and M. Tomoroga

University 'Politehnica' Timisoara, Electronics and Telecommunications Faculty, Timisoara, Romania

Abstract— **The paper presents an experimental method of ultrasound image filtering using newly developed mathematical morphology filters with spatially variant parameter - Amoeba filter. The speckle form of B-mode ultrasound is modeled in its dependence on depth and radial angle in the image. The adaptive filter parameter is varied according to local speckle model as observed on typical sensor images. Median adaptive filtering is performed in a sequence after the proposed amoeba filter noise form adjustment in image areas. The results are compared with direct fixed width median filter. Further extensions of the method are discussed based on results so far obtained.**

Keywords— **Ultrasound imaging, speckle filtering, morphological filters, ameba filters**

I. INTRODUCTION

The visualization of anatomical structures in medical practice relies very much on the experience of the physician. One characteristic of the ultrasound image is the scatter texture of the image referred to as speckle noise. Speckle noise reduces the image contrast, obscures and blurs anatomical details, decreasing the image quality.

One source of the speckle non-uniformity is the radial and angular depth ultrasound beam forming difference in an image. Modern ultrasound equipment has made significant progress in beam tracking techniques in hardware and software to homogenize the image.

Speckle form factor differences in different areas of the image remains a reality that impedes visualization of anatomical structures [7]. The speckle form was used by authors [5], to identify successive image positions.

Image enhancements while preserving organ anatomical margins, has been intensively studied for many years and is known to be a difficult problem [4], [6].

The simplest method in use is an edge-preserving filter, like median filter of appropriate width. The effectiveness of such an approach is hindered by the varying form of the speckle at different locations in the ultrasound image.

Recently a new class of morphological spatially variant filters has been proposed [1,2]. The domain was and still is under intense development in recent years, both on theoretic aspects as well as practical implementation [2].

The present paper explores the effectiveness of the spatially variant filters in the reduction of the speckle interference in interpretation of the ultrasound images, a problem still in search for a better solution [7].

II. BACKGROUND OF ULTRASOUND IMAGE FILTERING AND STATE OF THE ART IN MEDIAN FILTERING

A. Speckle Noise Problem in Ultrasound Imaging

According to recent literature median filtering is among the best methods to remove speckles form the image before processing or visualization. The property that makes median filter attractive for reducing speckle effect is the edge preserving property.

During the study it was found that the use of direct median filtering on ultrasound images, the most valued property of the median filter, edge preservation, is not really holding true.

At the same time the local speckle averaging for distinct and easy observation of different tissue layers leaves room for improvement.

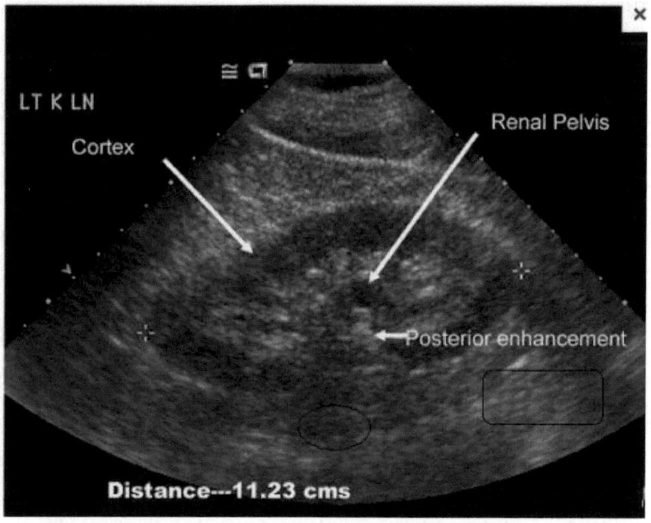

Fig. 1 Sample Ultrasound Image with selected areas of different speckle forms

IFMBE Proceedings 44,
DOI: 10.1007/978-3-319-07653-9_52, © Springer International Publishing Switzerland 2014

A reduced window size for median filter gives better results but is not appropriate for the distal radial and large axial deviations due to larger spread of the speckle noise in this areas of the image.

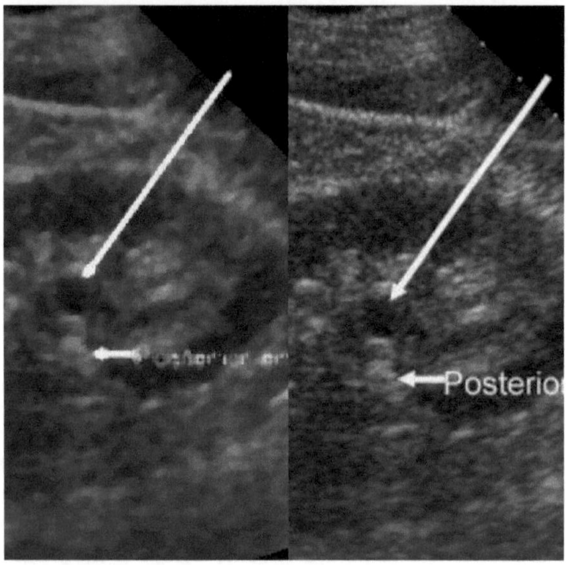

Fig. 2 Direct median filter used uniformly across the sample image

In the following the paper presents a novel ultrasound image speckle filtering scheme. In a first step a spatially variant morphological parameter is determined for specific speckle areas in a image. In a second step a median filter adjusted according to the first step parameter is used to filter out speckle noise from the image.

B. The Speckle Form Dependence on Location in Image

According to literature, the complexity of beam forming and its reflection on tissue areas in modern array ultrasound is well understood [9]. From the raw signals received, using hardware and software processing, the image is obtained and optimized for speckle problem containment.

The speckle effect is inherently linked to the physics and technology and total elimination from ultrasound images is a distant goal. For reducing the influence of speckle in the image visualization process, a variable axis elliptic model was found to be a cover for the area and form of speckle in different areas of a B-mode ultrasoud image.

The vertical axis of the ellipse was found to be relative constant with depth and angle of departure from image symmetry axis. The horizontal axis was found to be very angle dependent with a variation of one in two from image symmetry axis to maximal radial extension of the exploring beam.

Based with the speckle form model observed the adaptive amoeba filter parameters have been scaled. Each location received a set of amoeba parameter weights dependent on position in radial and angular direction.

The construction of the adaptive model of the ameoba filter has been thus founded on solid experimental basis from specific clinical cas images.

The novel ultrasound image smoothing method proposed was augmented with a second stage meant to preserve anatomical reflectivity density. An intuitive different grid scales processing filter was designed to optimize local smoothing to larger area variations covering anatomical details.

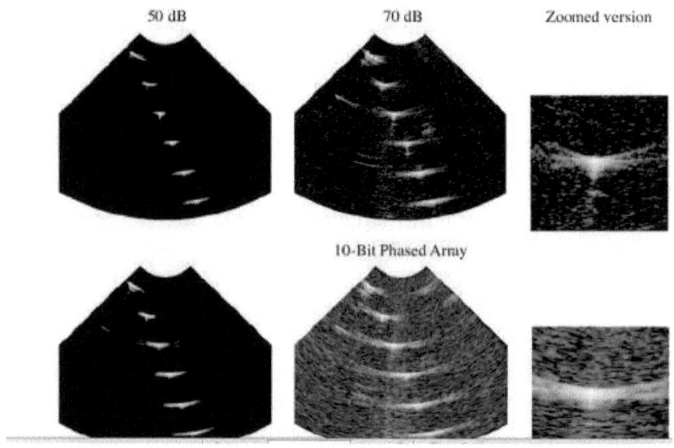

Fig. 3 Speckle form based on ultrasound technology dependence [9]

The coordination of the two levels of adaptive filtering was found to be essential in the application phase of the use of the novel filter to ultrasound images.

III. Morpphological Ameoba Filtering Experiments

In the present experiments with the proposed amoeba filter used a direct euclidean amoeba distance formula. Recent research shows a very large horizon, in the yet distant resolution for a method choose and optimize the distance formula of ameoba filters [11,12].

For the target application of kidney ultrasound images, the filtering of the variable form speckle noise the amoeba distance computations used polar coordinates. This choice followed the speckle distribution model as determined for B-mode ultrasoud images.

The amoeba distance formula used was on a 8-neighbour form – vertical for depth and horizontal for image off symmetry angle. Exploration order can not be always parallel to the orientation axis of the speckle model in the area, but it was found that this detail does alter the result. The correct shape is finally reached up to or less then maximal model area of the local ameoba form.

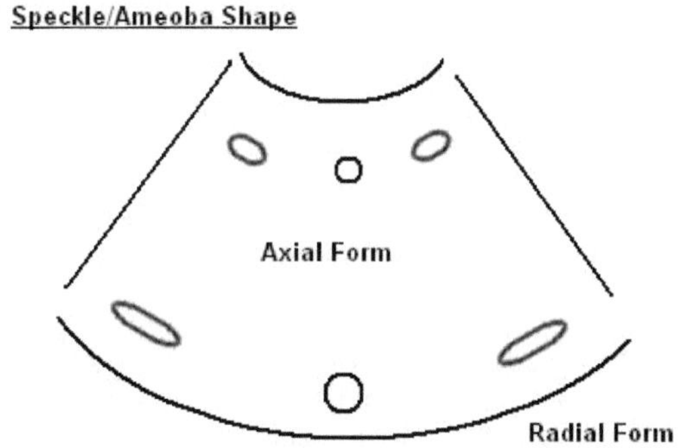

Fig. 4 Speckle and Ameoba form factor changes in the image

The ameoba distance was calculated in the classical way:

- given a pixel **P** in directions using 8-neighbour vicinity a sequence of **k** pixels is determined;
- **k** is smaller or equal to **H**, the maximal amoeba distance;
- the value of **k** is determined by limiting the cumulative euclidean distance added to a penalizing function on intensity;
- on the area determined this way the filtering procedure is then applied.

The distance formula depending on the adjusting parameter has a first term of counting euclidean path and a penalizing term depending on the image pixel intensity **G**.

$$D(a) = SUM_k (1 \ + a * (G_k)) \qquad (1)$$

The adjusting parameter **a** was found crucial to the determination of the ameoba behavior in image processing.

Table 1 Adaptive Ameoba form and resolution trials

	Radial Axis value	Angular Axis Value
Vertical Image Axis	n	2n
Angular Skew -30 degees	2n	4n

A sample image ad-hoc value was used to test the hypothesis of the experiments conducted to validate the experiments.

In order to find a best find a sequence of processing morphological succession of filters several approaches have been studied:

1. Extraction by 'top hat' of local maxima to locate local individual speckles
   - limit the 'hat' radius to extract isolated speckles only
   - do ultimate erosion to locate local maxima location
2. Find amoeba limit parameters for each local speckle location
3. Do radial median filtering with parameter found in step 2.

The blurring effect of the 'top hat' removal filter in the sequence is visible in the preliminary results. Further refining of the filtering sequence followed.

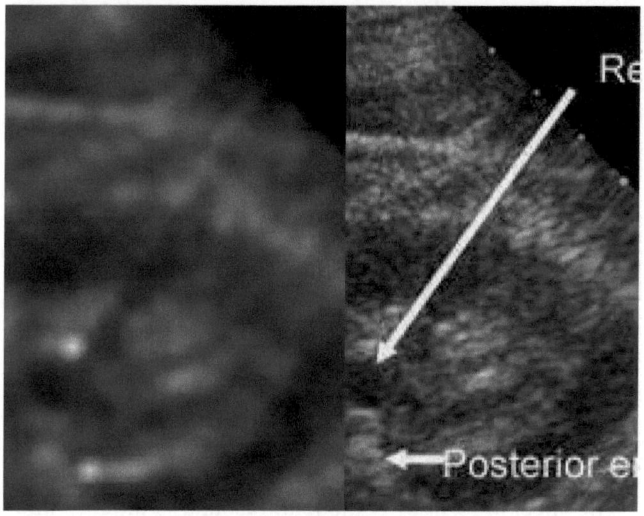

Fig. 5 Speckle removal using the median filter before ameoba selection

The experiments conducted have shown that the task of matching ameoba distance calculations are very much dependent on the sensor technology used.

IV. Results of Experiments on Clinical Case Imges

The positive results reported in the paper are that the adaptive structuring element form is crucial in the filtering scheme and the proposed algorithms and new morphological filters are on the right track.

For the kidney imaging target application, the filtering of the variable spread speckle in ultrasound images has been defined and explored in polar coordinates show promising results.

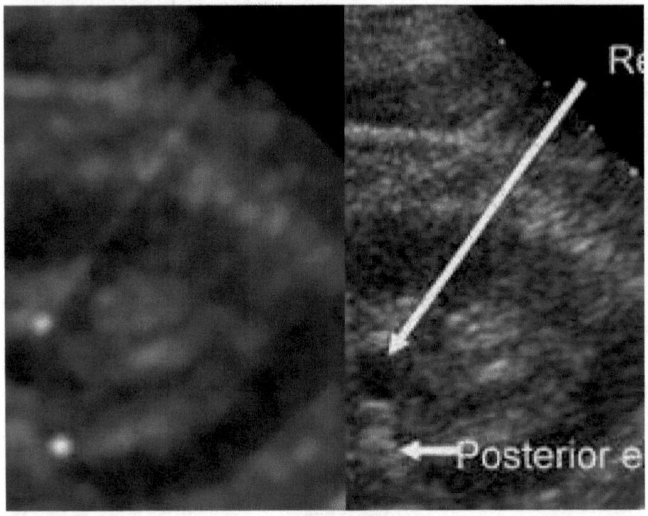

Fig. 6 Speckle removal using the median filter after ameoba selection with ad-hoc parameter values chosen

There are two optimizing parameters. The intrinsic parameter is the speckle noise form, which is dependent on the location in the image and the clinical application case with specific anatomic tissue variations to be visualised.

V. Conclusions

A new method of ultrasound image filtering using recently developed mathematical morphology filters with a spatially variant parameter - Amoeba filter.

The speckle form of B-mode ultrasound is initially modeled in its dependence on depth and radial angle.

The adaptive filter parameter is varied according to local speckle model as observed in experimental images. In the experiments conducted as reported in this paper a simple per case basis of the varying parameter smoothing was used. More elaborate geometrical measures need to be investigated.

Median adaptive filtering have been tried by different morphological filter sequence after the amoeba specific image location parameter setting. The results are compared with direct fixed width median filter.

Further extensions of the method are needed to optimized and leverage the initial results demonstrated so far.

Conflict of Interest

The authors declare that they have no conflict of interest.

References

1. Czerwinski, R.N.;Jones, D.L.; O'Brien, W.D., "Ultrasound speckle reduction by directional median filtering," Image Processing, 1995. Proceedings., International Conference on , vol.1, no., pp.358,361 vol.1, 23-26 Oct 1995,
2. R. Lerallut, É. Decencière, F. Meyer, Image filtering using morphological amoebas, Image and Vision Computing, Volume 25, Issue 4, April 2007, Pages 395–404
3. N. Bouaynaya, D. Schonfeld, Theoretical Foundations of Spatially-Variant Mathematical Morphology Part II: Gray-Level Images, IEEE TRANSAC. ON PAMI, VOL. 30, NO. 5, MAY 2008, pp:1-14
4. T. Loupas, W.N. McDicken, and P.L. Allan, An adaptive weighted median filter for speckle suppression in medical ultrasound images", IEEE Trans. Circuits Syst. , vol.36, No.1, pp.129-135, Jan.1989
5. Eom KB. Speckle reduction in ultrasound images using nonisotropic adaptive filtering.Ultrasound Med. Biol. 2011, 37(10), pp: 1677-88
6. A. Rakotomamonjy, P. Deforge, and P. Marche, Wavelet-based speckle noise reduction in ultrasound B-scan images, Ultrason. Imag. , vol. 22, No.2, pp.73-94, April 2000
7. Michailovich O.V, Tannenbaum A. Despeckling of Medical Ultrasound Images, IEEE transactions on ultrasonics,ferroelectrics, and frequency control,2006, Vol 53
8. J. L. Mateoa,A Fernández-Caballeroa, Finding out general tendencies in speckle noise reduction in ultrasound images, Expert Systems with Applications, Vol 36, Issue 4, May 2009, pp: 7786–7797
9. H. S. Bilge, Delta-sigma subarray beamforming for ultrasound imaging, Turk J Elec Eng & Comp Sci, Vol.18, No.6, 2010, pp: 1003- 1019
10. M. Welk, M. Breus, O. Vogel, Morphological Amoebas are Self-Snakes, Journal of Mathematical Imaging and Vision, 2010
11. Shuo Yang, Jianxun Li, Image restoration using new spatially-variant morphological filters, 2013 IEEE Region 10 Conference, 22-25 Oct. 2013, pp.1 - 4
12. A. C. Jalba and J. B. T. M. Roerdink. An efficient morphological active surface model for volumetric image segmentation. In M. H. F. Wilkinson and J. B. T. M. Roerdink, editors, Mathematical Morphology and Its Application to Signal and Image Processing, volume 5720 of Lecture Notes in Computer Science, pages 193–204. Springer, Berlin, 2009

Author: Ioan Jivet
Institute: University 'Politehnica' Timisoara
Street: V Parvan No 2
City: Timisoara
Country: Romania
Email: ioan.jivet@upt.ro

Automatic, Simultaneous, Non-invasive Measurements of Flow and Area in the Human Pulmonary Arteries from MRI Images

A. Lungu[1], J. Wild[1], Andy Swift[1], David Capener[1], David Kiely[2], and D.R. Hose[1]

[1] University of Sheffield, Cardiovascular Science Department, Sheffield, South Yorkshire, UK
[2] Pulmonary Vascular Disease Unit, Sheffield, South Yorkshire, UK

Abstract— **Pulmonary hypertension (PH), a disease with a high mortality rate, is currently diagnosed by invasive right heart catheterization (RHC). Quantification of wave reflections can offer information about the status of the pulmonary circulation in health and disease, and can be achieved by simultaneous measurement of flow and pressure at the same anatomical site. In practice such measurements are obtained using different acquisition techniques which needs to be synchronized in order to satisfy the simultaneity criterion. We hypothesis that combining the advantages of mathematical modelling with non-invasive Magnetic Resonance Imaging (MRI) measurements of flow and anatomy could offer totally non-invasive modalities for characterizing PH. Our preliminary work was focused on the development of automatic tools to determine accurately flow Q(t) and area A(t) measurements directly from MRI DICOM images, ultimately to support a novel characterisation protocol although the latter is beyond the scope of this paper.**

Keywords— **MRI, non-invasive, pulmonary arteries, segmentation, flow**

I. INTRODUCTION

PH is a disease characterized by increased values of the mean pulmonary arterial pressure (mPAP >25mHg), measured at rest by invasive RHC [1]. One cause of PH is increased pulmonary vascular resistance (PVR) from narrowing of distal vessels and decrease of the vessel compliance (C) that leads to the increase in the right ventricular afterload and ultimately right heart failure and death. A 0D-model of impedance could be used to model the changes in the overall resistance of the system (R_{total}) and C. Additional information about the dynamics of the pulmonary system can be added using a 1D model based on the wave transmission theory. In essence, important physiological characteristics of the overall status of the pulmonary circulation can be determined by computational modelling. But, regardless of the model level of complexity, the results rely on the accuracy and repeatability of flow and pressure measurements. Our analysis protocol requires simultaneous measurements of flow (Q(t)) and pressure (p(t))[2] or radius (r(t)) at the same site. Often, in clinical practice, the measurements are performed using different techniques, at different intervals of time and are highly dependent on the operator.

The solution proposed to overcome these issues relies on computing Q(t) and r(t) directly from MRI DICOM images of the main pulmonary arteries. The MRI acquisition is non-invasive and can offer accurate and simultaneous measurements of flow and anatomy as input data for the mathematical models.

II. MATERIALS AND METHODS

This paper describes a semi-automatic method to extract the flow and area, as functions of time over the entire cardiac cycle, directly from MRI DICOM images of the main pulmonary arteries. The semi-automatic method to extract the area was compared with the gold standard, manual segmentation, and the inter- and intra-operator variability was tested.

A. MRI Acquisition

MRI images of the main (MPA), right (RPA) and left (LPA) pulmonary arteries were acquired on a GE HD x 1.5T scanner using two spatially and temporarily registered MRI sequences: a phase contrast (PC) sequence to extract the flow and an anatomical cine sequence for determining the area.

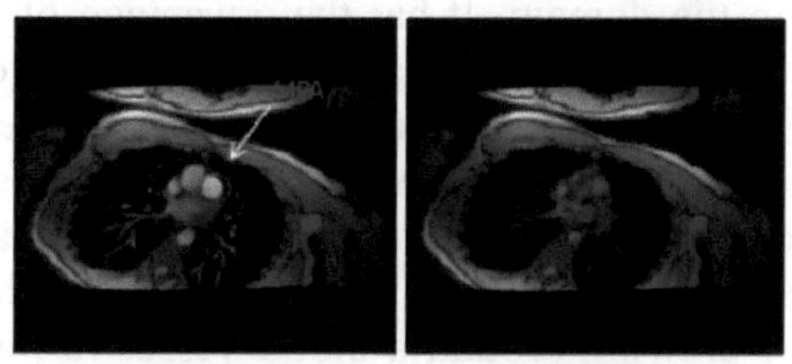

Fig. 1 Typical PC magnitude of the MPA during the peak systole (left), and the late diastole (right)

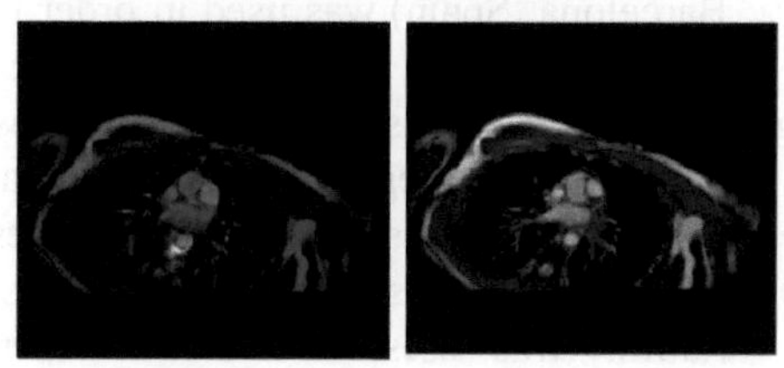

Fig. 2 Typical bSSFP images of the MPA during the peak systole (left) and late diastole.(right)

S. Vlad and R.V. Ciupa (eds.), *International Conference on Advancements of Medicine and Health Care through Technology*, IFMBE Proceedings 44,
DOI: 10.1007/978-3-319-07653-9_53, © Springer International Publishing Switzerland 2014

The Phase Contrast [3] sequence is a widely used routine in the clinical practice for blood flow quantification. The output of this sequence always includes a phase image, containing information about the velocity, and a magnitude image used for the anatomical orientation [4]. Because the sequence captures the phase shifts in the magnetic field caused by the movement of the blood, during diastole, when the blood flow is reduced, the images become more difficult to segment. Due to the high SNR and better blood vessel delineation a bSSFP (balanced Steady State Free Precession) sequence [5] was chosen for imaging the dynamic radius change. The images are acquired very quickly and they give a high level of anatomical detail, making them a better choice in tracking the contour of the vessel. Figures 1 and 2 show examples of typical PC-magnitude and bSSFP images of the MPA, during the peak systolic and late diastolic periods. Note that during systole, the vessel in the PC image can be easily distinguished, whereas during diastole, when the blood flow through the vessel is reduced this becomes much more difficult. In the bSSFP images, the blood vessel is well defined, making this technique a better choice obtaining accurate area changes during the diastole.

The two sequences were registered spatially in the same slice, pixel size (256x 128 matrix dimensions, 480x 288 mm FOV) and temporally using the same number of cardiac images (40) with the same retrospective gating during breath-hold, 8 views per gate and 10% arrythmia rejection. All the images were acquired orthogonal to the vessel during breath hold.

B. Manual Segmentation

The manual segmentation is considered to be the gold standard in the domain. It has the advantage of human rationality. The human eye can distinguish image artefacts from the real anatomical structure and can ignore them. On the other hand, even this advantage is not a consistent one because different operators have different criteria and they can be subjective in their judgment. Also, the manual process of drawing around a blood vessel for 40 slices is time consuming.

The open source framework, GIMIAS (Universitat Pompeu Fabra, Barcelona, Spain) was used in order to segment all three pulmonary arteries. Four operators, one specialist (radiologist) and three non-specialists (two of whom had previous experience of the segmentation of other anatomical structures from MR images) segmented the arteries from the given DICOMs. From the resulting segmentations the inter-operator variability was assessed. One of the operators also segmented the arteries three times, in order to assess the intra-operator variability.

C. Automatic Segmentation

The manual segmentation suffers from reproducibility (intra-operator variation), inter-operator variation, and the cost associated with the long duration of the process. Some of these disadvantages could be overcome using automatic segmentation. The method used for the automatic segmentation of the pulmonary arteries was developed in Matlab (R2011b, The MathWorks Inc.) using the departmental registration toolkit, ShIRT (Sheffield University Registration Toolkit) [6] to morph images over a time series and effectively track the motion and deformation of the region of interest (ROI).

During the registration, the mapping function (u,v) specifies how a given anatomical point from one image, defined by a set of coordinates x, y will 'move' to another set of coordinates x',y' in the second image (eq.1).

$$\begin{aligned} x' &= u(x,y) + x \\ y' &= v(x,y) + y \end{aligned} \tag{1}$$

The resulting mapping function (u,v), would be used further to relate each point from the drawn ROI with the corresponding point in the moved image.

The automatic segmentation process, named due to the minimum input of the operator, involves drawing the vessel contour in just one image, called the fixed image, chosen by the operator from the time series data (40 images in one series). Three different approaches (cases) of extracting the blood vessel position and area automatically were evaluated. These were dictated by the choice of the fixed image:

i) Fixed image corresponding to the peak systole image.

The timeframe where the PA was fully expanded was chosen as a fixed image. A contour of the blood vessel was manually drawn in the source frame, and the rest of the frames, considered moved images, were registered one by one into the fixed one.

ii) Fixed image corresponding to an average image of the entire time series of images.

An average image was created from all the frames. Then, the rest of frames were registered, and the result (40 registered images) was averaged again, creating a new fixed image where all the original MR frames were registered as moved images. The rationality of the *registered average* was that, an average can work as a denoising filter, reducing some artefacts, but cannot necessary guarantee the correct position of the vessel. That is why an intermediate step of registration was necessary.

iii) Successive registration of each image in the time series

In the third case of segmentation, all the images played a dual role: fixed and moved image. More precisely, the algorithm starts with first frame as a fixed image and second frame as moved image. After manually defining the borders of the PA in the first frame, the images were registered, and a new ROI, corresponding to the second frame was obtained. On the next time step, the previous moved image was used as fixed image and the third frame from the sequence was used as the target (moved) image. Instead of drawing again around the artery wall, the ROI generated from the previous time-step was used. The algorithm was then continued until the last slice. A graphical explanation of the process it has been represented in figure 3.

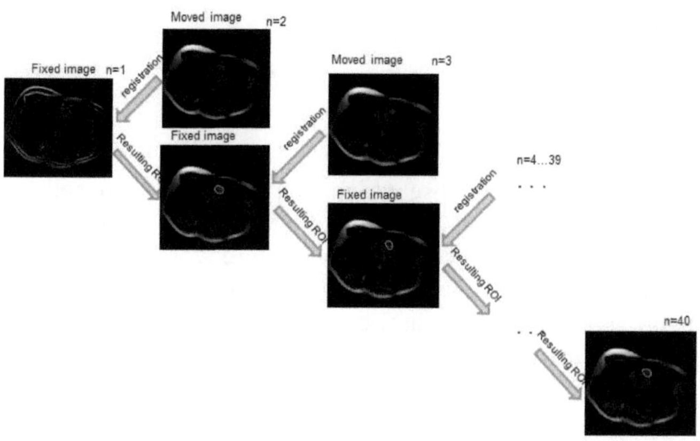

Fig. 3 Registration of successive images in time series

D. Flow Computation

Using a velocity encoding (venc) of 150 cm/s, the blood flow velocity (v) was computed for each pixel using the phase shift determined from the PC images (eq.2)[4].

$$v = \frac{phase\ shift\ X\ venc}{\pi} \tag{2}$$

Prior to computing the blood flow through the arteries, the blood vessels were isolated using the mask resulting from the area segmentation. The masks are binary images with the same dimensions as the flow images, with the pixel values 0 outside the arterial wall and 1 inside.

At each time step, the average velocity inside the vessel was multiplied by the average corresponding area resulting in the average blood flow over the entire cardiac cycle for the main, right and left pulmonary arteries. In the results sections the computed results were compared against the results from the scanner report card for each of the branches.

III. Results

A. Manual Segmentation

A.1 Intra-operator Variability

The first operator manually segmented three times the MPA, LPA and RPA. For each branch, the mean area variation, with the corresponding standard deviation, was plotted for each time step. Figure 4 shows the mean area of the three segmentations for the MPA with the corresponding SD at each of the 40 time instances.

Although the left and right branches of the pulmonary trunk are less affected by the movement of the heart or breathing artefacts [7] , due to the smaller size compared to the main artery, the LPA and RPA are more difficult to segmented and the standard deviation increases.

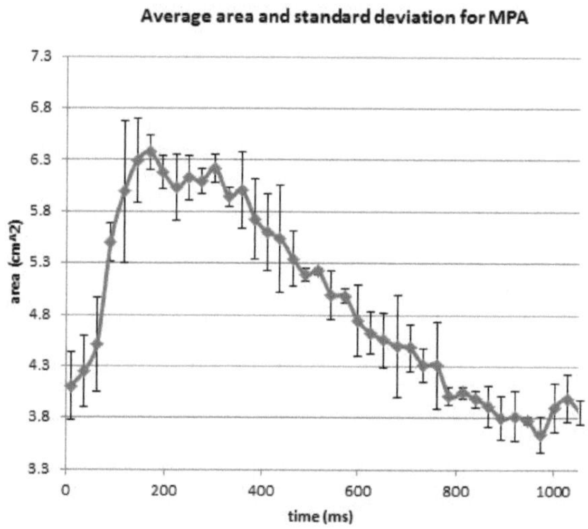

Fig. 4 Average area and the standard deviation for the MPA

A.2 Inter-operator Variability

The inter-operator variability was tested using the manual segmentation of four operators: two operators with previous experience in segmenting other anatomical structures, an unexperienced operator and a specialist (radiologist). Using the same method for expressing the error (one standard deviation of the mean), it was noted that the inter-operator variability was greater than the inter-operator variability.

From figure 5 it can be noticed that three from the operators were consistent in their estimation of the vessel size. Operator 3, totally inexperienced, is less consistent between the cases. This raises the question of the effect of experience and training: how much the inter-operator variability will decrease if all of them were adequately trained in how to segment the vessel.

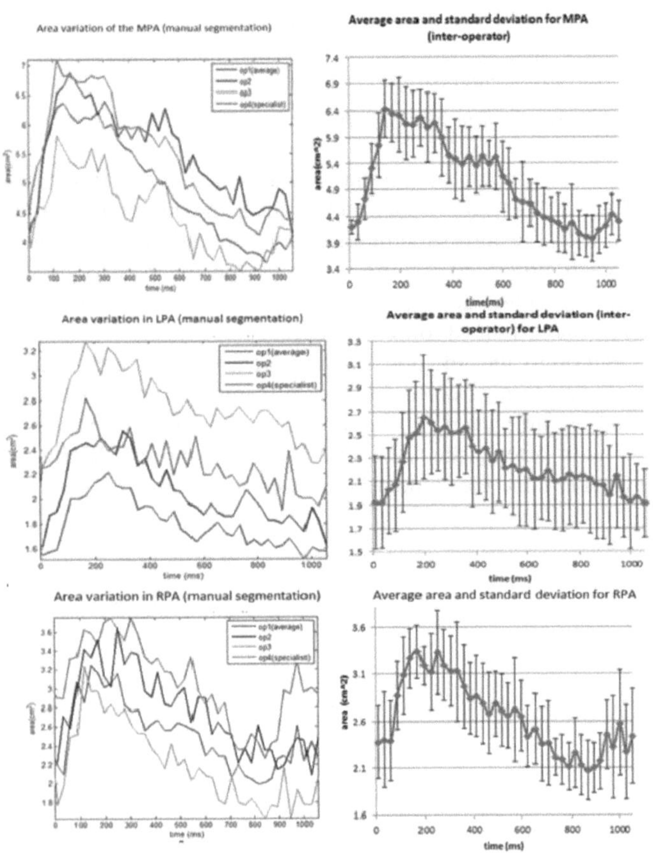

Fig. 5 Area variation obtained for each operator (left column) and average area and standard deviation (right column)

If the quality of the manual segmentation is judged by its temporal smoothness it might be argued that the specialist produces the 'best' segmentation of the MPA. The small dimensions of the RPA and LPA appear to cause difficulty even for the specialist. More important, it is noted that for the MPA three out four operators found the maximum amplitude of the area in the same range of values but for the other two branches the inter-operator variability increases.

B. Automatic Segmentation

For the automatic segmentation, three different approaches were used according to the choice of the target (fixed) image. All three area curves determined automatically are positioned in between ± 1SD of the 'manual' area mean, for all of the arteries. They have smoother character than the manual area results. Also, the area changes over time in the MPA follows the reported trend from invasive measurements reported in literature [8].

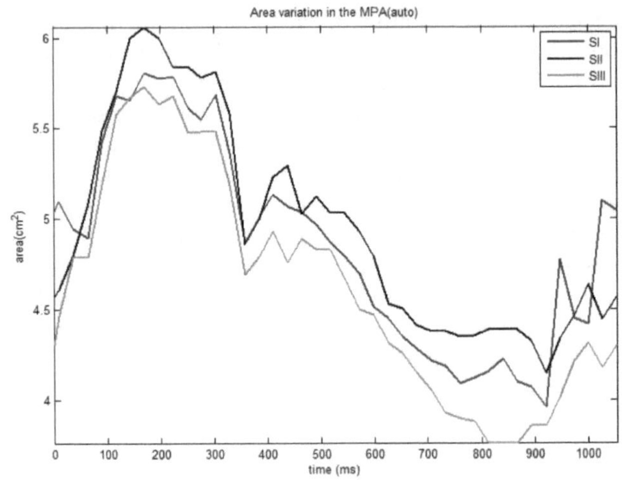

Fig. 6 Area variation of the MPA, after using automatic segmentation algorithms. Red- "peak systolic case", Blue-"average image case", Green- "successive time steps registration case"

It is difficult to choose which from the three proposed automatic segmentations offers the better representation of the real behavior of the vessel. For our future work, the decision was taken to use the second proposed protocol (the average image used as fixed image) based on the smoothness of the resulting curve.

C. Flow Quantification

Having the area of the blood vessel at every time step and the masks to isolate the velocity information from the phase contrast images, the flow variation during a cardiac cycle was computed for each of the three pulmonary arteries.

The flow waveforms computed based on the areas automatically determined from the 3 automatic segmentation protocols in the MPA are similar. The differences in the maximum amplitude come from the differences in maximum area amplitude, since the average flow depends on the average area at each time step (figure 7). For the left and right branches similar results were obtained.

The amplitude of the flow is directly influenced by the area mask that is applied. Although the flow derivation is tolerant to errors in area during diastole (when flow is low), it is important to identify the correct region of the image, corresponding to the cross-section of the vessel, in systole. It should be noted that an accurate area assessment in diastole remains important for pressure calculations, even if it is less important for the flow derivation.

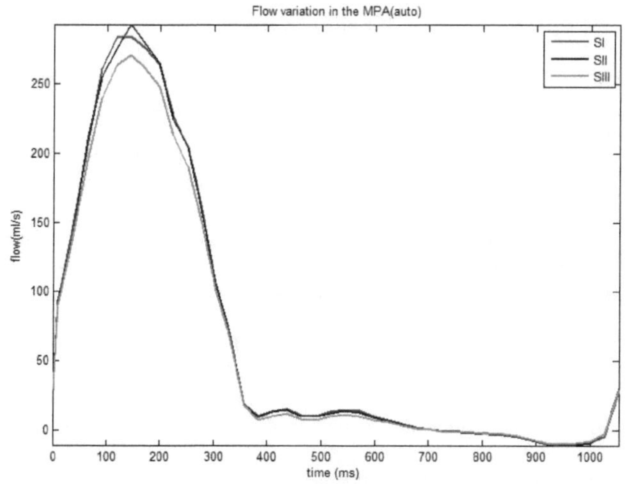

Fig. 7 Flow variation of the MPA, after using automatic segmentation algorithms. Red- "peak systolic case", Blue-"average image case", Green- "successive time steps registration case"

The importance of vessel tracking and placing the mask in the correct position, achieved by our proposed protocol, was emphasized through a direct comparison of our flow results with the ones obtained from the MRI scanner report. A screen shot of the report can be seen in figure 8. As it can be noted from figure 8 and table 1, the flow from the two branches added together does not satisfy continuity, which dictates that all the flow entering the MPA should go out through the LPA and RPA, since there are no other side branches.

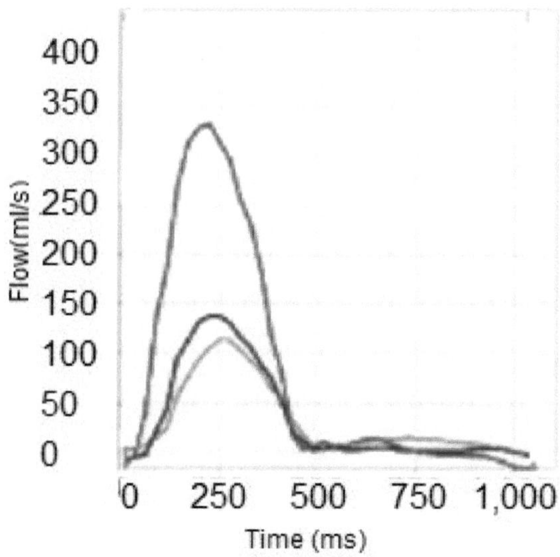

Fig. 8 Flow variation in MPA (red), RPA (green) and LPA (blue), during a cardiac cycle, exported from MR scanner

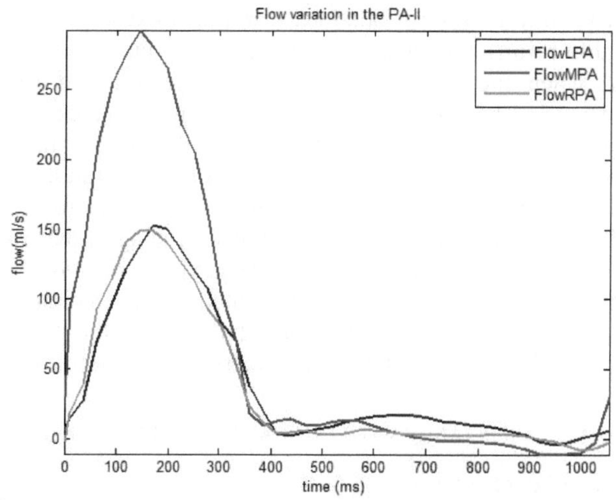

Fig. 9 Flow variation in MPA (red), RPA (green) and LPA (blue), during a cardiac cycle, computed using our scanner independent tool

Table 1 Comparison between the maximum flow values for MPA, LPA and RPA computed directly from the DICOMs and with scanner's built in algorithms

	MPA[ml/s]	LPA[ml/s]	RPA[ml/s]	LPA+RPA[ml/s]
Computed flow	292,5	152,8	148,9	301,7
Scanner's results	338,9	141,6	120,3	261,9

Computing the flow directly from the DICOM images, using the segmentation method that in the current example gave the smoothest MPA area variation, under-predicts the maximum flow in the main artery and over-predicts those in the left and right branches, when compared with the scanner's result. However it is noted that the sum of the LPA and RPA flows as reported by the native software in the scanner is 20% lower than the MPA flow (table 1). Using our own protocol, the error is less than 3.2 % for this case, which perhaps suggests that it might be more accurate in analyzing the flows in the arteries.

IV. CONCLUSIONS

Manual segmentation has the advantage of the human eye and judgment, being able to distinguish artefacts or to infer the location of an anatomical structure based on experience or intuition. On the other hand, this process is time consuming regardless of the operator experience. The automatic segmentations of the principal pulmonary arteries were comparable with the manual ones performed by the specialist, even smoother, and were performed in significant less time.

The flow waveform obtained using area extraction gave reliable results for all three pulmonary arteries. More than that, when the sum of flow through the left and right branches has been checked against the total flow, the results obtained directly from the DICOM MRI images had a smaller error in comparison with the MR scanner results.

Developing tools to extract accurate, simultaneous flow and area measurements from MRI DICOM images, that will overcome the problems regarding data synchronization and clinical operator dependency, represented our first step in the process of non-invasively inferring the status in the pulmonary circulation in health and pulmonary hypertension.

V. Compliance with Ethical Requirements

A. Conflict of Interest

Angela Lungu is a PhD student funded by the Engineering and Physical Science Research Council EPSRC.

B. Statement of Informed Consent

The results are based on the analysis of images from one volunteer, under the local ethical committee approval reported in section C. The individual gave informed consent for the imaging protocol and for the use of the anonymized images in this research study.

C. Statement of Human and Animal Rights

This study was performed under the auspices of the local ethical committee, approval number STH14070.

Acknowledgment

This research is funded by the Engineering and Physical Science Research Council, EPSRC.

References

1. Galie, N., et al., (2011), *Guidelines for the diagnosis and treatment of pulmonary hypertension (vol 30, pg 2493, 2009).* European Heart Journal,. **32**(8): p. 926-926.
2. van de Vosse, F.N. and N. Stergiopulos, (2011) *Pulse Wave Propagation in the Arterial Tree.* Annual Review of Fluid Mechanics, Vol 43,. **43**: p. 467-499.
3. Markl, M., P. Kilner, and T. Ebbers,(2011) *Comprehensive 4D velocity mapping of the heart and great vessels by cardiovascular magnetic resonance.* Journal of Cardiovascular Magnetic Resonance,. **13**.
4. Donald W. McRobbie, E.A.M., Martin J. Graves and Martin R. Prince, (2003), *MRI from picture to proton.* 1st ed. Vol. 1. 2003, Cambridge: Cambridge : Cambridge University Press,. 360.
5. Chavhan, G.B., et al.,(2008) *Steady-state MR imaging sequences: physics, classification, and clinical applications.* Radiographics,. **28**(4): p. 1147-60.
6. Barber, D.C. and D.R. Hose, (2005), *Automatic segmentation of medical images using image registration: diagnostic and simulation applications.* J Med Eng Technol,. **29**(2): p. 53-63.
7. Lotz, J., et al.,(2002) *Cardiovascular flow measurement with phase-contrast MR imaging: Basic facts and implementation.* Radiographics,. **22**(3): p. 651-671.
8. Greenfield, J.C. and D.M. Griggs, (1963) Relation between pressure and diameter in main pulmonary artery of man. Journal of Applied Physiology,. **18**(3): p. 557-&.

Author: Angela Lungu
Institute: University of Sheffield
Street: Beech Hill Road
City: Sheffield, S10 2RX
Country: UK
Email: mdp11al@sheffield.ac.uk

Structured Light Based Imaging Architecture for Guided Fracture Reduction

F. Neaga[1], I. Raus[2], R. Moga[3], D. Moga[3], S. Vlad[3], N. Stroia[3], and M. Munteanu[3]

[1] Sălaj County Hospital, Zalău, Romania
[2] "Dr. Constantin Papilian" Military Emergency Hospital of Cluj-Napoca, Romania
[3] Technical University of Cluj-Napoca, Romania

Abstract— **This paper introduces a structured light based imaging architecture able to serve for the development of an affordable guided fracture reduction system. The 3D models of the bones in the healthy limb are used for the preoperative alignment of the proximal and distal segments of the fractured bone using algorithm for automated registration. A structured light setup performs the reconstruction of 3D information needed for the intraoperative guidance in order to support the fracture reduction in accord with the preoperative alignment.**

Keywords— **Structured light, fracture reduction, registration**

I. INTRODUCTION

It is well-knonw that deformities due to malalignment in fracture reduction, can produce secondary degenerative joint disease and might even require surgical revision. For example, in the case of intramedullary nailing approach of femoral shaft fractures in adults, investigated in [1], the most widely documented malunions (occurring due to angulation, periaxial rotation and leg length discrepancies), the ranges of tolerances for malalignment have been documented as $5-15^\circ$ of varus/valgus angulation, 15° of flexion/extension angulation,$1-1.5cm$ in limb length and 15° of periaxial rotation.

In the last decades, the field of orthopaedic surgery benefited from several technologies that have been introduced in order to facilitate the correct bone alignment in fracture reduction and the accurate insertion of screws and nails. The widespreading of the computerized tools and software environments favoured the introduction of mechanical and robotic guidance systems based on tracking. Computer assisted orthopaedic surgery (CAOS) is very important among these technologies. There are two types of navigation technologies: image guided and non-image (surgeon defined anatomy) guided procedures. As pointed out in [2], in orthopaedic trauma surgery, CAOS based on image guided tracking has much more applications, since the introduction of the fluoroscopic navigation in 1999, but better clinical outcome of CAOS can be obtained by the use of other imaging techniques: CT, MR and optical images, and their combination (image fusion).

The traditional approach required the use of intraoperative x-ray. An improvement was made by the introduction of C-Arm fluoroscopy that allows the surgeon to obtain in vivo radiographic images. As indicated in [3] there are some difficulties of this technique associated with the nonuniform exposure variation across the field of view, the varying contrast and exposure from shot to shot. Moreover, the distortion pattern and camera parameters are orientation dependent and vary from unit to unit and session to session, requiring preoperative calibrations and use of predefined orientations.

The electromagnetic tracking systems are designed to determine the position and orientation of special sensors attached to surgical tools using a computerized control unit that powers and controls an electromagnetic (EM) field generator and can identify the tool location [4].

The computerized optical tracking systems have already proven results in the clinical environment. They are remarked for the high degree of accuracy that can be provided and for the possibility of combined 3D visualization/exploration/analysis offered by the integration with standardized CT and MRI imaging.

The procedures involved with fracture reduction as well as with the insertion of different internal fixtures can benefit from the 3D reconstruction of the fractured bones in two ways: pre-operatively, for surgical planning, and intra-operatively, where the ability to track/register the bone segments in real-time might be crucial (see the branching of Fig. 1 according to [5].

The solutions of computerized optical tracking rely on establishing (through calibration procedures and appropriate image processing algorithms) the correct relations (transformations) between several spaces: the coordinates of the surgical space, patient, and instrumentation. Some imaging sensors (cameras), active or passive markers connect to a computer running the appropriate software in order to provide real-time feedback to the surgeon.

According to [5], the reduction process based on an image guided surgery approach goes through several important phases:

- acquisition of 2D X-ray images to form a patient-specific model;
- pre-operative 3D reconstruction;

S. Vlad and R.V. Ciupa (eds.), *International Conference on Advancements of Medicine and Health Care through Technology*, IFMBE Proceedings 44,
DOI: 10.1007/978-3-319-07653-9_54,

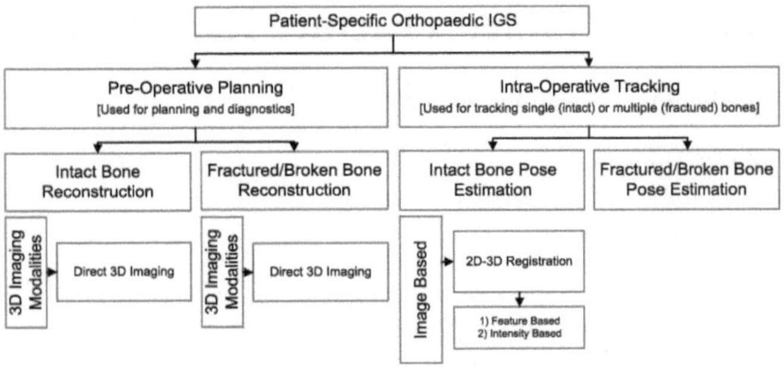

Fig. 1 Branching of orthopaedic image guided surgery approaches according to [5]

- simulation based planning of the reduction path with the pre-visualization and result inspection;
- intra-operative guidance using the 3D model for improved accuracy.

The approach investigated in this paper avoids the intra-operative fluoroscopy (see Fig. 2) by using a structured light based imaging architecture able to support real-time intra-operative guidance.

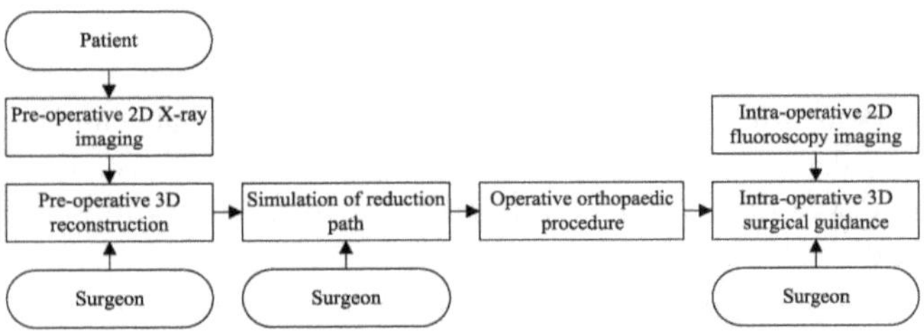

Fig. 2 Overview of the reduction process as described in [5]

II. Proposed Method

An important class of methods is based on the location and the orientation of a dynamic reference frame (DRF) [6] [7]. These methods use tracking systems consisting of image sensors and light-emitting diodes (LEDs). There are successful experiments made in image-guided surgery with such setups in two configurations: the active configuration, when the emitters are mounted on the DRF, and the passive configuration, when infrared light is emitted from the camera unit and reflected from some spheres mounted on the DRF.

In the first case, the tracking software compares the location of the LEDs in images and determines the location and orientation of the DRF relative to the camera, while in the second case the light reflected from the spheres is used in order to determine the location and orientation of the DRF.

Since the overall precision of an image-guided surgery system depends heavily on the accuracy of the optical tracking system, is important to point out its main error sources: quantization error of image sensor, imperfect optics, and inaccuracies of the mechanical fixtures. The study described in [8] measured the jitter of such setups, ie. quantifies the deviation of repeated measurements from the mean in the case of a stationary DRF, concluding that the configurations investigated have jitter less than $0.11mm$.

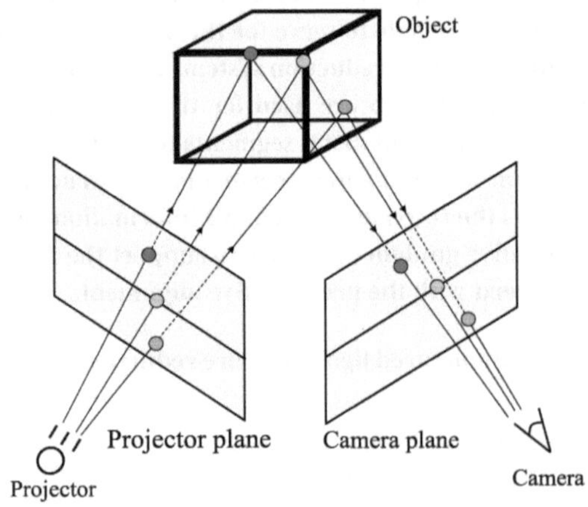

Fig. 3 Basic setup for structured light triangulation

The method proposed in this paper was designed as an alternative to these methods, considering the following:

- there are available software frameworks for structured light processing with proven functionality;
- the precision of the structured light based 3D reconstruction was demonstrated in many application areas;
- currently both LCD based light projectors and laser based projectors are available at low costs.

The use of structured light in medical applications is mainly reported in 3D shape reconstruction applications like structured light-based surface topography [9], volume and shape estimation [10], and reconstruction of bone surface by applying shape-from-shading to a sequence of endoscopic images [11].

It is therefore possible to define the architecture of an affordable image-guided surgery system that would combine preoperative CT imagery with intraoperative, structured light based, 3D reconstruction for providing an optical tracking based alignment as part of a computer assisted fracture reduction system.

Using T letter shaped rigid fixtures, with one screw arm, it is possible to have a rigid fixture of an external reference body to the bone segments (see Fig. 4). If a cube is used as external body, than the structured light techniques permit to have a passive DRF as cube (DRFAC).

The main steps of the proposed approach are summarized in what follows.

1. Based on X-ray images, the mounting of the two DRFAC fixtures is performed on the distal and proximal segments.
2. A 3D DICOM data set is acquired preoperatively using CT for both.
3. The bone and the fixtures are segmented from the surrounding soft tissue. 3D reconstruction is performed for the proximal and distal segments of the fractured bone as well as for the corresponding bone of the healthy limb (see Fig. 5).
4. The reflected mesh of the healthy bone (RMHB) is represented in a coordinate space defined in relation to the coordinate space of the DICOM data set.
5. The automatic alignment of the proximal and distal segments is done through registration algorithms using RMHB, determining the two transforms that optimally map the distal mesh (DM) and proximal mesh (PM) onto RMHB.
6. The relative position of the distal and proximal DRFAC is computed, to serve as a reference for the intraoperative image based tracking.
7. The 3D reconstruction of the two cubes is done intraoperatively in real-time, using structured light, and their relative position is computed, compared with the reference position determined at point 6.
8. The appropriate guidance is provided to the surgeon in order to minimize the positioning error, i.e, reach the optimal alignment between DM and PM simulated preoperatively at point 5.

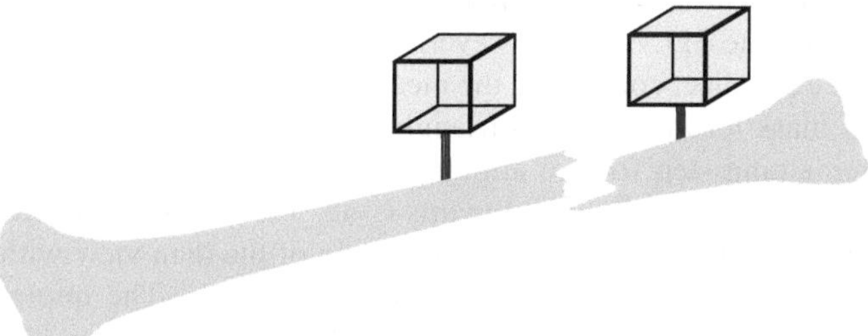

Fig. 4 The two cubes rigidly attached to the proximal and distal segments

III. REGISTRATION METHODS

The problem of registering two views can be stated as follows: for a given pair of views, D (data-view) and M (model-view), representing two scans of the same object, estimate the

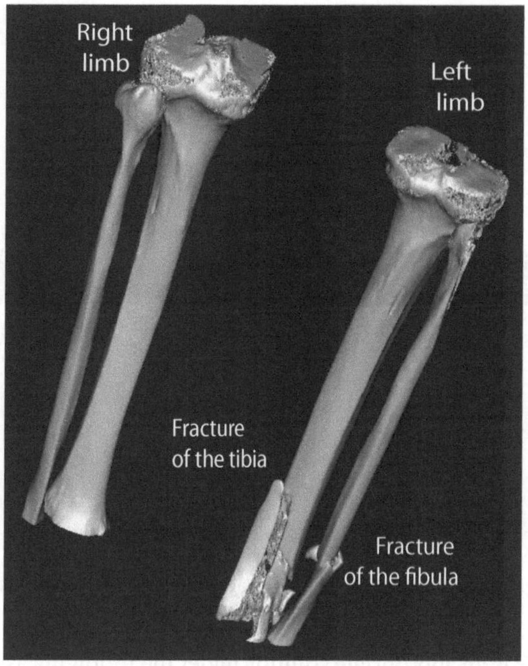

Fig. 5 3D reconstruction of the healthy limb and of the tibia and fibula of the fractured limb

parameters $\mathbf{a}$ of the transformation $T(\mathbf{a},D)$ which best align D to M [12]:

$$\mathbf{a}^* = argmin_a E(T(\mathbf{a},D),M) \quad (1)$$

where E is the error function and measures the alignment or the registration error.

One standard registration method is the ICP (*Iterative Closest Point*) algorithm with the overall aim of estimating a rigid transformation with parameters $\mathbf{a}^* = (\mathbf{R},\mathbf{t})$. The error function is [12]:

$$E_{ICP}(\mathbf{a},D,M) = \sum_{i=1}^{N_d} ||(\mathbf{R}\mathbf{d}_i + \mathbf{t}) - \mathbf{m}_j||^2 \quad (2)$$

where $(\mathbf{d}_i, \mathbf{m}_j)$ are corresponding points. For a data point $\mathbf{d}_i \in D$, the corresponding model point $\mathbf{m}_j \in M$ is computed such that:

$$j = argmin_{j \in \{1,\ldots,N_m\}} ||(\mathbf{R}\mathbf{d}_i + \mathbf{t}) - \mathbf{m}_j||^2 \quad (3)$$

The value $e_i^2 = ||(\mathbf{R}\mathbf{d}_i + \mathbf{t}) - \mathbf{m}_j||^2$ is the square of the residual.

The ICP algorithm starts from an initial estimate of the registration parameters. Each iteration consists on two main steps: closest point computation and rigid transformation estimation. The algorithm stops if the change in the error function value between two successive iterations is lower than a threshold.

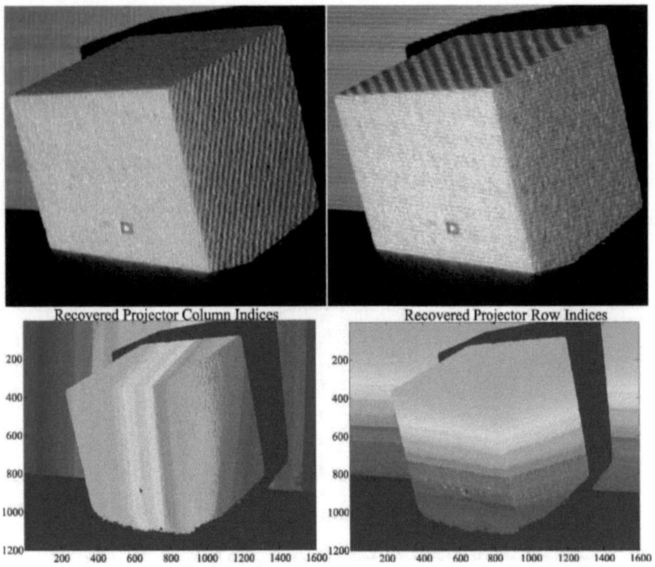

Fig. 6 Gray code structured light images used in cube reconstruction

ICP is an appropriate solution under the following assumptions [12]: ▷ The two views are close to each other. If not, it will probably converge to a local minimum. ▷ The two views fully overlap or the data-view is a subset of the model-view. Two other important issues associated with the ICP algorithm are the computation speed and the accuracy.

A variant of the ICP algorithm is the *Levenberg-Marquardt ICP* (LM-ICP) which models the registration as a Levenberg-Marquardt approach to a general optimization problem. The optimization function is defined such as outlier rejection and speed are taken into account. The LM-ICP problem formulation is defined as for the ICP algorithm. The error function [12],

$$E(\mathbf{a}) = \sum_{i=1}^{N_d} (e_i(\mathbf{a}))^2,\ e_i(\mathbf{a}) = ||\mathbf{R}\mathbf{d}_i + \mathbf{t} - \mathbf{m}_j|| \quad (4)$$

is written in the form $E(\mathbf{a}) = ||\mathbf{e}(\mathbf{a})||^2$, where $\mathbf{e}(\mathbf{a}) = \{e_i(\mathbf{a})\}_{i=1}^{N_d}$ is the residual vector.
The distance transform can be formulated such as to simplify the computation of the derivatives of E [12]:

$$D_\varepsilon(\mathbf{x}) = min_j \varepsilon^2(||\mathbf{m}_j - \mathbf{x}||) \quad (5)$$

where $\mathbf{x} \in X$ and X is a discrete grid representing the volume which encloses the model-view. By combining equations (4) and (5), the registration problem becomes: $E(\mathbf{a}) = \sum_i^{N_d} D_\varepsilon(T(\mathbf{a}, \mathbf{d}_i)))$. The goal of each iteration is to choose an update to the current estimate $\mathbf{a}_k$, $\mathbf{x}_{LM}$, so that setting $\mathbf{a}_{k+1} = \mathbf{a}_k + \mathbf{x}_{LM}$ reduces the registration error.

The basic stepts of the LM-ICP algorithm are listed in what follows in accord with [12] and [13]:

1. Set $\lambda \leftarrow \lambda_0$
2. compute distance transform $D_\varepsilon(\mathbf{x})$
3. set $\mathbf{a}_k \leftarrow \mathbf{a}_0$
4. compute $\mathbf{e}_k = \mathbf{e}(\mathbf{a}_k)$
5. compute the Jacobian matrix J
6. repeat
   7. compute update $\mathbf{a}_{k+1} = \mathbf{a}_k - (J^T J + \lambda I)^{-1} J^T)\mathbf{e}_k$
   8. compute $\Delta E = E(\mathbf{a}_{k+1}) - E(\mathbf{a}_k)$
   9. $if\ \Delta E > 0\ then$ increase λ, *else* decrease λ, *goto* 4.
10. $if\ ||\mathbf{e}_k|| > cst.\ goto$ 3

The tests performed on several fractured bones (femur, tibia, fibula) proved that the appropriate choice of the initial estimate of the registration parameters is very important for producing fast an correct results with LM-ICP. This motivated the development of a pre-alignment method that would bring the data in such appropriate starting position relative to the model.

For pre-alignment of the two views, the following methods were used: *central axes alignment* and *cross-section alignment*.

For aligning the central axis of the data with respect to the central axis of the model, Rodriguez's formula for three dimensional rotation was used [14]:

$$\mathbf{x}' = ((\hat{\mathbf{r}}\,\hat{\mathbf{r}}^t) + sin(\theta)(\hat{\mathbf{r}}\times) - cos(\theta)(\hat{\mathbf{r}}\times)(\hat{\mathbf{r}}\times))\mathbf{x} \quad (6)$$

In this formula, $\hat{\mathbf{r}}$ is a unit vector representing the rotation axis, $\mathbf{x}$ is the vector to be rotated about $\hat{\mathbf{r}}$ by the angle θ and $\hat{\mathbf{r}}\times$ is the cross-product matrix for $\hat{\mathbf{r}}$:

$$\hat{\mathbf{r}}\times = \begin{bmatrix} 0 & \hat{r}_z & \hat{r}_y \\ \hat{r}_z & 0 & -\hat{r}_x \\ -\hat{r}_y & \hat{r}_x & 0 \end{bmatrix} \quad (7)$$

The central axis is computed along the Z direction by dividing the 3D view into several slices of equal length and, for each slice, computing the mean value between the centers of mass for all the mesh triangles located in that slice. The remaining step for pre-alignment consists of rotation about the central axis. For solving this issue, a second method was applied which aligns the cross-section of the data view with respect to the cross-section of the model view. The implemented algorithm can be summarized as follows:

- divide the two views into several slices;
- for each slice: compute the **longest chord** by first searching the furthermost point from the center and then searching the furthermost point with respect to this point;
- select the slice with the maximum **longest chord** in the first quarter of slices;
- align the vectors formed by the two most distant points on the slice contour.

IV. EXPERIMENTS

Experiments were made using *Materialise Mimics* environment for 3D reconstruction from CT images and *Matlab* for registration and 3D reconstruction from structured light images.

The experiments on the 3D cube reconstruction were made using a series of Gray code structured light images generated in Matlab and then projected on the cube [15]. The extraction of the 3D point was done with the *mlStructuredLight* framework (available at the website mentioned in [15]) using previous calibration of the camera and of the projector based on the *Camera Calibration Toolbox* for Matlab of Bouguet [16].

The functionality implemented for registration consists in the following main steps:

- allows the user to select the STL files (model and data) consisting in a list of triangular surfaces that describe the bone surface meshing;
- allows the user to select start points from the data and model view (first or last point);
- performs pre-alignment (central axes alignment followed by cross section alignment);
- applies the LM-ICP algorithm on the pre-aligned data.

The testing of this functionality was performed on a series of experiments with real bone data. A part of a bone as 3D body was firstly selected to be aligned with the whole bone as 3D body in order to validate the correctness of the procedures. Next, distal and proximal segments from the fractured limb were aligned on the reflected 3D representation of the similar bone of the healthy limb.

An example of the model (reflected fibula of the healthy limb) and the data (distal segment of the fractured fibula) are presented in Fig. 7 and 8, respectively. The alignment of the central axes and the transformed data after pre-alignment are presented in Fig. 9 and 10. The results obtained after registering the pre-aligned data using LM-ICP are presented in Fig. 10.

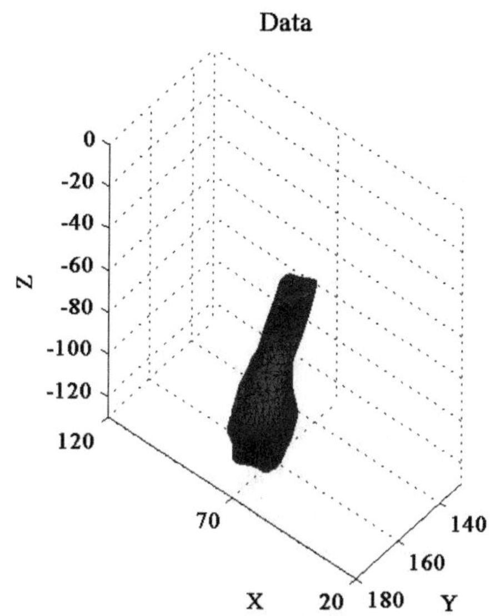

Fig. 8 Data view (3D reconstruction for the distal segment)

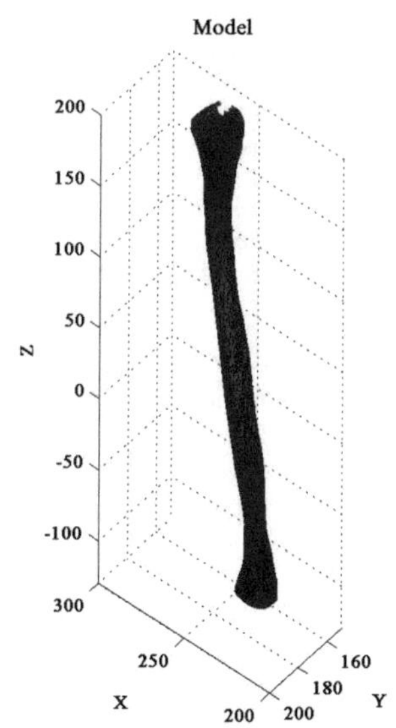

Fig. 7 Model view (3D reconstruction for the fibula of the healthy limb)

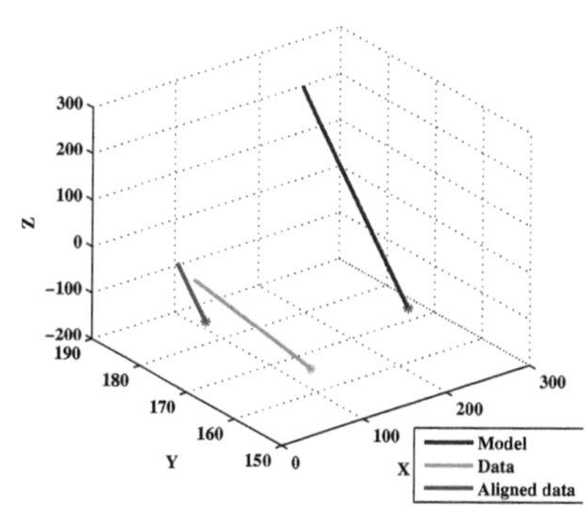

Fig. 9 Central axis alignment

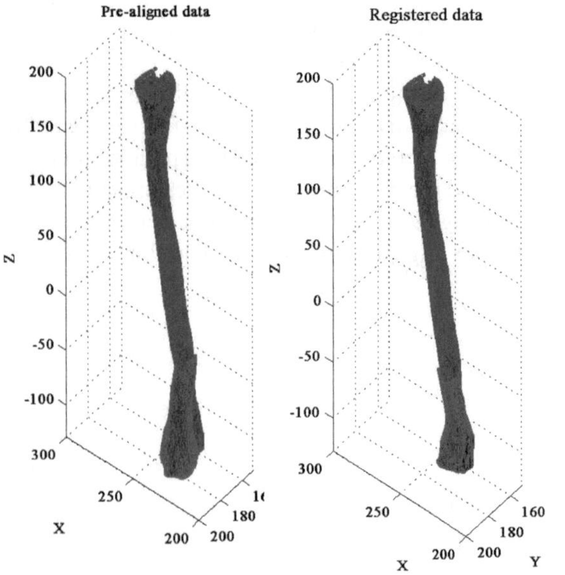

Fig. 10 Pre-aligned distal segment and registered distal segment

V. CONCLUSION

The 3D reconstruction from CT images and registration of the distal and proximal fragments based of the 3D reconstruction of the corresponding bone of the healthy limb can be used for the preoperative simulation and validation of the alignment for a correct fracture reduction. The structured light images can provide the basis for intra-operative alignment procedures in which external bodies rigidly attached to the proximal and distal segments are replacing active or passive DRFs. The experiments performed in Matlab have proven execution times in the order of few seconds, suggesting an optimized C++ implementation can work in real-time for providing the needed intraoperative guidance. An imaging architecture combining preoperative CT images and structured light based reconstruction may serve for the development of an affordable guided fracture reduction equipment.

CONFLICT OF INTEREST

The authors declare that they have no conflict of interest.

REFERENCES

1. Crookshank Meghan. *Current limitations in computer-assisted surgery of femoral shaft fractures and the use of intraoperative CT to improve characterization of fracture malalignment.* PhD thesisInstitute of Biomaterials and Biomedical Engineering, University of Toronto 2012.
2. Kwok Sui Leung . Computer assisted orthopaedic surgery: present status and future perspectives *Chinese Medical Journal.* 2010;123:2967–2968. DOI: 10.3760/cma.j.issn.0366-6999.2010.21.002.
3. Joskowicz Leo, Milgrom Charles, Simkin Ariel, Tockus Lana, Yaniv Ziv. FRACAS: A System for Computer-Aided Image-Guided Long Bone Fracture Surgery *Computer Aided Surgery.* 1998;3:271–288.
4. Moore Chris, Heotis Charles, Ritchey Nick. The Utilization of Electromagnetic Tracking to Facilitate Distal Targeting During Intramedullary Nailing *Bone & Joint Science.* 2012;3.
5. Gamage Pavan. 3D Reconstruction of Patient Specific Bone Models for Image Guided Orthopaedic Surgery Master's thesisDepartment of Mechanical Engineering, The University of Auckland New Zealand 2012.
6. Westphal Ralf, Winkelbach Simon, Gösling Thomas, et al. Telemanipulated Long Bone Fracture Reduction in *Medical Robotics* (Bozovic Vanja. , ed.)InTech 2008. http://www.intechopen.com/books/medical_robotics/telemanipulated_long_bone_fracture_reduction.
7. Westphal Ralf. *Sensor-Based Surgical Robotics: Contributions to Robot Assisted Fracture Reduction.* PhD thesisCarl-Friedrich-Gauß-Fakultät, Technische Universität Carolo-Wilhelmina zu Braunschweig 2007.
8. Khadem Rasool, Yeh Clement C., Sadeghi-Tehrani Mohammad, et al. Comparative Tracking Error Analysis of Five Different Optical Tracking Systems *Computer Aided Surgery.* 2000;5:98–107.
9. Wojciech Glinkowski, Slawomir Paśko, Katarzyna Walesiak, Robert Sitnik, Andrzej Górecki. Merging 3D optical measurement system (structured light-based surface topography) and digital radiograms - the technique and preliminary results *Scoliosis.* 2013;8. O24.
10. Silva Jorge A., Paiva Ana C., Restivo André, Campilho Aurélio C., Pontes J. Laranja. 3-D Surface Characterization Using a Structured Light Technique *Electrónica e Telecomunicações.* 2000;3.
11. Chenyu Wu , Srinivasa G. Narasimhan , Branislav Jaramaz . Shape-from-Shading under Near Point Lighting and Partial views for Orthopedic Endoscopy in *Workshop on Photometric Analysis For Computer Vision (PACV 2007)* 2007.
12. Castellani Umberto, Bartoli Adrien. 3D Shape Registration in *3D Imaging, Analysis and Applications* (Pears Nick, Liu Yonghuai, Bunting Peter. , eds.):221–2643D Imaging, Analysis and Applications 2012. ISBN: 978-1-4471-4062-7.
13. Fitzgibbon Andrew W.. Robust Registration of 2D and 3D Point Sets in *BMVC*:662–670 2001.
14. O´Brien James. *3D Transformations and Rotations.* University of California, Berkeley. Lecture Notes.
15. Lanman Douglas, Taubin Gabriel. *Build Your Own 3D Scanner: 3D Photography for Beginners.* Brown University 2009. ACM SIGGRAPH 2009 Course Notes.
16. Bouguet Jean-Yves. Camera Calibration Toolbox for Matlab http://www.vision.caltech.edu/bouguetj/calib_doc/index.html.

Water as a Third Compartment within the Skin's Stratum Corneum

N.M. Birlea[1], S.I. Birlea[2], and E. Culea[1]

[1] Physics Department, Technical University of Cluj-Napoca, Cluj-Napoca, Romania
[2] Electrical & Electronic Engineering, School of Engineering and Informatics, National University of Ireland Galway, Galway, Ireland

Abstract— **In this position paper we present our view of how water is distributed inside the skin's stratum corneum to create its electrical properties. The existence of a finite electrical resistance of the skin, especially for direct current, implies a continuous domain of water from the surface of the skin to the inner of the body. We propose water as a third compartment in stratum corneum that interpenetrates the other two compartments: intercellular lipids and corneocytes. We suppose that water exchange between the two generally accepted compartments, intercellular lipids and corneocytes, takes place at the junction between corneodesmosomes and lamellar extracellular lipids. We present the evidences from scientific literature sustaining such a view for water distribution in stratum corneum. This assumption could explain some electrical properties of the skin and why skin's permeability to hydrophilic solutes is better predicted by models that imply a substance transport through corneocytes and lipid bilayers in series.**

Keywords— **skin model, water distribution, permeability, transdermal drug delivery, electrical resistance**

I. Introduction

The electrical properties of the skin are important in many medical and non medical applications, such as electrical stimulation (muscle, functional, analgesic or transcranial) [1], drug delivery (mainly iontophoresis) [2], and also in the electrical assessment of skin condition (hydration, cancer) [3] or skin permeability to various substances [2], electrodermal response to various stimuli [1], or acupoint detection and assessment [4], to name a few.

The problem we pose here is why the electrical current, especially direct current, passes through skin. This issue is not trivial because such a phenomenon is conditioned by the existence of a continuous domain of water that contains ions the movement of which generates an electrical current from the surface of the skin to the tissues underneath.

In this position paper we present our view of how water is distributed inside the skin to create its electrical properties. First, we review the results from scientific literature concerning the structure of the skin, mainly its *stratum corneum* (SC), related to water distribution and electrical properties. Then we discuss how the SC components cooperate to manage SC water and the implications of our supposition for describing the electrical behavior and permeability to hydrophilic solutes of the skin. Finally, conclusions are drawn.

II. Epidermal architecture

The skin's water distribution is determined by its functions and structure, which are closely related to each other. The skin's main function is to protect our body from external factors. It has two main layers: the epidermis, on the top, and the dermis, at the bottom.

The epidermis consists of closely packed cells, keratinocytes, organized into several functionally different strata: basal, spinous, granular, lucid, which form the viable epidermis, and *stratum corneum* (SC), the outermost 15-20 layers of dead epidermal cells, the corneocytes [5]. The barrier function of the skin resides primarily in the stratum corneum, it is the shield that protects our inside from outside factors.

The SC is the barrier to the passive diffusion of water out of the skin, allowing us to live in air without suffering from dehydration, and is a barrier against foreign organisms or molecules. This barrier capacity is a function of the structural organization and physical state of the SC.

The structure of the SC was compared to a wall made of bricks (*corneocytes*) and mortar (*intercellular lipids*) in so called "brick and mortar" model [6]. The corneocytes are filled with hydrophilic keratinous filaments and surrounded by an inner *cornified envelope* with an external covalently bound lipid layer. The keratin filaments are cross-linked into tight bundles by filaggrin and this gives the characteristic flattened shape to the corneocytes. The densely packed corneocytes form a resistant network because they are interconnected by the *corneodesmosomes*, transmembranar glycoproteins linked with the keratin cytoskeleton [5].

The corneodesmosomes are evenly distributed around the cell surface in the deepest layers of SC, *SC compactum*, while they are found only at the edges of corneocytes at the outer SC, *SC disjunctum*. Loss of corneodesmosomal components in the corneocytes central areas starts at the bottom of SC and progresses to the surface, resulting in the formation of SC disjunctum and, finally, in desquamation [7]. The different degradation rate of the central and peripheral corneodesmosomes seems to be related to the *tight junctions* (transmembrane proteins that join adjacent membranes

S. Vlad and R.V. Ciupa (eds.), *International Conference on Advancements of Medicine and Health Care through Technology*, IFMBE Proceedings 44,
DOI: 10.1007/978-3-319-07653-9_55, © Springer International Publishing Switzerland 2014

together) that surround peripheral corneodesmosomes and inhibit the access of proteases [8]. So the interconnected corneocytes provide mechanical and chemical protection and together with intercellular lipid surroundings, (~10wt% of dry SC [9]) confer water impermeability to the skin.

The hydrophobic lipid compounds (~50 wt% ceramides, 35 wt% cholesterol and 15 wt% free fatty acids, approximately 1:0.9:0.4 molar ratio) tightly fill the *intercellular space* between corneocytes [10]. These intercellular lipids are organized into *lamellar lipid bilayers* of different periodicity ~13 nm (orthorhombic) and 6 nm (hexagonal) oriented parallel to the surface of the corneocytes and they are considered to form the only continuous structure and the traffic of substances across the skin always has to pass through these regions [11]. For this reason, the organization in the lipid domains is very important for the skin barrier function.

The actual skin barrier models accept the two-compartment structure of the SC (corneocytes–bricks and intercellular lipids–mortar) and focus on the explanation of molecular arrangements of intercellular lipids [12]: *stacked monolayer model* – lipid monolayers between pairs of bilayers; *mosaic domain model* – crystalline domains held together by lipids in a liquid crystalline state; *single gel-phase model* – single and coherent lamellar gel phase without liquid phase; *sandwich model* – a central liquid crystalline domain between two crystalline layers, to name a few. The cement formed by these lipids protects the body from external attacks and also from water loss, an essential feature for the adequate functioning of the inside of the body.

The control of the insensible loss of tissue water across the skin (TEWL–transepidermal water loss) is a very important barrier function of the SC *in vivo*. The non-negligible TEWL appears difficult to explain on basis only of the solid SC lipids [13]. The existence of a lipid fluid phase could allow for the TEWL, for the high elasticity of the skin and for the enzymatic activity in the SC intercellular space that is unlikely to take place in a crystalline phase. For clarifying these issues, extracted SC lipids, isolated corneocytes and whole SC were investigated at different relative humidities (water contents) [13] by means of isothermal sorption microcalorimetry (25°C) and relaxation and wideline ^{1}H NMR. They found that the uptake of water in SC is strongly dependent on the hydration of both the lipids and the corneocytes: at low relative humidities corneocytes take up more water than SC lipids do, while at high relative humidities (>80%) swelling of SC lipids is more pronounced than that of corneocytes. Also, their NMR data clearly have shown the coexistence of fluid and solid lipids.

Another NMR study [14] found that the water added to dry SC, first enters the corneocytes, until ~30% H2O, then water begins to accumulate in hydrated lipid regions. Water was found to exchange between these two domains on a time scale of few hundred milliseconds. Recent sorption studies on SC [15] found similar data with [13] and showed that water enters more rapidly compared to its exit at relative humidities <50%, with sorption time constants having a triphasic behaviour during absorption, but not during desorption.

High-resolution cryo-scanning electron microscopy studies also find that water can penetrate intercellular lipids that form cisternae and networks of spherical particulates [16]. Tan et al. [16] have discerned three rough stages of SC hydration as function of time: stage I. 0-2 h, a SC small expansion (10–20%); stage II. 2-8 h, further swelling of the SC (~50%) and occurrence of small gaps between corneocytes; stage III. 4-10 h, a 300 to 400% expansion of the SC and occurrence of ruptures. They found that the hydrated SC returns to normal (compact packing of corneocytes, without ruptures, dilations or cisternae) after 2–3 h at ambient conditions.

This observation has led them to the hypothesis that the conformations of skin lipids are based on the lipid–water phase diagram: as the water content in the SC returns to the natively hydrated levels, the intercorneocyte lipids again form extended structures. This statement is consistent with an older research on cosmetics and the structure of the SC where the facilitated transdermal transport is identified as a cause for structure-induced irritation due to changed conformations of the SC lipids, changes related to the phase diagram of various substances from the skin and cosmetic substances that facilitated liquid crystal layered structure or crystal structure of the lipids from SC [9]. All these studies point in the same direction, water exists in intercellular space of the SC.

The water is not uniformly distributed throughout SC. A noninvasive method that could determine water and other substances in SC as a function of skin depth is Raman spectroscopy [17]. These measurements confirm the existence of a water gradient in SC, from an inner 60-70 wt% to an outer 20-30 wt% of water usually over 10-20 μm of SC. This water gradient can be used to modulate the transport of drugs through skin like a permeability switch [18], e.g. at high degrees of skin hydration, equivalent with a low water gradient, the transport across skin increases abruptly and the phenomenon is reversible, i.e. the drug traffic nearly stops when the water gradient is high again.

Not only the water distribution but also the water absorption in SC is not uniform [19]. Richter et al. [19] reveal three different hydration zones within the SC: the outermost zone (massive swelling and loosening of intracellular filament packing), the middle zone (the most compact, with the smallest thickness variation) and near *stratum granulosum* the live-dead transition zone (with the highest hygroscopic potential and free unbound water content). They conclude that the SC itself is subdivided into three functional zones with individual water penetration and binding potentials and the middle zone hosts the functional SC barrier, because it is the least affected by hydration.

This finding is sustained by an earlier in vivo experiment [20]. Here the rate of transepidermal water loss (TEWL) and the electrical impedance spectra of the skin were recorded sequentially in vivo in human subjects as layers of the SC were progressively removed by the serial application of adhesive tape strips. The removal of the outermost SC layer had the largest effect on the skin low-frequency impedance, in contrast, TEWL changed little as the outer SC layers were stripped off, but increased dramatically when 6-8 μm of the tissue had been removed (Fig. 1). This strong effect of the first strippings on skin impedance at low frequency was also observed by other investigators [21].

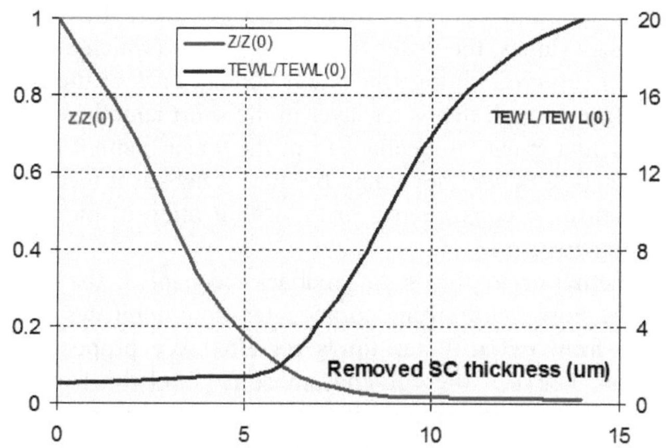

Fig. 1 The changes of the relative electrical impedance (red) and relative transepidermal water loss – TEWL (blue) versus the thickness of removed SC by tape stripping (schematic redrawn after [20])

The special importance of the SC in creating the electrical properties of skin is clearly shown for *in vitro* measurements on SC from human abdominal skin samples obtained after cosmetic surgery [22, 23]. These studies found that the resistance and capacitance of human SC depended nonlinearly on electrical current density, from 13 μA/cm² to 13 mA/cm². The electrical signal was applied as square-wave pulses (500 Hz) of monopolar constant current (5ms anodic, 5ms off, 5 ms cathodic, 5ms off). The human SC samples, exposed for 1h to the electrical current, presented perturbations of the intercellular lipid structure, aggravated with increasing current density, as shown by the electron micrographs and the X-ray diffractograms. Also was observed an increase in the SC hydration level as a result of electrical current application. Similar changes were found *in vivo* in the ultrastructure of human skin after iontophoresis, using cryo-scanning, transmission and freeze fracture electron microscopy [24].

At a higher current density (0.13 mA/cm²) the resistances were lower by a factor of two than the resistances at 13 μA/cm², the decrease was faster than the resolution of the voltage-sampling system (10 μs), and a second slower decrease of the resistances was observed, faster during the first minutes of application, then the resistances approached a rather constant level. During the experiment the voltage across the SC decreased from 10 to 1 V and then remained virtually constant. The activation energy of the resistance was only 0.37 kcal/mol at this current density [22].

For the lowest current density (13 μA/cm²) the resistance and capacitance values remained constant as a function of time, the voltage across SC was about 1V, and the activation energy of ion transport across human SC was 5.4 kcal/mol. Authors considered that this activation energy suggests the presence of highly conductive pathways [22].

The existence of a linear domain of the skin impedance at low voltage and low measuring currents (~10 μA/cm²) was also proved by in vivo experiments [25], but the boundary value between the linear and the nonlinear region was dependent on the measuring conditions and on the test subject. For this sinusoidal measuring signal they also observed slow and rapid variations of the skin impedance, especially for low frequencies and large currents, similarly with those reported by for square-wave electrical pulses [26].

The source of the electrical nonlinearity is SC, as proved by tape stripping experiments [21, 26, 27]. It is worth noting that Lykken [27] was able to separate the skin contribution and the inner body contribution to electrical parameters taking into account that the former depends on the electrode area and the later do not. Lykken also proposed 0.5-1 V as the boundary value between the linear and the nonlinear domain.

The skin has not the same electrical conductivity in every point on its surface. The higher conductivity is related to skin appendages: sweat pores and hair follicles [28], but also to *localized transport regions* (LTRs) which have a much greater surface density than appendages [29]. Two hydrophilic penetration pathways through the SC are probably related to LTRs: a low resistance inter-cluster pathway (between clusters of corneocytes) and a high resistance inter-corneocytes pathway (between the intercellular lipid lamellae) [30].

The radius of most abundant transepidermal hydrophilic pathways is of the order 10 nm, but much narrower (≤0.4 nm, water evaporation pathway) or much wider (~100 nm, inter-corneocytes-cluster pathway) pores may exist in the skin [30].

The size-distribution or density of the artificially created nanoporous pathways through the skin depends on the perturbation type applied to the skin [31]: chemical, ultrasonic, electric, but also depends on model assumptions used to deduce this information [30]. The density of natural intercellular hydrophilic pores in normal skin is estimated to be $\sim 10^7$ pores/cm² and this number increases to $\sim 10^9$ for "mild" perturbations of the skin [32]. Electricity is such a mild perturbation with various effects on skin, depending on electrical signal characteristics. When skin is stimulated with short electrical pulses (<5 ms) new LTRs appear far from appendages, but for pulses with lower voltages but longer duration (U_{skin}<30 V, τ>100 ms) LTRs often coincide with sweat ducts [33].

Any electrical measuring process is a perturbation applied to the skin, but as already mentioned a voltage under 1 V across the skin or a current density less than 10 μA/cm² will not modify SC structure. This is the linear domain of the electrical properties of the skin. Greater current densities or voltages will create a nonlinear dependence between skin impedance and current or voltage. For high voltages the nonlinearity is due to the electroporation of the appendageal macropores or of the SC [34]. For medium voltages and short pulses the skin electrical nonlinearity has not a so clear explanation.

A possible mechanism that could explain the nonlinearity at low voltage is the electrical conduction through a pore as described by the Nernst-Planck model [35]. This is the same model used in electroporation theory [36], but here it is explicitly shown the asymptotic behavior of the current density of pore vs. applied voltage. The main result is that the nonlinear current density as a function of voltage has two linear regions: one at low voltage with a quasi-ohmic, slow rising linear current density, and the other at high voltage with a non-ohmic, fast rising linear current, whose slope is that of the bulk current density, but shifted relative to it by a threshold voltage. The ohmic domain from low voltage is consistent with the aforementioned results.

III. Discussion

The issue of SC hydration, that means to find the site(s) at which water is sequestered in the SC, is a non-trivial, current and much-debated subject [37]. The mechanisms of hydration of the individual building-blocks (lipids and corneocytes) and whether these components have independent or cooperative roles in the hydration of SC are still open questions. It is clear from the experimental evidence presented that water exists both in the corneocytes and extracellular lipids.

The extracellular lipids are considered the sole continuous regions of the SC, and the molecules that pass through the skin barrier must be mainly transported through them [11, 13]. This paradigm seems to be incorrect as more and more scientists recognize that corneocyte phase transport plays a significant role [14, 38] and lateral diffusivities (transport along the lipid sheets) are several orders of magnitude higher than the diffusivity calculated from transbilayer hopping (transport across the lipid sheets). The same idea arises from skin's permeability prediction [39], where the best predictions were from models that modeled the aqueous pathway as consisting of transfer across lipid-corneocyte-lipid-corneocyte in series.

All of these suggest a cooperative mechanism between corneocytes and extracellular lipids. Nakazawa et al. [40] propose such a mechanism for water content adjustment in SC. They observed that X-ray diffraction peak width for short lamellar structure (6 nm) in the intercellular lipid matrix is narrowest at 20-30 wt% water content in the human SC, which means maximum order. When the water content in the SC deviates from 20-30 wt % to either lower or higher values, the water from corneocytes (which acts as a water reservoir) brings the water content back at the normal state through the water layer in the short lamellar structure. This regulation mechanism of the water content at the skin surface is very appealing because it acts as a feedback mechanism, a consequence of the stabilization of the short lamellar structure.

Whether or not this is the feedback mechanism, the problem of how water from corneocytes communicates with water from extracellular lipids remains. We propose the junction between the corneodesmosomes and the lamellar extracellular lipids as the place where water exchange between the two compartments of the SC occurs. This supposition is sustained by many images from the literature [7, 8, 16, 41, 42] that show the close proximity of the ends of lamellar lipid sheets with corneodesmosomes (Fig. 2).

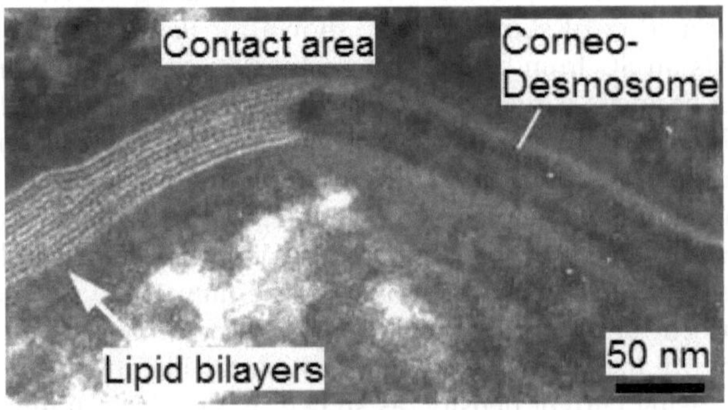

Fig. 2 The close proximity of the ends of lipid bilayers and the corneodesmosome suggests that this is the place where the water from the two compartments communicates (adapted after [42])

Aforementioned skin's permeability models lead to the same conclusion: there is cooperation between the two compartments and hydrophilic solutes must pass through extracellular lipids, mainly along lipid sheets, [38, 39] as well as through corneocytes. In addition, the models for electrical properties of skin at moderate voltages [34, 43] offer more reasonable values of the porated fractional area and electropores dimensions for the "straight-through model" relative to the "tortuous model". Here the "straight-through model" implies the lipid-corneocyte straight-through route, whereas "tortuous model" implies only the lipidic inter-bilayer pathways.

The electrical measurements on tape stripped skin show the large impact of the first stripped layers [20, 21, 25] on the skin low-frequency impedance (which is dominated by electrical resistance). This behavior can be explained by our hypothesis because the outermost SC layers contain few corneodesmosomes and the electric current path is mainly through tortuous extracellular lipids. Progressively removing these layers, the electric current has access to layers that contain more corneodesmosomes and consequently more electrical "shortcuts" through corneocytes and lower resistance.

As generally accepted, the extracellular lamellar lipids seal the space between corneocytes. To do so, the intercellular lipids adhere to the corneocyte-bound lipid envelope, which function as a scaffold for the organization of the extracellular lamellar bilayers, as needed for barrier function of SC [44]. This arrangement allows a very good sealing around corneocytes and corneodesmosomes. Such a sealing works well even if the parts (corneocytes) are slightly moving, especially if the extracellular lipids have elasticity and act as a self-healing material.

The role of corneodesmosomes in water management in the SC can also be seen from a pathologic dryness of the skin, "winter xerosis", in which the surface of corneocytes from the outer SC has an increased number of corneodesmosomes compared to those of normal skin [45]. This fact sustains the idea that corneodesmosomes have a very important role in water preservation in our body.

IV. Conclusions

In our view the skin's stratum corneum consists of three compartments which are extended over its entire thickness: corneocytes, intercellular lipids and water. While two of these compartments, corneocytes and intercellular lipids, can be clearly separated, the water compartment interpenetrates both. The major problem remaining is to find the place where water from corneocytes and intercellular lipids makes contact.

We propose the corneodesmosomes as the main link between water from inside the corneocytes and water from intercellular lipids. This assumption can explain the behavior of electrical resistance of the skin when SC is progressively removed. It also explains the more reasonable values of the skin's permeability to hydrophilic solutes of the models that take into account a substance transport through extracellular lipids and corneocytes, in series, and along rather than across the lipid bilayers.

Conflict of Interest

The authors declare that they have no conflict of interest.

References

1. Malmivuo J, Plonsey R. (1995). Bioelectromagnetism: principles and applications of bioelectric and biomagnetic fields. Oxford University Press, New York.
2. Li SK et al. (1998) Characterization of the transport pathways induced during low to moderate voltage iontophoresis in human epidermal membrane. Journal of Pharmaceutical Sciences 87(1) 40-48.
3. Ollmar S, Nicander I. (2005) Within and beyond the skin barrier as seen by electrical impedance, p335 in Bioengineering of the skin: water and stratum corneum. edited by Joachim Fluhr et. al. 2nd ed., CRC Press 2005
4. Ahn A C, Martinsen Ø G. (2007). Electrical characterization of acupuncture points: technical issues and challenges. The journal of alternative and complementary medicine, 13(8), 817-824.
5. Proksch E, Brandner JM, Jensen JM. (2008) The skin: an indispensable barrier. Exp Dermatol 17(12):1063-1072.
6. Elias P M (1983) Epidermal Lipids, Barrier Function, and Desquamation, Journal of Investigative Dermatology 80(6 Supplement) 44s-49s
7. Haftek M, Callejon S, Sandjeu Y, et. al. (2011) Compartmentalization of the human stratum corneum by persistent tight junction-like structures. Exp Dermatol 20(8):617-21.
8. Igawa S, Kishibe M, Murakami M, et. al. (2011) Tight junctions in the stratum corneum explain spatial differences in corneodesmosome degradation. Exp Dermatol 20(1):53-7.
9. Friberg SE (1990) Micelles, microemulsions, liquid crystals, and the structure of stratum corneum lipids, J Soc Cosmet Chem 41(3) 155-171.
10. Norlen L, Plasencia I, Bagatolli L (2008). Stratum corneum lipid organization as observed by atomic force, confocal and two-photon excitation fluorescence microscopy. International journal of cosmetic science 30(6), 391-411.
11. Bouwstra JA et al. (2003) Structure of the skin barrier and its modulation by vesicular formulations. Prog Lipid Res 42(1):1-36.
12. Kessner D, Ruettinger A, Kiselev MA, et al. (2008) Properties of ceramides and their impact on the stratum corneum structure: a review. Part 2: stratum corneum lipid model systems. Skin Pharmacol Physiol 21(2):58-74.
13. Silva C L, Topgaard D, Kocherbitov V, et al. (2007) Stratum corneum hydration: Phase transformations and mobility in stratum corneum, extracted lipids and isolated corneocytes. Biochim Biophys Acta 1768(11):2647-2659.

14. Laule C, Tahir S, Chia CL, et al. (2010) A proton NMR study on the hydration of normal versus psoriatic stratum corneum: linking distinguishable reservoirs to anatomical structures. NMR Biomed. 23(10):1181-90.
15. Johnsen GK, Martinsen ØG, Grimnes S. (2010) Sorption studies of human keratinized tissues, J Phys: Conf Ser 224:012094 doi: 10.1088/1742-6596/224/1/012094.
16. Tan G, Xu P, Lawson LB, et al. (2010) Hydration effects on skin microstructure as probed by high-resolution cryo-scanning electron microscopy and mechanistic implications to enhanced transcutaneous delivery of biomacromolecules. J Pharm Sci 99(2):730-740.
17. Egawa M, Tagami H. (2008) Comparison of the depth profiles of water and water-binding substances in the stratum corneum determined in vivo by Raman spectroscopy between the cheek and volar forearm skin: effects of age, seasonal changes and artificial forced hydration. Br J Dermatol 158(2) 251-60.
18. Björklund S, Engblom J, Thuresson K, Sparr E. (2010) A water gradient can be used to regulate drug transport across skin. J Control Release 143(2):191-200.
19. Richter T, Peuckert C, Sattler M, et al. (2004) Dead but highly dynamic–the stratum corneum is divided into three hydration zones. Skin Pharmacol Physiol 17(5):246-57.
20. Kalia YN, Pirot F, Guy RH. (1996) Homogeneous transport in a heterogeneous membrane: water diffusion across human stratum corneum in vivo. Biophys J 71(5):2692-700.
21. Yamamoto T, Yamamoto Y. (1976) Electrical properties of the epidermal stratum corneum. Med Biol Eng 14(2) 151-158.
22. Craane-van Hinsberg WHM, Verhoef JC, Junginger HE et al. (1997) Electroperturbation of the human skin barrier in vitro (I): the influence of current density on the thermal behaviour of skin impedance. Eur J Pharm Biopharm 43(1)43-50.
23. Craane-Van Hinsberg IW, Verhoef JC, Spies F et al. (1997) Electroperturbation of the human skin barrier in vitro: II. Effects on stratum corneum lipid ordering and ultrastructure. Microsc Res Tech 37(3):200-213.
24. Fatouros DG, Groenink HW, de Graaff AM et al. (2006) Visualization studies of human skin in vitro/in vivo under the influence of an electrical field. Eur J Pharm Sci. 29(2):160-170.
25. Yamamoto T, Yamamoto Y. (1981) Non-linear electrical properties of skin in the low frequency range, Med Biol Eng Comput 19(3) 302-310.
26. van Boxtel A (1977) Skin resistance during square-wave electrical pulses of 1 to 10 mA, Med Biol Eng Comput 15(6) 679-657.
27. Lykken DT (1970) Square-wave analysis of skin impedance. Psychophysiology 7(2) 262-275.
28. Trommer H, Neubert RHH. (2006) Overcoming the stratum corneum: the modulation of skin penetration. A Review. Skin Pharmacol Physiol 19(2):106–121.
29. Scott ER, White HS, Phipps JB. (1992) Direct imaging of ionic pathways in stratum corneum using scanning electrochemical microscopy, Solid State Ionics 53-56(Part 1) 176-183.
30. Cevc G (2004) Lipid vesicles and other colloids as drug carriers on the skin, Adv Drug Deliv Rev 56(5) 675-711.
31. Polat BE, Figueroa PL, Blankschtein D et al. (2011) Transport pathways and enhancement mechanisms within localized and non-localized transport regions in skin treated with low-frequency sonophoresis and sodium lauryl sulfate. J Pharm Sci 100(2):512-29.
32. Cevc G, Vierl U. (2010) Nanotechnology and the transdermal route: A state of the art review and critical appraisal. J Control Release 141(3) 277-299.
33. Pliquett U, Gusbeth Ch, Nuccitelli R. (2008) A propagating heat wave model of skin electroporation. J Theor Biol 251(2):195-201.
34. Chizmadzhev YA, Indenbom AV, Kuzmin PI, et al. (1998) Electrical properties of skin at moderate voltages: contribution of appendageal macropores, Biophysical Journal 74(2) 843–856.
35. Bîrlea NM, Bîrlea SI, (2012) The current-voltage relation of a pore and its asymptotic behavior in a Nernst-Planck model. Journal of Electrical Bioimpedance 3: 36–41.
36. DeBruin K A, Krassowska W. (1999) Modeling electroporation in a single cell. II. Effects of ionic concentrations. Biophys J. 77(3): 1225–1233.
37. Elias P M (2012). Structure and function of the stratum corneum extracellular matrix. J Invest Dermatol 132(9) 2131-2133.
38. Wang T F, Kasting G B, Nitsche J M. (2006). A multiphase microscopic diffusion model for stratum corneum permeability. I. Formulation, solution, and illustrative results for representative compounds. Journal of pharmaceutical sciences, 95(3), 620-648.
39. Chen L, Han L, Lian G. (2013). Recent advances in predicting skin permeability of hydrophilic solutes. Advanced Drug Delivery Reviews, 65(2), 295-305.
40. Nakazawa H, Ohta N, Hatta I. (2012). A possible regulation mechanism of water content in human stratum corneum via intercellular lipid matrix. Chemistry and physics of lipids 165(2), 238-243.
41. Lin T K, Crumrine D, Ackerman L D, et al. (2012). Cellular changes that accompany shedding of human corneocytes. Journal of Investigative Dermatology, 132(10), 2430-2439.
42. Wertz P W, (2000) Lipids and barrier function of the skin, Acta Derm Venereol, Supp 208: 7-11.
43. Chizmadzhev Y A, Zarnitsin V G, Weaver J C, Potts R O. (1995). Mechanism of electroinduced ionic species transport through a multilamellar lipid system. Biophysical journal 68(3), 749-765.
44. Elias P M, Gruber R, Crumrine D et al. (2013) Formation and functions of the corneocyte lipid envelope (CLE). Biochimica et Biophysica Acta (BBA)-Molecular and Cell Biology of Lipids.xxx
45. Rawlings AV, (2003) Trends in stratum corneum research and the management of dry skin conditions, Int J Cosmet Sci 25(1-2) 63–95.

Author address:

Author: Nicolae-Marius Bîrlea
Institute: Technical University of Cluj-Napoca
Street: Daicoviciu 15
City: Cluj-Napoca
Country: Romania
Email: mbirlea@phys.utcluj.ro

Evaluating SAR Distribution on the Human Head during MRI Examination as Function of Frequency

C. Marincaş[1], A. Nicu[1], C. Csutak[2], and R.V. Ciupa[1]

[1] Technical University of Cluj-Napoca, Electrotechnics and Measurements Department, Cluj-Napoca, Romania

[2] "IuliuHatieganu" University of Medicine and Farmacy of Cluj-Napoca, Cluj-Napoca, Romania

Abstract— **The present paper aims to evaluate the specific absorption rate (SAR) distribution in human head during MRI examinations. Numerical calculations of the SAR distribution into the human head during the Magnetic Resonance Imaging (MRI) proceedings were performed in SEMCAD X software based on the Finite Difference Time Domain (FDTD) method. The SAR distribution due to human head exposure to radio frequency radiation during MRI revealed areas with increased values. Based on our work, exposure threshold values could limit the number of investigations using MRI. Thus, research made during the preparation of this paper and the results obtained are very important both for the medical world as well as the legislative involved in the issue.**

Keywords— **MRI safety, SAR, FDTD, SEMCAD X**

I. Introduction

The physiologic and thermoregulatory responses of the human head exposure to radio frequency (RF) radiation are directly depending on the amount of the absorbed energy. Knowing that Specific Absorption Rate (SAR) distribution produced during a Magnetic Resonance Imaging (MRI) investigation is a function of variables such as: frequency, the type of RF coil used, the configuration of the anatomical region exposed, the present paper focuses on SAR distribution into the human head during MRI examination. Numerical calculations of the SAR distribution into the human head during the MRI proceedings were performed in SEMCAD X software based on the Finite Difference Time Domain (FDTD) method. The obtained results are in perfect agreement with the dispersion character of biological tissues.

Magnetic Resonance Imaging (MRI) is a non invasive technique which provides stabile and reliable information of brain structure. It is a direct multiplanar imaging modality, has an excellent tissue contrast resolution and a high sensitivity for brain water [1].

MRI is the most sensitive imaging modality for detecting brain abnormalities, even during the early stages of the disease. It is exquisitely sensitive for white matter disease, for evaluation of the posterior fossa, the sellaturcica and pituitary gland; has a great value in evaluation of congenital malformations of the brain. When the blood-brain barrier is damaged, enhancement occurs with gadolinium contrast agent, the degree of enhancement is greater with the MR scans compared to the Computed Tomography (CT) scans [2].

Precise numbers of the MRI examinations are not available; some marketing studies suggested that between the introduction of clinical MRI in the early 1980 and the end of 2007 more than 400.000.000 diagnostic MRI studies were performed. The 1.5 [T] operating systems have been the standard for high-performance MRI. During the recent years the development of the higher filed strength systems for clinical and research use increased significantly. In particular 3 [T] systems are now in use in many clinical centers for examinations of soft tissues and brain. A few research centers have 7 [T] magnets, or individual prototype systems with 8 [T] and 9.4 [T] magnets. The anatomic details are most relevant with these high field magnets [3].

The electromagnetic field energy generated by the RF coil in the MRI imaging is unevenly absorbed by the exposed tissues depending on their dielectric properties (relative permittivity, electrical conductivity and relative permeability). In MRI examinations of the brain using a standard head coil, the produced energy will be found mostly in the cephalic extremity of the examined patient. To assess the amount of energy absorbed by the tissue the notion of SAR (Specific Absorption Rate) was introduced.

SAR is defined as the dosimetric measure characterizing the energy rate absorbed by biological tissues when exposed to a radiofrequency electromagnetic field. The absorbed energy is converted into heat, and therefore it is necessary to monitor SAR, in order to not affect the involved tissue.

$$\mathrm{SAR} = \frac{\sigma E^2}{\rho}, \tag{1}$$

where: E is the electric field [V/m], σ is the electrical conductivity [S/m] and ρ is the density [kg/m^3]. The unit of SAR is watts per kilogram [W/kg] [4].

In MRI, SAR depends on several variables such as: operating frequency of the RF coil, the RF pulse sequence used (90° vs. 180°), the repetition time, the type of coil used to transmit RF pulse sequences, the tissue volume located in transmitting coil, the configuration of the anatomical region exposed and other factors, but in a smaller proportion [5].

S. Vlad and R.V. Ciupa (eds.), *International Conference on Advancements of Medicine and Health Care through Technology*, IFMBE Proceedings 44,
DOI: 10.1007/978-3-319-07653-9_56,

The SAR distribution in human head exposed to electromagnetic field has been estimated in the scientific literature through numerical and experimental calculations [6] – [8]. The models used in these studies are very different, taking into account from a few too many tissue types, from simple geometries to enhanced ones, thus the results obtained sometimes differs.

II. MATERIAL AND METHODS

Due to the progress in computer technology, the Finite-Difference Time-Domain (FDTD) method can be used in numerical calculation of the electromagnetic field interaction with the realistic human head during the MRI proceedings [9]. Our model was implemented in SEMCAD X.

SEMCAD X is a 3D wave electromagnetic and thermal simulation platform suitable for MRI coils, medical implant devices and other design applications. The program offers a user friendly interface and the simulations are performed in graphic mode.

In order to examine the head through MRI investigation a Birdcage coil is used. Depending on the static magnetic field of the equipment, a RF coil is to be implemented in order to obtain the resonance phenomena:

$$\omega_0 = \gamma B_0, \quad (2)$$

where (ω_0 is the precessional frequency [MHz] (Larmour frequency), B_0 is the static magnetic field [T] and γ is the gyro magnetic ratio of a certain nuclear spin [MHz/T]).

The analysis for the SAR behavior of the biological tissue during the MRI investigations was realized for the magnetic fields of 1.5 [T], 3 [T], 7 [T] and the resonance frequencies of 64 [MHz], 128 [MHz] and 300 [MHz]. There are three types of coils in general: transmission - reception coils, transmission coils and reception coils. For the SAR behavior analysis of the tissue the transmission coil is used.

The design of the low-pass birdcage RF coil with 8 longitudinal elements (legs) (length=180 [mm], end-rings diameter=240 [mm]) implemented in SEMCAD X is presented in figure 1.

The RF coil design proposed by the SEMCAD developers was used in the model [10]-[11].

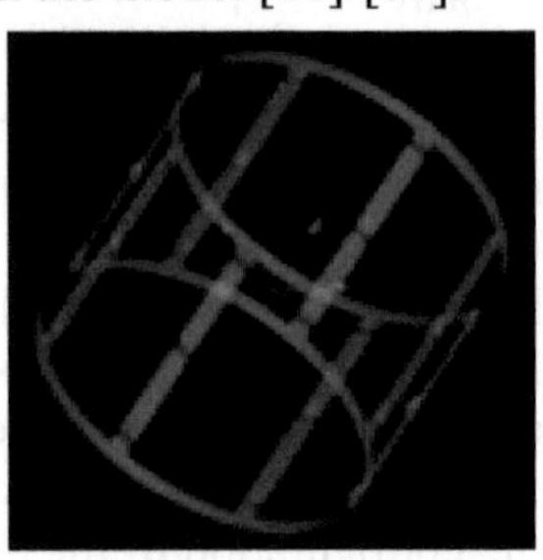

Fig. 1 Low-pass birdcage RF coil design

In the middle of each leg - segment a current source (red) and at the very end of the elements capacitors (blue) were implemented. The numerical values for the capacitors used are with respect to the work frequency: 32.4 [pF], 8 [pF] and 1.48 [pF]. A sinusoidal waveform with an amplitude of 1 [A] was used for the current sources. Each signal was dephased with 1/8*period.

The human model utilized for simulation is a male from the virtual family with the following characteristics: male, 34 years, 1.77 [m], 72.4 [Kg], 77 tissues, available in virtual family developed by IT'IS Foundation, Switzerland (www.itis.ethz.ch/itis- for-health/virtual-population/human-models/duke/). In our paper we used the 2 [mm] voxel resolution for Duke.

Duke was introduced into the RF coil (figure 2) and boundaries were used to truncate de torso. The simulations were performed according to the parameters that were already established and the simulation time was 30 periods.

Meshing was accomplished using the automatic grid generation model adapted to detail additional requirements: increased details for X and Y axis of the coil to eliminate possible problems that could be caused by the curvature of the coil and for three axes in the case of the skull to increase resolution in the brain.

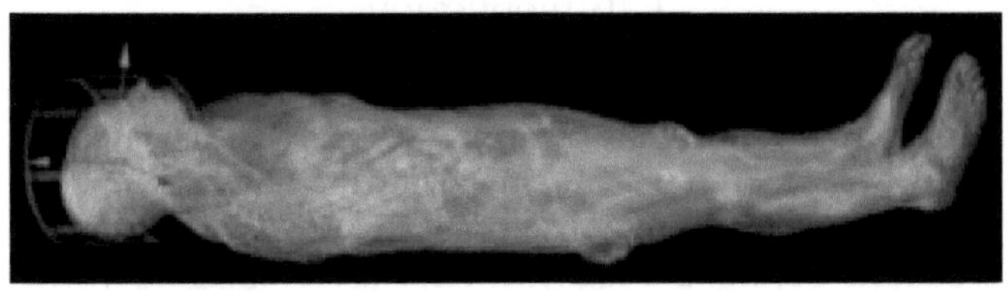

Fig. 2 Model positioning into the RF coil.

III. RESULTS

For the specific model tissues one can import the tissue properties that characterize the model for each resonance frequency. The results obtained regarding to the resonance frequency are separated in 3 cases:

1. 64 [MHz] Resonance Frequency

After discretization for 64 [MHz] resonance frequency case it was obtained a number of 224*243*189=10287600 cells. The results obtained after the simulation of the SAR distribution in the head are presented in figure 3.

All the values are db normalized. The maximum value is 3.53 [mW/g] and it is situated in the anterior segment of the right maxillary sinus mucosal. One can observe increased values of SAR in the soft parts of the nose base, the suboccipitale region (more obvious in the left paramedian region) or in the subarachnoid space over the falxcerebri.

2. 128 [MHz] Resonance Frequency

After discretization for 64 [MHz] resonance frequency case it was obtained a number of 211*225*177=8403070 cells. The results obtained after the simulation of the SAR distribution in the head are presented in figure 4.

All the values are db normalized. The maximum value is 3.8 [mW/g] and it is situated at the cerebrospinal fluid level from the left cerebellar hemisphere. After viewing the 3D SAR distribution, other areas with increased SAR values were discovered as follows: subocular region in the right, gray-matter fronto-parieto-occipital bilateral soft parts of the nose base and suboccipitale region.

3. 300 [MHz] Resonance Frequency

After discretization for 300 [MHz] resonance frequency case it was obtained 227*226*169=8670040 cells. The results obtained after the simulation of the SAR distribution in the head are presented in figure 5.

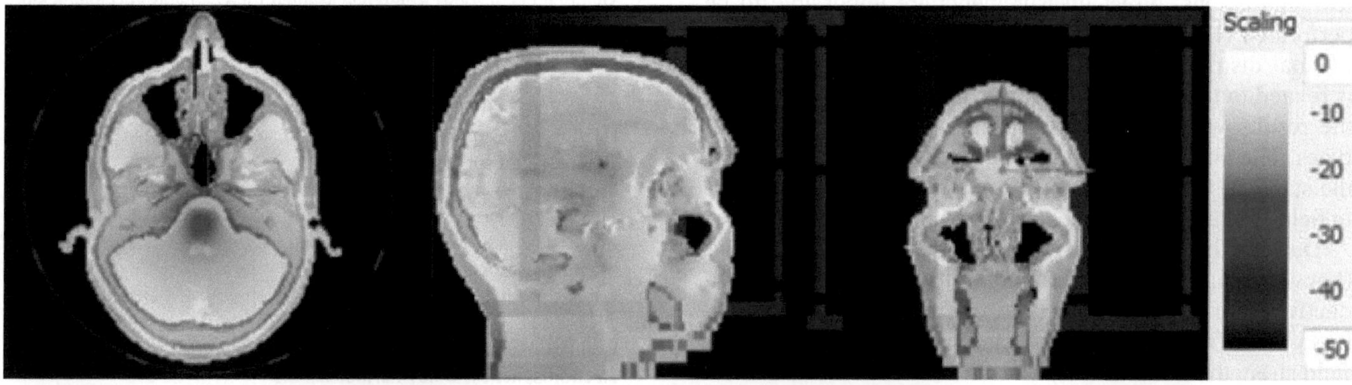

Fig. 3 SAR (64 [MHz]) distribution in axial, sagittal and coronal plane

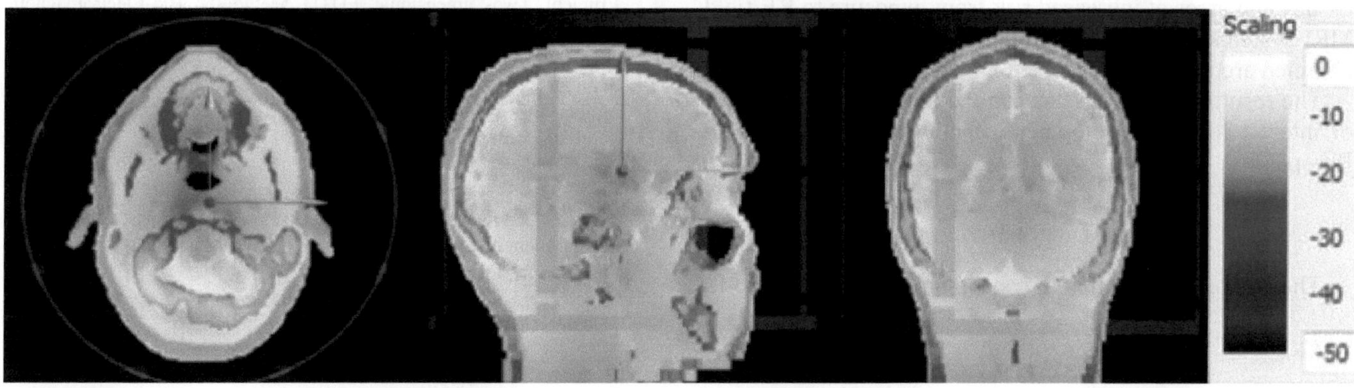

Fig. 4 SAR (128 [MHz]) distribution in axial, sagittal and coronal plane

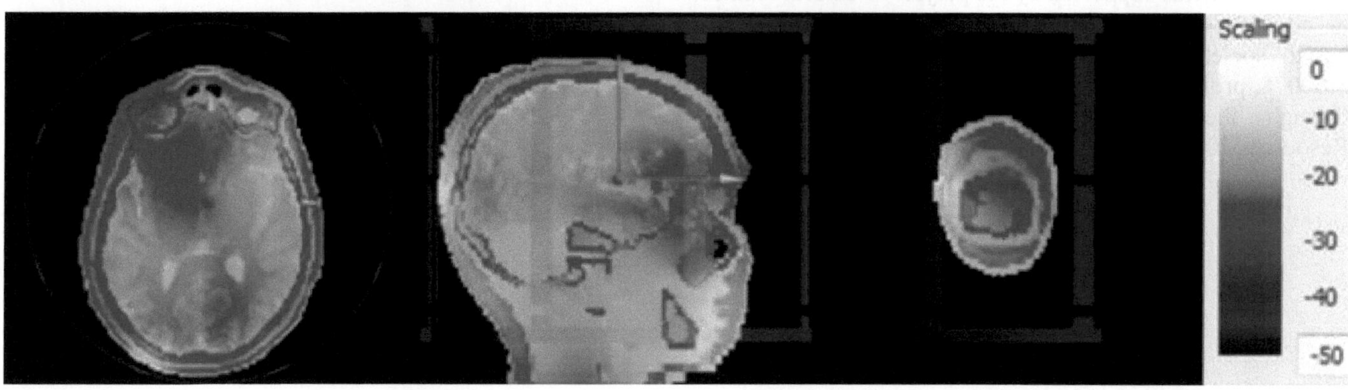

Fig. 5 SAR (300 [MHz]) distribution in axial, sagittal and coronal plane

All the values are db normalized. The maximum value is 8.63 [mW/g] and it is situated subcutaneously, in the left occipital region. After 3D visual appreciation, the high values of SAR were recorded at the left bucal region and the soft parts in the right suboccipital area.

IV. Conclusions

The possibility to evaluate the interaction between electromagnetic fields and biological tissues is given by numerical simulations; direct measurements are impossible to be performed. Besides the advantage of evaluating SAR and thermal distribution in biological tissues another advantage is related to the design of RF coils: to ensure high quality of the results without carrying out a large number of prototypes. The aim in designing these types of coils is to respect the standards and limitations on exposure to electromagnetic fields by minimizing adequate bond SAR value.

Due to the dispersion properties of biological tissues (knowing that the relative permittivity and electrical conductivity are nonlinear functions of frequency) SAR distribution is different in MRI systems with different magnetic field strength.

Our study showed the dispersed nature of biological tissues and areas at increased risk from exposure to RF field MRI systems. In normal conditions, the temperature values obtained are within the accepted limits.

The results reported in this paper addresses a certain area of interest for the development of clinical environment in Europe.

Conflict of Interest

The authors declare that they have no conflict of interest.

Acknowledgment

This work was supported by the project "Doctoral studies in engineering sciences for Developing the knowledge-based society SIDOC" contract no. POSDRU/88/1.5/ S/60078, project co-Funded from the European Social Fund through the Sectorial Operational Program Human Resources 2007 -2013.

References

1. Suzuki M, Kawasaki Y, Takayanagi Y, Nakamura K, Takahashi T (2012) Structural MRI- based classification: possible contributions to clinical diagnosis of schizophrenia. Psychiatria et Neurologia Japonica, 114(7):807-11
2. Edelman R, HesselinkJ, Zlatkin M (2005) Clinical Magnetic Resonance Imaging, 3-rd Ed. Elsevier
3. Scott W (2009) Atlas, Magnetic Resonance Imaging of the Brain and Spine, 4-th Ed., Lippincott Williams & Wilkins, Philadelphia,.
4. http://www.icmet.ro/SAREMF.pdf, accessed 2013
5. Shellock FG., (2009) Reference Manual for Magnetic Resonance Safety, Implants, and Devices. Biomedical Research Publishing Group, Los Angeles, CA
6. Baker KB, Tkach J, Hall JD, Nyenhuis JA, Shellock FG, Rezai AR (2005) Reduction of Magnetic Resonance Imaging-Related Heating in Deep Brain Stimulation Leads Using a Lead Management Device. Neurosurgery
7. Baker KB, Nyenhuis JA, Hrdlicka G, Rezai AR, Tkach JA, Shellock FG (2005) Neurostimulation Systems: Assessment of Magnetic Field Interactions Associated With 1.5- and 3-Tesla MR Systems, Journal of Magnetic Resonance Imaging
8. Cabot E, Lloyd T, Christ A, Kainz W, Douglas M, Stenzel G, Wedan S , Kuster N (2012) Evaluation of the RFHeating of a Generic Deep-Brain Stimulator Exposedin 1.5 T MagneticResonance Scanners, Bioelectromagnetics, Wiley Periodicals,Inc
9. Qiang R, Wu D, Chen J, Wang S, Wilton D, Kainz W (2006)An Efficient Two-Dimensional FDTD Methodfor Bio-Electromagnetic Applications, IEEE Transactions on Magnetics DOI 10.1109/TMAG.2006.871947
10. Schmid& Partner Engineering AG (2012), SEMCAD X Reference Manual
11. Schmid& Partner Engineering AG, (2011), SEMCAD X Tutorial

Cristinel Marincas
Department of Electrical Engineering and Measurement
Faculty of Electrical Engineering
Technical University of Cluj-Napoca, Romania
E-mail: Cristinel.Marincas@et.utcluj.ro

Evaluation of Thermal Distribution in the Head Following Exposure to an Electromagnetic Field Generated by a MRI Birdcage-Type RF Coil

C. Marincaş[1], A. Nicu[1], C. Csutak[2], and R.V. Ciupa[1]

[1] Technical University of Cluj-Napoca, Electrotechnics and Measurements Department, Cluj-Napoca, Romania
[2] "IuliuHatieganu" University of Medicine and Farmacy of Cluj-Napoca, Cluj-Napoca, Romania

Abstract— **The present paper aims to evaluate the thermal distribution in the head following exposure to an electromagnetic field generated by a Magnetic Resonance Imaging (MRI) birdcage-type Radio Frequency (RF) coil. The paper presents numerical calculations of the thermal distribution in the head using Finite Difference Time Domain (FDTD) method. The direct effect obtained due to human head exposure to radio frequency radiation is heating of the exposed tissue, but in usual exposure conditions, the temperature rise was situated in the accepted limits. Tissue heating from exposure to RF waves generated by the transmitter coil during MRI examination is one of the most important issues related to patient safety. After thermal modeling using SEMCAD X and compared with the SAR distribution obtained after the electromagnetic simulateon, the body's thermoregulatory ability was outlined, using the established boundary conditions for the background, internal regions of air and blood vessels. The obtained results revealed that numerical modeling (that was experimental validated in the final form) is suitable for medical product evaluation (eg. RF coils) in order to respect the safety regulations imposed by law.**

Keywords— **MRI safety, RF heating, FDTD, SEMCAD X**

I. INTRODUCTION

MRI examination is one of the most important techniques for head investigations. As a technique that does not use ionizing radiation it is suitable to be used without the restrictions of age or the number of previous examinations.

One of the issues related to patient safety during MRI examination is tissue heating from exposure to RF waves generated by the transmitter coil. In this sense, at world level, minimum requirements for the safety of magnetic resonance equipment used in medical diagnosis were established. Limits for exposure imposed by the international standard IEC 60601-2-33 are referred to those adopted in the European Community:

Limits for Whole Body Heating during MRI:

- *Normal mode limit (suitable for all patients) - 0.5 [°C] or 2 [W/kg];*
- *First level controlled mode (requires medical supervision) - 1.0 [°C] or 4 [W/kg];*
- *Second level controlled mode - greater than 1 [°C] or 4 [W/kg] (requires Institutional Review Board (IRB) approval).*

Localized Heating during MRI:

- *Head normal mode limit – 38 [°C] or 3.2 [W/kg] averaged over the head mass;*
- *Torso normal mode limit – 39 [°C] or 10 [W/kg] over any 10 grams of tissue;*
- *Extremities normal mode limit – 40 [°C] or 10 [W/kg] over any 10 grams of tissue;*
- *No first level for head, torso or extremities.*

Averaging time: 6 minutes.

During the MRI examination, the tissues are exposed to the electromagnetic field generated by the RF transmitter coil. Most of the energy is absorbed by the exposed tissue and then turned into heat as a result of resistive losses. The thermal response of tissues exposed during MRI examination depends on several factors: physiological (body's thermoregulatory capacity), physical (SAR - Specific Absorption Rate, duration of exposure, etc.), and environmental (environmental conditions of the MRI system, etc.). The human body dissipates heat by convection, conduction, radiation and evaporation in order to maintain thermal equilibrium. If the body's thermoregulatory ability does not handle the amount of the absorbed energy, heat accumulation areas appears at the exposed tissues level [1].

Even if a human subject has an effective thermoregulatory system by which the values of the temperature are in ranges imposed by standards and limitations, its exposure will be limited by appropriate SAR.

II. MATERIAL AND METHODS

To evaluate the thermal distribution in the head during an MRI examination (1.5 [T], 3 [T] and 7 [T] strength), using a standard RF coil we used numerical simulation environment SEMCAD X v.14.8 Aletsch developed by Schmidt& Partner Engineering (SPEAG) Switzerland (www.speag.com). Thermal simulations are based on the results obtained in a previous study that evaluates the distribution of SAR in the head, in the same conditions of exposure. Details of the simulation environment SEMCAD X and on results obtained in the evaluation of SAR distribution in the head using a RF coil operating frequencies of 64 [MHz], 128 [MHz] and 300 [MHz], corresponding 1.5 [T] MRI systems, respectively 3 [T], 7 [T], are presented in [2]. Phantom of

S. Vlad and R.V. Ciupa (eds.), *International Conference on Advancements of Medicine and Health Care through Technology*, IFMBE Proceedings 44,
DOI: 10.1007/978-3-319-07653-9_57, © Springer International Publishing Switzerland 2014

study is identical to that of the previous study, Duke (male, 35 years) with a resolution of 2 [mm], available in virtual family developed IT'IS Foundation, Switzerland (http://www.itis.ethz.ch/itis- for-health/ virtual-population/human-models/duke/).

Pennes thermal simulation model was needed to describe the heat transfer related to bloodstream, thus the Pennes bio-heat equation was used:

$$\rho \cdot c \cdot \frac{\partial T}{\partial t} = \nabla \cdot (k \nabla T) + \rho Q + \rho S - \rho_b c_b \rho \omega (T - T_b), \quad (1)$$

where: k [W/(m°C)]-the tissue thermal conductivity, S - Specific Absorption Rate [W/kg], ω [kg/(m^{3}s)]- the blood perfusion rate, Q [W/m^3] - the metabolic heat generation rate, ρ [kg/m^3]–the tissue density, ρ_b [kg/m^3] – blood density, c_b[J/(kg°C)] – the bloodspecific heat, T_b [°C]-temperature of blood.

Only the increase representation of the temperature was set, and as a source for thermal simulation reference to electromagnetic simulation was made. There were established three boundary conditions for: environment, internal regions of air and blood vessels. Types of boundary conditions that we have available in thermal simulation are: Neumann (flux flow determines whether inside or outside the solid, zero involving the two solid insulation), Dirichlet (fixed temperature is given interface) and mixed (effects modeling is as close convection - cooling due to the cooling effect due to blood or body ambient air). Thermal solver can be used to calculate the absolute temperature or temperature variation, depending on the initial conditions of temperature settings for different regions and border conditions. If the initial temperatures are set to zero then only the calculate temperature rise will be computed [3][4].

It has been set as a mixed type of outdoor temperature limit of zero and six, heat transfer among all tissues and the environment. For each: the esophageal lumen, trachea and pharynx lumen, and all tissues was chosen as one of Neumann boundary at zero heat flux, if arteries and veins have been chosen as the outside temperature limit Dirichlet type zero.

III. RESULTS AND DISCUSSIONS

1. 64 [MHz] Resonance Frequency

The maximum increased temperature of 0.113 [°C] was registered at the soft parts of the nose base. Excepting the maximum value, thermal distribution corresponding to the SAR for the same value of the resonance frequency (64 [MHz]), increased temperatures were registered in the sub-occipital region, respectively in the subarahnoid region alongside the falxcerebri (figure 1).

The reason the two values of maximum SAR or temperature, do not match is because the maximum SAR is only a punctate area. Following SAR mediation by 1 [g] or 10 [g] of tissue one can observe that the maximum area is recorded for the corresponding maximum thermal simulation.

2. 128 [MHz] Resonance Frequency

The maximum increased temperature is 0.102 degrees Celsius and has a right subocular disposal. Elevated temperatures were registered at the soft parts of the nose base and the top right region of the mouth. Discrete temperature rise was observed in the suboccipital region, respectively in the parietal subarahnoid space, adjacent vertex(figure 2).

Analyzing the SAR distribution for 128 [MHz] was observed that the maximum temperature values do not correspond to the maximum SAR limitations. The reason for maximum mismatch is similar to that specified for 64 [MHz]. There are anatomical areas where increased temperature values correspond to those of the increased SAR as follows: the soft parts of the nose base and the suboccipital region. Representing the SAR averaged over 1 [g] and 10 [g] helps us observe the most important areas with elevated SAR and the most extensive areas that have accumulated energy generated by the RF coil. Another important aspect of representation is the average SAR that it suggests areas predisposed to thermal heating. Through 1 [g] mediation, increased value is recorded in the soft parts of the nose and through 10 [g] mediation maximum values was recorded in the white matter and cerebrospinal fluid adjacent vertex. These figures show that a large amount of energy is absorbed in the soft parts of the nose and gray matter. The cerebrospinal fluid of vertex site is the most extensive area with increased SAR. An explanation of the fact that the highest temperature region is not found in areas with increased SAR may be due to boundary conditions imposed on the environment, internal regions of air and blood vessels.

3. 300 [MHz] Resonance Frequency

The value of the increase temperature is obtained for 0.11 degrees Celsius and is in the area of the left occipital subcutaneous tissue. Significant temperature area is also obtained in the oral cavity mainly on the left (figure 3). After analyzing the SAR distribution at 300 [MHz], it was found that maximum temperature corresponds to the maximum SAR limitations. Also areas with SAR distribution averaged over 1 [g] and 10 [g] of tissue are found in regions with increased temperatures. The fact that increased SAR regions overlap the increased temperature is due to the fact that the frequency of 300 [MHz] characterized by a increased SAR are not greatly affected by the boundary conditions imposed.

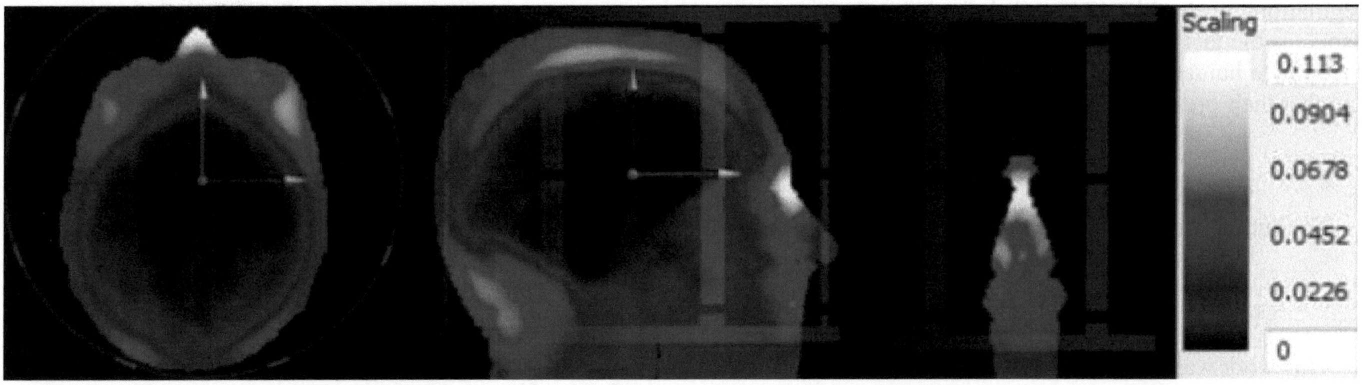

Fig. 1 Temperature distribution in the three planes of section (axial, sagittal and coronal) passing through the maximum value of the resonant frequency of 64 [MHz]

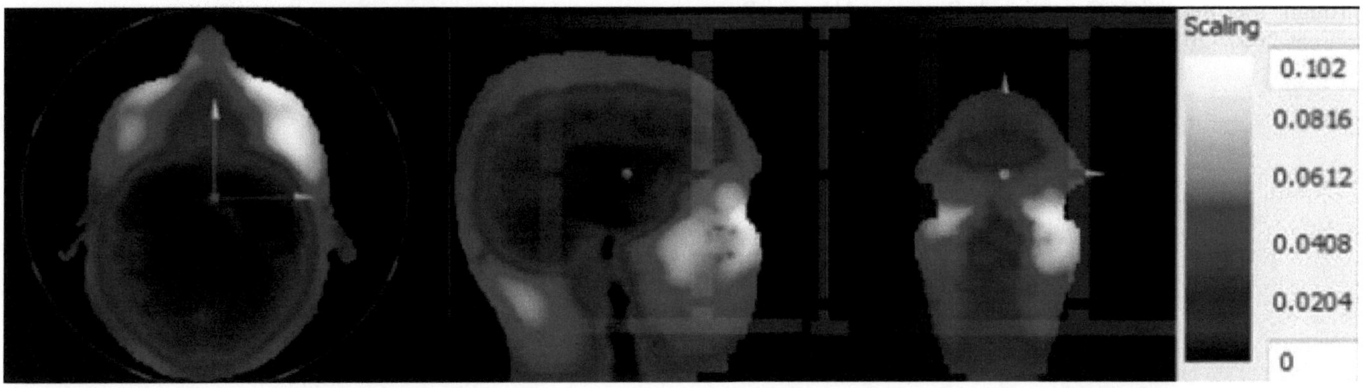

Fig. 2 Temperature distribution in the three planes of section (axial, sagittal and coronal) passing through the maximum value of the resonant frequency of 128 [MHz]

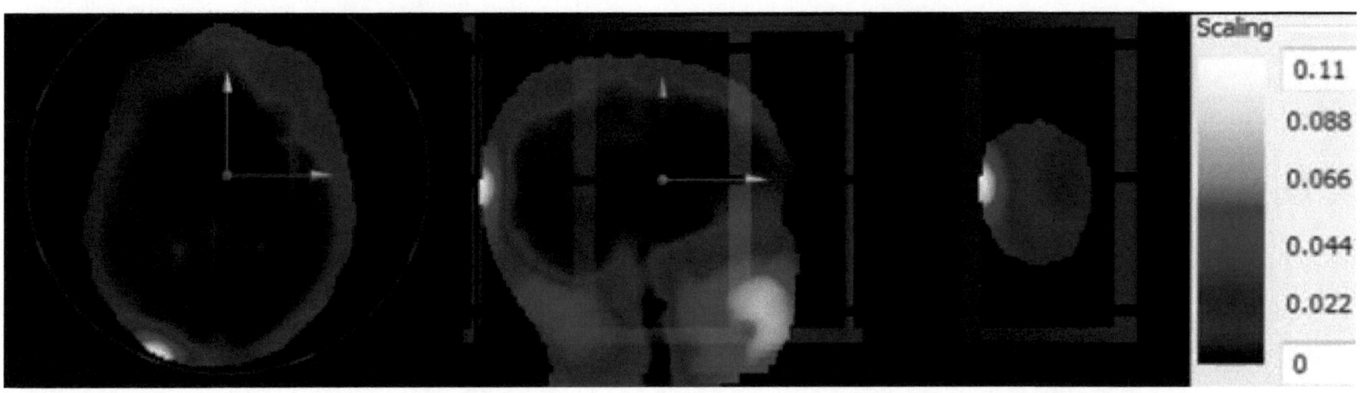

Fig. 3 Temperature distribution in the three planes of section (axial, sagittal and coronal) passing through the maximum value of the resonant frequency of 300 [MHz]

IV. Conclusions

Following evaluation of temperature distribution in the head, after exposure to an electromagnetic field generated by a birdcage-type RF coil, it can be observed that areas with increased temperatures do not fully correspond to those characterized by an increased SAR. Thermal analysis is necessary because it also captures the thermoregulatory ability of the body and thus ensures meeting all safety regulations in the MRI RF coil design. Another important aspect is the fact that thermal simulations can assess the risk faced by a human subject in medical metal implants, knowing that their presence enhance local SAR.

Conflict of Interest

The authors declare that they have no conflict of interest.

Acknowledgment

This work was supported by the project "Doctoral studies in engineering sciences for Developing the knowledge-based society SIDOC" contract no. POSDRU/88/1.5/S/ 60078, project co-Funded from the European Social Fund through the Sectorial Operational Program Human Resources 2007 -2013.

References

1. Shellock F G, (2009) Reference Manual for Magnetic Resonance Safety, Implants, and Devices, Biomedical Research Publishing Group, Los Angeles, CA.
2. Marincas C, Nicu A I, Csutak C and Ciupa R V (2014), Evaluating SAR distributionon the human head (during MRI examination) as function of frequency, MediTech 2014, (in press).
3. Schmid & Partner Engineering AG (2012), SEMCAD X Reference Manual
4. Schmid & Partner Engineering AG,(2011), SEMCAD X Tutorial

Cristinel Marincas
Department of Electrical Engineering and Measurement
Faculty of Electrical Engineering
Technical University of Cluj-Napoca, Romania
E-mail: Cristinel.Marincas@et.utcluj.ro

Assessment of the Need for Protection against Electromagnetic Radiation of Personnel Onboard Warships

G. Marin[1,2], G. Samoilescu[1], A. Baciu[3], D. Iorgulescu[1], and S. Radu[1]

[1] Electrical Engineering Department, Naval Academy, Constanta, Romania
[2] Research Center for Navy, Constanta, Romania
[3] Romanian Nautical College, Mogosoaia, Romania

Abstract— **The biological effects of electromagnetic fields on human factor have been widely studied. This paper intends to evaluate the necessity of protection against electromagnetic radiations in the case of a warship with various types of transmitters: HF, VHF, and UHF communication stations, various types of radars operating in the frequency range of 1 – 10 GHz, and direct beam transmitters – fire control systems, electronic warfare systems, etc.**

In order to analyze the impact of electromagnetic radiation on seafarers onboard naval ships, first there need to be identified the potentially dangerous areas, located in the proximity of emitting antennas. The safety distance to the radiation field is computed with Friis transmission formula in the free space, and potentially dangerous areas are located at lower ranges from the emission source. There were performed a series of electromagnetic field measurements, for frequency range 20-2000 MHz, in areas often transited by crew members and situated at insufficient range from all the antennas.

Even though electric field levels did not indicate reasons for concern, an extensive study must be further performed, with measurements in multiple frequency ranges and in various configurations of operating transmitters.

Keywords— **Biological effects, Electromagnetic radiation, Modeling and simulation, Ship electromagnetic environment**

I. Introduction

The issue of protecting the human factor against the exposure to electromagnetic fields has been extensively treated by specialists [1-7]. In 1967, the American National Standards Institute (ANSI), based on the U.S. Navy standards, determined that the maximum power density that the human body can withstand is 10 mW/cm^2, for a limited period of six minutes, in the frequency range 10 MHz - 100 GHz [6]. Since the '80s, these rules have been drastically revised. Further studies have showed that the energy absorbed by tissues depends on frequency, polarization field, and the physical dimensions of the irradiated body. Other norms issued in 1982 limited the level of absorption, indicating a maximum value of 0.4 W/kg in the first 6 minutes of exposure. Moreover, these rules were correlated with frequency, being more restrictive if the frequency is greater than 10 MHz, and even more restrictive for frequencies between 30 and 300 MHz, with a threshold value of 1 mW/cm^2.

The terminology describing these phenomena also changed, replacing the power density with the specific absorption rate (SAR) and further widening the range of frequencies considered to be harmful, down to 10 kHz (10 kHz-300 GHz).

The biological effects of electromagnetic fields on human factor have been widely studied, for various frequency ranges and power densities [2-4]. Analyzing the impact of electromagnetic radiation on seafarers onboard naval ships, a distinction need be made between ionizing radiation - interacting with living matter and electrically charging organic molecules, and non-ionizing radiation, generating local heating effects, with adverse effects in particular conditions. In order to determine the exposure of personnel on board ships, electromagnetic field measurements were performed at various points on board a naval ship. Given the complex phenomena of harmful interference onboard, due to the density, diversity and high power electrical and electronic equipment, the research is oriented mainly towards higher energy density areas in the vicinity of the antennas.

II. Review of Studied Biological Effects of Electromagnetic Field

The harmful effects of electromagnetic radiation consist of physical and chemical changes in tissues or destruction of atoms order in crystalline solids. During the electromagnetic radiation interaction with tissues, it causes harmful biological effects with or without thermal effect. The degree of destruction depends on factors such as field intensity, frequency, energy level, polarization and duration of exposure. After the electromagnetic radiation penetrates the tissue, its dielectric and conductive properties modify energy absorption and propagation of incident energy [2].

High danger is posed by thermal effects, depending on the intensity and frequency of the incident energy. This is more prominent in the range 100-3000 MHz. When electromagnetic energy is absorbed by tissues, it generates heat. If the heat cannot be dissipates as quickly as it is absorbed, internal body temperature will rise.

S. Vlad and R.V. Ciupa (eds.), *International Conference on Advancements of Medicine and Health Care through Technology*, IFMBE Proceedings 44,
DOI: 10.1007/978-3-319-07653-9_58,

Table 1 Diagram of harmful biological effects of microwaves

Frequency	Absorption rate of incident energy	Biological effects
200 MHz	Up to 40% of the incident energy	Energy penetration in the tissues. Radiation is not detected by the human sensory system. Depth heating of tissues.
1 GHz	Between 20-100% of the incident energy.	Varying degrees of radiation penetration. Energy absorption both in depth and by the superficial tissue (according to tissue characteristics).
3 GHz – 10 GHz	Up to 40% of the incident energy	Direct heating of tissues, detected by the sensory system. Energy absorption on skin surface. Remaining percentage of energy is reflected from skin surface.

The body's ability to dissipate heat depends on various factors such as: air flow in the respective environment, air humidity and temperature, the body's metabolism, clothing, radiant field power density, the amount of absorbed energy and the exposure time. The knowledge obtained from laboratory experiments [2] on the effects of radiation in the frequency range 200 MHz -10 GHz is summarized in Table 1.

Some of the observed non-thermal effects consist of less significant changes in blood properties, as a result of exposure to electromagnetic energy [5]. Some people can hear a buzz caused by exposure to microwave radiation.

III. THE ELECTROMAGNETIC ENVIRONMENT ONBOARD A WARSHIP

Sources of electromagnetic interference onboard warships cover a wide frequency range from 50 Hz to 20 GHz, and include generators and electric converters, electric motors and drive facilities, radio and radar systems, telecommunications systems, computer network, source of discharges, mobile radiotelephones [6].

The main sources of radiation on board are the communication antennas radiating through all metallic structures nearby. Figure 1 illustrates the frequency bands used in military applications, relative to the international standard bands and the civil and industrial applications.

There are three types of onboard transmitters:

- Stationary - multidirectional transmission in HF, VHF, UHF;
- Rotating - 2D and 3D radars, some of which emit high power pulse energy (air surveillance, sea surface surveillance, navigation radars);
- Direct beam - fire control systems, electronic warfare radars, satellite communication antennas.

The most difficult issue is presented by HF antennas, because they must be installed in areas inaccessible to personnel while operated. VHF and UHF antennas, placed at height do not pose any problems in terms of personnel radiation (there is though the risk of secondary radiators).

However, HF transmitting antennas with frequencies between 2 - 30 MHz must be at 1.20 m (horizontally) and 2.40 m (vertically) far from all superstructure areas occupied by personnel. HF antennas radiating less than 250 W need to be at least 3.60 m far from welded superstructures [6].

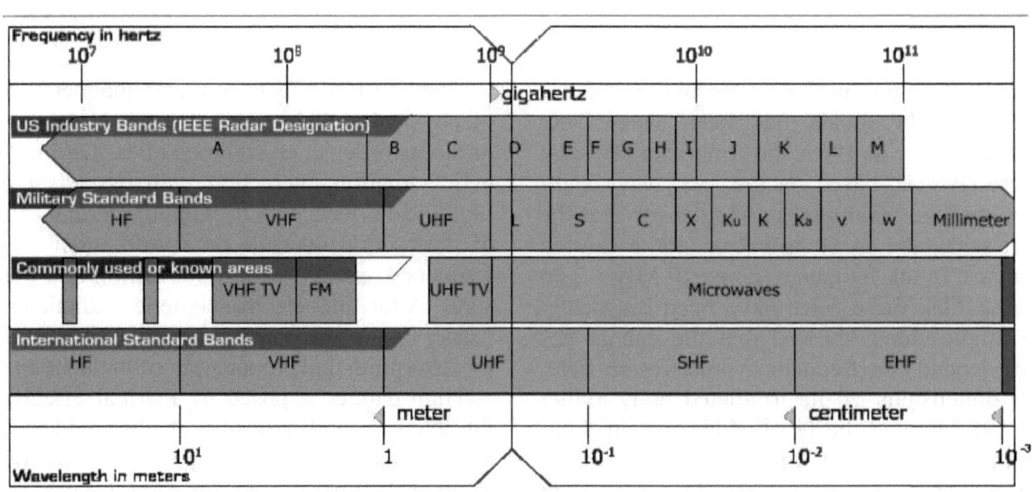

Fig. 1 Frequency bands for military, civil and industrial applications

Radar antennas (rotating transmitters) are generally installed at heights on masts or supports in areas occupied by people. They are a source of risk, causing personnel intermittent exposures to intense radiation.

Third type transmitters emit direct beams and are usually mounted next to crew occupied areas. It is required for these areas to be shielded from radiation, even though the transmitters are generally fitted with beam disruption on areas not of interest. They pose difficult issues for personnel protection [5].

IV. Calculation of Safety Distance to Radiation Field

Near field (the Fresnel region) is defined as the area of space with coordinates are between 0 and λ/2π. The far-field region extends from the end of the Fresnel region. There is no strict delimitation of the two areas.

The assessment of power density in the far-field region is relatively simple. Antenna gain and transmission diagram do not depend on the distance from antenna. Therefore, the far field on power density axis is given by the transmission formula in free space [6]:

$$W_d = \frac{P_t G_o}{4\pi\, d^2} \tag{1}$$

where:

W_d is the power density in a given point of observation, [mW/cm^2];
G_o - antenna gain in the far field;
P_t - average transmitted power [mW];
d - distance from the antenna to observation point [cm].

Equation (1) does not include the effects of ground reflection, which, if any, may cause an increase of power density value of 4 times than the one in free space.

Substituting in equation (1) W_d = 10 mW/cm^2, there is determined the minimum safety distance for personnel working in the far field area:

$$d = \sqrt{\frac{P_t G_0}{40\pi}} \quad (cm) \tag{2}$$

The average transmitted power P_t can be determined if the maximum power P_{t_max} is known:

$$P_{t\,(ave)} = P_{t\,\max} \times r_e \tag{3}$$

where r_e denotes the transmission rate and is computed with relation:

$$r_e = \frac{l_p}{p_p} = l_p \times f_r \tag{3}$$

The quantities in equation (3) denote:

l_p – pulse width (μs);
p_p – pulse repetition period (μs);
f_r – pulse repetition frequency.

Usually, for stationary antennas the safe distance is approximately 5 meters, while for the rotating ones, it is 2 meters.

V. Measurement the Electromagnetic Field on Board a Warship

The ship chosen for research is a frigate with main dimensions: length L = 145 m, width B = 15 m, draft T = 5 m. Starting from the ship plans study, there can be identified areas of potential danger to the embarked personnel. Figure 2 is illustrates the analyzed ship, on which there are marked the positions of radar antennas and other high power antennas. Potentially dangerous areas are the bridge deck and antennas deck, situated immediately above the bridge.

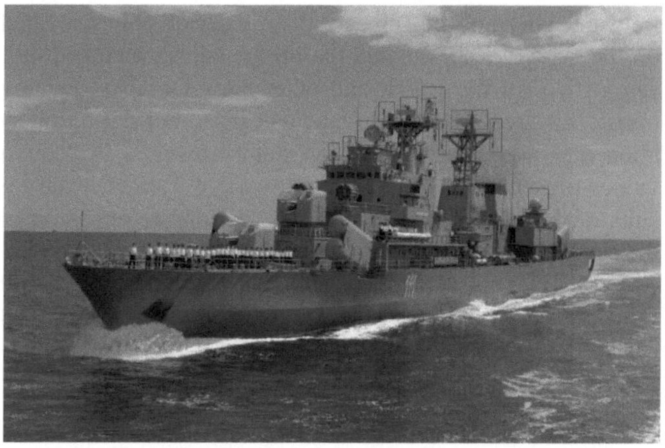

Fig. 2 The analyzed warship with highlighted antenna positions

The research consisted in measurements of the radiation field were performed outside the bridge, on the respective deck, during the operation of VHF communication stations and the surveillance radar.

Table 2 Main field values measured outside the bridge

Case	Frequency [MHz]	Electric field strength [V/m]	Electric field level [dBμV/m]	Power density [W/m²]	Power density [μW/cm²]
VHF station	97,0000	0,2480	107,8891	0,0002	0,0163
	98,0000	0,3045	109,6707	0,0002	0,0246
	99,0000	0,1511	103,5879	0,0001	0,0061
	103,0000	0,1463	103,3041	0,0001	0,0057
	104,0000	0,3808	111,6140	0,0004	0,0385
	105,0000	0,3722	111,4149	0,0004	0,0367
	106,0000	0,1863	105,4039	0,0001	0,0092
	107,0000	0,1374	102,7570	0,0001	0,0050
Radar	1925,0000	0,1837	105,2831	0,0001	0,0090
	1926,0000	0,2123	106,5387	0,0001	0,0120
	1932,0000	0,1415	103,0121	0,0001	0,0053
	1933,0000	0,1297	102,2597	0,0000	0,0045
	1934,0000	0,1575	103,9454	0,0001	0,0066
	1935,0000	0,2824	109,0184	0,0002	0,0212
	1936,0000	0,2167	106,7155	0,0001	0,0125
	1938,0000	0,1809	105,1487	0,0001	0,0087
	1939,0000	0,2197	106,8384	0,0001	0,0128
	1940,0000	0,1536	103,7253	0,0001	0,0063
	1942,0000	0,1454	103,2501	0,0001	0,0056
	1947,0000	0,1435	103,1357	0,0001	0,0055

In the first stage, there were measured values of electric field intensity and power density in a set of points located on the bridge deck, outside the bridge superstructure [8,9]. The officer of the watch and other crew members usually transit this area. The measurements carried out during operation of a VHF communication station resulted in 8 main values presented in the first eight rows of Table 2. The results of the 12 measurement points, during the emission of the surveillance radar, are given in the last 12 rows.

The device used for measurements is a portable electric field meter with isotropic probe, with frequency range 30 MHz – 3 GHz.

VI. Results discussion

The measurement points are located at distances of 1 - 5 m from each other, and at ranges from 10 - 20 m from the radiating antennas. In order to determine the electric field in the bridge deck on a larger area, simulation by finite element method was used. The electric field was simulated with specialized software [10] on a circular area with radius of 10 m from the central point. The boundary condition imposed on the circular edges is a Dirichlet condition with null potential.

Figures 3 and 4 present the electric field distribution in two different situations: operation of a VHF communications station and of the surveillance radar, respectively. The frequency ranges for the two situations are: 90-110 MHz in the first case, and 1.9-2 GHz in the second case, respectively. Electric field strength E (V/m) values are situated in the range 0.019 - 0.3808 V/m in the first case, and between 0.0141 - 0.2824 V/m, in the latter, respectively.

Maximum limits for occupational exposure to electromagnetic fields required by ICNIRP for the frequency range f = 400 - 2000 MHz, are given by the following set of relations [12]:

$$\begin{aligned} E(V/m) &= 3 \times f^{1/2} \\ H(A/m) &= 0.008 \times f^{1/2} \\ B(\mu T) &= 0.01 \times f^{1/2} \\ S(W/m^2) &= \frac{f}{40} \end{aligned} \tag{5}$$

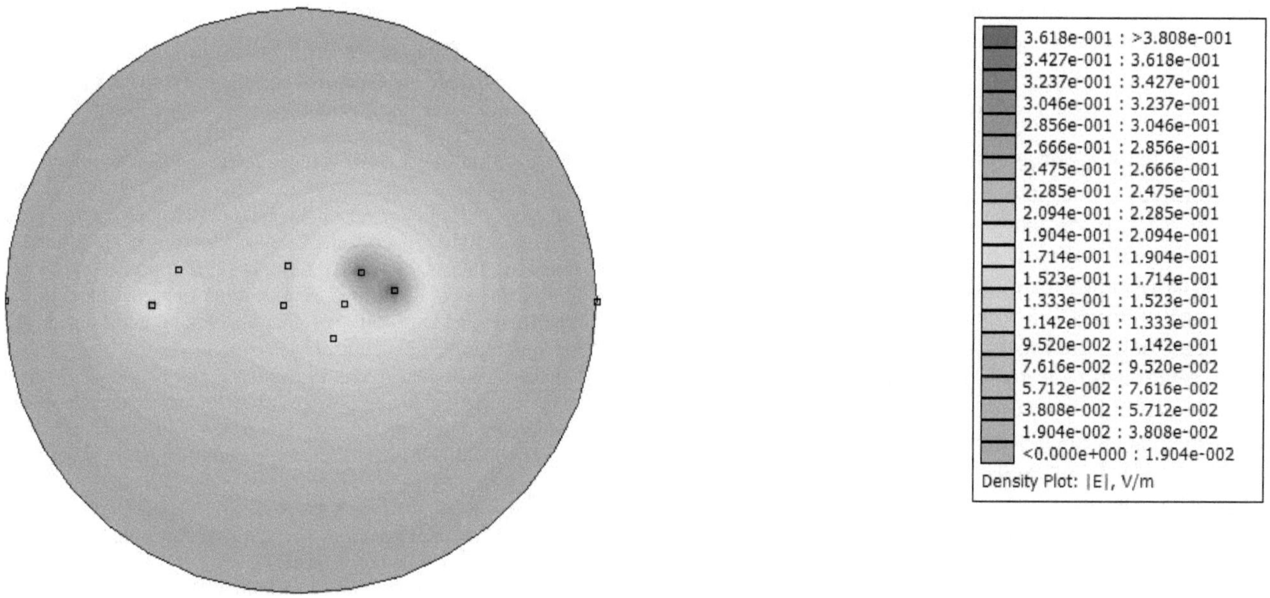

Fig. 3 Electric field distribution during the operation of a VHF communications station, frequency 90-110 MHz

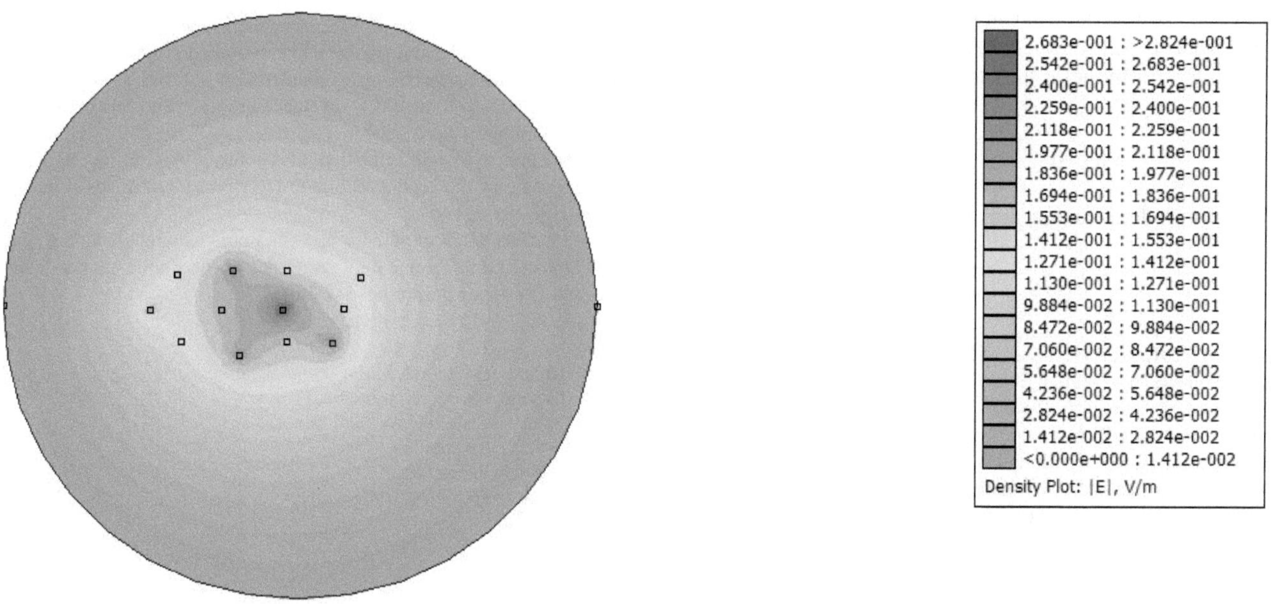

Fig. 4 Electric field distribution during the operation of surveillance radar, frequency 1.9-2 GHz

where E is the electric field strenght, H is the magnetic field strenght, B denotes the magnetic flux density, S is the power density, and f is igven in MHz [12].

Replacing f with the value of 1000 MHz, we obtain the following limits of electric and magnetic field:

E = 94.86 V/m, H = 0.25 A/m, B = 0.31 μT, and S = 25 W/m^2, respectively.

According to military standard STANAG 2345, the maximum allowed power density is approximately S = 30 W/m^2, for the average exposure duration of 6 minutes [13].

Regarding the electric field, personnel exposure is not considered dangerous in the analyzed area outside the bridge. There were not found any values higher than the power density limits of 25 or 30 W/m^2.

Electric field values in the simulation area were definitely below the limits imposed by the ICNIRP or STANAG 2345 or other regulations [12-17].

VII. CONCLUSIONS

Due to the large number of radiation generating devices and the limited space, the electromagnetic environment onboard the ship is probably among the most dangerous areas, from the point of view of electromagnetic radiation .

The available area for mounting transmission and reception antennas onboard is about 10 x 90 m. Due to limited space, contact fields are most likely in the Fresnel region, in which the relationships between radiation models and field intensity are difficult to predict.

Although measurements have not indicated field levels higher the standard imposed limits, it is recommended to take measures for the protection of personnel working in areas near radar and communications antennas, by reducing exposure time, or even prohibiting crew presence on antenna deck throughout transmission.

Further studies need to be performed, for the complete assessment of electromagnetic radiation from various types of emitters: communication antennas, various radar antennas, and direct beam transmitters, employing novel techniques in electromagnetic interference problems.

CONFLICT OF INTEREST

The authors declare that they have no conflict of interest.

REFERENCES

1. Ianoz, M. (2012) A review of studies on Health Effects of Electromagnetic Fields, ICPE-CA 9th CEM Workshop, Sibiu, Romania
2. Zamfirescu, M., Sajin, I., Rusu, I., Sajin, M., Kovacs, E. (2000) Biological Effects of Radiofrequency and Microwaves Electromagnetic Radiations, Medical Publishing House, Bucharest
3. Crist, A., Klingenbock, A., Samaras, T., Goiceanu, C., Kuster, N. (2006) The Dependence of Electromagnetic Far-Field Absorbtion on Body Tissue Composition in the Frequency Range from 300 MHz to 6 GHz, IEEE Trans. Microw. Theory Techn., vol. 54, no. 5
4. Schwan, H. P., Foster, K.R. (1980) RF-Field Interactions with Biological Sistems: Electrical Properties and Biophysical Mechanisms, Proc. IEEE, p.104
5. Calotă, S.V., Deliu, N., Licurici, M., Ferastraeru, C., Contulescu, A. (1998) Studiu privind expunerea profesională la radiaţii neionizante de înaltă frecvenţă şi riscul pentru sănătate, Public Health Institute, Bucharest
6. Sotir, A., Moşoiu, T. (1997) Electromagnetic Compatibility, Military Publishing House, Bucharest
7. Gary, C. (1993) Les effects biologiques des champs magnétiques. Que peut direl`électricien à ce sujet?, Revue "Energetica", p. 41, nr.2-B
8. Baciu, A., Jula, N., Sotir, A., Marin, G. (2013) Simulation of Radiation Field Effects on a Maritime Ship upon an Electric Model of the Human Body, 2nd Int. Conf. on Nanotechnologies and Biomedical Engineering, Chişinău, Republic of Moldova
9. Miclaus, S., Bechet, P. (2007) Estimated and measured values of the radiofrequency radiation power density around cellular base stations, Rom. Journ. Phys., vol. 52, nos. 3–4, p. 429–440, Bucharest
10. Meeker, D. (2009) Finite Element Method Magnetics. User's Manual (femm 4.2)
11. Marin, G., Radu, O., Curca, E., Roca, M., Baciu, A. (2012) Cercetări privind influenţa câmpului magnetic asupra factorului uman, Research Center for Navy Worshop, Constanta
12. *** ICNIRP – Guide Lines For Limiting Exposure To Time-Varying Electric, Magnetic And Electromagnetic Fields (Up To 300 GHz)
13. *** NATO Standard: STANAG 2345 – Evaluation and Control of Personnel Exposure to Radio Frequency Fields – 3 kHz to 300GHz
14. *** Human Exposure to Electromagnetic Frequencies of 10 kHz-300 GHz Frequency Domain, Romanian Standard Project: SR EN 50166-2, IRS, Bucharest (according to standard EN 50166-2/1994)
15. ***Directive 2004/40/EC of the European Parliament and of the Council of 29 April 2004
16. ***Council Recommendation of 12 July 1999 on the limitation of exposure of the general public to electromagnetic fields (0 Hz to 300 GHz), 1999/519/EC
17. *** 96/98/EC Norm for Air and Sea Radio Communication Apparatus, Transposed in Romania by the Order of the Public Works, Transport and Housing Minister no. 582/2003

Author: Georgiana Marin
Institute: Research Center for Navy
Street: 4 Stefanita Voda
City: Constanta
Country: Romania
Email: georgiamarin01@gmail.com

Study on the Influence of Electromagnetic Field Produced by a Medical Equipment on the EEG Signals

C. Luca[1], A. Sălceanu[2], and R. Ciorap[3]

[1] Technical University "Gh.Asachi", Faculty of Electrical Engineering, Iasi, Romania
[2] UMF "Gr.T.Popa", Faculty of Medical Bioengineering, Iasi, Romania

Abstract— **Many researches have been done in the last years upon the various effects of electromagnetic fields (EMF) on biological signals. There are several studies involving subjects who perform various tasks while being exposed to EMF, concluding that some aspects of cognitive function and some distinctive parts of brain physiology may be affected by the exposure to EMF. This paper aims to study the influence of electromagnetic field produced by a medical equipment on the EEG signals processed in real time.**

Keywords— **medical device; electromagnetic interferences; biological signals**

I. INTRODUCTION

Electromagnetic compatibility (EMC) is the ability of two systems or different electronic devices to function properly, one close to the others, in an environment with electromagnetic traffic.

In the hospital setting there are many causes that lead to the existence of electromagnetic radiation. Hospitals are equipped with some types of equipment, such as electrosurgery or microsurgery units which produces electromagnetic radiation and equipments such as EKG (Electrocardiograph) or EEG Monitor (Electroencephalography), which are very sensitive to electromagnetic disturbances.[1]

A preterm infant can be born with a weight varying between 500 gr and 2200 gr, so requiring a long-care and a long time spent in a heating system type . All these patients incurred medical investigations (EEG continuous monitoring, vital signals and EKG monitoring, x-rays) that is performed with the patient in the incubator to ensure continuously heat and humidity needed to support it.

The main problem of a new born preterm is the loss of heat and very quickly dehydration. That's why Neonatal Intensive Care Units use specific medical equipment to provide thermal comfort to a newborn. Such type of equipments are: airshield incubator, radiant warmer or cot warmed up.

While doing echoimaging, there is no question of an electro-magnetic compatibility, in terms of biological signals such as EEG and EKG , artefacts produced by the existence of a disruptive electromagnetic field could induce a possible wrong diagnosis.[2]

II. EQUIPMENT REQUIRED

To study the influence of the electromagnetic field produced by a medical device on EEG signal collected in real time, we used biological signal simulators.

In investigating the effect of MFs in the head and neck areas, investigating the effect of MFs on the brain signals of people who are exposed to MFs is one of the most common methods because the EEG records are very fast, noninvasive,and inexpensive method for the diagnosis of brain responses to external stimuli. [3]

EEG measures voltage fluctuations resulting from ionic current flows within the neurons of the brain.[4] In clinical contexts, EEG refers to the recording of the brain's spontaneous electrical activity over a short period of time, usually 20–40 minutes, as recorded from multiple electrodes placed on the scalp.[5]

One approach to deal with MFs effect on the central nervous system is monitoring their possible negative effects. Therefore, there is no appropriate evidence in the evaluation of the brain signals that explain communication between changing of EEG (by exposure to MFs) and possible negative or positive effects.[3]

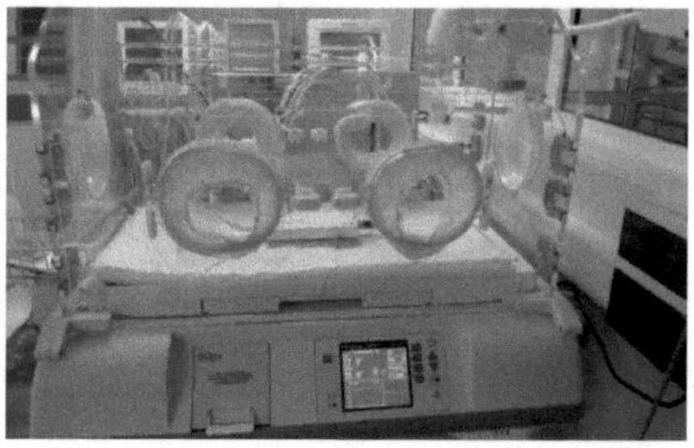

Fig. 1 The Airshield Isolette C2000 (SN: ZT17334)

The tests were carried out in the Department of Neonatal Intensive care level III of the Clinical Hospital "Cuza Voda Iasi", using an Airshield Isolette C2000 Drager, used as heating support for the patient. In all departments of Neonatal Intensive care Units there are these early types of airshields.

S. Vlad and R.V. Ciupa (eds.), *International Conference on Advancements of Medicine and Health Care through Technology*, IFMBE Proceedings 44,
DOI: 10.1007/978-3-319-07653-9_59, © Springer International Publishing Switzerland 2014

The equipments used for the study are: an Airshield Isolette C2000 Drager and Braintz type III-Electroencephalograph. Isolette C-2000 is manufactured in 2004 and provides thermal comfort of the newborn. In terms of electromagnetic compatibility this equipment has the following technical specifications:

Table 1 Technical specifications Airshield Isolette C2000 Drager[6]

Standards	Emissions	Immunity
EN 60601-1 EN60601-2 EN60601-2-19	Emission RF-class A IEC61000-3-2 class A	**Power frequency** 50/60 Hz: IEC60601test: 3A/m Compliance test: 3A/m Conducted RF IEC61000-4-6 Test **IEC60601**: 3Vms and 20Vms (150Hz-80MHz) Compliance test: V1 = 3Vms and V2=10Vms RF radiated IEC61000-4-3 Test **IEC60601**: 10V/m (80MHz-2,5GHz) Compliance test: E1= 10V/m

Braintz type III Electroencephalograph is a system of continuous EEG monitoring of newborn. Signal collection is done with the help of five electrodes: two electrodes for the left hemisphere, two for the right hemisphere and a reference electrode. Deling with the newborn, the EEG monitor is used for secondary brain damage in conditions such as subarachnoid hemorrhage. Brain hemorrhage is the most common pathology in new born preterm.

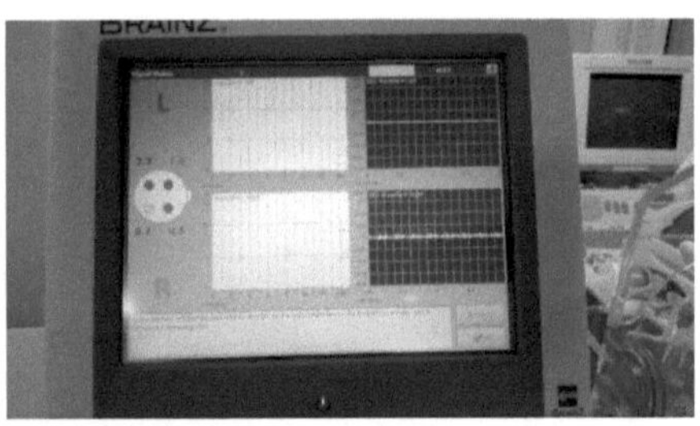

Fig. 2 Braintz type III Electroencephalograph

III. Mode of work

For a patient in an intensive care unit monitoring of the important vital biological signals is essential. The collection of these signals is carried out under the conditions in which these patients in intensive therapy are surrounded by a variety of medical equipment, sources of disturbing signals (airshiel units, neonatal ventilator, phototeraphy lamp, vital signs monitors).

These disruptive electromagnetic field sources are much stronger in case of a newborn in an intensive care unit, owing to the fact that these patients require to ensure thermal comfort. The Airsheild used in our measurements doesn't have an alternative battery in case of power failure.

Measurements protocol that we established is the following:

- Airshield Isolette C-2000 (Serial Number: ZT17434, manufactured in 2004) is warmed up to a temperature of 37,9°C and 50% umidity

- On the Electroencephalograph Braintz type III (serial number:1177, manufactured in 2010) we attached an EEG simulator signal type Natus. This type of simulator gives us a linear signal without artefacts or pathology.

-The EEG signal Simulator is being placed inside the Airshield and we start monitoring.

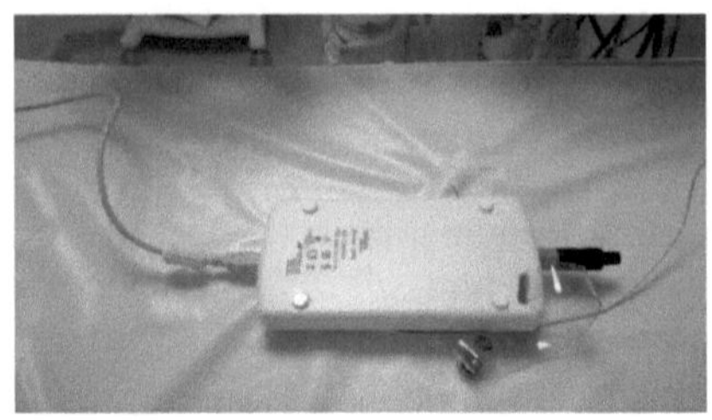

Fig. 3 EEG simulator signal type Natus

-After aproximaly 20 minutes of monitoring, we have simulated a power failure and we closed de Airshield.

-After 10 seconds of power failure we get start the airshied. In this time the EEG monitoring continues.

-We also used a mobile phone to create a controlled electromagnetic field. We measured the EEG signal with the mobile phone in call and off call near EEG simulator.

IV. Measurements and Results

After registering the brain activity, signals were processed in AnalyZe 2.0 program. For a better observation of the signal, the processing it was done over a period of 30 minutes, 15Hz timing signal.

The EEG is typically described in terms of rhythmic activity and transients. The rhythmic activity is divided into bands by frequency.[7] To some degree, these frequency bands are a matter of nomenclature (i.e., any rhythmic activity between 8–12 Hz can be described as "alpha"), but these designations arose because rhythmic activity within a certain frequency range was noted to have a certain distribution over the scalp or a certain biological significance.[8]

Most of the cerebral signals observed in the scalp EEG falls in the range of 1–20 Hz (activity below or above this range is likely to be artifactual, considering standard clinical recording techniques,[9]

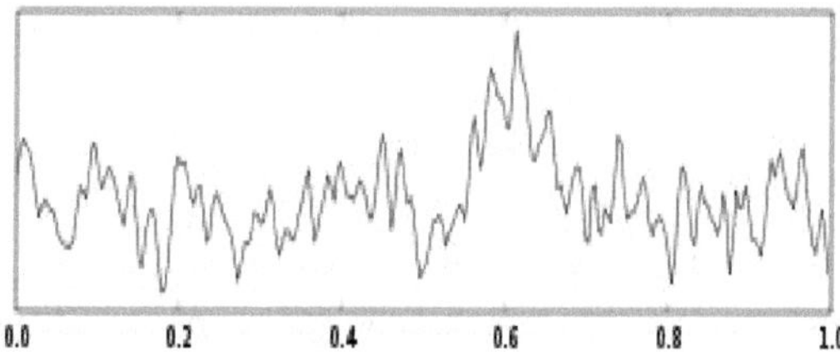

Fig. 4 Normal brain activity

It was noticed that over a period of 2 minutes of recording the brain activity using the Natus simulator, some disruptive signals appear with a maximum value of -10μV .

We can exclude the possibility of noise due to "the patient" because Natus simulator of EEG signal behaves like a normal patient in terms of brain activity. This fact proves that the influence of the electromagnetic field generated by the environment in which takes place the measurements is significant.

The measurements were performed on an artificial "patient", called TEST-EMF and we marked the events occurred over the monitoring like on/off the airshield.

Processing has been carried out from several points of view, to be able to consider the existance of electromagnetic field.

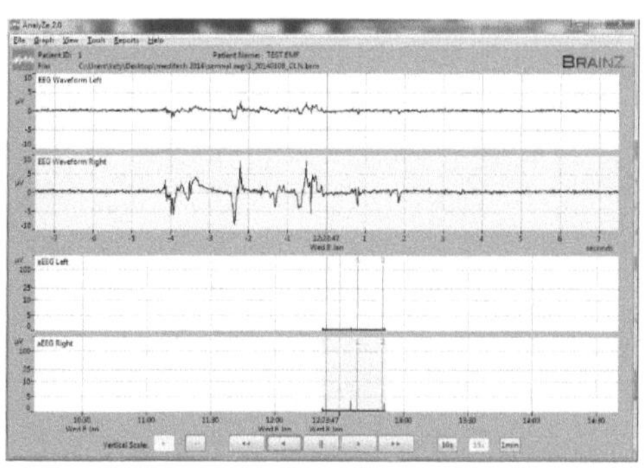

Fig. 5 EEG signal processed in Analize 2.0

Two minutes after the beginning of monitoring, using a mobile phone as disturbtive unit, we noticed the appearance of a significant perturbation which reach -10μV on the right hemisphere and -5μV on the left one. Notice that the right hemisphere is more affected than the left, although the signal Simulator used excludes the possibility of the existence of a difference signal between the two hemispheres.

They often study the possible negative effects of the MFs, especially the AC power (50/60 Hz). However, in practice, it is observed that MFs in some cases have had a positive effect on some diseases such as improving the standing balance by exposure to MF with 200 μT in the head and the neck areas [10] and reduction of tremors in the quality by exposure to MF with 1000 μT, while the negative effect of MFs in some diseases, especially epilepsy, is partly confirmed 11].

After about 20 minutes of monitoring we simulate a power failure and we close de Airshield. At this time we don't observe any disturbing signal.

After 10 minutes of power failure we get on the airshied.In this time the EEG monitoring continues and we observe a disruptive signal on the right hemisphere which reach -10μV.

We also studied the signal impedance on the two hemispheres, noticing a higher value in the right one.

It is clear that our device is very susceptible to interference from outside sources. The first problem that we observed is with 50-60 Hz power-line noise due to the fact that we observe a disruptive signal on the right hemisphere which reach -10μV after 10 seconds of power failure of airshield.

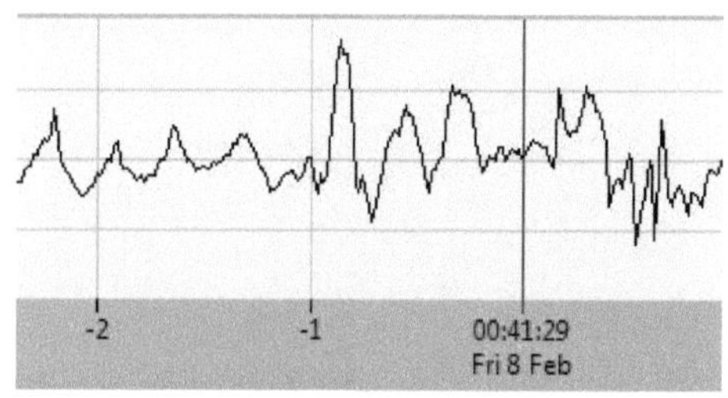

Fig. 6 60 Hz Noise Corrupting an EEG Signal

V. Conclusions

As results of the studies carried out within the framework of this work, appear some questions on how the collection procedure of biomedical signals in neonatal intensive care wars. These units utilize a wide range of top quality medical equipment and the electromagnetic field has a high level and significantly influences the quality of sensitive signals such as EEG (electroencephalography), EKG (electrocardiograph) or SpO_2 (oxygen partial saturation in the blood).

It requires special attention in the study of these signals disrupted clinic, in order to delineate true crises such as seizures from an electromagnetic influence.

This paper aimes to warn on the existence of electromagnetic fields in a neonatal intensive care units that must be considered by the professionals working in the area.

Conflict of Interest

The authors declare that they have no conflict of interest.

References

1. Smith J, J Alexander v. Kramarenko,Uner Tan , EFFECTS OF HIGH-FREQUENCY ELECTROMAGNET, Intern. J. Neuroscience, 113:1007–1019, 2003Copyright 2003 Taylor & Francis0020-7454/03
2. Cook MR, Graham C, Cohen HD, Gerkovich MM. A replication study of human exposure to 60-Hz fields: effects on neurobehavioral measures. Bioelectromagnetics 1992;13:261–85.
3. Andrew A. Marinoa,b,*, Erik Nilsena, Andrew L. Chesson Jr.c, Clifton Frilota, Clinical Neurophysiology 115 (2004) 1195–1201Effect of low-frequency magnetic fields on brain electrical activity in human subjects
4. Argiro e. Maganioti, Charalabos c. Papageorgiou,WI-FI ELECTROMAGNETIC FIELDS EXERT GENDER RELATED ALTERATIONS ON EEG IC FIELDS ON HUMAN EEG: A BRAIN MAPP STUDY,
5. Niedermeyer E. and da Silva F.L. (2004). Electroencephalography: Basic Principles, Clinical Applications, and Related Fields. Lippincot Williams & Wilkins. ISBN 0-7817-5126-)
6. User Manual , Incubator Air-Shields Isolette C2000 Drager, Part number Revisions Date, 85 990 05 1 October 2004, 2004 by Draeger Medical Infant Care, Inc. ALL RIGHTS RESERVEd
7. Bell GB, Marino AA, Chesson AL. Frequency-specific blocking in the human brain caused by electromagnetic fields. Neuroreport 1994;5(4): 510–2.
8. Swartz, Barbara E. (1998). "The advantages of digital over analog recording techniques".Electroencephalography and Clinical Neurophysiology 106 (2): 113–7. doi:10.1016/S0013-4694(97)00113-2. PMID 9741771.
9. Millet, David (2002). "The Origins of EEG". International Society for the History of the Neurosciences (ISHN).
10. Dobson J, St. Pierre TG, Schultheiss-Grassi PP, Wieser HG, Kuster N. Analysis of EEG data from weak-field magnetic stimulation of mesial temporal lobe epilepsy patients. Brain Res 2000;868: 386–91.
11. Seyed Ali Shafiei1, Seyed Mohammad Firoozabadi2*, Kazem Rasoulzadeh Tabatabaie3, Mojdeh Ghabaee4 Iranian Journal of Medical PhysicsVol. 9, No. 2, Spring 2012, 141-152 Received: November 27, 2011; Original Article Evaluating the Changes in Alpha-1 Band Due to Exposure to Magnetic Field

Author: PHD Student **Luca Cătălina**
Institute: Technical University "Gh.Asachi" / Faculty of Electrical Engineering
Street: Bd. Profesor Dimitrie Mangeron, no. 21- 23, 700050
City: Iasi
Country: Romania
Email: luca.katalina@yahoo.com

Experimental and Computational Study of the Temperature Distribution at the Surface of a Metallic Implant Exposed to High Frequency Electromagnetic Fields

B. Ilie[1] and D. Rafiroiu[2]

[1] Computer and Electric Engineering Dept., "Lucian Blaga" University SIBIU, Romania
[2] Measurement and Electrotechnics Department, Technical University, Cluj-Napoca, Romania

Abstract— **The dramatically increase in number of the portable devices with radiofrequency (RF) transponders built-in, wireless devices, like mobile phones, smart phones, tablets and so on, and the use of this kind of equipments in the vicinity of the human body rise a strong question about their safety, especially for persons wearing metallic implants like the vascular stents in the head and neck region.**

This paper presents experimental and computational studies, aiming to assess the variation of the temperature at the surface of a conductive cylindrical implant in RF electromagnetic (EM) field, both in open air and in biological tissue. The implant heating source was considered to be the EM RF radiation field exclusively. The biological heat source was completely ignored.

With the implant located 5mm deep inside biological tissue and a 2W power emitted by the radiation source, a maximum temperature increase of 1.2°C was found at the surface of the implant. However, in non-uniform EM field, closer to the radiation source, a higher temperature increase of 1.6°C was found at the surface of the implant. The spatial distribution of the temperature at the surface of the implant was studied experimentally, using a limited number of temperature transducers and computationally, using an RF+thermal coupled model implemented in Comsol 4.3.b.

Keywords— **Metallic implant, Radio Frequencies field, heating**

I. Introduction

The number of people carrying portable devices with wireless capabilities is dramatically increasing nowadays. Therefore, the phenomena involving human tissues heating in RF EM field has become an intensively studied topic.

Many people have studied this problem both experimentally and computationally, in different contexts (MRI, cellphones) [1-5]. Different numerical methods (FDTD, FEM) have been used.

With regard to energy absorption in the tissue surrounding the metallic implants, a worst case scenario has been identified. The absorption is evidently highest when the longest dimension of the implant and the RF field source (antenna) are parallel [1].

In such cases, two phenomena occur. First, a conductive object in the tissues may cause a notable local enhancement of the EM field, thus increasing the power absorption in the tissue and its temperature. Secondly, the passive conductive implant is heated due to the currents induced by the RF EM field.

Using FDTD method, Olteanu at al [5] have simulated the heating of cylindrical stent implanted in a human head and exposed to an 835 MHz EM radiation. The temperature distribution around the implant is shown in Fig. 1.

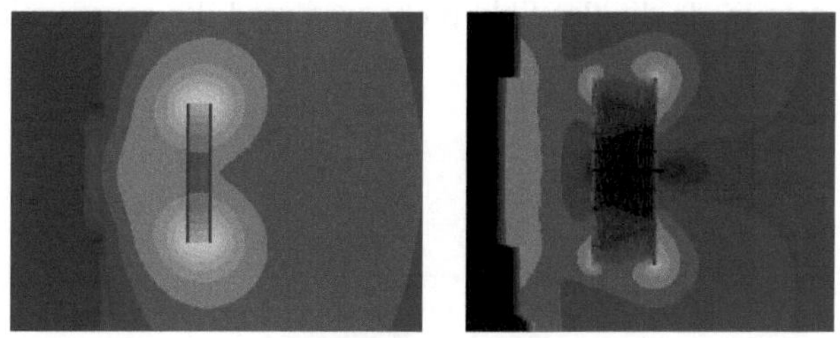

Fig. 1 Temperature distribution arround a cylindrical stent, when exposed to an 835 MHz EM radiation[5]

II. Experimental setup

This paragraph describes the experimental setup used for measuring the temperature at the surface of a cylindrical implant when exposed to a uniform RF EM field.

A. Uniform Electromagnetic Field Generation

For this purpose, a Transverse ElectroMagnetic (TEM) cell [6] was used. The TEM cell IFI Model CC-104 SEXX shown in Fig. 2 has a relatively uniform field distribution.

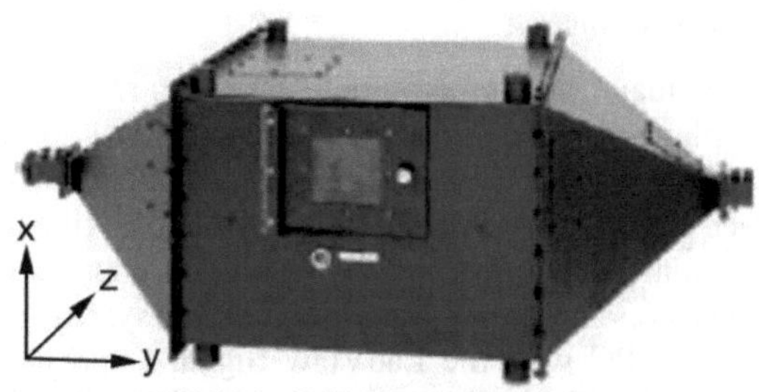

Fig. 2 TEM cell and the coordinate system

IFMBE Proceedings 44,
DOI: 10.1007/978-3-319-07653-9_60, © Springer International Publishing Switzerland 2014

The cell was fed by a RF generator HAMEG 8134-2 through a RF power amplifier OPHIR 5150F at a frequency of 850MHz. The RF field was measured by using a RF Rhode-Schwartz analyzer, type FSH3, with appropriate sensors. During the measurements, the SWR ratio was below 1.2. The configuration of the measuring system is depicted in Fig.3

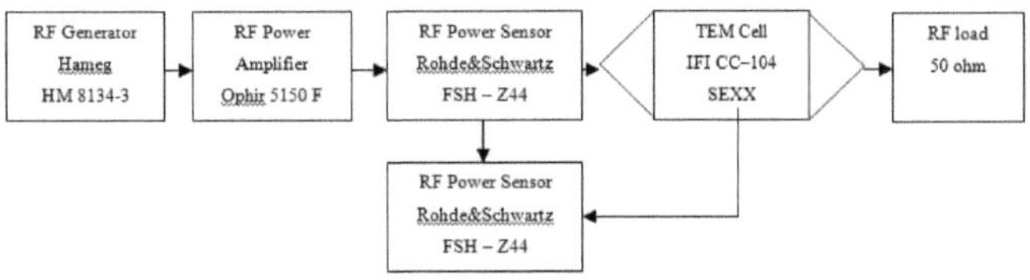

Fig. 3 RF field measuring system

B. Field Strength Measurement in the TEM Cell

To measure the electromagnetic field inside the cell, a custom made dipolar field probe was used. Its construction is shown in Fig. 4.

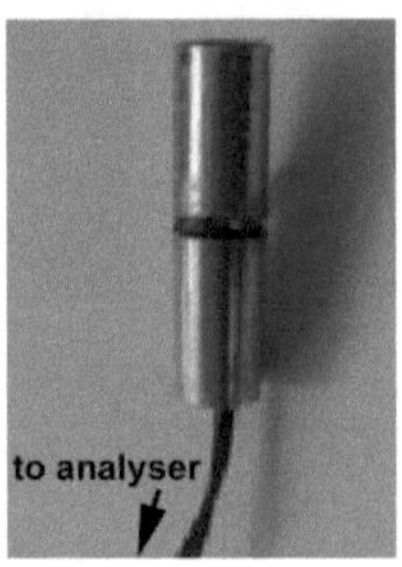

Fig. 4 The dipolar field probe

The field probe was used to check the field uniformity inside the cell. The results of these measurements are presented in section III. Later on, the field probe was replaced by a cylindrical metallic implant on whose surface the temperature was measured. The metallic implant is a 0.2mm thick cylindrical shell, 5.4mm in diameter and 20mm long.

C. Discrete Points Temperature Measurement at the Implant's Surface

To evaluate the temperature distribution at the surface of the implant, a measuring system was added to the field measuring system. The new measuring system consists of a data acquisition system from NI (USB6215), with 16 electrically isolated channels, 16 bit resolution/channel and 250 ksample/sec. The temperature acquisition system was connected to a PC with the LabView Signal Express software installed. The block diagram of the resulting EM field and temperature measuring systems is illustrated in Fig. 5.

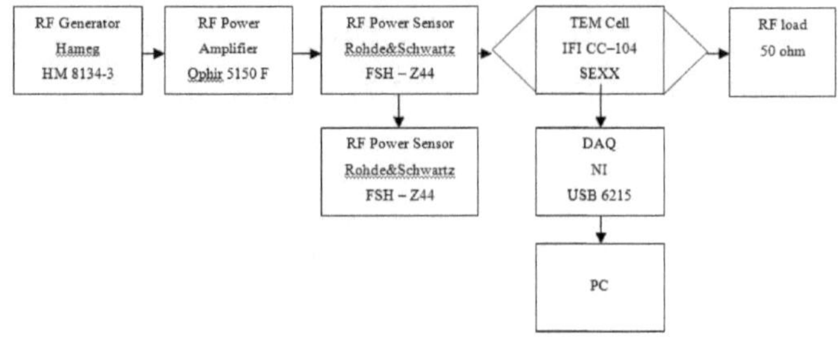

Fig.5. RF filed and temperature measuring system

For measuring temperature at the surface of the implant, 6 small thermistor sensors were used: NTCS0402E3103LT sensors, with 10kΩ resistance, 1% tolerance, 5s thermal time constant and 1x0.5x0.5 mm in size. The arrangement of the 6 thermistors on the surface of the implant is shown in Fig.6.

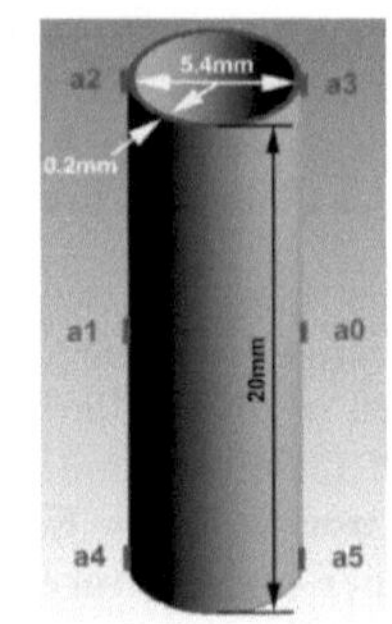

Fig. 6 Arrangement of thermal sensors on the surface of the implant

III. EXPERIMENTAL RESULTS

A. Field Power Measurement with the Dipole Probe

After choosing a point, approximately in the center of the TEM cell, the field probe was placed there and used to measure the field along each of the three axes, in air. The values of the output power of the dipolar field probe measured along each of the three directions (P_x, P_y, P_z), for different values of the input power of the TEM cell P_{in} [W] are presented in Table 1.

Table 1 EM power measured by the field probe along each direction, in air, for different input powers

P_{in} [W]	P_x[W]	P_y[W]	P_z[W]
1	0.58	0.057	0.16
2	1.14	0.11	0.32
3.95	2.29	0.23	0.64
7.94	4.57	0.45	1.28
15.84	9.12	0.91	2.57

The same kind of measurement was made inside of biological tissue (a piece of fresh meat) at 5mm and at 15mm from the surface, respectively. Tables 2 and 3 show the measured output powers, for different values of the input power of the TEM cell, at 5 mm and 15 mm deep inside the biological tissue.

Table 2 EM power measured by the field probe along each direction, at 5mm inside biological tissue, for different input powers

P_{in} [W]	P_x[W]	P_y[W]	P_z[W]
1	0.51	0.0083	0.0058
2	1.02	0.016	0.012
3.95	1.99	0.033	0.023
7.94	3.89	0.077	0.047
15.84	7.41	0.15	0.059

Table 3 EM power measured by the field probe along each direction, at 15mm inside biological tissue, for different input powers

P_{in} [W]	P_x[W]	P_y[W]	P_z[W]
1	0.023	0.0003	0.0029
2	0.048	0.0007	0.0069
3.95	0.097	0.0015	0.015
7.94	0.19	0.0033	0.032
15.84	0.38	0.0069	0.066

B. Temperature Distribution at the Implant Surface

According to Tables 1-3, the greatest power is always absorbed with the dipole oriented along the x axis. Therefore, the dipolar field probe was replaced by the dipole-like implant fitted with temperature sensors and oriented along the x axis. This allowed us to measure the temperature distribution at the surface of the implant, corresponding to a 2W input power, in air, at 5 and 15 mm deep inside the biological tissue, respectively. A0 to A5 are the temperature values recorded by each of the 6 temperature sensors placed on the surface of the implant according to Fig. 6. Each temperature value was recorded in time, until the steady state temperature was reached. Thereafter, the power supply to the TEM cell was interrupted and the temperature measurement continued until the ambient temperatures of 23.8°C in air and 22°C in tissue were reached again. Figures 7-9 show the temperature histories recorded, in every case.

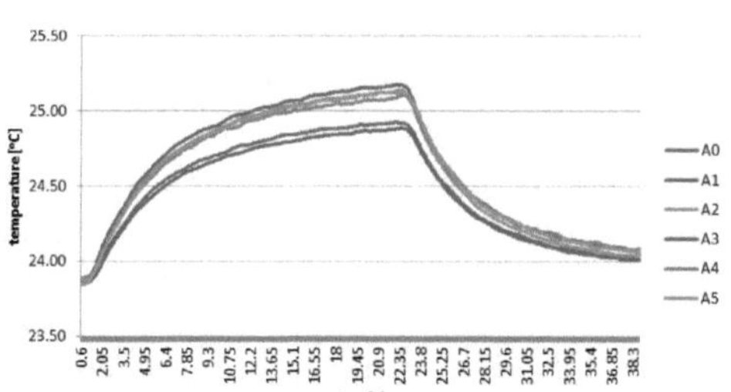

Fig. 7 Temperature histories on the implant surface in air, for a 2W input power of the TEM cell

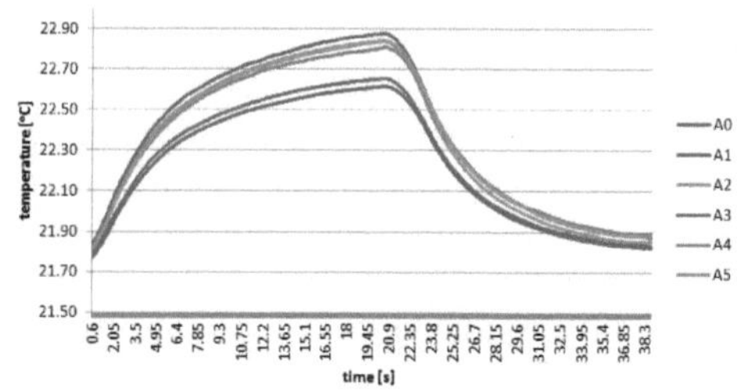

Fig. 8 Temperature histories on the implant surface, at 5mm deep inside the biological tissue, for a 2W input power of the TEM cell

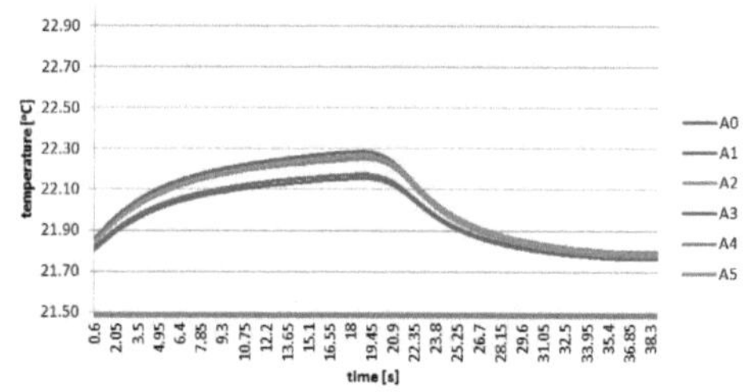

Fig. 9 Temperature histories on the implant surface, at 15mm deep inside the biological tissue, for a 2W input power of the TEM cell

IV. PASSIVE METALLIC IMPLANT IN NON-UNIFORM RF EM FIELD: NUMERICAL SIMULATION

However, the RF EM field is not always uniform and the temperature distribution at the surface of a passive metallic implant and in the biological tissue that surrounds it could be affected by the proximity of the EM field source. A typical example is a vascular stent placed close to the surface of the body and affected by the radiation of a cell phone.

A. Model Setup

This typical scenario was simulated using Finite Element Method (FEM), in Comsol 4.3.b. The modelled system consists of a 95 mm radius, low conductivity sphere mimicking the human head and a dipolar antenna mimicking the cell phone. Inside the sphere, a cylindrical metallic shell identical with the one used in our experimental study (see Fig. 6) was placed. The material properties of the conductive sphere (the head) and the implant are given in Table 4. The sphere properties correspond to the average values in the human head.

Table 4 Material properties used in the model

Property	head	implant
ε_r	56	1
μ_r	1	1
σ [S/m]	0.84	1.000.000
ρ [kg/m^3]	1030	6450
Cp [J/kg/K]	3710	545
k [W/m/K]	0.528	16

The antenna is oriented along the y axis, placed at 10 mm away from the surface of the head and consists of two thin metallic rods that have a sinusoidal voltage applied between them. The length of each rod (arm) is one quarter of the wavelength, $\lambda/4=0.0897$ m. The antenna operates at the frequency of 835 MHz. The diameter of each arm is $\lambda/40$. The geometry of the model is shown in figure 10.

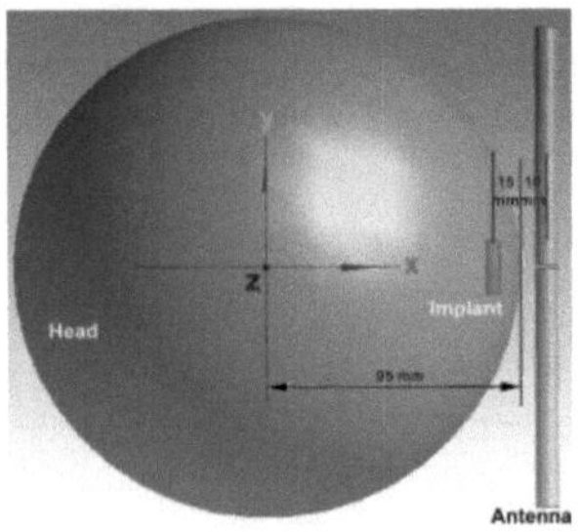

Fig. 10 The geometry of the model

The arms were considered to be Perfect Electric Conductors (PECs). They are excited by a cable type lumped port having the characteristic impedance of 75Ω. The terminal's voltage is variable, according to the required input power: $V_0=12.5$V for $P_{in}=1$W and $V_0=19.45$V for $P_{in}=2$ W.

The sphere and the antenna are surrounded by air and to avoid EM wave reflection, a spherical Perfectly Matched Layer (PML) 0.35m in radius and 0.1m thick was used.

As per the heat transfer problem, the implicit thermal insulation condition was applied everywhere on the outer surface of the sphere and at its interface with the metallic implant. The model was initialized at a 0°C temperature, everywhere in the sphere and in the implant.

B. Simulation Results

A total number of 6 scenarios have been simulated.

First, the head was considered without implant and the source power of the antenna was 1W and 2W respectively. Figure 11.a shows the temperature distribution at the surface of the head corresponding to an input power of the antenna, $P_{in}=1$W.

For a better view of the temperature distribution inside the head, temperature was plotted along two lines parallel to the ox axis. Both lines start from the oy axis and end on the surface of the head. One of the lines starts at y=0.0m and the other at y=0.01m (the implant's extremity used in the subsequent simulations). Figure 12 shows these temperature distributions.

Table 5 shows the values of total power P and of the powers P_x, P_y and P_z absorbed by the head along each of the three directions. The maximum SAR value in head is also indicated in table 5.

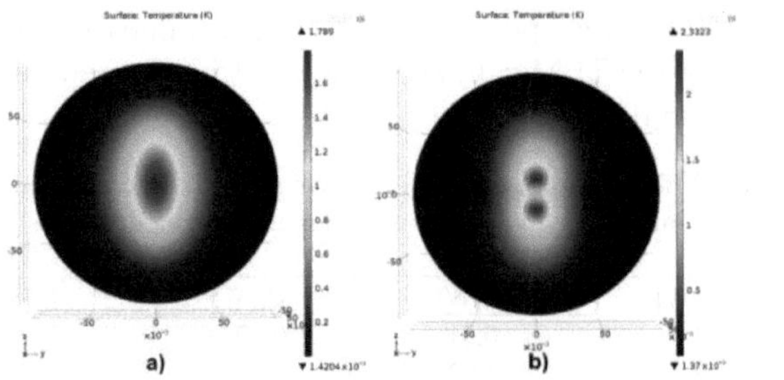

Fig. 11 Temperature distribution at the surface of the head, for $P_{in}=1$W: a) without implant, b) with implant at 5mm

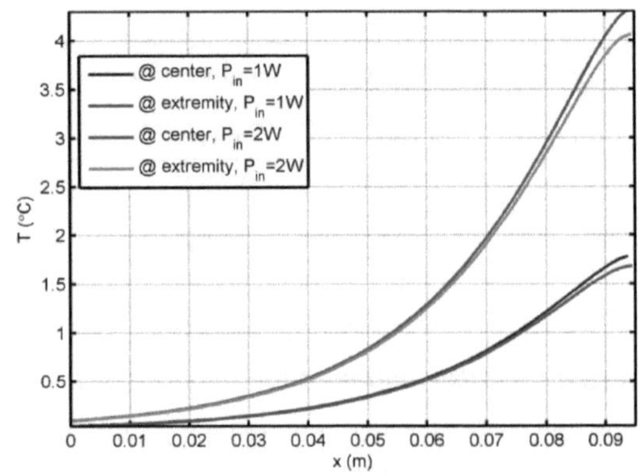

Fig. 12 Temperature distribution along the ox axis and along a line that will pass through the implant's extremity, for $P_{in}=1$W and $P_{in}=2$W respectively

Table 5 Power absorbed by the head and the maximum SAR value in the head, without implant, for different input powers of the antenna

P_{in}	1 W	2 W
P (W)	0.666	1.614
P_x (W)	0.841	2.037
P_y (W)	-2.2e-4	-5.34e-4
P_z (W)	1.7e-3	4.2e-3
SAR_{max} (W/kg)	18.5	44.7

Secondly, the implant was placed at 5mm and 15mm deep inside the head. Simulations were run for the 1W and the 2W input power, respectively. Figure 11.b shows the temperature distribution at the surface of the head, with the implant at 5mm and the input power of 1W.

The temperature distributions along the two parallel lines inside the head, with the implant at different depths and for different input powers of the antenna are represented in figure 13. The upper panel's graphs correspond to the 5mm deep implant and the second's to the 15mm deep implant.

The values of the total power absorbed by the head with implant and of the powers absorbed along each direction are presented in table 6. The maximum SAR values are also indicated in table 6. In all cases, the greatest power absorbed by the head is P_x and the smallest is P_z. The negative absorbed powers suggest that the head loses power along the respective directions. More dramatic is the increase of the maximum SAR value in the head with implant (table 6), compared with the head without implant (table 5): a 1000 times.

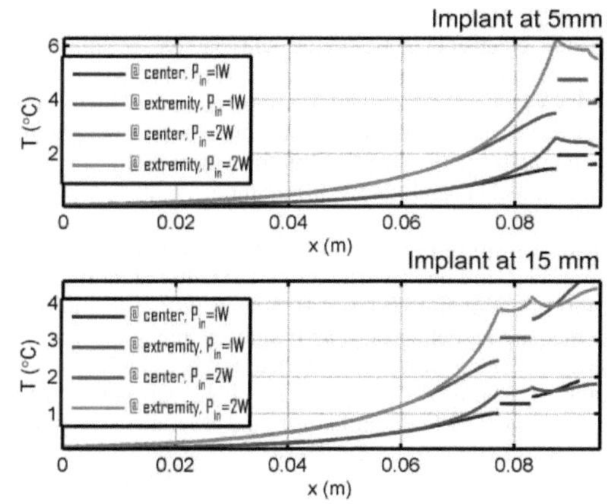

Fig. 13 Temperature distribution along the ox axis and along a line that passes through the implant's extremity, for different positions of the implant and for different input powers of the antenna

Table 6 Power absorbed by the head and the maximum SAR value in the head, with the implant at different depths, for different input powers of the antennca

P_{in}	1 W	2 W
	With implant at 5 mm	
P (W)	0.619	1.497
P_x (W)	0.849	2.057
P_y (W)	-1.07e-4	-2.58e-4
P_z (W)	-3.07e-4	-7.44e-4
SAR_{max} (W/kg)	11,260	27,262
	With implant at 15 mm	
P (W)	0.653	1.582
P_x (W)	0.823	1.993
P_y (W)	-2.42e-4	-5.85e-4
P_z (W)	7.83e-4	1.9e-3
SAR_{max} (W/kg)	5,695	13,790

As our entire work mostly focuses on the implant's temperature, rather than on the head's temperature, the implant's surface temperature was plotted in figure 14, for each position of the implant and for the antenna's input power of 1W. The most relevant characteristics of the temperature distribution at the surface of the implant are the non-uniformity and the maximum value. Clearly, when the implant is closer to the head's surface, its temperature gets higher values and its distribution is more uniform than when it is farther to the surface.

These characteristics can be correlated with the temperature distribution inside the head (see Fig. 13) and with the power absorbed by the implant. Table 7 shows the values of total power P and of the powers P_x, P_y and P_z absorbed by the implant along each of the three directions. The maximum SAR values at the surface of the implant are also indicated in table 7.

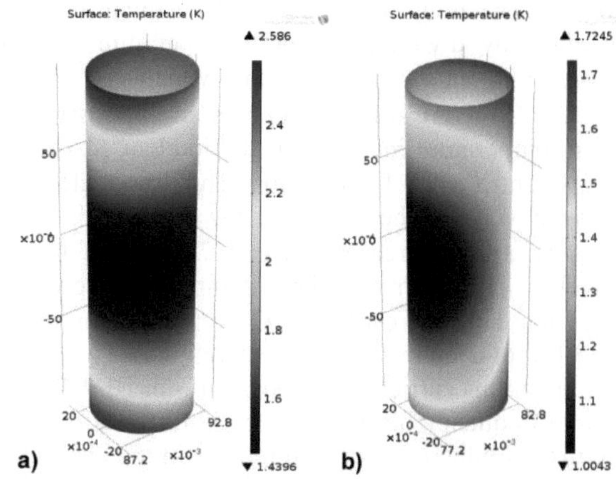

Fig. 14 Temperature distributions at the surface of the implant for the input power of the antenna 1W: a) implant at 5mm and b) implant at 15mm

Table 7 Powers absorbed by the implant and the maximum SAR value at the surface of the implant, for different input powers of the antenna

P_{in}	1 W	2 W
	With implant at 5 mm	
P (W)	3.91e-4	9.47e-4
P_x (W)	4.72e-2	0.114
P_y (W)	-1.89e-5	-4.57e-5
P_z (W)	-4.63e-6	-1.13e-5
SAR_{max} (W/kg)	6,105	14,782
	With implant at 15 mm	
P (W)	2.66e-4	6.44e-4
P_x (W)	2.16e-2	5.23e-2
P_y (W)	2.24e-5	5.42e-5
P_z (W)	1.8e-5	4.36e-5
SAR_{max} (W/kg)	5,657	13,697

A simple comparison between the values that are given in tables 6 and 7 shows that most of the power is absorbed by the head tissue surrounding the implant. However, when the implant is close to the head surface, the maximum SAR values in the head are almost twice as big as the maximum SAR values at the surface of the implant. This suggests that, when the implant is very close to the head surface, the point with the maximum SAR value in the head moves away from the implant's surface and come closer to the head surface.

V. Conclusions

The measurements carried out in our experiment show the temperature variation at six measuring points on the surface of the implant. When the implant was in air and the input power of the TEM cell was 2W, the maximum (steady state) temperature increase at the implant's extremity was of 1.45°C while in the middle, the maximum temperature increase was of 1.0°C. A rough approximation of the temperature gradient along the length of the implant (oy axis) can be made by dividing the total temperature variation along the implant to its length, which is, 0.45°C /0.02m=22.5°C/m. At different depths in the tissue, the maximum temperature increases at the implant's extremity were 1.2°C and 0.4°C, for the 5mm and 15mm deep implant, respectively. In the middle of the implant, the maximum temperature increases were 0.77°C and 0.32°C, respectively. The corresponding temperature gradients along the implants were of 21.5°C/m and 4°C/m for the 5mm and 15mm deep implant, respectively.

The simulations carried out in non-uniform HF EM field, at the same frequency but in a biological tissue with different electrical conductivities (fresh muscle in the experiment and brain in the simulation), revealed higher temperature increases and higher temperature gradients. These differences could be explained by the higher conductivity of the brain tissue (0.84 S/m) as compared to the fresh skeletal muscle's which is about 0.68 S/m at the 800MHz frequency [8]. Another thing that could explain these differences between the experimental and the numerical simulation results is the difference between the conductivities of the implant. In the experiment, the implant was made of brass with conductivity 15.9×10^6 S/m [9], while for the simulation the electrical properties of the Nitinol alloy were used. Brass is 16 times more conductive than the nitinol alloy. Finally, for the experiment, rectangular voltage impulses were used to power the TEM cell whereas in the simulation, a sinusoidal voltage was considered. However, most the difference might be due to the proximity of the RF field source and its non-uniformity, in the simulated scenario.

To conclude, we may say that in real life, the implant is heated by both the RF EM field and the biological heat source. In the current study, no biological heat source was accounted but we definitely have to consider it in our next investigations, together with the blood flow effects.

References

1. Virtanen H, Keshvari J, Lappalainen R. (2006) Interaction of radio frequency electromagnetic fields and passive metallic implants--a brief review. Bioelectromagnetics. Sep;27(6):431-9.
2. Matikka Virtanen H, Keshvari J, Lappalainen R. (2010) Temperature changes associated with radiofrequency exposure near authentic metallic implants in the head phantom--a near field simulation study with 900, 1800 and 2450 MHz dipole. Phys Med Biol. 7;55 (19):5867-81.
3. Olteanu M, Rafiroiu D. (2011) Temperature Increase due to Specific Absorption Rate Enhancement around Metallic Stent Implants. EHB,
4. J. Ruoff, C. Würslin, H. Graf, F. Schick (2012) Resolution adapted finite element modeling of radio frequency interactions on conductive resonant structures. Magn Reson Med, 67(5):1444-52
5. Olteanu M, Marincaş C, Rafiroiu D. (2012) Dangerous Temperature Increase from EM Radiation around Metallic Implants. ACTA ELECTROTEHNICA, 53:2, 175-181,
6. M. Popovic, S. C. Hagness, A. Taflove, (1998) Finite-Difference Time-Domain Analysis of a Complete Transverse Electromagnetic Cell Loaded with Liquid Biological Media in Culture Dishes, IEEE Trans. on BME, 45:8, 1067–1076 .
7. M. Morega, S. Micläuş, A. Machedon. (2008) Analysis of the electromagnetic field in a controlled enclosure for biological dosimetry part 1. Design and validation of the numerical model. Rev. Roum. Sci. Techn. – Électrotechn. et Énerg., 52:2, 225–235.
8. D. Miklavcic et al, Electrical Properties of Tissues. In Wiley Encyclopedia of Biomedical Engineering, 2008
9. http://www.tibtech.com/conductivity.php

Corresponding author:

Author: Beriliu Ilie
Institute: "Lucian Blaga" University
Street: Bulevardul Victoriei ,10
City: Sibiu
Country: Romania
Email: Beriliu.Ilie@ulbsibiu.ro

A Numerical Simulation of the Electrical Monitoring of the Brachial-Ulnar-Radial Arterial Hemodynamic

A.M. Morega[1,2], C. Savastru[1], and M. Morega[1]

[1] University POLITEHNICA of Bucharest, Department of Electrical Engineering, Bucharest, Country
[2] "Gh. Mihoc – C. Iacob" Institute of Statistical Mathematics and Applied Mathematics Romanian Academy, Bucharest, Romania

Abstract— **Blood pressure measurement (BPM) is a standard method of investigation for the cardiovascular activity. In this study we are concerned with its usage for the evaluation of the flow in the brachial-ulnar-radial tree. First, we consider a standard piezoelectric transducer (PZT) usable in BPM. Next, we build a mathematical model that sums up the blood flow-vessel-muscle-PZT interactions to investigate the BPM information and analyze it numerically. Finally, we present a lumped circuit equivalent that may conveniently be used to analyze the cardiovascular activity monitored through BPM methods.**

Keywords— **Brachial blood pressure, applanation tonometry, arterial flow, vessel wall deformation, piezoelectric transducer, numerical simulation, finite element**

I. INTRODUCTION

Hemodynamic phenomena of the cardiovascular flow are accompanied by changes in human body expressed by variations of pressure in the arterial tree. A safe, non-invasive and fast way to observe the index of cardiovascular performance is the arterial blood pressure measurement that offers an accurate central pulse pressure waveform [1-7]. The brachial artery is a suitable place to measure blood pressure because its proximity to the aorta, that provides for a good correlation of the heart rate to the aortic pressure and also the close position of the vessel with the skin [1].

Blood pressure monitoring systems sense changes in the hemodynamic process based on pressure transducers, when over the artery act forces in order to flatten the area of interest [3-5]. Piezoelectric transducers (PZTs), among others, have proved the accuracy and sensitivity needed for blood measurements, provided that some imposed conditions are met [8]: a) the artery needs a solid nearness structure in order to be flattened, b) sensors dimensions are reduced compared to the flattened area, c) the artery wall and the skin can be considered an ideal membrane.

In this study we propose a mathematical model aimed at investigating, through numerical simulation, the hemodynamic of the brachial-ulnar-radial arterial tree as perceived by a set of PZTs. Based on this information, we introduce equivalent hydrodynamic impedances. The dynamics of these quantities bear the main features of the arterial flow, which may be useful in interpreting the cardiovascular activity. The PZT device in this study is a concept sensor inspired from commercial instruments intended for blood pressure measurements. The measuring technique, to the best of our knowledge, is proposed for the first time here.

II. THE PIEZOELECTRIC TRANSDUCER

Fig. 1 shows a schematic view of the simplified PZT: a flat cylinder of 8 mm radius and 2 mm height, with a central piezoelectric disc (PZD), surrounded by foam and capped by an aluminum disk. The device converts the mechanical stress induced by the blood flow (via the arm) into an electrical signal. When the vessel wall expands, during the acceleration phase of the blood flow, the piezoelectric disc is compressed against a (presumably) rigid holder (*e.g.*, a cuff), which results in a voltage drop that may be conditioned and used for monitoring purposes.

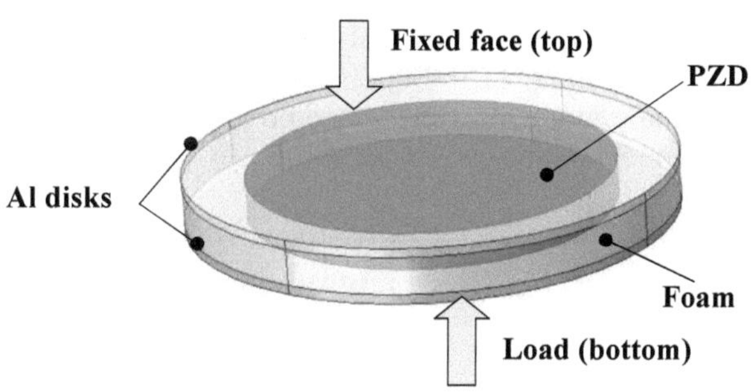

Fig. 1 Schematic view of the simplified piezoelectric device used for blood pressure monitoring. The Al discs act as armatures.

The piezoelectric conversion is based on the relation between the stress, strain, electric field, and electric displacement field in strain-charge form [9]

$$\begin{aligned} \varepsilon &= s_E\sigma + d^T\mathbf{E}, \\ \mathbf{D} &= d\sigma + \varepsilon_0\varepsilon_{rT}\mathbf{E}, \end{aligned} \qquad (1)$$

where σ [Pa] is the stress, ε is the strain, d is the coupling matrix, s_E [Pa^{-1}] is the compliance matrix, $(\cdot)^T$ is

S. Vlad and R.V. Ciupa (eds.), *International Conference on Advancements of Medicine and Health Care through Technology*, IFMBE Proceedings 44,
DOI: 10.1007/978-3-319-07653-9_61, © Springer International Publishing Switzerland 2014

the transposition operator, $\varepsilon_0 = 1/(4\pi \cdot 9 \cdot 10^9)$F/m is the electrical permittivity of the free space, ε_{rT} is the relative permittivity, **D** [C/m^2] is the electric flux density (electrical displacement), and **E** [V/m] is the electric field strength. All parts of the device (Al disks, foam, PZD) are isotropic.

As the PZT works under relatively slowly varying stress (at the pulse rate of the circulatory system) and the PZD is an elastic linear material with small deformations, the electrical part of problem may be assumed static, decoupled, described through the mathematical model

$$-\nabla(\varepsilon_0 \varepsilon_r \nabla V) = \rho_v, \tag{2}$$

where V [V] is the electric potential and ρ_v [C/m^3] is the electrical charge volume density.

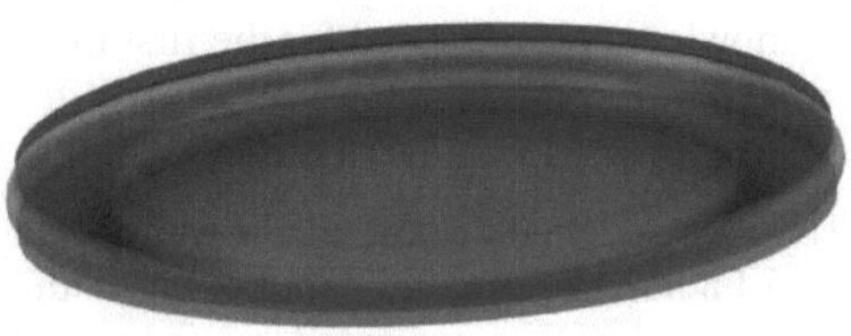

Fig. 2 PZT deformation, magnified 3e7 times for better viewing

The boundary conditions are (mechanical): prescribed displacement for the face that contacts the skin (the arm surface under the PZT is flattened, pre-stressed through fastening); the opposite face is fixed; the lateral side is free, and (electrical): floating potential for the face that contacts the skin; the opposite face is grounded; electrical insulation (zero charge density) for the lateral side.

The mathematical model was solved numerically, in the finite element technique [10]. Fig. 2 shows the deformation at a specific time moment, which corresponds to the beginning of the hemodynamic cycle (Fig. 4.b).

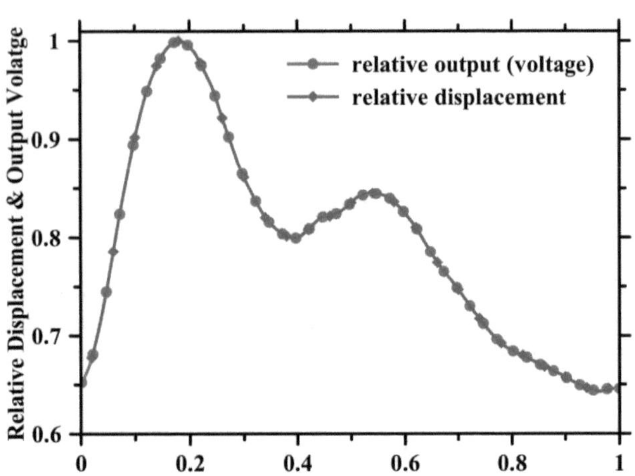

Fig. 3 Piezoelectric sensor, boundary: total displacement

Fig. 3 shows the mechanical excitation and the electrical response. This representation, in nondimensional values (both quantities are divided by their respective maximum values of the order $O(10^{-7})$ m, for displacement, $O(10^{-4})$ V for voltage), shows off that in this study PZT behaves as a linear device hence may provide for a convenient monitoring of the hemodynamic flow.

III. The Hemodynamic-Structural-Piezoelectric Model

In this study we are concerned with the hemodynamic flow in the brachial-ulnar-radial arterial sub-tree, and the associated structural deformations of the blood vessels that are transmitted through the arm to a set of PZTs that convert the flow dynamics into electrical signals to be monitored.

We use numerical simulation therefore there is a concern about simpler, excessively idealized computational domains, which are prone to produce less meaningful results. On the other hand, the anatomy of the regions of interest is usually complex enough and poses significant difficulties to numerical modeling when detailed, image-based reconstruction approach is used to build the computational domain [10].

Here, as in [11], we rely on a simpler CAD solution (built using [13]) that is convenient to the numerical simulation while rendering the main details of the anatomical structure under investigation.

A. The Hemodynamic Flow

The brachial artery and its downstream tributaries (radial and ulnar arteries) belong to the group of relatively large size blood vessels that are considered of *resistive* type [11]. The mathematical model that describes the viscous, laminar, incompressible, pulsatile flow in the brachial-radial-ulnar arterial system is made of [12]

momentum balance (*Navier – Stokes*)

$$\rho\left[\frac{\partial \mathbf{u}}{\partial t} + (\mathbf{u}\cdot\nabla)\mathbf{u}\right] = -\nabla p + \eta\nabla^2\mathbf{u}, \tag{3}$$

mass conservation

$$\nabla \cdot \mathbf{u} = 0. \tag{4}$$

Here **u** [m/s] is the velocity field, p [N/m^2] is the pressure field, $\rho = 1060$ kg/m^3 is the mass density, and η [Pa·s] is the dynamic viscosity. We use the power law type of fluid, where $\eta = m\gamma'^{n-1}$, γ' is the shear rate tensor, m = 0.017 Pa·s^n, and n = 0.708 are model parameters, that is credited to solve the discrepancies among published values of the viscosity measured using different techniques [12].

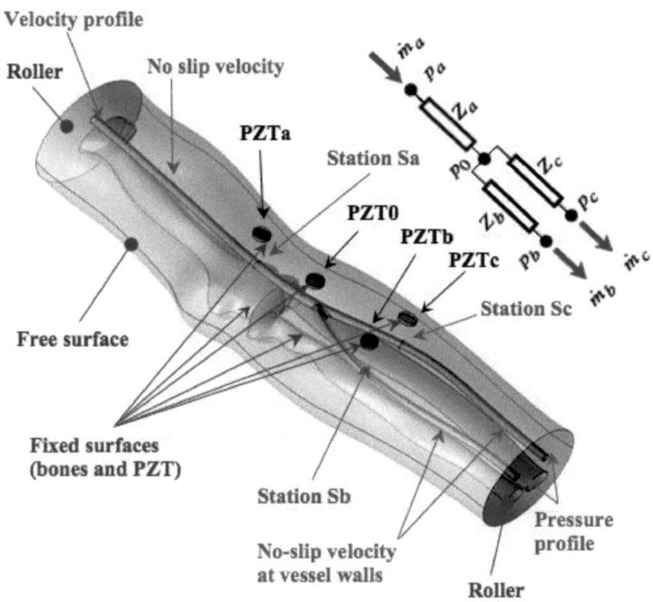

a. The computational domain, and the boundary conditions for flow and structural interactions. Sa, Sb and Sc are stations used to monitor the flow.

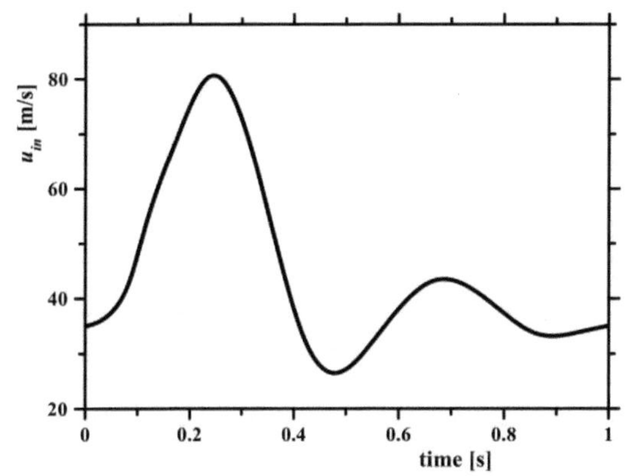

b. The inlet velocity profile [12], [15].

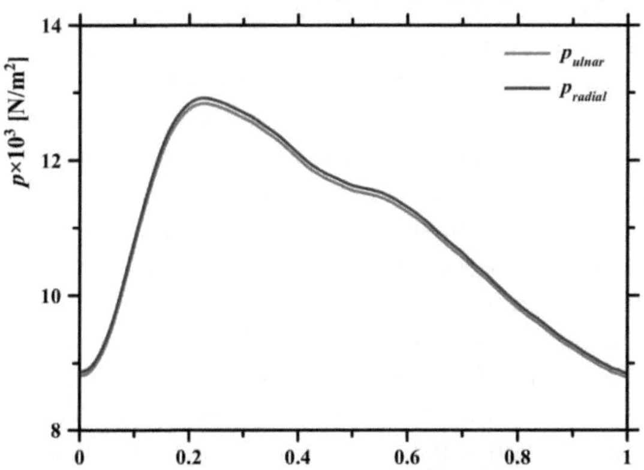

c. The outlet pressure profiles [12].

Fig. 4. Computational domain and boundary conditions in the hemodynamic and structural problems

The boundary conditions (BCs) that close the model are (Fig. 4): no-slip velocity conditions at the walls; prescribed uniform pressure conditions at the radial and ulnar outlets (Fig. 4,c), and uniform velocity profile at the brachial inlet (Fig. 4,b). They correspond to a cardiac rhythm of 100 bpm.

The arterial vessels have relatively large cross sections, they oppose little resistance to the flow therefore the pressure drops are small. The structural model introduced next represents the load with the total stress distribution that is computed in the fluid-dynamics analysis.

B. The Structural Model for the Arm

The walls of the arteries and the muscular tissue are hyperelastic materials [12], [14,15]. Their constitutive laws are defined using a strain energy density function, W. The stress, S is the derivative of W with respect to Green-strains, E, $S = \partial W/\partial E$. The strain energy density model used here is neo-Hookean (isotropic model)

$$W = \frac{1}{2}J^{-\frac{2}{3}}\left(I - \frac{1}{3}\bar{I}_1 C^{-1}\right) + \frac{1}{2}\kappa \cdot J(J-1)C^{-1}, \quad (5)$$

where $J = \det(\mathbf{F})$ is the relative variation of the volume; $\mathbf{F}$ is the deformation gradient; $C = \mathbf{F}^T\mathbf{F}$ is the right Cauchy-Green tensor, and $I_1 = \mathrm{trace}(C)$. For the muscle, the initial shear modulus is $\mu = 719{,}676$ Pa, the initial bulk modulus is $\kappa = 14{,}393{,}520$ Pa, which corresponds to the Poisson's ratio $\nu = 0.45$ [12], [14].

The BCs that close the model are given in Fig. 3. The bones are a rigid structure hence no deformation may occur. At the inlet and outlet cross-sections of the arterial walls the BCs are of "roller" type. The total stress upon the vessel walls, solved for in the first step, is used as BC load in the structural analysis of the arterial walls deformations produced by the pulsatile flow.

C. The PZT Model

The stress propagated by the arm to the PZTs is used as load, and the voltages produced by the sensors deformations are recorded to monitor the blood flow dynamics.

Here, unlike in (1), the piezoelectric conversion is based on the relation between the stress, strain, electric field, and electric displacement field in stress-charge form [9]

$$\begin{aligned} \sigma &= c_E \varepsilon - e^T \mathbf{E}, \\ \mathbf{D} &= e\varepsilon + \varepsilon_0 \varepsilon_{rS} \mathbf{E}, \end{aligned} \quad (6)$$

where e [C/m²] is the coupling matrix, and c_E [Pa] is the elasticity matrix. The upper faces of the PZTs (opposed to the skin-PZTs interfaces) are fixed, to simulate the effect of the cuff. The model (3)-(6) was FEM solved.

We used the following solution strategy: the hemodynamic problem was solved first. Then, using the load field on the vessels walls thus obtained, the structural problem of the blood vessels and surrounding tissue was modeled. Finally, the PZT problem was solved using the stress field on the interfaces PZT-skin.

The outcomes of this three-step scheme are the PZT voltages that monitor the dynamics of the blood flow. As will be shown, they may be used to compute circuit lumped parameters (Fig. 4,a), dynamic quantities that may be useful in interpreting the cardiovascular hemodynamic.

IV. Results and Discussion

The hemodynamic of the brachial flow is seen through the velocity field (streamlines, arrows) and deformations (Fig 5.). The flow structure shows recirculations downstream the bifurcation, which evolve cyclically in time. The bifurcation region is also the region of a higher gradient of pressure, which may produce higher local stresses in the vessels walls. This region is of particular interest in atherosclerosis evolution, and its study makes the object of a vast body of literature, *e.g.* [17], and it is also the subject of our future work. Fig. 6 shows the pressure at Sa,Sb,Sc (Fig. 4,a) obtained thorough numerical simulation.

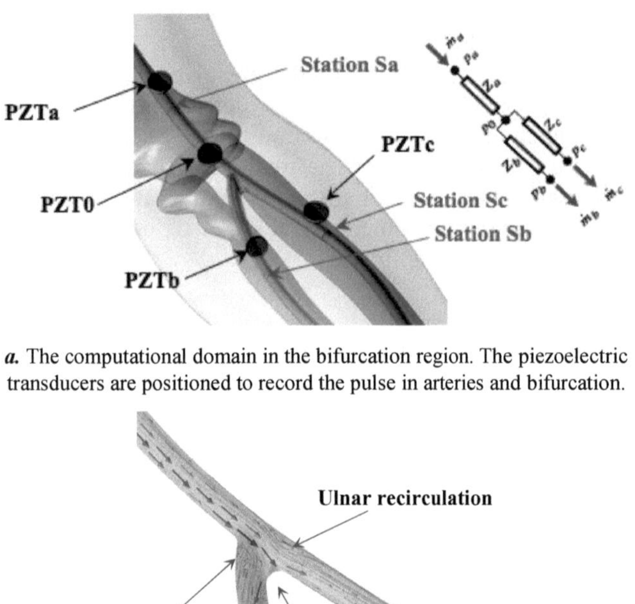

a. The computational domain in the bifurcation region. The piezoelectric transducers are positioned to record the pulse in arteries and bifurcation.

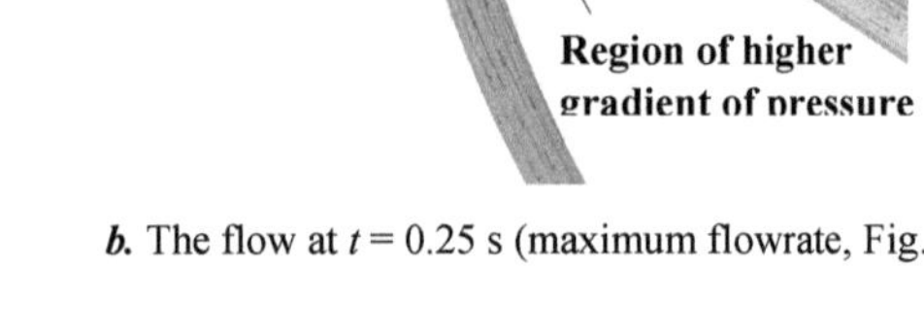

b. The flow at $t = 0.25$ s (maximum flowrate, Fig. 4,b).

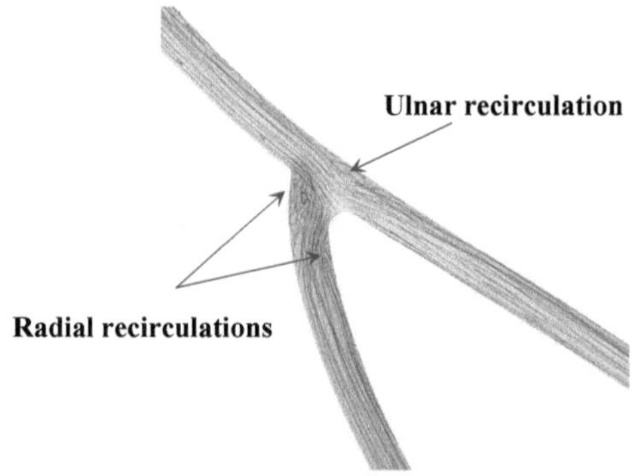

c. The flow at $t = 0.5$ s (minimum flowrate, Fig. 4,b).

Fig. 5 The flow in the brachial-radial-ulnar as shown through streamlines and arrows of velocity. The surface color is proportional to pressure

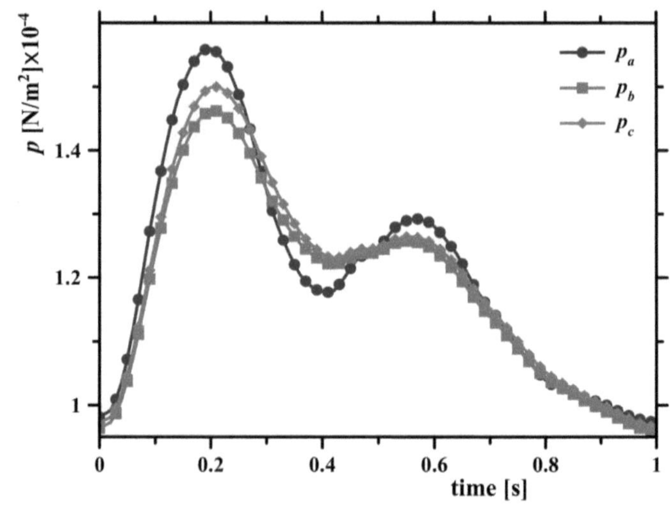

Fig. 6 Average pressures at Sa, Sb, Sc (Fig. 4,a) during the cardiac cycle

In the brachial artery, the early systolic wave ($t \sim 0.2$ s) is presumably associated with the fast rise in pressure at the beginning of systole, which is augmented by the reflected compression wave from the bifurcation [6]. The following decay in local pressure is associated with a forward-traveling expansion wave, while the reduction in pressure at the end of systole occurs in association with another forward-traveling expansion wave ($t \sim 0.4$ s). Similar pressure dynamics are noticed in radial and ulnar arteries due to the reflected waves produced there by the hand.

The numerical simulation of the PZT sensing is shown in Fig. 7 and Fig. 8. Apparently, the PZTs responses follow closely the dynamics revealed by the pressure while providing for a very convenient (numerical and experimental) monitoring method. Using the PZTs outputs, the differential voltages that correspond roughly to each arterial branch (brachial, radial, ulnar) of the arterial tree of concern may be obtained (Fig. 8).

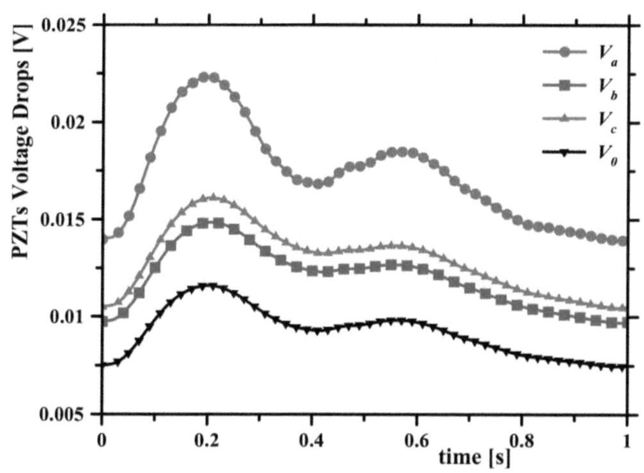

Fig. 7 PZTs voltage outputs

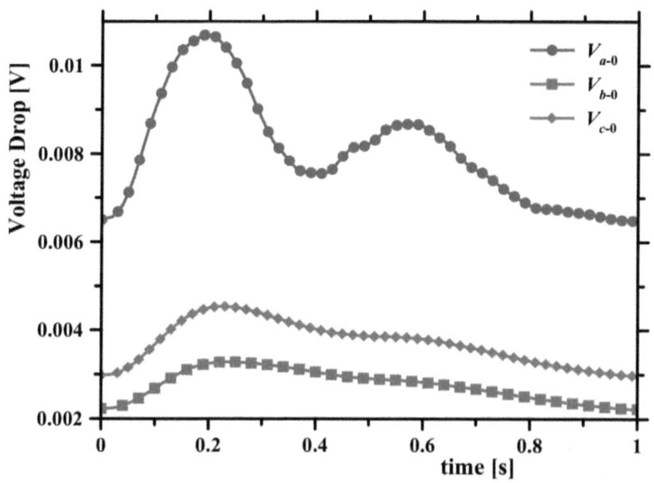

Fig. 8 Voltage drops on the brachial artery, radial and ulnar ramifications

This information is used next to introduce and compute a set of hydrodynamic circuit lumped impedances that define an equivalent star circuit (Fig. 3,a, Fig. 5,a).

A. A Lumped Parameters Perspective to the Hemodynamic Flow

Assuming that the voltage output of the sensors is linear and proportional to the local pressure and using the mass flow rates in the arteries we conjecture that $\tilde{V} = \tilde{p}$, and define the computational impedance

$$\tilde{Z} = \tilde{p} / \tilde{\dot{m}} . \quad (7)$$

Here $\tilde{V} = V / V_{\max}$ is nondimensional voltage, V [V] is the PZT output and $V_{\max}$ [V] its maximum value, $\tilde{p} = p / p_{\max}$, p [N/m^2] is the average value of the local pressure (at Sa, Sb, Sc) and p_{max} its maximum value; $\tilde{\dot{m}} = \dot{m} / \dot{m}_{\max}$ is the nondimensional mass flow rate (inlet and outlets to the computational domain) and $\dot{m}_{\max}$ its maximum value.

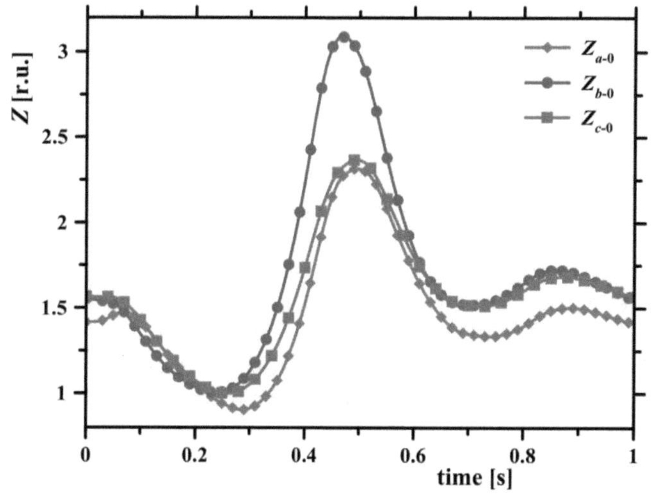

Fig. 9 The dynamic impedances of the brachial, radial and ulnar arteries

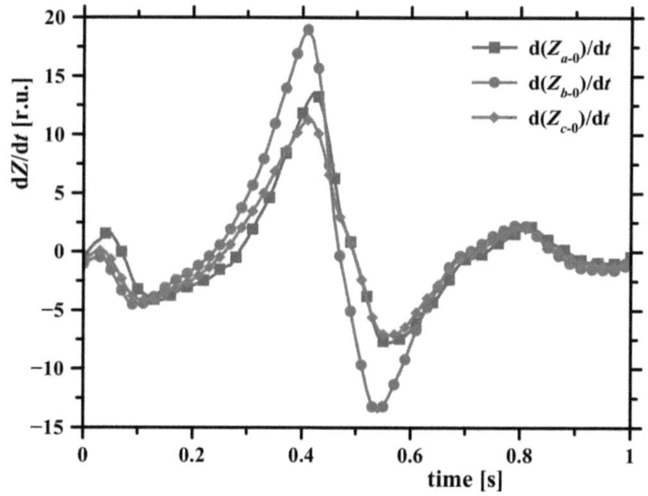

Fig. 10 Time derivatives of the impedances in Fig. 9

In this study, the mass flow rates in (7) are obtained by numerical simulation. However they may be obtained experimentally too, *e.g.* [18,19].

Fig. 9 shows the dynamic impedances (7) for the brachial, radial, and ulnar arterial segments, and Fig. 10 shows their time derivatives. The particular moments $t = 0.2$ s and $t = 0.4$ s, previously noted, are clearly seen in Fig. 10. As in the cardiometry monitoring techniques, *e.g.* [20], the relevance of the impedance derivative is key in better outlining events in the hemodynamic cycle, *e.g.* at $t \sim 0.55$ s and $t \sim 0.85$ s. Their significance and interpretation may make the object of a future research.

V. CONCLUSIONS

In this study we investigated the pulsatile blood flow in the brachial artery and its ulnar and radial tributaries to understand its blood pressure monitoring (BPM) aspects, the flow-vessel-muscle structural interactions that may occur in the brachial bifurcation, and the PZT sensing of the brachial-radial-ulnar hemodynamic.

Recirculation regions emerge downstream the bifurcation, in the ulnar and radial arteries, and their amplitudes depend on the phase in the cardiovascular cycle. The pressure highest gradient and deformation occur in the bifurcation, at the brachial-radial-ulnar junction. Although this region is less prone to plaque deposition, its vicinity with the recirculations in the radial and ulnar artery – more likely favorable for plaque deposition – may transform the bifurcation in a region exposed to vascular fracture.

The mechanical deformations of the blood vessels and arm are negligibly small. The pressure fluctuations in the arteries propagate through the arm to be sensed by the PZTs. For the working conditions assumed in this study the electrical response of the PZT is linear, which makes it fit for an accurate, convenient monitoring the dynamics of the pressure field in the arteries.

The lumped parameters – dynamic hydrodynamic impedances – and their associated time derivatives provide for a circuit, more convenient approach in the analysis of the cardiovascular activity as observable based on BPM technique.

ACKNOWLEDGEMENTS

The work was conducted in the Laboratory for Electrical Engineering in Medicine, affiliated with the BIONGTEH platform at UPB.

CONFLICT OF INTEREST

The authors declare that they have no conflict of interest.

REFERENCES

1. Patvardhan E, Heffernan KS, et al (2011). Augmentation index derived from peripheral arterial tonometry correlates with cardiovascular risk factors, NCBI, 253758, DOI: 10.4061/2011/253758
2. Non-Invasive blood pressure monitor with augmentation index, HEM 9000AI, Omron.
3. Hiroshi M., Clinical assessment of central blood pressure, Curr Hypertens Rev. 2012, DOI: 10.2174/157340212800840708
4. Shantanu S, GhatakAn S Inexpensive Arterial Pressure Wave Sensor and its application in different physiological condition, 2005, arXiv:physics/0512071
5. DynaPulse Analysis Center http://www.dynapulse.com/
6. Zambanini A, Cunningham SL, Parker KH, Khir AW, Thom SAMcG, Hughes AD Wave-energy patterns in carotid, brachial, and radial arteries: a noninvasive approach using wave-intensity analysis", Am J Physiol Heart Circ Physiol 2005, 289, pp. 270–276
7. Quick CM, Berger DS, Noordergraaf A Constructive and destructive addition of forward and reflected arterial pulse waves", Am. J. Physiol Heart Circ. Physiol 280, 2001, pp. 1519–1527
8. Webster JG (2006) Encyclopedia of medical devices and instrumentation 2nd ed., 6
9. Comsol Multiphysics, v. 3.5a (2010) – v. 4.3b (2013).
10. Morega AM, Dobre AA, Morega M Numerical simulation of magnetic drug targeting with flow – structural interaction in an arterial branching region of interest, Comsol Conf., Versailles, France, 17-19 Nov. 2010
11. Feijóo RA Computational methods in biology, 2nd Summer School LNCC/MCT, Petrópolis, January 2000
12. Morega AM, Savastru C, Morega M Numerical simulation of flow dynamics in the brachial-ulnar-radial Arterial System, IEEE International Conference on e-Health and Bioengineering, EHB 2013, November 21-23, 2013, Iasi, Romania.
13. SolidWorks (2010).
14. Elert G The Physics Hypertextbook-Viscosity. physics.info
15. Bangash M.Y.H., Bangash F.N., Bangash T. Trauma. An engineering analysis with medical case studies investigation, Springer, ISBN 3-540-36305-X, 2007.
16. Taylor C., Hughes TJR, Zarins C, Finite element modeling of three-dimensional pulsatile flow in the abdominal aorta: Relevance to atherosclerosis, Annals of Biomedical Eng., vol. 26, 1998, pp. 975–987
17. Deng X, King M, et al. Localization of atherosclerosis in arterial Junctions, ASAIO Journal, vol. 41, pp. 58–67, 1995. [PubMed: 7727823].
18. Özcan H, Öztekin PS, Zergeroğlu AM, Ersöz G, Fıçıcılar H, Üstüner E Doppler ultrasound evaluation of the structural and hemodynamic changes in the brachial artery following two different exercise protocols, Diagnostic and Interventional Radiology, vol. 12, 2006, pp. 80-84
19. http://www.ti.com/product/afe5808
20. Morega AM, Dobre AA, Morega M Numerical simulation in electrical cardiometry", OPTIM 2012, 13th International Conference on Optimization of Electrical and Electronic Equipment, 24-26 May 2012, Brasov, Romania, paper RD-005282, IEEE-eXplore.

Author: Alexandru M. Morega
Institute: University POLITEHNICA of Bucharest
Street: Splaiul Independenţei no. 313, sector 6
City: Bucharest
Country: Romania
Email: alexandru.morega@upb.ro

$TPPS_4$ Controlled Release from PVA Hydrogels in Photodynamic Therapy of Cancer

R.M. Ion[1,2] and S.C.F. Patachia[3]

[1] ICECHIM, Nanomedicine Research Center, Bucharest, Romania
[2] Valahia University, Materials Engineering Department, NANOMEC Research Center, Targoviste, Romania
[3] Transilvania University of Brasov, Design Product and Environment Faculty, Brasov, Romania

Abstract— **Hydrogels are hydrophilic polymer networks whose applications are based on their ability to retain large amounts of water. They can be used as drug carriers structures with applications in the controlled release of active substance. In this paper, the PVA hydrogels (synthesized by freezing-thawing cycles) were subjected for loading $TPPS_4$ in order to be tested in photodynamic therapy model cells. Hydrogel loading procedure with $TPPS_4$, sorption experiments, the retention efficiency of porphyrins on the PVA hydrogel and controlled release of $TPPS_4$ from the PVA hydrogel have been achieved and discussed. Endothelial cell line, HUVEC, as adherent cells line model in photodynamic therapy, were grown on the surface of hydrogels mentioned, and monitorized by microscopic techniques, following the cellular membrane integrity. Also, the influence of $TPPS_4$ forms on hydrogel properties was analyzed.**

Keywords— **$TPPS_4$, PVA hydrogels, HUVEC cells, photodynamic therapy**

I. INTRODUCTION

Nowadays, the hydrogels have important biomedical applications, among them, hydrogels from poly (vinyl alcohol) (PVA) being one of the most applied due to their advantages: water soluble, non-toxic, non-carcinogenic and biodegradable [1]. These hydrogels have an increasingly interest for controlled release applications, and the kinetics of the entrapped drugs from such hydrogels can be monitored by the regulation of the water uptake of the polymer or by crosslinking it [2-5].

Today there is a growing need for the development of controlled release formulations in the pharmaceutical industry, especially in complex therapeutic areas such as oncology. In this direction, a stabilization of the porphyrin in the hydrogel matrix represents a step forward in photodynamic therapy (PDT). 5,10,15,20-tetra-sulfonato-phenyl porphyrin ($TPPS_4$) is a photo-sensitizer used mainly in the photodynamic therapy of various types of cancer (skin cancer, eye cancer, non small cell lung cancer not treatable by chemotherapy or cobalto-therapy), but also in cancer diagnosis (functionalized $TPPS_4$ accumulates specifically in tumors and the fluorescence resulting from irradiation can be used to detect tumoral tissue) and in the treatment of viral infections such as herpes simplex infection [6].

In photodynamic therapy the photo-sensitizer reacts by exposure to light source producing an excited state able to transform the molecular oxygen into singlet oxygen – highly reactive with the undesirable tissue cells and make efficient the applied treatment [6]. The excited meta-stable, singlet state O_2 destroys the cancer cells via two distinct mechanisms: a) direct disruption of cell function by breaking of the cell wall or destruction of the cell mitochondria, and b) constriction of the vascular network in the tumor that preventing nutrients to the tumor [7, 8].

In this paper, the PVA hydrogels (synthesized by freezing-thawing cycles) were tested for loading with $TPPS_4$. Hydrogel loading procedure with $TPPS_4$, sorption experiments, the retention efficiency of porphyrins on the PVA hydrogel, and controlled release of $TPPS_4$ from the PVA hydrogel have been achieved and discussed. Endothelial cell line, HUVEC, as adherent cells line and photodynamic therapy model, were grown on the surface of hydrogels mentioned, and monitorized by microscopic techniques, following the cellular membrane integrity. Also, the influence of $TPPS_4$ forms on hydrogel properties was analyzed.

II. EXPERIMENTAL PART

A. Materials and Methods

Poly (vinyl alcohol) hydrogel: The PVA solution was prepared by dissolving PVA 90-98 (degree of polymerization of 900 and a degree of hydrolysis of 98%) polymer powder in distilled water under continued magnetic stirring for 3 hours at 90°C. The PVA hydrogel has been prepared from a 13% wt. PVA solution by 3 consecutive cycles of freeze (-20^{0}C, 12 hours) and thaw (20^{0}C, 12 hours), by using a cryostat [9]. The resulting hydrogel has been conditioned in distilled water.

Loading experiments protocol: $TPPS_4$ loading on the PVA hydrogels has been achieved directly immersing the pre-weighed PVA hydrogel tablet (1.5 g) in 5 mL of 10^{-3} M $TPPS_4$ solution and kept 30 minutes for loading.

Measurement of the retention efficiency of porphyrins on the PVA hydrogel: The retention process of the porphyrins

S. Vlad and R.V. Ciupa (eds.), *International Conference on Advancements of Medicine and Health Care through Technology*, IFMBE Proceedings 44,
DOI: 10.1007/978-3-319-07653-9_62,

on PVA hydrogels has been monitored by UV-VIS spectrometry with a Specord M400 Spectrophotometer. The retention efficiency (normalized to the swollen hydrogel mass) has been calculated according to the formula:

$$RE(\%) = \frac{m_{Porphyrin\_retained}}{m_{Porphyrin\_initial} \cdot m_{hydrogel}} \cdot 100 \quad (1)$$

where:

$m_{Porphyrin\_initial}$ is the initial amount of porphyrin to be found in the solution, and $m_{Porphyrin\_retained}$ is determined from the difference between the initial and the remaining amounts of porphyrin after retention [10].

Controlled release experiments: Release experiments were carried out by using a $TPPS_4$-loaded PVA hydrogel, rinsed thoroughly after loading with distilled water, and then placed in the appropriate quantity of medium (distilled water). An aliquot of the medium was taken at the fixed time interval of 24 h. The amount of released porphyrin has been determined spectrophotometrically. Due to the photosensitivity of $TPPS_4$, all vessels were completely protected from light influence with aluminium foil.

HUVEC cells tests: The HUVEC human cell endothelial line from ombilical vein HUVEC–C (ATCC - Nr. CRL-1730) [11]. Endothelial cell line, HUVEC, adherent cell line was grown on the surface of hydrogels mentioned. Hydrogels have been punched in ϕ1cm and transferred to culture plates. Hydrogels have been rebalanced in specific culture medium and the cells were seeded.

Fluorescence microscopy: Labeled cells were observed in situ either on the optical scatter imaging microscope platform, which was also fitted with an epifluorescence modality, using an inverted microscope (Eclipse T300, Nikon) with epifluorescence, to monitor fluorescence emission. With a 10 nm band pass interference filter an incident red beam λ = 590 nm, has been obtained.

Intracellular localization study: We determined the intracellular localization of our compound $TPPS_4$ with a LSM510 laser scanning confocal microscope (Carl Zeiss, Germany) mounted on an upright fluorescence microscope (Nikon E600) equipped for the observation and acquisition of images in the interferential contrast mode (DIC). Cells were seeded in flasks and allowed to grow at 37°C and 5% CO_2 up to 50–70% confluence. The medium was then removed and the cells were washed twice with phosphate buffered saline (PBS) and incubated at 37°C and 5% CO_2 in PBS containing the appropriate dye [12]. For each compound we optimized the proper working concentration (2 to 10 μM) and the suitable incubation time (15 min to 1h).

III. Results and Discussion

The experimental data reveal that $TPPS_4$ has a high affinity for PVA hydrogels. One can also observe from the sorption curves that the sorption equilibrium is reached fast (in 5 min in most cases). The sorption mechanism of $TPPS_4$ onto the PVA hydrogel can be interpreted as having two components: physi-sorption and chemi-sorption. In physi-sorption, the porphyrin is encapsulated into the pores of the nanostructured hydrogels, by a mechanism mainly controlled by diffusion [13]. The chemi-sorption mechanism consists of the hydrogen bonding between the –OH groups of the poly(vinyl alcohol) and the pyrrolic nitrogen of the porphyrin molecule [14].

$TPPS_4$ shows distinct behaviour when in contact with the PVA hydrogel. The aspects of the hydrogels with retained porphyrins are depicted in Fig. 1 (a). During the sorption of $TPPS_4$ from the water-based solution onto the hydrogel, a transition from the green to a red colour has been observed, due to the transformation of aggregated form of $TPPS_4$ into a monomeric one [1], [15] (Fig. 1 (b)).

The main absorption band is located at 416 nm and is assigned to monomeric form of $TPPS_4$. The aggregated forms could be identified by the new Soret band (490 nm), by reduction of those four Q bands (515, 545, 585 and 645 nm) of monomeric form into only two red shifted bands (658 and 708 nm) and by reducing the molar absorption coefficients of these new bands, as a sign of the oligomerization [6].

The retention efficiency, calculated with eq. 1, is 71,7%. The retention efficacy in the case of $TPPS_4$ shows a strong retention capacity of the PVA 90-98 hydrogel [16].

The remaining concentration in $TPPS_4$ solution after 10 min is decreasing from 10^{-3} mol/L to $0.3*10^{-3}$ mol/L, so is almost half of the concentration loaded into the PVA hydrogel, Fig. 1 (c).

The controlled release experiments were carried out by using a $TPPS_4$-loaded PVA hydrogel, rinsed thoroughly after loading, with distilled water, and then placed in the appropriate quantity of medium (distilled water). The amount of $TPPS_4$ released at different periods of time t, (M_t), and that obtained after equilibrium was reached, (M_∞) have been determined by VIS spectrophotometry. The ratio M_t/M_∞ has been plotted against time to obtain the release profile (Fig. 1 (d)). From Fig. 1(d), it could be noted a non-Fickian release of $TPPS_4$ from the PVA hydrogel matrix. This could be explained by the effect of ionic $TPPS_4$ on the PVA network and of the water state into the gel.

The release ratio was 68% of the total encapsulated $TPPS_4$ into the gel.

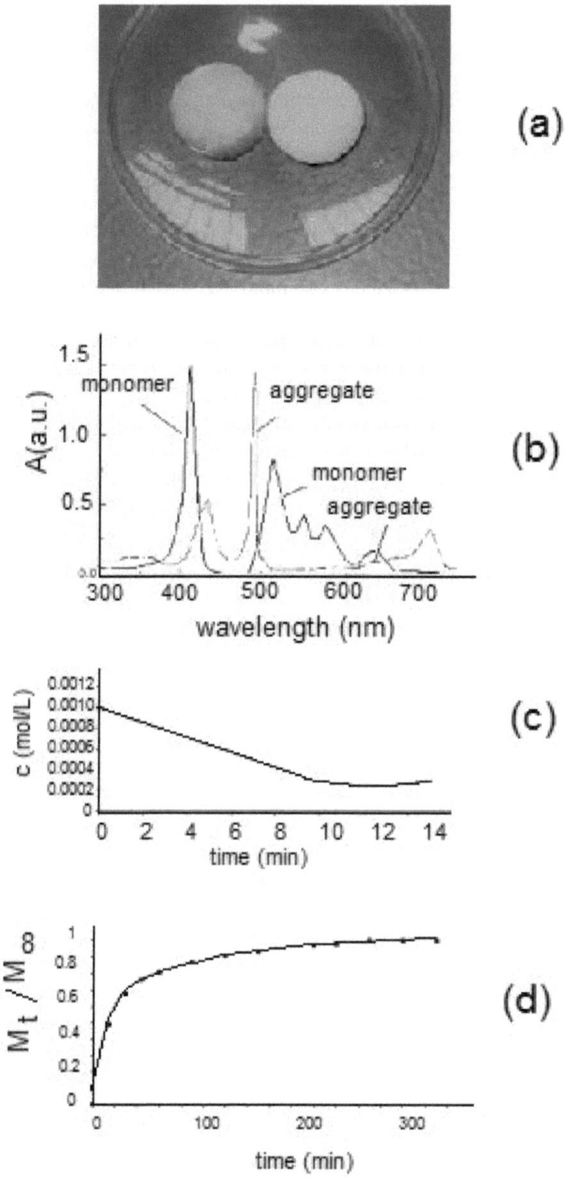

Fig. 1 Aspect of PVA hydrogel with (left) and without $TPPS_4$ hydrogel (right)(a), $TPPS_4$ absorption spectra changes during the adsorption on PVA hydrogel(b), kinetics of $TPPS_4$ loading in PVA hydrogel (c) and kinetic of $TPPS_4$ release from the PVA hydrogel (normalized to encapsulated $TPPS_4$ amount)(d)

These results could be well correlated with the SEM microscopy images obtained from PVA 90-98 samples loaded with $TPPS_4$. SEM analysis showed a high loading with $TPPS_4$ porphyrin (visible as small microgranules on the surface of the gel) (Fig. 2).The SEM microscopy put into evidence interconnected pores with a size distribution in the range of 80-950 nm. This structure allows for the retention of $TPPS_4$ porphyrin.

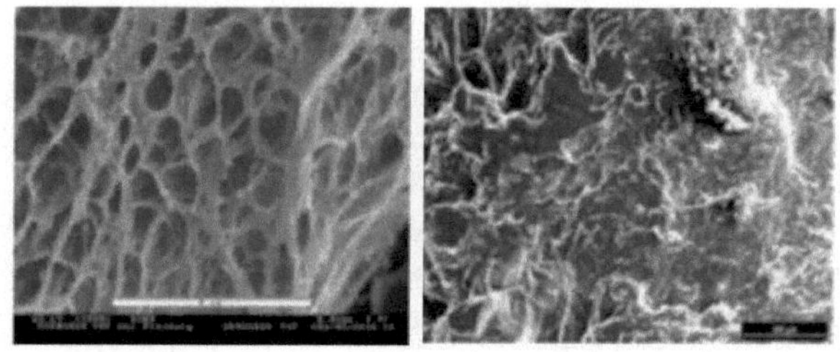

Fig. 2 SEM images of PVA 90-98 hydrogel (left) and of $TPPS_4$ porphyrin-loaded PVA 90-98 hydrogel(right)

HUVECs were selected in our experiments as an *in vitro* model to assess the vascular toxicity of $TPPS_4$. In Fig.3 is observed a networked structure of the hydrogel and non-adherent HUVEC cells (left). The tested hydrogels show promising characteristics applying for some *in vitro* experimental systems on cellular lines, at short times, not modifying the cellular functionality. After 24h the used cell line adhered to the hydrogel structure and expanded compared to control sample (right).

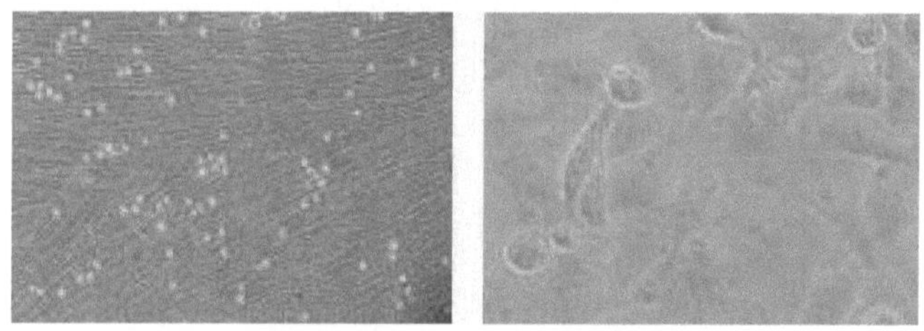

Fig. 3 Phase contrast micrographs of HUVEC with $TPPS_4$-PVA hydrogel (left-1 h after cell seeding and right- 24 h after cell seeding)

For this purpose HUVEC cells pre-incubated with $TPPS_4$ were illuminated with red light. PDT led to a dramatic change in the morphology of these endothelial cells. To examine mitochondrial structure in HUVECs treated with $TPPS_4$ in PVA for 24 h, MitoTracker Red FM (1 μM) was added after twice PBS washing. After a short incubation period of 15 minutes, the fluorescence images are visble for mitochondria. The photosensitizer accumulated in mitochondria and its fluorescence emission is detected in red region (~590 nm), before (left) and after PDT protocol. A deformation of the cells, as a sign of the cellular death, is observed after PDT (right), Figure 4.

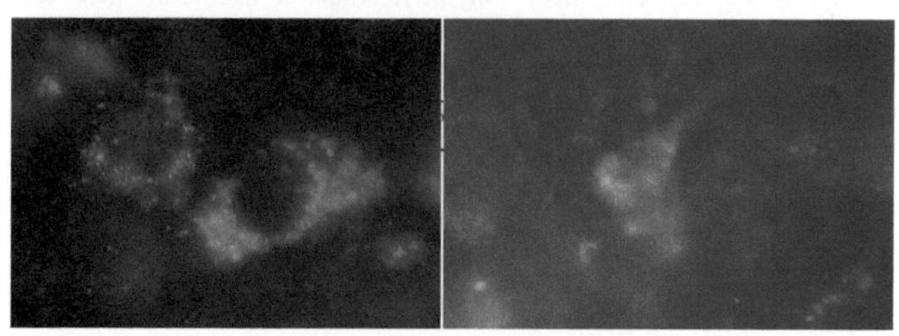

Fig. 4 Laser scanning confocal microscopy of HUVEC before (left) and after (right) the PDT protocol

IV. Conclusions

In this paper, the PVA hydrogels (synthesized by freezing-thawing cycles) were tested for loading with $TPPS_4$. Hydrogel loading procedure with $TPPS_4$, sorption experiments, the retention efficiency of porphyrins on the PVA hydrogel, and controlled release of $TPPS_4$ from the PVA hydrogel have been achieved and discussed. The properties of the hydrogel can be determined precisely by VIS spectrophotometry and SEM. Endothelial cell line, HUVEC, as adherent cells line and photodynamic therapy model, were grown on the surface of hydrogels mentioned, and monitorized by microscopic techniques, following the cellular membrane integrity. Also, the influence of $TPPS_4$ forms on hydrogel properties was analyzed. We can conclude that PVA hydrogels represents an efficient encapsulation vehicle for porphyrins, and have a good sorption profile for this porphyrin, and is better suited for the preparation of controlled-release vehicles.

Acknowledgment

We acknowledge the contribution of PhD. Eng. Varga Stefan to some experimental work.

Conflict of Interest

The authors declare that they have no conflict of interest.

References

1. Varga S, Patachia S, Ion RM (2007) Development of controlled release devices for photodynamic therapy of cancer Pollack Periodica 2: 131-140
2. Varga S, Patachia S, Ion RM (2007) Nanostructured PVA hydrogel materials as vehicles for the encapsulation and controlled release of porphyrin-based cancer therapeutics, Bulletin of the Transilvania University of Brasov: Supplement Bramat 4: 153-160
3. Hassan CM, Peppas NA. 2000) Structure and applications of poly(vinyl alcohol) hydrogels produced by conventional cross-linking or by freezing/thawing methods. Adv Polym Sci. 153:37-65.
4. Patachia S, Ion RM, Varga S et al (2007) Porphyrin encapsulation in nanostructured hydrogels. J.Optoel. Adv. Mat. 9(6): 1816-1820
5. Petrisor G, Ion RM, Brachais CH, et al. (2012) Designing Medical Devices Based on Silicon Polymeric Material with Controlled Release of Local AnestheticsJ. Macromol. Sci. Part A 49(5):439-444
6. Ion RM,Planner A, Wicktowicz K, et al. (1998) The incorporation of various porphyrins into blood cells measured via flow cytometry,absorption and emission spectroscopy Acta Biochimica Polonica 45:833-847
7. Neagu M, Manda G, Constantin C et al. (2007) Synthetic porphyrins in experimental photodynamic therapy induce a different antitumoral effect, J.Porphyrins and Phthalocyanines, 11: 58-65
8. Ion RM (2012) The Use of Phthalocyanines and Related Complexes in Photodynamic Therapy, in Photosensitizers in Medicine, Environment and Security, Springer, 2012, pp. 315-349
9. Lozinsky VI. Cryotropic gelation of poly(vinyl alcohol) solutions. Russ Chem Rev. 1998;67:573-586.
10. Petrisor G, Ion RM, Brachais CH, et al. (2012) In Vitro Release of Local Anaesthetic and Anti-Inflammatory Drugs from Crosslinked Collagen Based Device, J. Macromol. Sci. Part A 49(9):699-705
11. Gifford SM, Grummer MA, Pierre SA et al. (2004) Functional characterization of HUVEC-CS: Ca2+ signaling, ERK 1/2 activation, mitogenesis and vasodilator production. J. Endocrinol. 182(3):485-99
12. Ion RM, Fierascu RC, Neagu M. et al. (2010) Porphyrin (TPP)–Polyvinylpyrrolidone (PVP)–Fullerene (C60) Triad as Novel Sensitizer in Photodynamic Therapy. Science of Advanced Materials, 2: 1–7
13. Lozinsky VI, Plieva FM. Poly(vinyl alcohol) cryogels employed as matrices for cell immobilization. 3. Overview of recent research and developments. Enzyme Microb Technol.1998;23:227-242.
14. Takamura A, Ishii F, Hidaka H. (1992) Drug release from poly(vinylalcohol) gel prepared by freeze-thaw procedure. J Control Release 20:21-27
15. Boda D, Neagu M, Constantin C. et al. (2009) New Photosensitizers Versus Aminolevulinic Acid (ALA) In Experimental Photodynamic Therapy Of Actinic Keratosis – A Case Report, Analele Stiintifice ale Universitatatii „Alexandru Ioan Cuza, Sectiunea Geneticasi Biologie Moleculara, X: 61-69
16. Pop SF, Ion RM, Neagu M. et al. (2012) Sensitizer localization and immune response in photodynamic therapy of B16 cells, Laser Physics21(3):576-581.

Author of correspondence: Rodica-Mariana Ion
Institute: ICECHIM, Bucharest
Street: 202 Splaiul Independentei
City: Bucharest
Country: Romania
Email: rodica_ion2000@yahoo.co.uk

Preparation and Characterization of Anchoring Films Designed for the Biofunctionalization of Porous Titanium

A.M. Salantiu[1], P. Pascuta[2], V. Popescu[2], S. Simon[3], L. Muresan[4], and C.O. Popa[1]

[1] Department of Materials Science and Engineering, Technical University of Cluj-Napoca, 103-105 Muncii Avenue, 400641 Cluj-Napoca, Romania
[2] Department of Physics and Chemistry, Technical University of Cluj-Napoca, 103-105 Muncii Avenue, 400641, Cluj-Napoca, Romania
[3] Physics Faculty and Interdisciplinary Research Institute in Bio-Nano-Science, Babes-Bolyai University, 400084, Cluj-Napoca, Romania
[4] Faculty of Chemistry and Chemical Engineering, Babes-Bolyai University, 400084, Cluj-Napoca, Romania

Abstract— **In this study, porous titanium compacts obtained by the pressing-sintering route, previously modified by an anodic oxidation treatment, were coated with 3- Aminopropyltriethoxysilane (APTES) in order to facilitate a later immobilization of peptides in view of improving their biocompatibility. The surface of porous titanium before and after modification was characterized by X-ray photoelectron spectroscopy (XPS) and attenuated total refraction-Fourier transform infrared spectroscopy (ATR-FTIR). According to spectral analysis, after the bonding of APTES films on the anodized PM porous titanium surfaces, a new peak located around 1110 cm^{-1} attributed to siloxane groups suggests that the silane agent had been grafted onto the surface of the modified titanium substrate. Also, after the deposition of APTES films, significant changes were seen in the XPS spectrum, as the peaks corresponding to Ti disappeared, indicating a full silane coverage on the porous surface.**

Keywords— **porous titanium, silane, surface modification, anodic oxidation, coating, covalent attachment**

I. INTRODUCTION

The idea of covalently attaching a biomolecule to the surface of a metal substrate with the aim of triggering a specific cell response has great potential [1]. Over the last decades, the modification of metal substrates with organics has been widely approached [2]. A method commonly employed to covalently attach biomolecules onto hydroxylated surfaces is functionalization using an aminosilane reaction [1]. 3-Aminopropyltriethoxysilane (APTES) is one of the possibilities to be chosen as organic silane coupling agent for the introduction of chemically reactive bioactive groups on biomaterials substrates. Titanium possesses the best combination of mechanical and biocompatibility properties among the metals used in medicine [2]. However, the properties of titanium – base biomaterials, such as those used for bone implants, can still be improved by using porous structures. Thus, bone ingrowth provides a strong implant/bone bond, while the pores may be three-dimensionally interconnected to provide enough space for the attachment and proliferation of the new bone tissue and to facilitate the transport of body fluids [3]. Silane adsorption onto metal oxide surfaces can produce diverse molecular entities and conformations owing to the range of interactions between APTES and surface hydroxyls. Si–OH generated by the hydrolysis of APTES forms hydrogen bonds with the metal surface, then further dehydrates to form Si–O–Ti covalent bond with the metal substrate. Furthermore, the hydrogen-bonded molecules may self catalyze the condensation of the silanol with a surface hydroxyl group, forming covalent siloxaned bonds [2].In this study, the surface modification of porous titanium through anodic oxidation treatment was followed by the deposition of silane coupling agents and the effects were investigated by XPS and ATR–FTIR.

II. MATERIALS AND METHODS

A. Porous Titanium Sample Preparation

Commercially pure titanium powder (with a purity higher than 99.5%) obtained by the hydration-milling-dehydration process with the powder particles size lower than 150 μm was used to produce porous disc specimens with 11.5 mm diameter and about 2 mm height. The powder was pressed in a closed die with 400 MPa and sintered at 1100°C for 1 h in vacuum of 10^{-5} torr.

B. Porous Titanium Sample Anodic Oxidation

Anodic oxidation was performed at room temperature using a conventional three electrode cell with a porous titanium disc, sample pressed with 400 MPa, as working electrode, a platinum electrode as counter electrode and a saturated calomel electrode (SCE) as reference electrode.

A commercial potentiostat (PAR 2273) was used for electrochemical investigations. Prior to the oxide growth,

S. Vlad and R.V. Ciupa (eds.), *International Conference on Advancements of Medicine and Health Care through Technology*, IFMBE Proceedings 44,
DOI: 10.1007/978-3-319-07653-9_63, © Springer International Publishing Switzerland 2014

the porous titanium disc electrode was cleaned in an ultrasonic bath using distilled water.

The parameters for the anodic oxidation of porous titanium samples were 1V and 1h. 0.25 M H_2SO_4 aqueous solution served as electrolyte and was contained in the 300 cm^3 electrochemical glass cell. After the anodic oxidation, the samples were again rinsed with distilled water, dried at 60°C, and then heat treated at 550°C for 1h aiming to the crystallization of the as-formed amorphous titanium oxide.

C. Silanization of Anodized Porous Titanium Samples

Silanisation of porous titanium anodic oxidised samples was performed in 5% 3-Aminopropyltriethoxysilane (APTES) in toluene at room temperature, overnight. After cleaning in toluene and ethanol, the samples were cured at 110°C for 1 h. One hour of curing was selected, based on the silanization procedures described in the literature [4].

D. Characterization of Porous Titanium Surface Modification

The crystallographic characteristic of the oxide layer was investigated by X-ray diffraction (Shimadzu XRD 6000).

FTIR was used to confirm the structure of APTES films on the modified titanium substrate by using a Perkin-Elmer FTIR spectrometer equipped with an ATR accessory (PIKE MIRacle™).

The elemental composition of APTES films and the modification of titanium substrate were analyzed by XPS, using a SPECS PHOIBOS 150 MCD with an Al radiation source (hv=1486.6 eV) at a power of 250W. Dried samples were mounted for spectroscopy on molybdenum stubs using double-sided adhesive copper tape. The pressure in the analysis chamber was around 10^{-10} mbar. The following sequence of spectra was recorded: survey spectrum, C 1s, O 1s, Ti 2p, Si 2p, N 1s. A charge correction was performed using the C 1s peak at 284.6 eV.

III. Results

A. Crystalline Structure of Films Obtained after the Anodic Oxidation of Porous Titanium

Fig.1 shows the XRD patterns of as-prepared films after the anodic oxidation of porous titanium in 0.25 M H_2SO_4 for 1h at 1V and followed by heat treatment at 550°C. For the as-prepared sample presented in Fig. 1a, only the peaks for titanium were present. Several peaks attributed to anatase and rutile were detected in Fig. 1b for the sample anodized and then heat treated at 550°C.

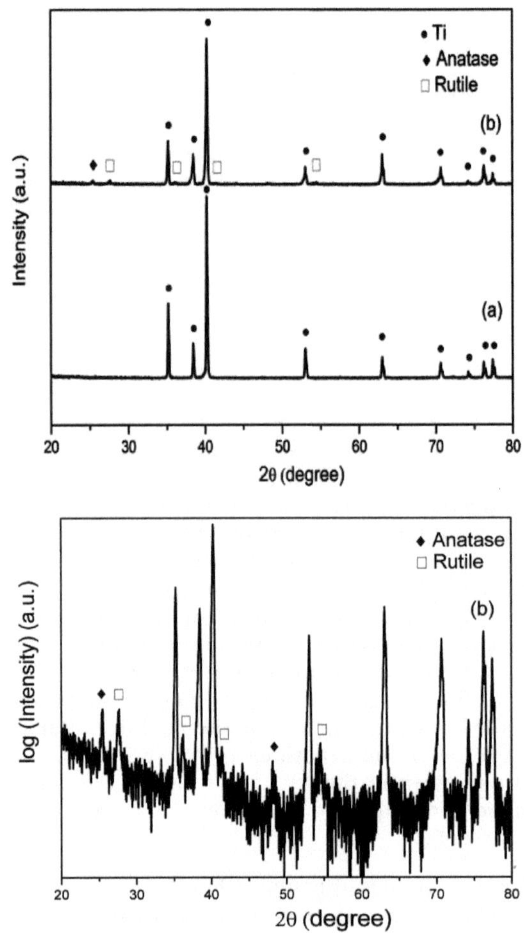

Fig. 1 XRD patterns for as-prepared anodic oxidation sample (a), and followed heat treatment at 550°C (b)

B. Fourier Transform Infrared Spectroscopy

Fig. 2 shows the FTIR spectra corresponding to samples in the two stages of surface conditioning (anodization and coating). In Fig. 2A (anodized film), the band between 900-500 cm^{-1} was due to the Ti-O vibration. FTIR spectra in the range 4000-500 cm^{-1} for APTES films prepared from toluene solutions are presented in Fig. 2B. Around 3400 cm^{-1}, the symmetric and asymmetric –NH stretch modes amino group in APTES were found to be weak in the spectra. Between 2800 and 3000 cm^{-1} several CH stretch modes of the APTES backbone and ethoxy groups are found.

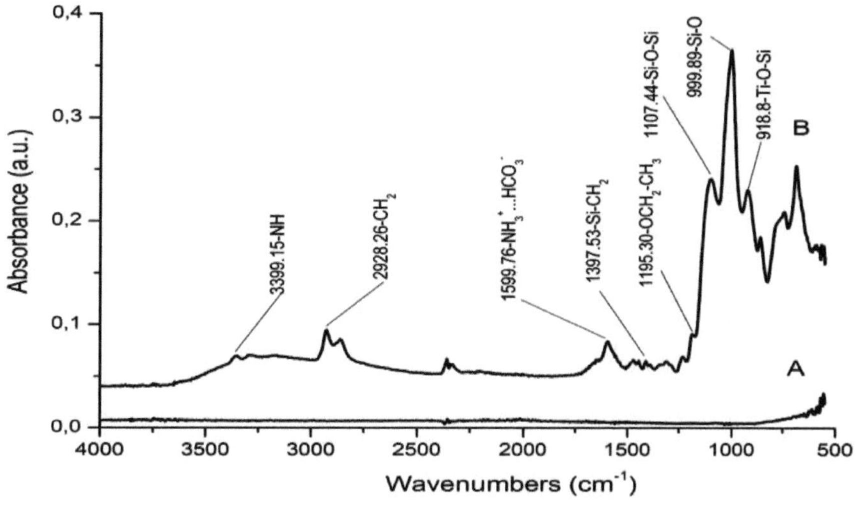

Fig. 2 FTIR spectra of anodic oxidation treated porous titanium (A), and followed APTES deposition on anodized titanium (B)

The most important structural information regarding APTES films is found between 1800-900 cm^{-1}. One dominating vibrational mode is found around 1600 cm^{-1}. Such vibrational mode arises when surface amino groups form bicarbonate salts in a reaction with atmospheric CO_2, as reported previously. Vibrational modes at 1397 cm^{-1} (-Si-CH_2) were not clearly observable in Fig. 2B. The mode near 1195 cm^{-1} arises from unhydrolyzed ethoxy moieties in APTES (-OCH_2CH_3). The peak located around 1107 cm^{-1} is attributed to Si-O moieties of polymerized APTES. The strong mode around 1000 cm^{-1} is attributed to siloxane groups (Si-O-Si) in polymerized APTES.

C. X-ray Photoelectron Spectroscopy

For further examination of both oxide layer and APTES films on treated samples, XPS analysis was employed.

XPS is a suitable method to obtain information regarding the different constituents on the surface (substrate, silane, other organic compounds).

In Fig. 3, the spectra of oxidized and silanized titanium surfaces are shown, expressing the observed constituents. The atomic concentration of elements expressed on the surface of titanium samples is given in Table 1.

Due to silanization, the titanium peak disappeared from the XPS spectra (Fig. 4), indicating full silane coverage of the surface. Thus, the siloxane layer was too thick for the bonding between silane and titanium substrate to be observed.

The O 1s spectrum shows a difference between the two surface modifications. The spectrum for anodic oxidation treated samples shows two peaks, one centred at 529.2 eV which corresponds to O 1s in the TiO_2 layer and another peak centred around 532 eV, which was attributed to the hydroxyl groups.

In the O 1s XPS spectrum for APTES films, only the peak at 532 eV was present.

In the C 1s spectrum, the main peak at 284.6 eV is associated with contamination due to various chemical species (C-C) and the peaks at 293 eV and 296 eV present on the surface of the oxide layer were attributed to the K $2p_{3/2}$ and K $2p_{1/2}$ XPS spectra.

Multilayers of APTES were attached to the anodized surface; these were directly occurring in the N 1s and in the Si 2p signals at 398.6 eV and 102.2 eV.

IV. Discussion

Ti spontaneously forms an oxide layer in air and in the body with a thickness of approximately 2-5 nm that provides a low corrosion resistance. Thus, it is recommended to thicken artificially the oxide layer, for instance by anodization, in order to improve the overall biocompatibility for endosseous implants.

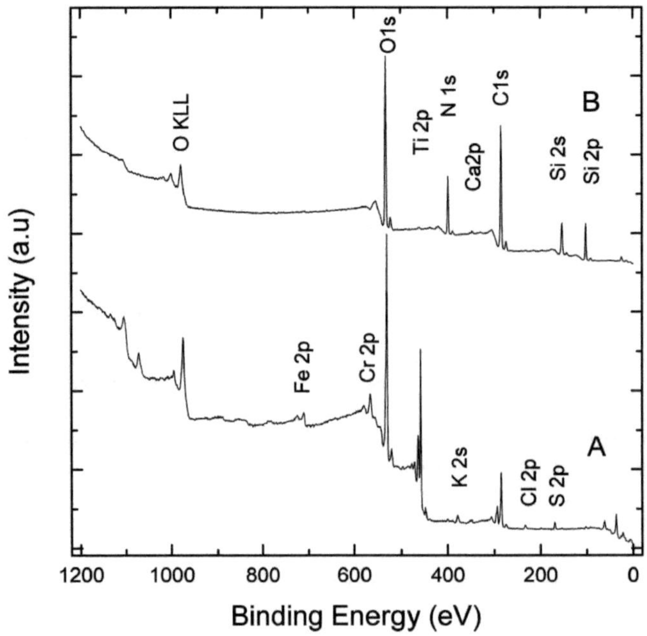

Fig. 3 XPS full spectra for anodic oxidation treated titanium (curve A), and followed APTES deposition (curve B)

Table 1 Atomic concentration of elements present on surface of titanium samples as determined by XPS [%]

	Fe	O	C	Cr	K	N	Cl	Si	S	Ca	Ti
(A) Surface$_{OX}$	1.1	49.6	29.6	0.7	2.5	0.7	0.2	---	2.3	---	13.3
(B) Surface$_{APTES}$	---	22.8	48.6	---	---	11.9	---	16.3	---	0.2	0.2

Oxidized surfaces change the properties of the titanium implants and play an important role during the dynamics of the osseointegration process.

With regard to the chemical properties, anatase is an important phase of titanium dioxide, since it is more reactive and thus more effective in forming bone-like apatite, as bioactive layer. On the other hand, rutile, the other stable phase of titanium dioxide, has also a positive effect in improving the biocompatibility of titanium surface [5].

The infrared spectra for deposited silane sample after the condensation reaction with the surface oxide layer of treated titanium showed strong ≡Si-O-Si≡ (siloxane) bands in the region 1130-1000 cm^{-1}. Also, corresponding ≡Ti-O-Si≡ bands could be seen at 900-1000cm^{-1}. The spectra showed strong siloxane signals when cured at a high temperature of 110°C.

This is showing the chemical nature of the coating–substrate bonding, as a major condition for stable adhesion. Subsequent attachment of bioactive molecules, such as RGD peptides, can be performed while the anchorage film is strongly chemically bonded on the substrate.

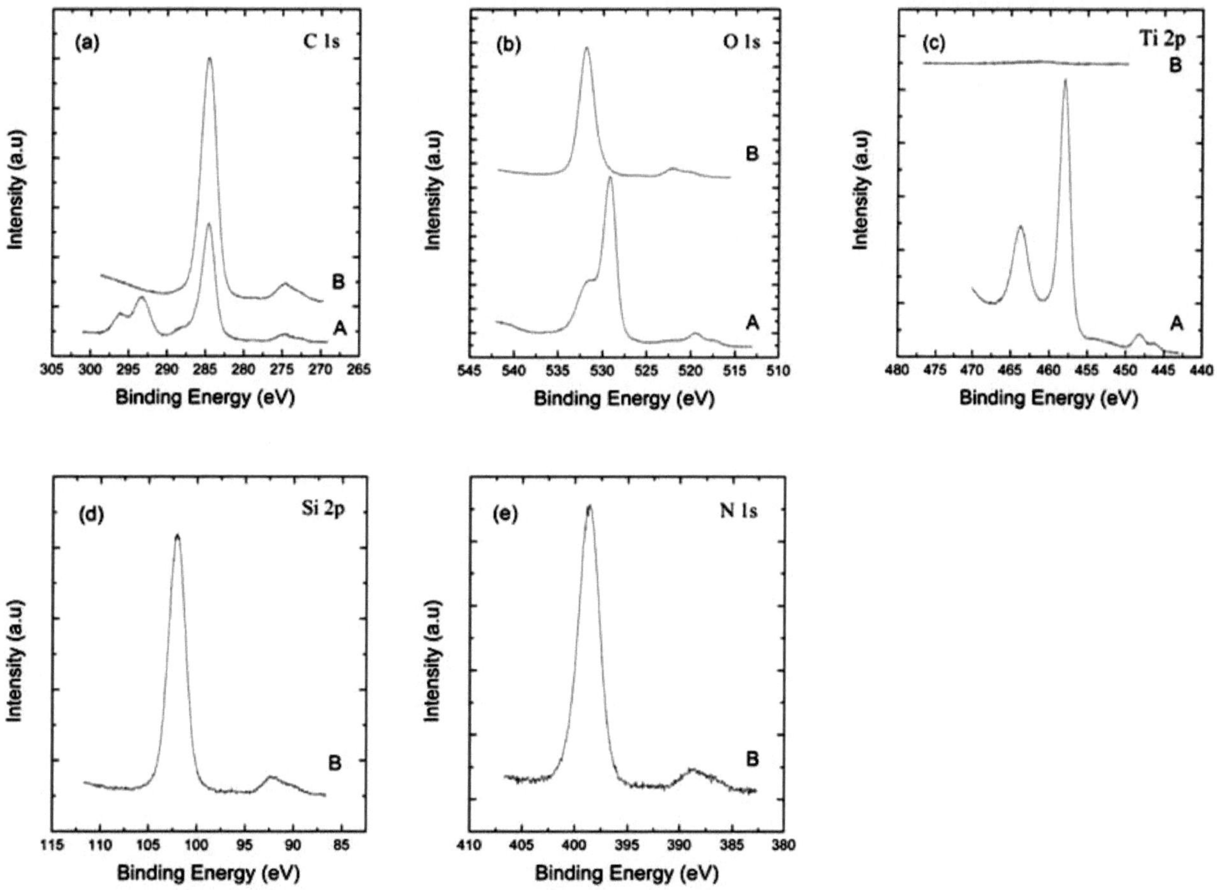

Fig. 4 XPS depth profiles of C 1s (a), O1s (b), Ti 2p (c), Si 2p (d) and N 1s (e) core-levels for APTES films grown on anodized porous Ti substrate

Due to silanization, the titanium peak disappeared from the XPS spectra, indicating full silane coverage of the surface. As shown in the XPS spectra, the presence of the Si-O-Si at 102.2 eV demonstrated again that the silane molecules were chemically bound to the titanium surface.

V. Conclusions

In this study, we demonstrated the way to produce appropriate anchoring layers in view of further deposition of bioactive phases onto porous titanium destined to endosseous implants.

APTES films were successfully grafted onto the porous surface of PM Ti compacts by the means of chemical bonding.

The stability of the resulted film is of major importance in view of further biofunctionalization of porous titanium with improved biocompatibility. The demonstrated nature of the organic-metallic bond is assuring the needed stability of the anchorage film in view of medical applications.

Acknowledgement

This work was financially supported by the project STEMREG PN-II-PT-PCCA-2011-3.1-0700.

Conflict of Interest

The authors declare that they have no conflict of interest.

References

1. Pegg E. C, Walker G. S, Sotchford C. A et al. (2008) Monofunctional aminosilanes as primers for peptide functionalization. Inc.J. Biomed Mater Res 90A: 947-958;
2. Tan G, Zhang L, Ning C et al. (2011) Preparation and characterization of APTES films on modification titanium by SAMs. Thin Solid Films 519: 4997-5001;
3. Vasconcellos L. M. R, Oliveira M. V, Alencastro Graça M. L et al. (2008) Porous titanium scaffolds produced by powder metallurgy for biomedical applications. Materials Research 11:275-280;
4. Matinlinna J.P, Areva S, Lassila L. V, et al. (2004) Characterization of siloxane films on titanium substrate derived from three aminosilanes. Surface and Interface Analysis 36:1314-1322;
5. Gligor I, Marcu T, Todea M, L. Cont et al. (2011) Surface conditioning of porous titanium for endosseous implants by chemical and heat treatments. Journal of Optoelectronics and Advanced Materials 13:879-882.

Synthesis of Nanoceria for Biomedical Applications

A. Balint[1], A. Mesaros[1], L. Mirea[2], V. Bogdan[3], and L. Perju-Dumbrava[2]

[1] Technical University of Cluj-Napoca, Department of Physics and Chemistry, Cluj-Napoca, Romania
[2] University of Medicine and Pharmacy, Department of Clinical Neurosciences, Cluj-Napoca, Romania
[3] University "Politehnica" Bucharest, Faculty of Applied Chemistry and Material Science,
1-7, Gh. Polizu Street, 011061, Bucharest, Romania

Abstract— **Due to the unique property of cerium to easily switch oxidation states between Ce^{3+} and Ce^{4+}, cerium oxide has gained a considerable interest in the field of biomedicine as potential antioxidant agent exerting neuroprotective effects, as well. This work reports on the solvothermal synthesis and characterization of ultrasmall (<10 nm) ceria nanoparticles using oleylamine as solvent and capping agent.**

Keywords— **Cerium oxide, ultra-small nanoparticles, solvothermal synthesis, antioxidant behavior, neurodegenerative diseases**

I. Introduction

The field of engineering has made a considerable progress in nanotechnology, particularly in materials science. Nanoparticles (NPs) have gained a large number of applications due to their specific properties derived from the low dimensionality. Among the functional materials synthesized at nanoscale, metal oxides have peculiar characteristics. The nature of the metal-oxygen bond, varying from nearly ionic to covalent or metallic, and the crystal structures, ranging from simple rock-salt to highly complex structures with modulable mechanical, thermal, electrical, magnetic, optical and chemical properties, are responsible for this behavior. The broad spectrum of properties render metal oxides technological applications in electronics, energy conversion and storage, surface coatings, gas sensing, medical science [1].

Cerium oxide (ceria, CeO_2) is a rare earth metal oxide with a stable cubic fluorite structure that contains cerium in two oxidation states cerium (III), and cerium (IV). Among lanthanides, cerium is quite distinctive since it has 4f and 5d partially filled electron subshells for potential excited states, resulting in a valence structure that may undergo significant changes depending on the chemical environment [2].

Lately, apart the catalytic, sensing and protective applications, cerium oxide nanoparticles are under investigation in the biomedical research field due to the special combination of properties, such as stability and intrinsic redox behavior [3].

Ceria particle size, shape, and surface chemistry can be also considered in connection to the unique redox behavior.

While bulk ceria particles mainly contain Ce^{4+} in the fluorite-type structure, cerium oxide nanoparticles (nanoceria) contain a large fraction of Ce^{3+} and oxygen vacancies, accordingly. The decrease in particle size and the oxygen vacancies generate lattice expansion, as a consequence of the increased surface to volume ratio, in constrast to other nanoparticles (e.g. metals), which show a decrease in lattice parameters with decreasing size [4]. These surface defects store, release and transport oxygen and oxygen vacancies rendering ceria oxygen buffering capabilities on which the antioxidant properties for terapeutic applications are based. The valence state and the oxygen defects allow ceria nanoparticles to act as auto-regenerative redox status modulators [5].

The major biomedical applications of nanoceria envisage neuroprotection (Alzheimer's disease, Parkinson's disease) [6, 7], antitumor effect [8] and diagnostic imaging [9]. Unlike materials, biological organisms have intrinsic mechanisms to fight against the free radical production. Organism aging and disease is the result of free radical generation which exceeds the inner antioxidant capacity, resulting in an oxidative stress. Since the brain and the central nervous system are the sites of the most heavy free radical production, high oxidative stress occurs. The antioxidant properties of cerium oxide nanoparticles allow them to decrease the accumulation of reactive oxygen species (ROS) and prevent subsequent ROS-induced apoptosis in normal cells [6].

Biochemically, ceria NPs have been shown to act as either a superoxide dismutase mimetic, converting superoxid to hydrogen peroxide (H_2O_2), or a catalase mimetic, converting H_2O_2 to water [10].

Over the last few years, the number of synthesis approaches to ceria oxide nanoparticles reported in literature has almost exploded, giving access to a large and rapidly growing collection of properties for specific applications. Ceria nanoparticles have been prepared either by coprecipitation [11], microemulsion [12], or hydrothermal [13] routes. Tarnuzzer et al. [14] prepared ultra-small cerium oxide nanoparticles from 2 to 5 nm and showed they could

S. Vlad and R.V. Ciupa (eds.), *International Conference on Advancements of Medicine and Health Care through Technology*, IFMBE Proceedings 44,
DOI: 10.1007/978-3-319-07653-9_64,

protect against radiation induced cell damage. Chen et al. [15] used similarly prepared cerium oxide nanoparticles to prevent retinal degeneration caused by reactive oxygen intermediates. Various surface agents (polyacrylic acid PAA, polyethylene glycol PEG, Dextran) have been used to sterically stabilize cerium oxide nanoparticles in biological media [16].

In this work we report on the synthesis and characterization of ultra-small CeO_2 nanoparticles as potential candidates for anti-neurodegenerative therapy. By using the solvothermal synthesis we have obtained ultrasmall (<10nm) ceria NPs surrounded by an organic shell of oleylamine. Our results demonstrate that it is possible to control the size, shape and the dispersion degree by varying the synthesis parameters.

II. Materials and Methods

The cerium acetylacetonate $Ce(C_5H_7O_2)_3.xH_2O$ and the oleylamine $C_{18}H_{37}N$ were purchased from Alfa Aesar. For the CeO_2 NPs synthesis, the solvothermal decomposition (heating-up process) of cerium acetylacetonate (2 mmol) dispersed in 50 ml oleylamine (OLA) was used. The solution was directly added into a three-neck round bottomed flask equipped with a condenser, a magnetic stirrer, thermograph and heating mantle. The mixture was slowly heated-up to reflux at around 320 °C and kept at reflux for 2 hours. A brown homogeneous colloidal suspension containing ceria NPs dispersed in OLA has been obtained. It has been noticed that these colloids are stable at room temperature. The addition of a 4:1 volume ratio mixture of ethyl acetate and ethanol to the final solution resulted in the separation of the CeO_2 NPs. Finally, the cerium oxide powder was obtained by drying the precipitate under vacuum.

In order to identify the crystalline phases and to estimate the average particle sizes, X-ray powder diffraction (XRD) and Transmission Electron Microscopy (TEM) investigations were performed. The XRD pattern of the sample was recorded on a Bruker AXS D8 Discover diffractometer (40 kV, 40 mA, $\lambda_{CuK\alpha 1}$=1,54056 Å). The TEM images and the selected area electron diffraction (SAED) patterns were obtained on a Tecnai G2 F30 S-TWIN transmission electron microscope at an accelerating voltage of 300 kV.

The chemical nature of the sample was estimated by Fourier Transform Infrared Spectroscopy (FTIR). The FTIR spectrum was recorded on a Bruker Tensor 27 Spectrometer. The obtained CeO_2 NPs were investigated by thermogravimetric and differential thermal analysis from room temperature up to 800 °C in air at a heating rate of 10°C/min by using a Mettler Toledo TGA/SDTA analyzer.

III. Results and Discussion

The thermal decomposition of different cerium salt precursors in high boiling organic solvents in the presence or absence of surfactants is an efficient one-pot method for the synthesis of cerium oxide monodisperse nanoparticles [17, 18]. The thermal decomposition process is reported to be accompanied by the formation of free radicals, which can undergo various reactions, such as: recombination, decay into smaller organic fragments, or to propagate the decomposition, by reacting with other intermediate complexes. The detailed decomposition mechanism of the process has not been established yet. In our experimental conditions, during the heating-up process, simultaneously with the cerium acetylacetonate decomposition, the oxidation from Ce^{3+} to Ce^{4+} and the formation of CeO_2 NPs takes place. The organic solvent molecules are physisorbed or chemisorbed on the surface of the nanoparticles. A schematic illustration for the formation of CeO_2 NPs by the solvothermal decomposition of cerium acetylacetonate using oleyamine as a solvent is presented below:

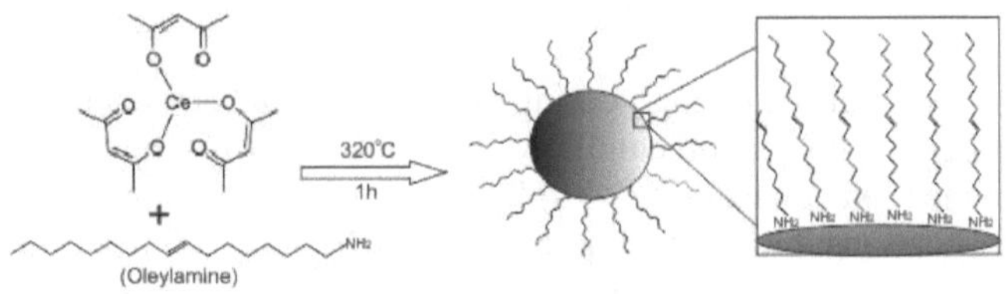

The structure of the nanoparticles was studied by X-ray diffraction – figure 1. All the reflections have been indexed with those of the pure cubic structure of CeO_2 (JCDD PDF 034-0394). No peaks belonging to any other phase have been observed in the XRD pattern, indicating the high structural purity of the sample. The peak broadening of the XRD patterns indicates the significantly small size of the crystallites. The average crystallite sizes of the sample have been calculated using Scherrer formula:

$$D_p = \frac{0.9 \cdot \lambda}{\beta \cdot \cos\theta}$$

where Dp is the average crystallite size, λ is the wavelength of the Cu Kα line, θ is the Bragg angle and β is the full-with at half-maximum (FWHM) of the diffraction peak in radians, resulting 7.6 nm.

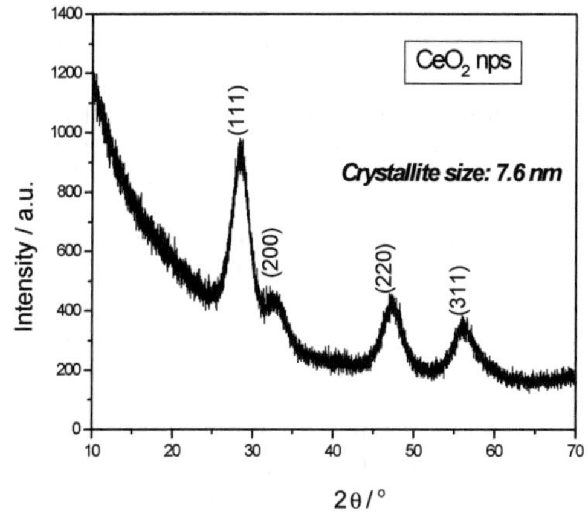

Fig. 1 XRD pattern of the CeO_2 NPs

The TEM and the high resolution transmission electron microscopy (HRTEM) images of the ceria NPs are presented in figure 2. The TEM investigation is more sensitive for heavier elements (cerium), and so it gives a highly intense response/contrast from the well-structured cerium oxide core. By analyzing the bright field image presented in figure 2(a), one can observe the presence of spherical-shaped, agglomerated, ultra-small CeO_2 nanoparticles, with an average size of 4±1 nm. The blurred zones around the ceria NPs can be attributed to the amorphous organic shell. A closer view into the crystal structure of CeO_2 NPs is achieved by the HRTEM image shown in figure 2 b. The polycrystalline nature is evidenced by the different atom plane orientation.

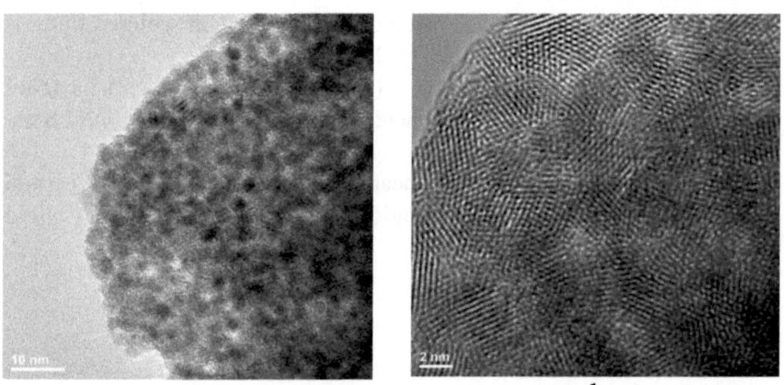

a b

Fig. 2 TEM bright field (a) and HRTEM (b) images of the CeO_2 NPs

The crystallite size value calculated from the XRD data is larger than the value obtained from the TEM images. This difference is indicative for the lower cristallinity degree due to the existence of the organic shell onto the nanoparticles surfaces. The discrepancy in the particles size from TEM and XRD measurements can be explained by the fact that the Scherrer formula underestimates the grain size since it ignores the broadening of the diffraction reflections also due to the microstrain in the lattice.

Further, TG and FTIR analysis were undertaken to get a more detailed insight view of the chemical composition of the as-prepared CeO_2 NPs.

To support the hypothesis of the adsorbed organic shell at the nanoparticle surface, thermo-gravimetric analyses were performed aiming to qualitatively study the bonding strength of the solvent molecules. A weaker bond (physisorbed specimens) exhibits weight losses at lower temperatures, while a stronger bond (chemisorption) is associated with weight losses at higher temperatures.

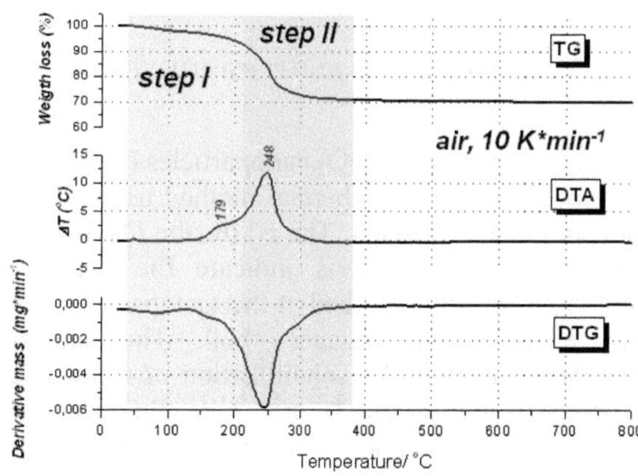

Fig. 3 DTA-TG analyses for the CeO_2 NPs

The TG-DTA-DTG curves are shown in figure 3. Below 200 °C, a slight weight loss of 5.5 % can be observed and attributed to the atmospheric humidity and, eventually, to organic solvent residues. In the temperature range 200 – 350 °C, the second weight loss step accompanied by a 24.2 % weight loss is associated with the thermal decomposition of the chemisorbed oleylamine.

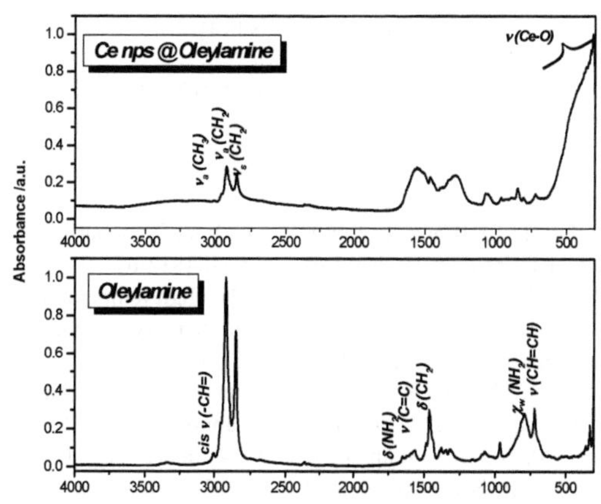

Fig. 4 FTIR spectra of oleylamine and CeO_2 NPs

FT-IR spectroscopy was used to better understand the chemical nature of the nanoparticles. Figure 4 presents the spectra corresponding to pure oleylamine and to the as-obtained CeO_2 nanoparticles. In both spectra one can observe the characteristic vibration bands of oleylamine: the band in the region 1330-1650cm^{-1} is due to the –NH_2 bending mode and the bands around 2929 cm^{-1} and 2850 cm^{-1} are for the methyl stretching. The ceria NPs IR spectrum presents a high intensity band at lower wavenumbers, below 630 cm^{-1}, attributed to the cerium-oxygen vibration ν(Ce-O) [19]. The broadening of the –NH_2 bending mode in the ceria NPs spectrum can be explained by the perturbation of the vibrational -NH_2 due to the interaction with the ceria core.

IV. Conclusions and perspectives

Ultra-small crystalline CeO_2 nanoparticles (<10 nm) have been prepared by the solvothermal method using $Ce(acac)_3$ and oleylamine as a solvent. The FTIR, the DTA-TG-DTG and the TEM investigations indicate the presence of oleylamine molecules adsorbed at the nanoparticles surface forming a protective organic shell. The oleylamine simultaneously ensures the solubilization of $Ce(acac)_3$ and the capping of the resulted ceria NPs obtained by this simple solvothermal synthesis. The nanoparticle dimensions make them adequate for their use as an effective antioxidant in neurodegenerative diseases. These results make the as-obtained ceria NPs proimising candidates for biochemical and in-vitro/in-vivo testing.

Acknowledgment

This work was supported by the European Community in the frame of the EUROTAPES project.

Conflict of Interest

The authors declare that they have no conflict of interest.

References

1. Niederberger M, Pinna N (2009), Metal Oxide Nanoparticles in Organic Solvents, Springer Verlag, ISBN 978-1-84882-671-7
2. Lee S S, Zhu H, Contreras E et al (2012), High temperature decomposition of cerium precursors to form ceria nanocrystal libraries for biological applications, Chem Mater 24: 424-432
3. Xu C, Qu X (2014), Cerium oxide nanoparticle: a remarkably versatile rare earth nanomaterial for biological applications, NPG Asia Materials 6, e90, doi:10.138/am.2013.88, 2014 Nature Publishing Group
4. Sahu T, Bisht S S, Das K R et al (2013) Nanoceria: Synthesis and Biomedical Applications, Current Nanoscience 9: 000-000
5. Gupta S, Brouwer P, Bandyopadhyay S, Patil S, Briggs R, Jain J., Seal S. (2005) TEM/SEM investigation of size and surface properties of nanocrystalline ceria, J. Nanosci Nanotechnol, 5: 1101-7
6. Estevez A Y, Erlichman J S, (2011) Cerium oxide nanoparticles for the treatment of neurological oxidative stress diseases book chapter in Oxidative Stress Diagnostics, Prevention and Therapy, Andreescu S et al; ACS Symposium Series, Am Chem Soc, Washington 1083:255-88
7. Singh N, Cohen C, Rzigalinski B A (2007), Treatment of neurodegenerative disorder with radical nanomedicine, Annal N.Y. Acad Sci 1122:219-30
8. Wason M S, Zhao J (2013), Cerium oxide nanoparticles: potential applicationsfor cancer and other diseases, Am J Transl Res 5(2):126-31
9. Buzea C, Blandino I I P, Robbie K (2007) Nanomaterials and naoparticles: sources and toxicity, Biointerphases, 2(4): MR17-MR172
10. Lee S S, Song W, Cho M et al, Antioxidant properties of cerium oxide nanocrystals as a function of crystal diameter and surface coating, Am. Chem.Soc. Nano 7(11):9693-9703
11. Uekawa N U, Wu M, Wu Y J et al (2002) Synthesis of CeO_2 spherical fine particles by homogeneous precipitation method with polyethylene glycol, Chem. Lett 8:854-855
12. Zhang J J, Wu X Wu Z Yet al (2001) Structural characteristics of cerium oxide nanocrystals prepared by the microemulsion method, Chem Mater 13:4192-4197
13. Ivanov V K, Kopitsa G P, Baranchikov et al (2009) Hydrothermal growth of ceria nanoparticles, Russion J Inorg Chem 54: 1857-1861
14. Tarnuzzer R, Colon J Patil S et al (2005) Vacancy engineered ceria nanostructures for protection from radiation-induced cellular damage, Nano Lett 5(12):2573-7
15. Chen J, Patil S Seal S et al (2006) Rare earth nanoparticles prevent retinal degeneration induced by intracellular peroxides, Nat Nanotechnol 1(2):142-50
16. Karakoti A S, Singh S Kumar A at al (2009) PEGylated nanoceria as radical scavenger with tunable redox chemistry, J Am Chem Soc 131(40): 14144–14145.
17. Jrishnan A, Sreeremya T S, Murray E et al (2013) One-pot synthesis of ultra-small cerium oxide nanodots exhibiting multi-colored fluorescence J Colloid Interf Sci 389:16-22
18. Devaraju M K, Liu X, Yin S et al (2012) A rapid solvothermal synthesis of cerium oxide hollow sphere and characterization, J Solid State Chem 194:43-47
19. Goharshadi E K, Samiee S, Nancarrow P (2011) Fabrication of cerium oxide nanoparticles: Caracterization and optical properties, J Colloid Interf Sci 355:473-480

Corresponding author:
Author: Amalia Mesaros
Institute: Technical University of Cluj-Napoca
Street: 28, Memorandumului Street
City: Cluj-Napoca
Country: Romania
Email: Amalia.Mesaros@chem.utcluj.ro

Reliability of Gait Parameters Depending on HJC Estimation Method

M. Krepelka, M. Toth-Taşcău and D.I. Stoia

Faculty of Mechanical Engineering, Politehnica University of Timişoara, Romania

Abstract— **The study investigates the effect of hip joint center (HJC) estimation methods on the angular parameters during gait analysis. Data analysis consisted of descriptive statistics such as mean and standard deviation (SD) used to characterize the gait cycle, while analysis of variance (ANOVA), data intraclass correlation coefficients (ICCs), Pearson product-moment correlations (r), and Bland and Altman methods were used as estimates of reliability. While the small sample size represents a limitation, the preliminary research suggests that the agreement between the data sets decreases with the increase of the HJC estimation error. Also, after evaluating the effect of mislocating the HJC, a method was tested to correct the initial gait data. This method yielded, in average, an approximately 8% increase of the ICC (0.8-28%), while the mean differences were taken down to zero.**

Keywords— **HJC, gait cycle, kinematic parameters, hip angle, biomechanics, reliability, ICC**

I. INTRODUCTION

With life expectancy increasing, there is now an emphasis on sustaining an active lifestyle. Gait analysis is more often used to assist in identifying diagnostic measures in gait disorders or monitoring of the rehabilitation process by determining changes in gait patterns [1].

Complex clinical gait analysis usually includes kinematics, kinetics and electromyography that are fundamental for the purpose of characterizing gait patterns.

A kinematic gait analysis evaluates the movement of the lower extremities, the angles of their segments and the way in which they alter during walking [2]. Joint angle analysis is important because it enables to quantify the functional range of motion of the joint, describing the orientation of a given segment in relation to another.

In order to assess the outcome of rehabilitation programs, clinical interventions or disease progression, reliable outcome measures are essential. In the case of kinematic gait analysis, reliability refers to the amount of change in angular displacements that is dependent to measurement error and not actual improvement or deterioration of the gait.

It is well documented that, in the case of measuring systems using body markers, skin movement artifacts cause measurement errors that may affect accuracy [3],[4].

Another variable that is important in the determination of accurate angular parameters and consequently joint loads is the hip joint center (HJC) estimation.

The hip joint center is a fundamental landmark in the identification of lower limb mechanical axis, being the point with respect to which hip joint moments are calculated.

Thus, errors in its location may lead to substantial inaccuracies both in joint reconstruction and in gait analysis.

In gait analysis hip joint center location is usually estimated noninvasively based on the distance between external markers placed over bony landmarks at the pelvis, or by radiographic methods [5], [6], [7].

The goal of this research was to test if the default setting of the measuring system, estimating the HJC at 20% offset from the external marker placed on the greater trochanter, can represent a reliable option for estimation of HJC coordinates in gait analysis.

To accomplish this, the default apparatus method was compared with two other estimation methods: the greater trochanter (GT) method [8] that places the HJC at one-quarter of the distance from the ipsolateral to the contralateral greater trochanter and the radiographic method.

This study aimed to quantify how mislocation errors affect the reliability of the results and to find a simple method to correct the results using statistical methods.

II. MATERIALS AND METHODS

A. Procedure

The measurements were realized in the Motion Analysis Laboratory of Politehnica University of Timişoara using Zebris measuring system CMS-HS that allows an objective three dimensional kinematic analysis of the human gait by means of analyzing the tracks of body surface markers.

The measuring method is based on the determination of spatial coordinates of miniature ultrasound transmitters, the spatial position of the markers being determined by triangulation [9].

The preliminary study was based on a healthy 30 year old female subject, with no previous history of musculoskeletal disease.

After the attachment of the ultrasound marker triplets and the definition of anatomic landmarks, the subject was advised to walk at a comfortable self-selected velocity and was allowed 5 minutes training time to get used to the marker attachments and walking range.

Under the mentioned condition, angular variation for each individual joint in all the possible movements

S. Vlad and R.V. Ciupa (eds.), *International Conference on Advancements of Medicine and Health Care through Technology*, IFMBE Proceedings 44,
DOI: 10.1007/978-3-319-07653-9_65,

(flexion-extension, adduction-abduction and rotation) were assessed in order to identify those influenced by the HJC location.

The study consists in three different scenarios: a default value of the hip distance of 60%, the value of 50% defined with the GT method and a value obtained using radiographic measurements (45%).

The radiographic measurements were made on an antero-posterior topogram of the subject that recently underwent a CT scan. The radiographical HJC location was estimated as the center of the optimal fit circle drawn over the femoral head. The distance between the two defined points yielded a ratio of 45% in relationship to the measurement of the distance between the skin points that are usually defined as the great trochanter position during gait analysis.

Three sessions of walking were recorded for each scenario in order to check the inter-trial reliability of kinematic gait parameters, with a sampling rate of 25Hz. Anatomical landmarks, marker position and calibration were kept unaltered during the analysis. From observing the data plots, the best cycle for each scenario was considered, resulting in 9 sets of data, paired for each scenario.

B. Data Analysis

Subsequent data analysis was done for the motions of interest, hip movements, using SPSS 20 (SPSS Inc, Chicago, IL).

The reliability of the angular pattern was assessed using Pearson's r for each pair, as an inter-class correlation coefficient. As product-moment correlations only reflects reliability in the sense of parallelism of scores between data sets and did not offer quantitative measures, furthermore, the degree of agreement between the measurements of each pair was evaluated using a hypothesis test for equivalence, the intraclass correlation coefficient (ICC) [10], and Bland-Altman statistics [11].

ICC(2,1) measures the extent of absolute agreement or interchangeability of the methods(or scenarios in this given case), which is based on the two-way random-effects ANOVA.

$$ICC\ (2,1) = \frac{MS_S - MS_E}{MS_S + (k-1)MS_E + \frac{k(MS_T - MS_E)}{n}} \quad (1)$$

where MS_S indicates subjects mean square, MS_E indicates error mean square, MS_T indicates the trial mean square, n is the size of the sample and k is the number of methods [10],[12]. Thus, the intraclass correlation coefficient then provides a scalar measure of agreement or concordance between all the methods.

Bland-Altman analysis, also known as the method of differences, has been used for measuring the degree of agreement [11]. With this method, the differences between the two settings (60% and 50%) and the radiological reference measurement are emphasized.

III. RESULTS AND DISCUSSIONS

As the gait cycles had different lengths (1.2-1.4 s), the kinematic data sets were time-normalized to present the angular profiles as proportion of cycle.

After cycle selection and time normalization we were left with 9 sets of measurements, 3 for each investigated motion of the hip, namely flexion/extension, adduction and rotation.

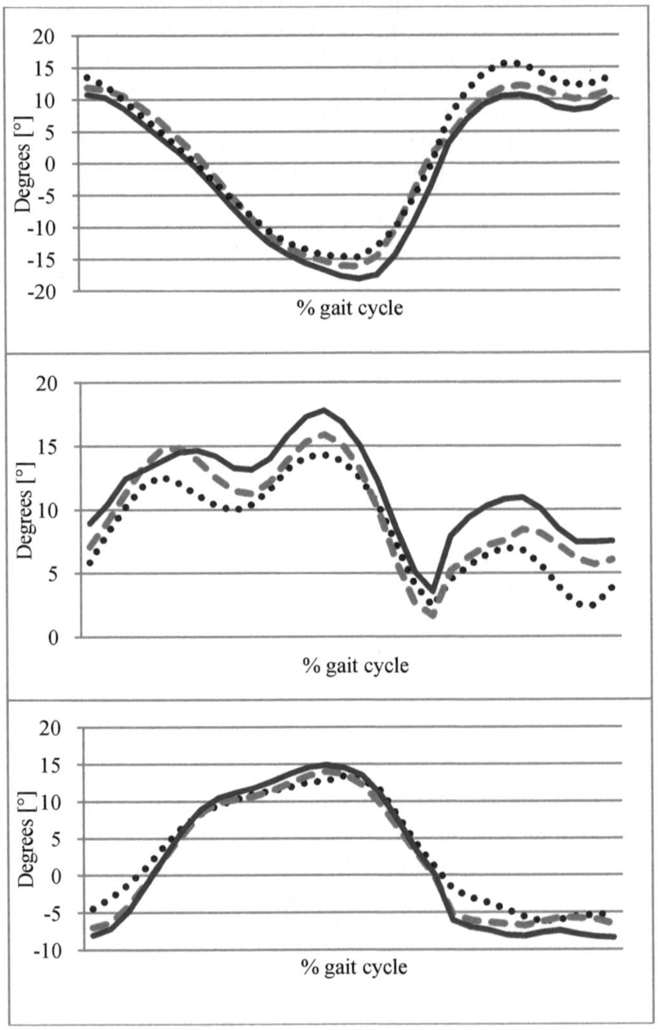

Fig. 1 Ang ular variation profiles for hip flexion-extension, hip adduction and hip rotation of the left limb

Table 1 Analysis results: Pearson's correlation, ICC and Bland-Altman statistics

Movement	Group	r	ICC	Mean diff	SD_{diff}
Flexion	45%-60%	0.992	0.956	2.911	1.370
	45%-50%	0.993	0.976	1.969	1.225
Adduction	45%-60%	0.958	0.749	-2.935	1.136
	45%-50%	0.976	0.892	-1.727	0.948
Rotation	45%-60%	0.993	0.956	1.332	2.082
	45%-50%	0.998	0.991	0.178	1.167

As stated before, Pearson's correlation coefficients give information about the degree of association between two sets of data, and not reliability.

As we can see in Table 1, the measurement pairs are highly correlated ($p<0.001$) despite a systematic difference of up to approx. 3° between scenarios. In this case, correlation reflects the extent to which measurements co-vary in identical testing situations. This is a measure that indicates a good agreement in time-dependent phases of gait between scenarios. This may be accounted for by the training previously undertaken by the subject.

ICC scores indicate strong (0.7-0.8) and excellent agreement (>0.8) between the tested pairs of measurements at 95% confidence interval.

Even though we notice that the overall results show a strong correlation, we could not conclude that the magnitude of the difference is acceptable in clinical use.

Thus, knowing that the data are linearly correlated, regression models were used to model the relationship between data pairs in order to predict the value of a variable from the value of another variable, using the formula:

$$Y = a + bX, \tag{2}$$

where Y is the predicted score, b is the slope of the line and a is the Y intercept.

These models were used as corrections for the data sets that are observed to have low agreement and, from these data sets predict new sets that closely resemble those of the radiological defined HJC.

After calculating the regression coefficients and new data sets were generated from the 50% and 60% scenario data on all considered movements. These sets represent predictions of the radiological results based on the results of the 50% and 60% after the correction, in this case noted 50%' and 60%'.

The predicted data sets were plotted against the 45% measurement set to illustrate the precision of the predictions, and consequently, the improvement in the amplitude disagreement of the measurements.

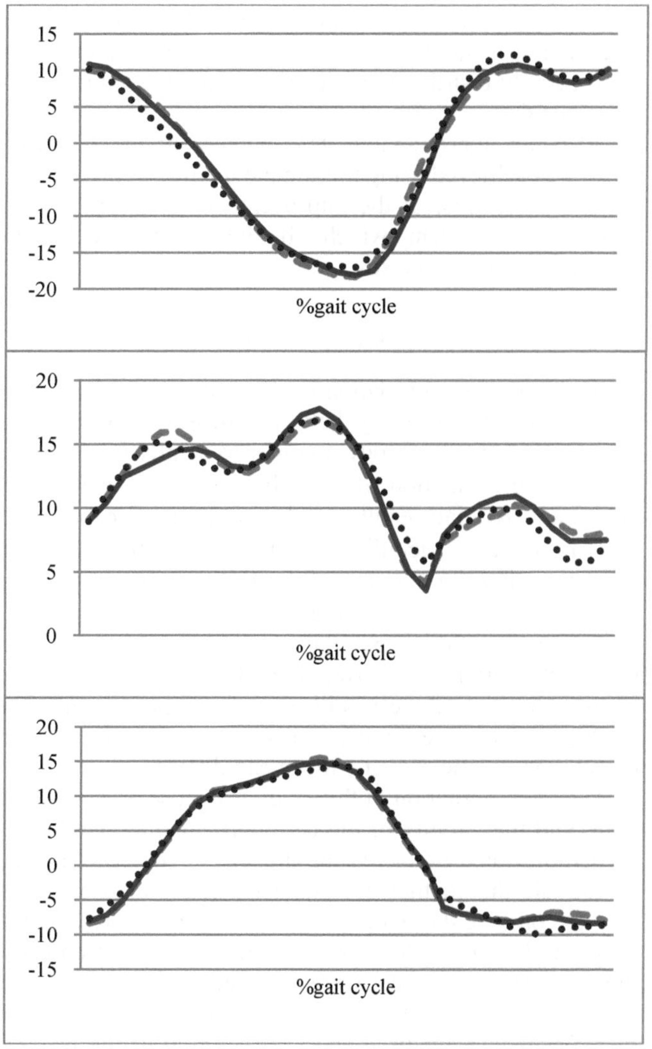

Fig. 2 Predicted angular profiles for hip flexion-extension, hip adduction and hip rotation of the left limb

The statistical calculations were redone for the new sets of predicted data in order to quantify the degree of agreement.

Table 2 Analysis results: Pearson's correlation, ICC and Bland-Altman statistics for the predicted data sets

Movement	Group	r	ICC	Mean diff	SD_{diff}
Flexion	45%-60%'	0.992	0.993	0	0.920
	45%-50%'	0.993	0.993	0	0.864
Adduction	45%-60%'	0.958	0.959	0	0.784
	45%-50%'	0.976	0.976	0	0.601
Rotation	45%-60%'	0.993	0.994	0	0.735
	45%-50%'	0.998	0.999	0	0.337

We notice that the mean difference of the newly generated data sets equal 0, suggesting that the prediction errors were equally distributed above and below the values of the reference data.

Also, an approximately 8% increase of the ICC (0.8-28%) was achieved using this simple method of prediction. As expected, most of the improvement was in the case of adduction movement, which, for the initial data, had the lowest correlation indexes.

IV. Conclusions

The intraclass correlation coefficient was used as an index of interchangeability between measures of the same patient, same methodology, in order to emphasize the influence of the estimation of HJC. In addition, the ICC and Bland and Altman results can be important for their clinical application, deciding whether the errors gave by misestimating the position of the HJC can be mistaken as changes occurred in the patient.

The results of this method of correction suggest that even though the differences between the three scenarios were not statistically high, there is still room for improvement using simple statistical regression. This is reflected by the high correlation coefficients and low mean differences.

The main limitation of this study is the use of a single patient, and the validity of the considered method could only be demonstrated by increasing the size of subjects. In order to validate this method for clinical use, it would be necessary to combine the findings with data from test-retest reliability studies. Knowing that the magnitude of difference is not a statistical decision, we would need to get a conclusive feedback regarding the clinical importance of the found differences gait analysis, and also research of the progression of the differences in the joints situated lower on the limb, i.e. knee and ankle.

If the differences within mean $\pm$ 1.96 SD are not clinically decisive, the methods of HJC position estimation may be used interchangeably.

Despite the study limitation of small sample size, the data provides preliminary evidence suggesting that as the estimation error of HJC increases, the agreement between the outcome measures decreases.

Future work will consist in growing a data base that would include patients of both genders and all ages, and, using non invasive methods, generate a mathematical formula that would help the examiner to better estimate the position of the joint center.

Conflict of Interest

The authors declare that they have no conflict of interest.

References

1. DeLisa J A (1998) Gait Analysis in the Science of Rehabilitation. DIANE Publishing, Washington, US
2. Oberg T, Karsznia A, Oberg K (1994) Joint angle parameters in gait : Reference data for normal subjects: 10-79 years of age. J Rehabil Res Dev 31:199-213
3. Benoit D L, Ramsey D K, Lamontage M et al. (2006) Effect of skin movement artifact on knee kinematics during gait and cutting motions measured in vivo. Gait Poisture 24:152-164
4. Leardini A, Chiari L, Della C U et al. (2004) Human movement analysis using stereophotogrammetry Part 3. Soft tissue artifact assessment and compensation. Gait Posture, 21:212-225
5. Seidel G K, Marchinda D M, Dijkers M et al. (1995) Hip joint center location from palpable bony landmarks- a cadaver study. J Biomech 28:995-998
6. Kirkwood R N, Culham E G, Costigan P (1999) Radiographic and non-invasive determination of the hip joint center location: effect on hip joint moments. Clin Biomech 14:227-235
7. Bell A L, Pedersen D R, Brand R A (1990) A comparison of the accuracy of several hip center location prediction methods. J Biomech 23: 617-621
8. O'Connor K M, Weinhandl J T (2010) Hip joint movements using a greater trochante method of locating the hip joint center, Conference Proceedings of the Annual Meeting of the American Society. 2010, pp 252-253
9. Zebris CMS-HS: Operating Instructions.
10. Shrout P E, Fleiss J L (1979) Intraclass correlations: uses in assessing rater reliability. Psychol Bull 36:420-428
11. Bland M J, Altman D G (1986) Statistical methods for assessing agreement between two methods of clinical measurement. The Lancet 327:307-310
12. McGraw K O, Wong S P (1996) Forming inferences about some intraclass correlation coefficients. Psychol Methods 1:30-46
13. Weir J P (2005) Quantifying test-retest reliability using the intraclass correlation coefficient and the SEM. J Strength Cond Res 19:231-240

Author: Dan Ioan Stoia
Institute: Politehnica University
Street: Bd. Mihai Viteazu nr.1
City: Timişoara
Country: Romania
Email: ionut@cmpicsu.upt.ro

Comparison of Vertebral Strengths Derived from FE Models of the Vertebral Body and the Vertebral Body with Posterior Elements

C-H. Lee[1], P. Landham[2], R. Eastell[1,3], M.A. Adams[2], P. Dolan[2], and L. Yang[1,3]

[1] Mellanby Centre for Bone Research, University of Sheffield, Sheffield, UK
[2] Centre for Comparative and Clinical Anatomy, The University of Bristol, Bristol, UK
[3] INSIGNEO Institute for in silico Medicine, University of Sheffield, Sheffield, UK

Abstract— **Vertebral fracture is the most common type of osteoporotic fracture and is associated with significant health and economic costs. In recent years, patient-specific vertebral body finite element (FE) models based on quantitative computed tomography (QCT) have been developed to investigate vertebral strength. Current models consider the vertebral body alone with loading restricted to pure compression. However, osteoporotic vertebral fractures are often associated with forward bending which concentrates loading on the anterior vertebral body leading to the typical wedge fractures observed in life. The purpose of this study is to compare the vertebral strengths derived from FE models with those measured experimentally under forward bending conditions. Sixteen cadaveric spinal units, each consisting of two vertebrae and an intervertebral disc (IVD), were scanned using clinical QCT. Specimens were then potted in dental cement and loaded on a materials testing machine to generate a wedge fracture. Custom codes developed and validated previously in MATLAB were used to generate FE models with an 8-node voxel mesh: one of the vertebral body alone ("VB"), and another of the vertebral body with posterior elements intact ("VB w/PE"). Artificial padding was generated at the inferior and superior endplates to represent the dental cement and facilitate the simulation of the forward-bending condition. Transverse-isotropic linear-elastic material properties were assigned to the vertebra, and the FE model was solved using ANSYS. Vertebral strength was defined in two different ways; i) the load that caused maximum Von Mises strain exceeding a yield strain of 0.78% (VM_ER), and ii) the load that caused maximum Von Mises stress exceeding a yield stress (VM_SR) in contiguous elements that occupied at least 244.14 mm³. Linear regression was used to compare FE- and experiment-derived vertebral strength data. This showed that there was a positive correlation between the strength measured experimentally and the strength derived from both FE models; VM_SR (r^2= 0.78 VB, r^2= 0.75 VB w/PE), VM_ER (r^2= 0.75 VB, r^2= 0.68 VB w/PE). The results of this study indicate that a simple vertebral body FE model under forward-bending conditions may be sufficient for the estimation of vertebral strength.**

Keywords— **Vertebral fracture, Finite element model, Patient specific, Osteoporosis, Vertebral strength**

I. Introduction

Vertebral fracture is the most common type of osteoporotic fracture and is associated with significant health and economic costs, both in the UK and throughout Europe. In recent years, finite element analysis has been used to improve assessments of fracture risk by integrating information about in vivo loading conditions with data on bone geometry and density obtained from QCT scans. This allows stress and strain to be calculated non-invasively and bone strength to be determined. Many researchers have developed continuum finite element models of the vertebral body that have been well validated [1-7]. However, only one-QCT-based model has been used routinely as a clinical research tool in osteoporosis studies in patients [3, 5]. As with previous FE models, this particular model has been used to investigate vertebral body strength under pure compressive loading which is generally representative of the standing posture. However, there are several limitations of such an approach. First of all, artificially removing the posterior elements in the model disrupts the continuity of the cortex and trabecular network and this may weaken the vertebral body causing strength to be under-estimated [8-10]. Secondly, osteoporotic vertebral fractures often occur during forward bending activities which concentrate loading on the anterior vertebral body, and it is this type of loading rather than pure compression that causes the anterior wedge fractures commonly observed in life. FE models of the vertebrae that simulate loading in flexed postures may result in different strength estimates than those that simulate pure axial compression, and this may impact on the prediction of fracture risk.

The aim of this project is to compare vertebral strengths derived from FE models of the vertebral body (VB) and the vertebral body with posterior elements (VB w/ PE), with those measured experimentally under forward bending conditions.

S. Vlad and R.V. Ciupa (eds.), *International Conference on Advancements of Medicine and Health Care through Technology*, IFMBE Proceedings 44,
DOI: 10.1007/978-3-319-07653-9_66,

II. Material and Methods

A. Specimen Preparation

Thoracolumbar spines (T11-L5) were obtained from cadavers (Female=5, Male=3; 74 - 97 years old) that had been donated for medical research. Two motion segments were dissected from each cadaveric spine at the University of Bristol. Prior to mechanical testing, these specimens were sealed in bags and transported to the University of Sheffield in a dry ice box for scanning. The specimens were scanned with a clinical QCT machine (LightSpeed VCT, GE Medical Systems, 120 kV, 60 mA/slice, 0.3867 x 0.3867 x 0.625 mm^3 voxel size) at the Northern General Hospital, Sheffield. A solid calibration phantom (Mindways, Mindways, SanFrancisco, CA) was used to calibrate Hounsfield unit (HU) values with bone mineral density.

B. Patient- Specific Finite Element Modelling

Custom codes, developed previously and written in MATLAB (Mathworks Inc., Natick, MA, USA), were used to support the full process of the image processing framework, and the finite element modelling and analysis. The commercial software ANSYS (ANSYS Inc., Canonsburg, PA, USA) was used as the main FE solver. The procedure in figure 1 is described briefly.

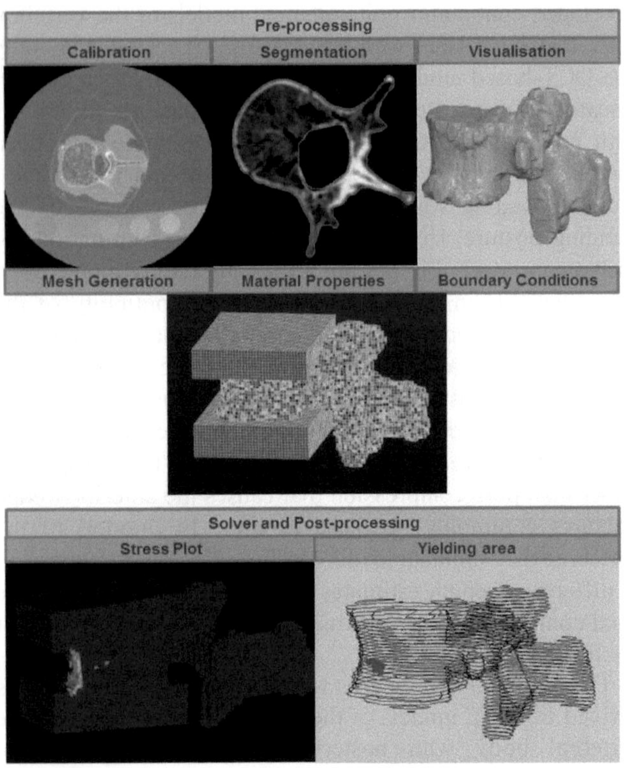

Fig. 1 The FE modelling procedure

The CT data were calibrated from Hounsfield units to density values using a hydroxyapatite phantom. The segmentation of the bone was carried out with thresholding and morphological operations such as open, close, dilate, erode and fill. The posterior parts were removed during segmentation for the vertebral body only model. Artificial cement paddings were generated at inferior and superior endplates (Figure 1, middle panel) for applying boundary conditions. The final masks of the CT images with the padding parts were rescaled to isotropic voxel size of 0.4 x 0.4 x0.4 mm^3 so that they could be directly converted into an 8-node voxel finite element model.

Material properties in table 1 were assigned into each element. First, empirical relationships between volumetric bone density and bone material properties were used to determine the elastic modulus and compressive yield limit for the vertebra [11]. The tensile yield limit [12], ultimate stress limit [2, 12, 13] and strain limit [14] of the vertebra were assigned according to the literature. Transversely isotropic linear-elastic material properties were considered and Poisson's ratios of 0.381 and 0.104 were assigned [15]. The mechanical properties of the artificial padding representing the dental cement were obtained from the manufacturer's manual (E=2000 MPa, v=0.3; Ultrahard Die Stone ISO-Type IV, Kerr).

Table 1 Material properties

Part	Properties	References
Vertebra	$E_z = -34.7 + 3230\rho_{QCT}$	Kopperdahl et al. 2002
	$E_x = E_y = 0.333E_z$ $v_{xy}{}^1 = 0.381$ $v_{xz}{}^1 = v_{yz}{}^1 = 0.104$ $G_{xz} = G_{yz} = 0.157E_z$ $G_{xy} = \frac{E_x}{2(1+v_{xy})} = 0.121E_z$	Ulrich et al. 1999
	$\sigma_{yc} = -0.75 + 24.9\rho_{QCT}$	Kopperdahl et al. 2002
	$\sigma_{yt} = \sigma_{yc} * 0.79$	Keaveny et al. 1994
	$\sigma_{uc} = 1.2 * \sigma_y$	Crawford 2003; Morgan and Keaveny 2001
	$\varepsilon_y = 0.0078$	Kopperdahl et al. 2002
	$\varepsilon_u = 0.145$	Morgan et al. 2003
Padding	$E = 2000\ MPa$ $v = 0.3$	Lewis 1997

A forward-bending loading condition was simulated to represent the mechanical test. The bottom surface of the lower padding was constrained in all degrees of freedom, and tilted displacement boundary conditions were applied on the top surface of the upper padding. The FE models were then solved using a commercial software package, ANSYS (ANSYS Inc., Canonsburg, PA, USA). Vertebral strength was defined in two different ways; i) the load that caused maximum Von Mises strain exceeding a yield strain of 0.78%, and ii) the load that caused maximum Von Mises stress exceeding a yield stress in contiguous elements that occupied at least a volume of 244 mm³. In this way the contiguous region containing the highest stress ratios, and thus having the greatest likelihood of being the site of initial failure was determined. Linear regression between FE- and experiment-derived vertebral strength was performed.

C. Experimental Data

The experimental tests were performed by the Spine Biomechanics Laboratory, University of Bristol [16]. The test procedures are described briefly here. The metal specimen holders were attached to baseplates and loaded via low-friction rollers attached to the upper base plate; the angle of the upper plate could be varied to allow complex loading to be applied to the motion segment. The experimental set-up can be seen in figure 2.

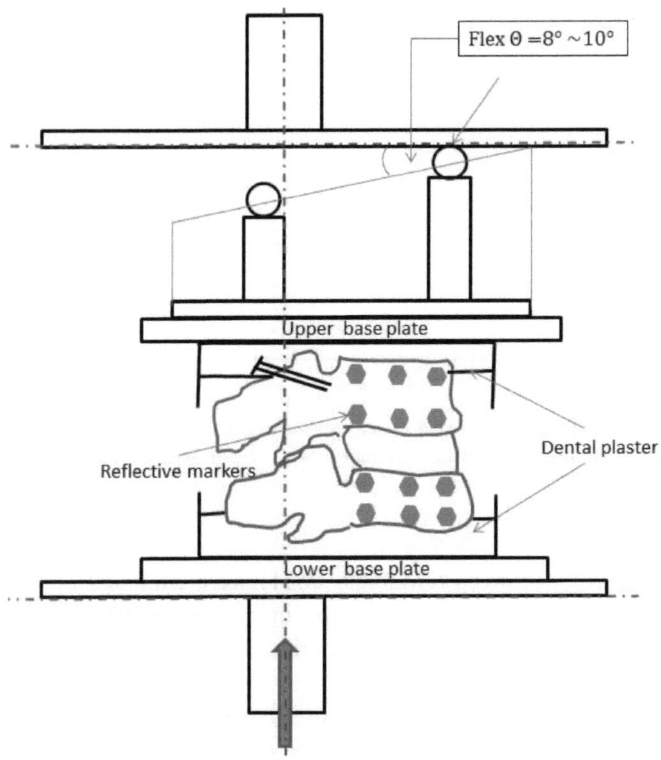

Fig. 2 Schematic view of the experimental test set up

Each motion segment was positioned in flexion in order to simulate a stooped posture. The motion segment was then compressed at a rate of 3mm/s while a graph of compressive load versus displacement was plotted in real time. Fracture was detected from a reduction in gradient (stiffness). The compressive force applied at this point was recorded as the yield strength. The compression loading cycle was then immediately repeated at 3mm/s so that the shift in the load displacement curve could be obtained. This loading technique usually creates an endplate fracture, often accompanied by fracture of the anterior cortex, of a single vertebra within the motion segment [16]. Fracture location was identified by taking a lateral radiograph, and was subsequently confirmed by dissection.

III. RESULTS

A. Stress and Strain Distribution

The von Mises stress and strain distribution on the FE models was similar in the both FE models; vertebral body alone and vertebra with posterior elements as shown in figure 3.

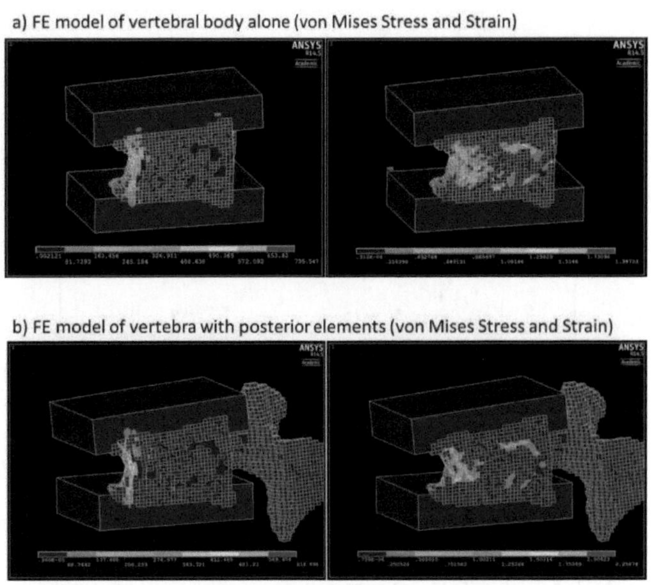

Fig. 3 von Mises Stress (left) and strain (right) plot of the FE models; a) Vertebral body alone, b) Vertebra with posterior elements

B. Correlation with Experimental Data

The experimental strength was positively correlated with the strength of the VB FE model (r^2= 0.78 VM_SR, r^2= 0.75 VM_ER), and the VB w/ PE FE model (r^2= 0.75 VM_SR, r^2= 0.68 VM_ER) as shown in figure 4 and figure 5.

Table 2 FE- and Experiment- derived vertebral strength (N)

Specimen	VB FE Strength		VB w/ PE FE Strength		Exp- Str.
	VM_SR	VM_ER	VM_SR	VM_ER	
0001	770	1212	815	1276	1104
0003	640	1214	689	1059	1600
0005	397	627	399	538	1180
0007	340	740	468	535	1685
0013	1633	2062	1654	1814	3090
0015	2116	2824	2025	2745	4412
0017	1503	1821	1327	1588	3399
0019	1353	1874	1260	1479	2906
0021	558	1301	616	1113	1861
0023	611	1031	569	938	1194
0025	1284	1942	1331	1601	1930
0027	1040	1807	1234	1664	2215
0031	999	1372	1003	1337	1319

a) FE model of vertebral body alone (VM_SR)

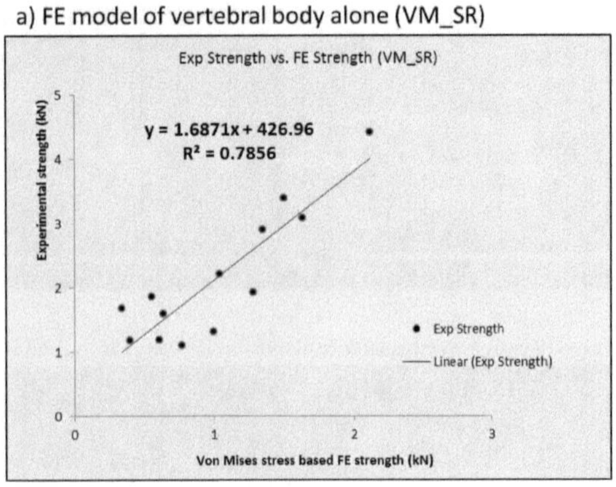

b) FE model of vertebral body alone (VM_ER)

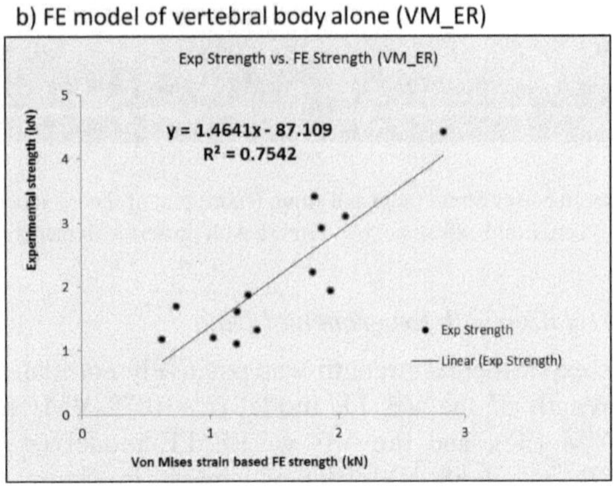

Fig. 4 Linear regression between Experiment- and FE-derived strength (FE model of vertebral body alone; a) von Mises Stress, b) von Mises Strain.

a) FE model of vertebra with posterior elements (VM_SR)

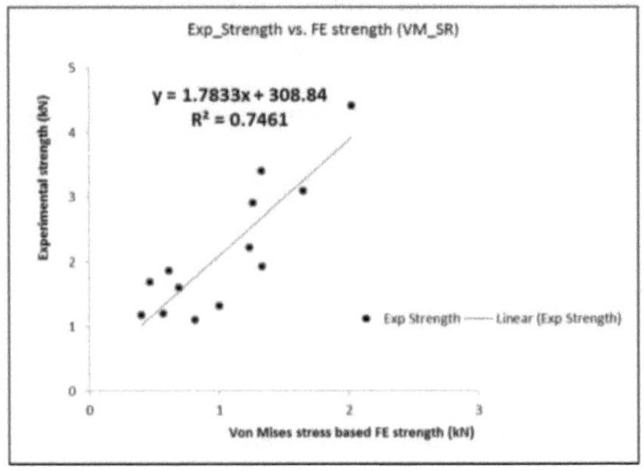

b) FE model of vertebra with posterior elements (VM_ER)

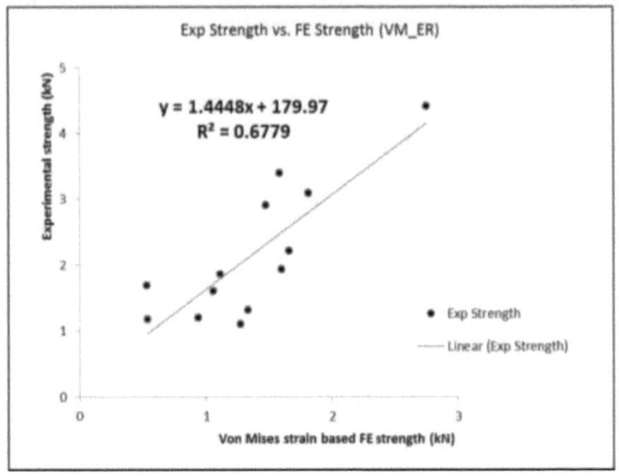

Fig. 5 Linear regression between Experiment- and FE-derived strength (FE model of vertebral with posterior elements; a) von Mises Stress, b) von Mises Strain

Two specimens (No.0009, 0011) were excluded due to poor image quality and one specimen (No. 0029) was discarded due to failure of the experimental test.

C. Correlation between VB Model and VB w/PE Model

Linear regression between the VB FE strength and the VB w/ PE FE strength was performed. Three specimens were discarded and, because each spinal unit has two vertebrae, this gave twenty six FE results that could be compared. The VB FE strength was strongly correlated with the VB w/ PE FE strength (r^2 =0.97 VM_SR; r^2 =0.96 VM_ER) as shown in figure 6.

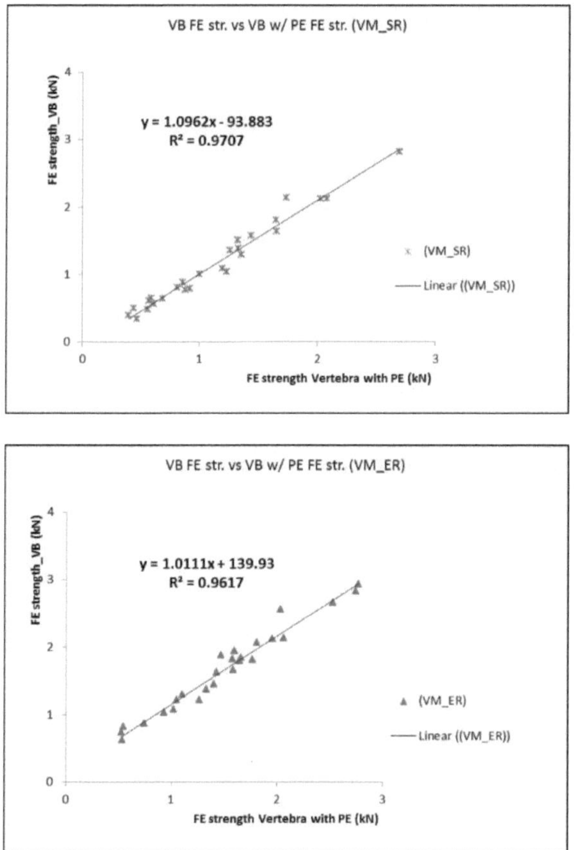

Fig. 6 Linear regression between VB FE strength and VB w/ PE FE strength; von Mises stress-based strength (top), von Mises strain-based strength (bottom)

IV. Discussion

This study was based on the premise that vertebral strength obtained from a FE model of the vertebral body alone could not represent the strength of an individual vertebra during forward bending. However, this study has shown that both models give results that are positively correlated with the experimental data (r^2= 0.68 - 0.79) and with each other (r^2= 0.96 – 0.97). This can be explained by the fact that, in flexion, most of the compressive load is borne by the anterior column of the spine, and very little is resisted by the neural arch [17, 18]. Consequently, in anterior bending, the effect of the posterior elements on vertebral strength is not high. However, if other daily activities such as extension or torsion are considered, then the posterior elements will play a much greater role. Finally, some limitations of this study should be noted. Firstly, neither of the two FE models take account of the intervertebral disc, which plays an important role in load distribution on the vertebral endplate, nor the ligament and muscle forces, and both consider only the specific forward bending condition (Θ = 8.5°). Secondly, the results of the FE models were compared with experimental data obtained by generating a wedge fracture in a single vertebral body of a spinal unit rather than in a single vertebra alone. Further work is in progress to generate and validate a FE model of the functional spinal unit (FSU) that consists of two vertebrae and the adjacent IVD.

V. Conclusions

The results of this study indicate that the strength derived from the simple vertebral body FE model under the forward-bending condition can be used to estimate the vertebral compressive strength instead of FE modelling of the vertebral body with posterior elements.

Acknowledgment

This research is funded by the NIHR-Biomedical Research Fellowship 2011-2013 scheme. The views expressed in this publication are those of the authors and not necessarily those of the NHS, the NIHR or the UK Department of Health.

Conflict of Interest

The authors declare that they have no conflict of interest.

References

1. Homminga J M, Weinans H, Gowin W et al. (2001) Osteoporosis Changes the Amount of Vertebral Trabecular Bone at Risk of Fracture but Not the Vertebral Load Distribution. Spine 26:1555-1560
2. Crawford R P, Cann C E and Keaveny T M (2003) Finite element models predict in vitro vertebral body compressive strength better than quantitative computed tomography. Bone 33:744–750
3. Keaveny T M, Donley D W, Hoffmann P F et al. (2007) Effects of Teriparatide and Alendronate on Vertebral Strength as Assessed by Finite Element Modeling of QCT Scans in Women With Osteoporosis. J Bone Miner Res. 22:149-157
4. Buckley J M, Loo K and Motherway J (2007) Comparison of quantitative computed tomography-based measures in predicting vertebral compressive strength. Bone 40:767-774
5. Melton L J, Riggs B L, Keaveny T M et al. (2007) Structural Determinants of Vertebral Fracture Risk. J Bone Miner Res. 22:1885-1892
6. Chevalier Y, Charlebois M, Pahr D et al. (2008) A patient-specific finite element methodology to predict damage accumulation in vertebral bodies under axial compression, sagittal flexion and combined loads. Comp Meth Biomech Biomed Eng. 11:477-487
7. Zeinali A, Hashemi-Malayeri B, Akhlaghpoor S and Nazemi M (2008) Noninvasive Prediction of Vertebral Body Compressive Strength Using Finite Element Method and An Image Based Technique. In: 4th Kuala Lumpur International Conference on Biomedical Engineering 2008 Springer Berlin Heidelberg

8. Eastell R, Cedel S L, Wahner H W et al. (1991) Classification of vertebral fractures. J Bone Miner Res. 6:207-215.
9. Wasnich RD (1996) A new, standardized approach to fracture risk interpretation. Hawaii Med J 55:141-143.
10. Jackson SA, Tenenhouse A, Robertson L et al. (2000) Vertebral Fracture Definition from Population-Based Data: Preliminary Results from the Canadian Multicenter Osteoporosis Study (CaMos). Osteoporos Int. 11:680.
11. Kopperdahl D L, Morgan E F and Keaveny T M (2002) Quantitative computed tomography estimates of the mechanical properties of human vertebral trabecular bone. J Orthop Res. 20:801-805.
12. Keaveny T M, Wachtel E F, Ford C M and Hayes W C (1994) Differences between the tensile and compressive strengths of bovine tibial trabecular bone depend on modulus. J Biomechanics 27:1137-1146
13. Morgan E F and Keaveny T M (2001) Dependence of yield strain of human trabecular bone on anatomic site. J Biomechanics 34:569–577
14. Morgan E F, Bayraktar H H and Keaveny T M (2003) Trabecular bone modulus–density relationships depend on anatomic site. J Biomechanics 36:897-904.
15. Ulrich D, Van Rietbergen B, Laib A and Ruegsegger P (1999) The Ability of Three-Dimensional Structural Indices to Reflect Mechanical Aspects of Trabecular Bone. Bone 25:55–60.
16. Luo J, Bertram W, Sangar D et al. (2010) Is kyphoplasty better than vertebroplasty in restoring normal mechanical function to an injured spine? Bone 46:1050-1057
17. Pollintine P, Przybyla AS, Dolan P, Adams MA (2004) Neural arch load-bearing in old and degenerated spines. J Biomechanics 37:197-204
18. Adams MA, Pollintine P, Tobias JH, Wakley GK, Dolan P (2006) Intervertebral disc degeneration can predispose to anterior vertebral fractures in the thoracolumbar spine. J Bone Mineral Res 21 9 1409-16

Author: Chu-Hee Lee
Institute: Mellanby Centre for Bone Research, University of Sheffield
Street: Beech Hill Road
City: Sheffield, S10 2RX
Country: UK
Email: chuhee.lee@sheffield.ac.uk

Author Index

Keyword Index

MIX
Papier aus verantwortungsvollen Quellen
Paper from responsible sources
FSC® C105338

If you have any concerns about our products,
you can contact us on
ProductSafety@springernature.com

In case Publisher is established outside the EU,
the EU authorized representative is:
Springer Nature Customer Service Center GmbH
Europaplatz 3, 69115 Heidelberg, Germany

Printed by Libri Plureos GmbH
in Hamburg, Germany